Exercise and Sport Sciences Reviews

Volume 25, 1997

EXERCISE AND SPORT SCIENCES REVIEWS

Volume 25, 1997

Editor

JOHN O. HOLLOSZY, M.D.

Professor of Medicine
Department of Internal Medicine
Washington University School of Medicine
St. Louis, Missouri

American College of Sports Medicine Series

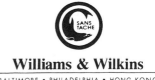

Williams & Wilkins

BALTIMORE • PHILADELPHIA • HONG KONG
LONDON • MUNICH • SYDNEY • TOKYO

A WAVERLY COMPANY

Accurate indications, adverse reactions, and dosage schedules for drugs are provided in this book, but it is possible that they may change. The reader is urged to review the package information data of the manufacturers of the medications mentioned.

RC
1200
.E94
V 25
July 1999

Printed in the United States of America
(ISBN 0-683-18333-8)

97 98 99
1   2   3   4   5   6   7   8   9   10

Preface

Exercise and Sport Sciences Reviews, an annual publication sponsored by the American College of Sports Medicine, reviews current research concerning behavioral, biochemical, biomechanical, clinical, physiological, and rehabilitational topics involving exercise science. The Editorial Board for this series currently consists of 13 recognized authorities who have assumed responsibility for one of the following general topics: athletic medicine, biochemistry, biomechanics, environmental physiology, epidemiology, exercise physiology, gerontology, growth and development, metabolism, molecular biology, physical fitness, psychology and rehabilitation. The organization of the Editorial Board should help foster the commitment of the American College of Sports Medicine to publish timely reviews in areas of broad interest to clinicians, educators, exercise scientists, and students. The goal for this Editorial Board is to provide reviews in each of these 13 areas whenever sufficient new information becomes available on topics that are likely to be of interest to the readership of *Exercise and Sport Sciences Reviews.* Further, the Editor selects additional topics to be developed into chapters based on current interest, timeliness, and importance to the above audience. The contributors for each volume are selected by the Editorial Board members and the Editor.

John O. Holloszy, M.D.
Editor

Contributors

Deborah J. Aaron, Ph.D.
Department of Epidemiology
University of Pittsburgh
Pittsburgh, Pennsylvania

Thomas P. Andriacchi, Ph.D.
Department of Orthopedic Surgery
Rush-Presbyterian-St. Luke's Medical Center
Chicago, Illinois

Bernard R. Bach, Jr., M.D.
Department of Orthopedic Surgery
Rush-Presbyterian-St. Luke's Medical Center
Chicago, Illinois

David B. Burr, Ph.D.
Departments of Anatomy and Orthopedic Surgery
Biomechanics and Biomaterials Research Center
Indiana University School of Medicine
Indianapolis, Indiana

Charles A. Bush-Joseph, M.D.
Department of Orthopedic Surgery
Rush-Presbyterian-St. Luke's Medical Center
Chicago, Illinois

James A. Carson, Ph.D.
Department of Integrative Biology
University of Texas Houston Health Science Center
Houston, Texas

Jean-Pierre Després, Ph.D.
Lipid Research Center
Laval University Medical Research Center
Ste-Foy (Quebec) Canada

Peter H. Fentem, M.B.Ch.B.
University Division of Stroke Medicine/Stroke Research Unit
Nottingham City Hospital (NHS) Trust
Nottingham, England

Mark Hargreaves, Ph.D., FACSM
School of Human Movement
Deakin University
Burwood, Australia

Gregory W. Heath, D.H.Sc., M.P.H., FACSM
Division of Adult and Community Health
Behavioral Surveillance Branch
National Center for Chronic Disease Prevention and Health Promotion and
    Centers for Disease Control and Prevention
Atlanta, Georgia

Debra E. Hurwitz, Ph.D.
Department of Orthopedic Surgery
Rush-Presbyterian-St. Luke's Medical Center
Chicago, Illinois

W. Larry Kenney, Ph.D.
Noll Physiological Research Center
The Pennsylvania State University
University Park, Pennsylvania

Ronald E. LaPorte, Ph.D.
Department of Epidemiology
University of Pittsburgh
Pittsburgh, Pennsylvania

Richard L. Lieber, Ph.D.
Departments of Orthopaedics and Bioengineering
University of California and V.A. Medical Centers
San Diego, California

Marius Locke, Ph.D.
School of Physical and Health Education
University of Toronto
Toronto, Ontario, Canada

Barbara J. Nicklas, Ph.D.
Division of Gerontology
University of Maryland School of Medicine
Baltimore V.A. Medical Center (GRECC)
Baltimore, Maryland

Bruce J. Noble, Ph.D.
University of Pittsburgh
Pittsburgh, Pennsylvania

Roberta J. Park, Ph.D.
Department of Human Biodynamics
University of California, Berkeley
Berkeley, California

Fredric J. Pashkow, M.D.
The Cleveland Clinic Foundation
Department of Cardiology
Cleveland, Ohio

Tina J. Patel, M.S.
Departments of Orthopaedics and Bioengineering
University of California and V.A. Medical Centers
San Diego, California

Jeffrey T. Potts, Ph.D.
Department of Internal Medicine & Physiology
University of Texas Southwestern Medical School
Dallas, Texas

Peter B. Raven, Ph.D.
Department of Integrative Physiology
Cardiovascular Research Institute
University of North Texas Health Science Center
Ft. Worth, Texas

Robert J. Robertson, Ph.D.
University of Pittsburgh
Pittsburgh, Pennsylvania

Robert A. Schweikert, M.D.
The Cleveland Clinic Foundation
Department of Cardiology
Cleveland, Ohio

Xiangrong Shi, Ph.D.
Department of Integrative Physiology
Cardiovascular Research Institute
University of North Texas Health Science Center
Ft. Worth, Texas

Bruce L. Wilkoff, M.D.
The Cleveland Clinic Foundation
Department of Cardiology
Cleveland, Ohio

Contents

1
Functional Adaptations in Patients with ACL-Deficient Knees

DEBRA E. HURWITZ Ph.D.
THOMAS P. ANDRIACCHI, Ph.D.
CHARLES A. BUSH-JOSEPH, M.D.
BERNARD R. BACH, JR., M.D.

CLINICAL ISSUES

Injury to the anterior cruciate ligament (ACL) is among the most frequent sports-related injuries [26]. It has been estimated that skiing alone accounts for more than 100,000 ACL injuries in the United States per year [22]. In addition, there has been a rapid increase in ACL injuries in women's sports, such as basketball, soccer, and volleyball. Thus, a better understanding of the functional changes associated with ACL injuries could be extremely important for future improvements in rehabilitation and surgical treatment methods.

Restoration of function in the short term and prevention of long-term pathological changes to the knee are among the primary goals in the treatment of the ACL rupture. In addition to initial functional losses that occur primarily during more stressful athletic activities, long-term degenerative changes to the knee have been demonstrated in subjects after loss of the ACL. The degenerative changes occur despite the fact that active athletic participation has been reduced or abandoned [13, 20, 25, 28].

It is often difficult to predict from passive physical examination of the knee which patients will be functionally impaired by the loss of this ligament and which patients will have minimal symptoms [1, 8, 18, 34, 36, 43]. Clinical studies [34, 36] report that approximately one-third of patients who had an ACL-deficient knee (ACLD patients) were able to pursue recreational activities; another one-third compensated but had to reduce many activities; and one-third had poor function even after discontinuing sport activities. Several studies [20, 28] have reported both degenerative changes and moderate or severe symptoms during stressful activities of daily living in some patients but not in others. Perhaps some individuals are better suited to functionally adapt to the loss of the ACL.

Loss of the ACL has been shown to influence the passive mechanics of the knee joint by decreasing overall stiffness of the knee or increasing instability of the knee [16, 22, 31]. However, it is possible to adapt dynamically [6, 12, 35] for the stability lost at the knee through muscular substitution during ambulatory activities. The number of surgical reconstructions of the ACL are increasing; yet, the management of an ACL-deficient knee still remains controversial. The variable natural history in the progression of degenerative joint disease in some patients and not in others suggests that some patients make appropriate functional adaptations for the loss of the ACL.

Although surgical and nonsurgical (rehabilitation) treatment modalities [1, 8, 18, 43] have demonstrated clinical improvement, the results are short term, and the long-term efficacy of various procedures to treat ACL deficiency is still unknown. Current methods of clinical examination do not always provide an adequate objective assessment of functional improvement. The ability to assess the probability of future degenerative changes associated with the loss of the ACL would be extremely valuable for treatment planning and the evaluation of various treatment modalities for the ACL-deficient knee.

CHAPTER OVERVIEW

This chapter focuses on the functional biomechanics of the ACL-deficient knee during the daily activities of walking and stair climbing, as well as on the more stressful athletic activities of jogging and side cutting. The mechanism of functional adaptations in ACLD patients is analyzed, and the clinical implication of the dynamic adaptations, as related to muscular substitution for the loss of the ACL, is examined. The functional biomechanics will be examined with regard to the issues dealt with below.

Muscular Substitution

Muscular substitution may provide one means of compensating for the loss of the ACL. Increased activity in muscles that act as synergists to the ACL and decreased activity in those that act as antagonists increase knee stability in the absence of the ACL. Studies have focused on the interaction between the ACL and the changing direction of pull of the quadriceps mechanism during knee flexion. It has been reported that quadriceps contraction produces strain in the ACL when the knee is flexed less than 45° and reduces strain in the ACL when the knee is flexed beyond 75° [4, 38] (Fig. 1.1A). When the knee is near full extension, the patellar ligament places an anterior pull on the tibia. In the absence of the ACL, the tibia would move forward until the forces could be balanced by secondary restraints to anterior displacement. As the knee flexes beyond approximately 45°, the orientation of the patellar ligament reverses direction during the quadriceps contraction and now places a posterior pull on the tibia. Thus, at deeper flexion angles, the contraction of the quadriceps acts to compensate for an absent ACL.

Quadriceps contraction induces not only an anterior displacement but also an internal rotation of the tibia [21]. The quadriceps axially deviate

FIGURE 1.1.

A, Mean passive normal, simulated quadriceps isometric, and simulated quadriceps isotonic strain patterns. Quadriceps contraction significantly increased ACL strain for knee flexion angles less than 45° and significantly decreased ACL strain for knee flexion angles greater than 75°. B, Mean passive normal and simulated hamstring isometric strain patterns. Hamstring contractions significantly decreased ACL strain for knee flexion angles greater than 75°. Reproduced from ref. 38.

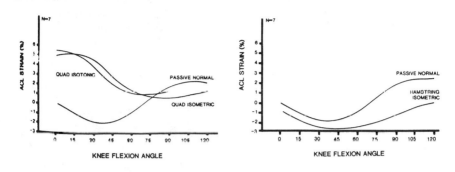

10–15° as they pass over the patella to the tibial tubercle, causing internal rotation of the tibia. This may further contribute to the pivoting phenomenon found in ACLD subjects.

The hamstrings are in a position to provide both rotatory stability and resistance to anterior drawer. Functionally, when the knee is flexed more than 75°, the hamstring contraction significantly reduces the strain in the ACL (Fig. 1.1B). When the knee is flexed less than 75°, the strain is reduced but not by a significant amount [38]. The ability of the biceps femoris to resist internal rotation greatly increases as the knee flexion angle increases [21]. Thus, it is reasonable to believe that hamstring substitution occurs among ACLD patients when the knee is flexed, which often occurs during more stressful athletic activities, such as twisting, pivoting, and stopping from a run.

This chapter reviews the use of muscular substitution (quadriceps and/or hamstrings) and its relationship to the angle of knee flexion. The following questions are examined:

- During activities of daily living, when the knee is near full extension, do ACLD patients tend to avoid quadriceps contraction or increase hamstring contraction?
- Is the nature of the functional adaptations during various activities related to the angle of knee flexion?
- Do ACLD patients who tolerate stressful activities increase hamstring contraction to compensate for the structural loss of the ACL?

Origin of compensations

Although the origin of the compensations during gait and other more stressful activities is unknown, several theories have been postulated. Compensations may originate from higher neurological centers (learned responses) or from more local peripheral mechanical and neurological receptors. It is not likely that patients instantaneously adapt to instability and the subsequent movement of the tibia during each step. It is more likely that adaptations occur before the instability generated from the muscle contraction, so that abnormal anterior drawer or strain on the secondary restraints does not develop. Side-to-side symmetry during activities suggests the dominance of a high neurological center as the stimulus whereas side-to-side asymmetry suggests a lower-level peripheral compensatory mechanism.

To address this issue, this chapter will examine the following question:

• During activities of daily living, are the functional adaptations present on the affected side also present on the contralateral (unaffected) side?

RATIONALE AND METHODS FOR FUNCTIONAL TESTING OF THE ACL-DEFICIENT KNEE

Functional testing offers the opportunity for objective and quantitative testing of patients with injuries to the ACL. It provides unique information not attainable through standard clinical examination, because the subject is tested under conditions that replicate activities of daily living, as well as more stressful sports activities. Information from functional testing has the potential to improve treatment [36, 37]. There are many measures that can be quantified during functional tests. Thus, it is important to select variables that focus on the measures that directly relate to the physical aspects of the problem. Functional analysis has focused on parameters associated with muscles that act as synergists or antagonists to the function of the absent ACL. It, therefore, provides a means of determining whether dynamic adaptations or muscular substitution can help explain the variable clinical history of patients with ACL injuries.

The technology and instrumentation to conduct functional testing is available from a number of sources with sufficient resolution to provide meaningful measurements. The ground reaction forces, limb segment masses, and inertia are used to calculate joint moments and forces. The basic components of the measurement system include a force platform, an optoelectronic system for motion measurement, a computer and, in some cases, muscle activity is monitored using fine wire or surface electrodes. The external moments are calculated along the axes of flexion-extension, abduction-adduction, and internal-external rotation. In addition, knee motion and temporal measurements are quantified. Moments are typically normalized to body weight (Bw) and height (Ht) or Bw and leg length to allow comparison among subjects of different sizes.

Previous studies [2, 3, 6, 10] have demonstrated that the external moments measured can be interpreted in terms of the loads on muscles, passive soft tissue, and joint surfaces. Mechanical equilibrium dictates that external forces and moments must be balanced by internal forces and moments. Internal forces generated by muscles, passive soft tissues, and joint contact forces create these internal moments. If muscles act only synergistically when balancing the external moments, then one can directly infer the internal muscle force in synergistic muscle groups. For example, the total force in the quadriceps needed to balance an external moment tending to flex the knee joint can be determined [2]. However, when antagonistic muscle activity is present, the external moment reflects the net balance between agonist and antagonist muscles. The force in the synergistic muscle group is greater under these conditions. The external moment can, however, be used to get a conservative estimate or lower bound on the synergist muscle force.

In many electromyographic (EMG) studies, only the duration and timing of the muscle activity is analyzed [9, 27, 41], whereas in others the magnitudes are analyzed [17, 29, 30, 40]. EMG activity is typically normalized to either the peak value during an activity or the peak value during a maximum voluntary contraction.

ADAPTATIONS DURING GAIT

Berchuck et al. [10] showed that the greatest change in gait in ACLD patients was the flexion-extension moment at the knee. This study examined the knee kinematics and kinetics of 16 ACLD patients and 10 control normals. The pattern of the flexion-extension moment during stance phase was interpreted in terms of the net quadriceps or net knee flexor demand (hamstrings and/or gastrocnemius) during stance phase. Typically, at heel strike, there was an external moment tending to extend the knee joint (demanding net knee flexor force); as the knee moved into midstance, the external moment reversed its direction (demanding net quadriceps force); as the knee passed midstance the moment again reversed its direction (demanding net flexor muscle force); and, finally, in the preswing phase, the moment tended to flex the knee (demanding net quadriceps muscle force) (Fig. 1.2). The ACLD patients walked in a manner that avoided the moment tending to flex the knee during the middle portion of stance phase (Fig. 1.2). This type of gait was interpreted as a tendency to avoid or reduce the demand on the quadriceps muscle and has been called a "quadriceps avoidance" gait [2, 10]. Despite the relatively low loads on the knee that occurred during level walking, 75% of the patients studied had the "quadriceps avoidance" gait whereas 25% had a normal biphasic flexion-extension

FIGURE 1.2.

The normal flexion-extension moment during the stance phase of level walking. Gait tended to oscillate between flexion and extension. In ACLD patients, the magnitude of the quadriceps demand (2*) was reduced or avoided during stance phase, as indicated in the figure.

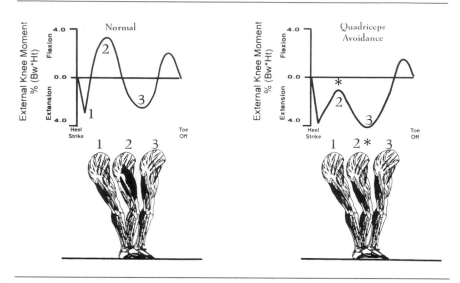

moment. The magnitude of the difference between the normal and ACLD patients during walking was large [more than 100%]. The external moment tending to flex the joint at heelstrike was also increased.

A follow-up study by Birac et al. [11] of 23 ACLD patients indicated that the emergence of the "quadriceps avoidance" pattern was related to time since injury. The "quadriceps avoidance" pattern was more common in patients who were further from their injury date. For example, 80% of those who were at least 6 years from their injury developed the "quadriceps avoidance" pattern, as compared to only 44% of those who were less than 1.5 years from their injury.

The findings from the EMG study by Limbird et al. [30] were consistent with the changes in the joint kinetics reported by Berchuck et al. [10] and Birac et al. [11]. EMG activity in 12 ACLD patients and 15 control normals was measured during normal- and fast-speed walking. The majority of the differences occurred at normal walking speeds during the transitions between swing to stance and stance to swing. During the loading transition, decreased rectus femoris, vastus lateralis and gastrocnemius, as well as increased biceps femoris and semitendinosus activity, was found. The net effect of this change in muscle activity is to generate a greater posterior force on the tibia during weight acceptance. During the stance to swing transition, greater quadriceps and less biceps femoris activity were found, which would have actually increased the anterior force on the tibia.

Beard et al. [9] demonstrated an increased duration in hamstring activity but no change in duration in quadriceps activity (Fig. 1.3). This study examined the EMG activity of the quadriceps (vastus medialis), hamstrings (semitendinosus and semimembranosus), and the gastrocnemius, along with the sagittal plane knee angle during gait, in 18 ACLD patients approximately 2 yr after initial injury and in 9 control normals. The knee angle during terminal extension was also significantly greater in the ACLD group, as compared to that of both the normals and their own contralateral side. The duration of hamstring activity was correlated with both the minimum knee flexion at heel strike and the terminal knee extension angle. The authors felt that the increased knee flexion angle during terminal extension may have facilitated the hamstring muscles in preventing anterior subluxation of the tibia with respect to the femur. However, at these knee angles the hamstrings are not efficient synergists to the ACL in preventing anterior translation [38]. Although increased duration of hamstring activity was demonstrated, the authors emphasized that this did not imply that the magnitude of the activity was increased.

Ciccotti et al. [17] used fine wires to study EMG activity in 8 ACLD patients who were 24–36 months postinjury and who had completed a 6-month rehabilitation program. The muscle activity was expressed as a percentage of the activity present during a maximum manual test. During walking, increased vastus lateralis activity during the loading response was observed. Increased rectus femoris during preswing, increased biceps femoris during terminal swing, increased tibialis anterior during terminal stance, and increased soleus during midstance were also noted. The authors attributed this preferential increase in vastus lateralis activity over that of the remaining quadriceps muscles as a mechanism for reducing internal rotation. However, in the absence of excessive patella subluxation it is unlikely that preferential vastus lateralis activity can effectively reduce internal rotation of the tibia on the femur. Moreover, Andriacchi et al. [4] demonstrated that the quadriceps muscles typically act synergistically. Ciccotti et al. also attributed the increased biceps femoris activity in terminal swing to a protective mechanism against the anterior tibial translation from quadriceps activity during the loading response whereas the preferential increase in the lateral hamstring at heelstrike was attributed to protecting the knee from pivoting. Likewise, increased tibialis anterior activity during terminal stance may have resulted in foot inversion in conjunction with dorsiflexion, which results in the tibia externally rotating. The study by Ciccotti et al. was designed to compare ACL-reconstructed patients with ACLD patients and control normals. The authors concluded that rehabilitation alone was not sufficient to restore normal gait patterns.

FIGURE 1.3.

Comparison of quadriceps, hamstrings, and gastrocnemius muscle activity duration in the control and in ACLD patients (n = 17). Duration of muscle activity is expressed as percentage of stance phase. *, significant difference. Reproduced from ref. 9.

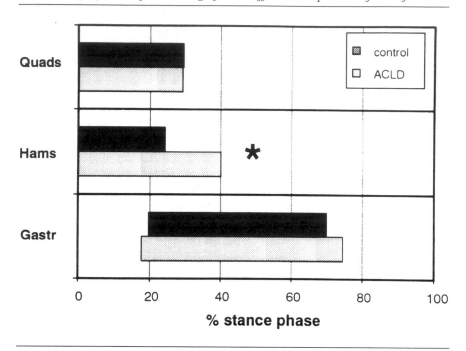

In contrast to the study of Ciccotti et al. [17] study, Shiavi et al. [40] demonstrated decreased quadriceps and hamstring activity. Muscle activity at approximately 1 yr after injury in 20 ACLD patients and 26 control normals was studied. A clustering analysis based on the Fourier transform of the average linear envelope of the muscle activity was used to identify patterns representative of the ACLD patients and patterns representative of the normals. During fast walking the ACLD patients had decreased rectus femoris activity both at heelstrike and at the end of stance. At fast speeds the ACLD patients lacked or had a decreased second phase of quadriceps activity during the latter part of stance, and the vastus lateralis had a lower intensity during the swing to stance transition and a major phase of shorter duration. The hamstrings had decreased activity during single-leg stance. The semitendinosus, biceps femoris, and medial gastrocnemius all had a delay in activity.

Lass et al. [29] measured EMG activity in 14 ACLDs and 16 control normals at approximately 46 mo after injury. The activity of the vastus lateralis and medialis and lateral and medial hamstrings and medial gastrocnemius started earlier than normal, and the duration of the vastus medialis and gastrocnemius was greater. Alterations in muscle timing, and not amplitude, were found.

Two studies, both with fairly small sample sizes demonstrated no differences in EMG activity during level walking. Carlsöö and Nordstrand [16] measured the kinematics and EMG activity in five normals and five ACLD patients at approximately 6 months after injury who showed no evidence of quadriceps atrophy. Although a decreased knee range of motion was measured, there was no change in the EMG patterns. Kålund et al. [27] measured EMG activity (onset and duration) during treadmill walking in nine ACLD patients at least 2–3 yr after injury vs. that of nine control normals. No differences were noted during level walking. However, during uphill walking the hamstrings were activated earlier in the ACLD patients, as compared to the controls.

Tibone et al. [41] also demonstrated no side-to-side asymmetries in EMG patterns of the quadriceps, hamstrings, and gastrocnemius during walking. Tibone et al. measured EMG activity (onset and duration), motion, and forces during walking, jogging, stair climbing, and two different cutting activities in 20 ACLD patients approximately 37 mo after injury. No control group of normals was evaluated. The only asymmetry occurred in the midstance vertical force during fast walking. The midstance vertical force was actually greater on the ACLD side, as compared to the contralateral side. The authors attributed this increase in force to a decrease in the upward rise of the center of gravity as the body passed over the single-stance limb.

The influence of strength deficits and functional adaptations during gait was examined by Czerniecki et al. [19], who measured tibiofemoral rotation during gait, using a triaxial goniometer, in 11 patients with ACL injuries approximately 32 mo after their injury and in 9 control normals. During treadmill gait, the total range of tibial rotation was not significantly different between the ACLD and normal groups, and the difference between the range of tibial rotation between the affected and unaffected side of the ACLD group was not significantly different from that of the normal subjects. However, when the ACLD patients were walking faster, the side-to-side difference between the range of tibial rotation of the ACLD patients was weakly correlated with the difference in quadriceps and hamstring strength.

Based on the various gait studies, a consensus can not be reached regarding the exact nature of the gait adaptations present in the ACLD patients. There was evidence that the adaptation consists of reduced quadriceps activity, increased quadriceps activity, increased hamstring activity, or reduced hamstring activity [9, 17, 29, 30, 40]. Others found no qualitative alterations in the EMG activity [16, 27, 41]. In interpreting the results, one must recall that increased duration in muscle activity alone does not reflect on whether or not the magnitude of the muscle forces is greater or less during this time period. In fact, during jogging Tibone et al. [41] correlated increased duration with decreased muscle strength.

From an anatomical viewpoint the hamstrings do not serve as effective synergists to the ACL when the knee is near full extension. Their ability, therefore, to compensate for the loss of the ACL during the loading response and midstance phases of gait would be limited. However, quadriceps contraction during these phases of the gait cycle would induce an anterior drawer, causing the quadriceps to act as an antagonist to the ACL. A decrease in quadriceps activity would, therefore, appear to be a more effective mechanism for reducing anterior drawer during this portion of the gait cycle.

Reports of quadriceps strength deficits among ACLD patients would also be more consistent with a reduction in quadriceps activity during walking, rather than with an increase in hamstring activity. Tibone et al. [41] demonstrated a 14% quadriceps deficit and a 4% hamstring deficit in ACLD patients, whereas McHugh et al. [32] also demonstrated a significant strength deficit on the involved side for both the quadriceps and hamstrings.

Several reasons may account for differences in the EMG results. The method of analysis used in determining the magnitudes, or even just the threshold used for determining whether a muscle is on or off, obviously had an impact on the results. Different normalization and thresholding techniques were used by the various investigators. For example, the on/off activity in the study of Tibone et al. [41] was based on a visual inspection of the EMG tracings, whereas Beard et al. [9] used a threshold of one-eighth of the maximum amplitude during the activity. This may have accounted for some of the discrepancies in results.

Limbird et al. [30] also noted that differences in walking speeds may account for the discrepancies among the various studies. Tibone et al. [41] also noted that differences in the force plate data during running were occasionally found with the initial trials and that these differences disappeared with subsequent trials. This suggests that as subjects perform trials repeatedly, a learning process occurs, until the activity is performed in a more consistent manner. Although walking is a routine activity, this is certainly a consideration for the less common activities, such as cutting or jogging, or perhaps, even walking on a treadmill.

Another possible cause of the contradictory EMG results is that although all the patient populations studied were ACLD patients, there still could have been many clinical and demographic factors that varied between the groups. For example, in the study by Ciccotti et al. [17], the patients were within 2 yr of injury, as opposed to those in the study of Birac et al. [11], who were longer term. Evidence that the "quadriceps avoidance gait" does not emerge until 3 yr after injury has been presented [11]. The extent of meniscal involvement or the amount of strength deficit of either the quadriceps or hamstrings are other factors that may be different between the study groups. The subsequent natural history of the patient may also influence adaptation. In some studies patients may have gone on for immediate reconstruction whereas in others they were able to function adequately without a reconstruction.

ADAPTATIONS AS RELATED TO KNEE FLEXION ANGLES

Jogging places greater demands on the knee joint than walking. The magnitude of the knee flexion moment (net quadriceps moment) was increased by more than a factor of 5 during jogging, as compared to that of level walking (Fig. 1.4) [6, 10]. Berchuck et al. [10] demonstrated that even though the net quadriceps demand was substantially greater than that during jogging, when compared to level walking the percentage change in the net quadriceps moment between ACLD and normal subjects was substantially less. ACLD patients only had a 24% reduction in the net quadriceps moment during jogging, as compared to more than 100% reduction during walking. The maximum net quadriceps moment during jogging occurred when the knee was at approximately 40° of flexion, as compared to 20° during level walking [10].

Several EMG studies have also demonstrated decreased quadriceps activity during jogging. Shiavi et al. [40] reported decreased vastus medialis and lateralis activity during early stance and increased vastus lateralis activity in the middle-to-late stance. Tibone et al. [41] demonstrated an earlier onset of vastus medialis obliquus activity on the affected side, as compared to that on the unaffected side. The earlier onset of the vastus medialis obliquus was associated with a strength deficit on the affected side. The authors believed that a weaker muscle must be activated earlier to achieve symmetric limb placement at heelstrike. The medial and lateral hamstring muscles were symmetrical, but the medial hamstrings were on for a greater duration than the lateral ones. The authors thought that the earlier cessation of the lateral hamstrings (biceps femoris longus) may have been associated with an anterolateral subluxation of the tibial plateau during midsupport. The vertical force was also reduced on the affected side, as compared to that on the unaffected side.

During ascending stairs, the maximum net quadriceps moment occurred at approximately 60° of flexion. Even though the moment during stair climbing was substantially larger than that of level walking, Berchuck et al. [10] found that ACLD patients had a greater than normal net quadriceps moment while climbing the stairs. Shiavi et al. [40] also reported increased vastus lateralis, biceps femoris, tibialis anterior, and rectus femoris activity during stair climbing. Tibone et al. [41] reported a premature cessation of vastus medial obliquus activity during stance on the affected side, as compared to that on the unaffected side, as the body weight was being raised after contralateral toe off. This was beneficial for decreasing the functional

FIGURE 1.4.

A comparison of the pattern of flexion-extension moments during level walking and jogging. The illustration shows the limb configuration during jogging.

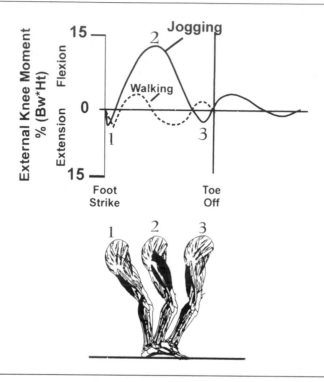

anterior drawer when the knee was near full extension. Similarly, the early onset of biceps femoris longus activity on the affected side, as compared to that on the unaffected side before initial contact, further protected the knee from excessive anterior tibial displacement.

The adaptations during the activities of daily living appeared to be dependent on the angle of knee flexion when the greatest net quadriceps demand occurred and not just on the magnitude of the net quadriceps demand. These observations suggested an interaction between the direction of pull of the patella ligament and the functional role of the ACL (Fig. 1.5). Thus, during level walking, when the maximum net quadriceps moment demand occurred between 0° and approximately 20°, there was a greater tendency for the quadriceps contraction to produce an anterior pull on the tibia. The adaptation to avoid quadriceps contraction eliminated this anterior force component when the knee was near full extension (Fig. 1.5). This mechanism may explain the large reduction in the net quadriceps moment

FIGURE 1.5.

A summary of the relationship between the adaptive mechanisms seen in ACLD patients. The adaptive mechanism appeared to be related to the orientation of the pull of the patellar ligament. The adaptive mechanisms were closely related to the angle of knee flexion and its associated effect on the direction of pull of the patellar ligament. AP, anteroposterior.

Activity	Knee Flexion Angle	Patellar Ligament Orientation	Functional Adaptation
	Angle @ Maximum Quadriceps Moment	AP Component on Tibia	% Change from Normal Net quadriceps Moment
Walking	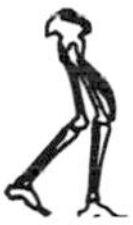 20°	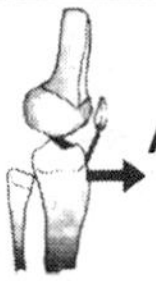 Anterior	144% Reduction
Jogging	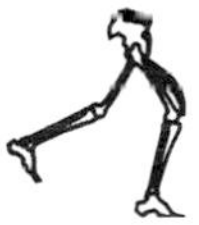 40°	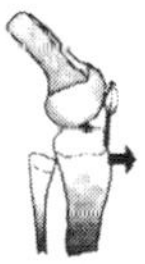 Anterior	24% Reduction
Stair Climbing	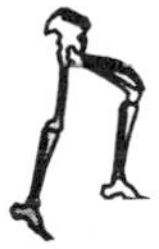 60°	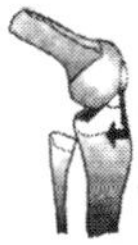 Posterior	42% Increase

seen among ACLD patients. Thus, the increased net quadriceps moment seen in ACLD patients during stair climbing suggested that there was an increased use of the quadriceps as a possible means of dynamic muscular substitution for the absent ACL when the knee was at greater flexion angles.

HAMSTRING FACILITATION DURING MORE STRESSFUL ATHLETIC ACTIVITIES

The typical normal pattern of the flexion-extension moment for both the run-to-stop and run-to-lateral side-step cut had a predominant moment tending to flex the knee (demanding net quadriceps forces) during the major portion of stance phase (Fig. 1.6). Andriacchi et al. [5] showed that ACLD patients had a higher net hamstring moment during the early portion of support phase in both the running and cutting and running-to-a-

FIGURE 1.6.

Typically, ACLD patients had a higher moment tending to extend the knee (demanding net hamstring forces) during early stance. The figures of the leg below the graph indicate the position of the knee joint. As knee flexion increases, the ability of the hamstrings to substitute for ACL function increases.

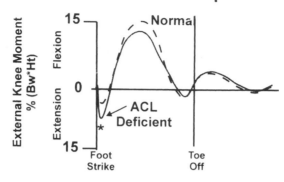

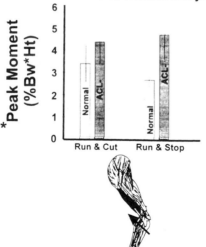

Increased Hamstring Muscle Force Can Dynamically Substitute for ACL During Stressful Activities

stop activities. It is possible that the patients activated the hamstring muscles to a greater extent in the early portion of this activity to dynamically stabilize the knee against the higher rotational and abduction-adduction loads that occurred during the middle portion of that activity [39]. The magnitude of the twisting and adduction moment components during cutting and stopping was substantially higher than that which occurred during activities such as level walking. These higher twisting moments may cause buckling of the knee, as often has been reported by ACLD patients [6].

During side step cutting, Branch et al. [12] demonstrated increased activity in muscles that were synergists to the ACL and a decrease in those that functioned as antagonists to the ACL. EMG activity during side step cutting of 10 ACLD subjects and 5 normal control subjects demonstrated increased lateral hamstring activity during the precut swing phase and increased medial hamstring and decreased quadriceps and gastrocnemius activity during the stance phase. The authors suggested that the increased lateral hamstring activity increased the external rotation of the tibia before foot plant, which decreases the pivot shift phenomenon. An increase in hamstring activity may be a desirable compensation for ACLD patients during stressful athletic activities. Ciccotti et al. [17], however, demonstrated no increased quadriceps or hamstring activity during cross-cutting and attributed this to the task not being a rote motion.

Tibone et al. [41] studied both the straight cut and a cross-cut. In the straight cut the reference limb is planted, and the cut is made to the opposite side whereas in the cross-cut the swing limb is brought across the front of the body, and the cut is made to the same side of the body as for the planted limb. Only 11 of the 20 subjects were able to perform the cutting activities without apprehension. The angle of cut was symmetrical for the straight cut but was less sharp for the cross-cut. Likewise, the forces during the cross-cut were reduced on the affected side, as compared to those on the unaffected side. The alteration in the cut angle may have reduced the amount of relative rotation between the tibia and femur.

SYMMETRIC OR ASYMMETRIC GAIT: ARE ADAPTATIONS LEARNED RESPONSES?

The previously mentioned study by Beard et al. [9] demonstrated that all but the terminal knee extension angle during gait was symmetric and not statistically different from that of the normal. Although the duration of hamstring activity was increased, as compared to that in the normal, it was not significantly different from that of the unaffected side. Symmetric EMG patterns were also found in the study by Tibone et al. [41]. Moreover, Berchuck et al. [10] demonstrated that the change in knee flexion moment was present on both sides during walking and jogging.

The adaptations reviewed in this chapter suggest a reprogramming of the locomotor process. For instance, the increased hamstring activity during the cutting activities is likely a method of adaptation that has been developed before a particular activity, because it requires anticipation of high loads that occur later in that activity. In most situations muscles cannot contract quickly enough to protect the knee from a sudden destabilizing force. However, if the muscle contracted before the initiation of the higher loads, the patient probably will not experience the symptoms associated with the instability, because the muscles have provided additional stability. It is more likely that the adaptation occurs before the instability generated from the muscle contraction, so that the abnormal anterior drawer or strain on the secondary restraints does not develop. Perhaps in patients who do not develop this adaptation, there is a continual strain on the secondary restraints to anterior drawer (menisci and collaterals), causing continued stretching of these structures and the eventual degenerative problems reported in some ACLD patients.

CLINICAL IMPLICATIONS OF FUNCTIONAL ADAPTATIONS

Do functional adaptations protect secondary restraints or dynamically substitute for the ACL? Mikosz et al. [33] used a mathematical model of the ligamentous knee joint to quantify the extent of unloading of the secondary restraints that occurs when subjects adapt their gait to the "quadriceps avoidance" pattern previously described. The typical characteristic of the functional adaptation observed in some ACLD patients was input into a three-dimensional mathematical model of the knee joint [3]. The model included a mathematical representation of the menisci, ligaments, joint capsule, osseous structures, patellar mechanism, and hamstring muscles. Motion and moments from level walking and jogging during the maximum net quadriceps moments were input into the model. The percent change in strain for all ligaments and capsule, along with the percent change in meniscal shear force between the patients who developed the adaptive gait ("quadriceps avoidance"), was compared to that of those who did not develop an adaptive gait (i.e., who maintained normal quadriceps-hamstring patterns).

The model predicted that ACLD patients who did not develop the "quadriceps avoidance" gait had a 55% increase in strain in the capsule, whereas patients with the "quadriceps avoidance" gait had an 18% decrease in strain in the capsule, when compared to that of normals. ACLD patients who did not develop the "quadriceps avoidance" gait had a 47% increase in medial meniscus shear force during level walking, whereas patients with the "quadriceps avoidance" gait had a 21% decrease in medial meniscus shear force, when compared to that of normals.

During jogging, ACLD patients who did not reduce their net quadriceps moment had a 70% increase in strain in the capsule, whereas patients who jogged with the reduced quadriceps moment had a 43% increase in strain in the capsule, when compared to that of normals. During jogging ACLD patients who did not reduce their net quadriceps moment had a 54% increase in the medial meniscus shear force, whereas patients who jogged with a reduced quadriceps moment had 29% increase in medial meniscus shear force, when compared to that of normals.

The results of this study demonstrated that the adaptive "quadriceps avoidance" gait seen in the majority of ACLD patients during level walking and the reduced quadriceps moments during jogging decreased the strain in the secondary restraints. Moreover, ACLD patients who walked with normal gait and jogging patterns substantially increased the strain in the secondary restraints.

The modifications in function identified in these studies [12, 41] are presumably adaptations produced by a subconscious protective mechanism to avoid the excessive anterior displacement of the tibia that can occur in the absence of the ACL. It is more likely that these adaptations are the result of repetitive experiences after the loss of the ACL. It is possible that reprogramming of the locomotor process occurs, such that the adaptations occur before instability and excessive anterior displacement result. This can be accomplished by altering the pattern of muscle contracture as part of an adaptive locomotor program. Thus, the adaptations anticipate the instability and, thus, avoid the abnormal displacement. This general locomotor reprogramming could be part of a learning process that takes place during the early stages after an ACL injury. It is necessary that the locomotor system be reprogrammed in a manner that anticipates instability before the occurrence of the episode that produces instability, because the latency time for muscle contraction is too slow to instantaneously respond to a rapid stimulus.

This reprogramming hypothesis has a number of implications toward the clinical management of ACLD patients. It provides the basis for an explanation as to why some patients adapt, whereas others do not develop an adaptive gait. Perhaps some patients do not have a sufficient kinesiological sense of the instability occurring at the knee to provide the appropriate control for modifications in the patterns of muscle firing. Some subjects may have an enhanced ability to fine tune the balance between the quadriceps and hamstring contractions, using a higher level of movement coordination. These adaptive mechanisms can be seen both during simple activities, such as walking, as well as during more stressful activities, such as the lateral side step cutting maneuvers.

These results suggest that the patients who are capable of adapting their function to the absence of an ACL can protect the secondary restraints, such as the medial meniscus, during level walking. Thus, even for the individual who reduces his or her sports-related activities, an adaptive gait may be important for protecting against long-term damage to the medial meniscus. A patient who does not develop an adaptive gait will cyclically apply an anterior force to the tibia during each step of walking. These cyclic loads can eventually stretch and damage the medial meniscus. Thus, over time, the degenerative joint changes seen in patients with ACLD patients are likely to be more prevalent among patients who do not develop an adaptive gait. Similarly, subjects who perform sports activities under more stressful conditions can protect against the rotational and translational stresses at the knee joint by increasing hamstring contraction as the limb is striking the ground. Again, this muscle contraction must occur before the destabilizing loads occur. As knee flexion increases, the ability of the hamstrings to compensate for ACL deficiency increases. It should be noted that to maintain the knee in this flexed position, one needs strong quadriceps to hold the knee flexed while maintaining cocontraction of the hamstrings. Again, the more coordinated athlete may adopt this process subconsciously, but perhaps rehabilitation and training could enhance these protective mechanisms. The significant role of the hamstrings in the ACLD patients during the stressful athletic activities further emphasizes the importance of hamstring strengthening in the rehabilitation process.

Testing of ambulatory function or gait analysis is particularly relevant to the ACLD population. The appropriate selection of treatment modalities, rehabilitation, and evaluation of patients after treatment can be greatly enhanced through the appropriate use of functional testing. These results suggest that all patients do not adapt in the same manner to the loss of the ACL. It has been shown in other studies [35, 42] that the nature of functional adaptations quantified during gait analysis can be extremely useful in the treatment planning and selection of patients for particular procedures. It is likely that clinical testing of ambulatory function during both activities of daily living and more stressful athletic activities will improve treatment outcome and rehabilitation of the ACLD population.

REFERENCES

1. Andersson, C., L. R. Odensten, L. Grood, and J. Gullquist. Surgical or non-surgical treatment of fracture rupture of the ACL: a randomized study with long-term followup. *J. Bone Joint Surg.* 71A:965, 1989.
2. Andriacchi, T. P. Dynamics of pathological motion: applied to the anterior cruciate deficient knee. *J. Biomech.* 23(1):99–105, 1990.
3. Andriacchi, T. P., G. B. J. Andersson, R. Fermier, D. Stern, and J.O. Galante. A study of lower limb mechanics during stairclimbing. *J. Bone Joint Surg.* 62A:749, 1980.
4. Andriacchi, T. P., G. B. J. Andersson, R. Örtengren, and R. P. Mikosz. A study of factors influencing muscle activity about the knee joint. *J. Orthop. Res.* 1:266–275, 1984.
5. Andriacchi, T. P., and D. Birac. Functional testing in the anterior cruciate ligament-deficient knee. *Clin. Orthop.* 40–47, 1992.
6. Andriacchi, T. P., G. M. Kramer, and G. C. Landon. The biomechanics of running and knee injuries. American Academy of Orthopaedic Surgeons: Symposium on Sports Medicine. G. Finerman (ed.) *The Knee.* St. Louis: C. V. Mosby, 1985, pp. 23–32.

7. Arms, S. W., M. H. Pope, R. J. Johnson, R. A. Fischer, I. Arvidsson, and E. Eriksson. The biomechanics of anterior cruciate ligament rehabilitation and reconstruction. *Am. J. Sports Med.* 12:8, 1984.

8. Barrack, R. L., J. D. Bruckner, J. Kneisl, W. S. Inman, and A. H. Alexander. The outcome of nonoperatively treated completed tears of the ACL in active young patients. *Clin. Orthop.* 258:192, 1990.

9. Beard, D. J., R. S. Soundarapandian, J. J. O'Connor, and C. A. F. Dodd. Gait and electromyographic analysis of anterior cruciate ligament deficient subjects. *Gait Posture* 4:83–88, 1996.

10. Berchuck, M., T. P. Andriacchi, B. R. Bach, Jr., and B. R. Reider. Gait adaptations by patients who have a deficient ACL. *J. Bone Joint Surg.* 72A:871, 1990.

11. Birac, D., T. P. Andriacchi, and B. R. Bach, Jr. Time related changed following ACL rupture. *Transactions of the 37th Annual Meeting of the Orthopedic Research Society.* 1991, vol. 1, p. 231.

12. Branch, T. P., R. Hunter, and M. Donath. Dynamic EMG analysis of anterior cruciate deficient legs with and without bracing during cutting. *Am. J. Sports Med.* 17:35, 1985.

13. Bray, R. C., and D. J. Dandy. Mensical lesions and chronic ACL deficiency: meniscal tears occurring before and after reconstruction. *J. Bone Joint Surg.* 71B:128, 1989.

14. Bresler, B., and J. P. Frankel. The forces and moments in the leg during level walking. *Trans. Am. Soc. Mech. Eng.* 48A:62, 1953.

15. Butler, D. L., F. R. Noyes, and E.S. Grood. Ligamentous restraints to anterior-posterior drawer in the human knee. *J. Bone Joint Surg.* 62A:259, 1980.

16. Carlsöö, S., and A. Nordstrand. The coordination of the knee-muscles in some voluntary movements and in the gait in cases with and without knee joint injuries. *Acta Chir. Scand.* 134:423–426, 1983.

17. Ciccotti, M. G., R. K. Kerland, J. Perry, and M. Pink. An electromyographic analysis of the knee during functional activities. II. The anterior cruciate ligament-deficient and -reconstructed profiles. *Am. J. Sports Med.* 22(5):651–658, 1994.

18. Clancy, W. G., J. M. Ray, and D. J. Zolton. Acute tears of the ACL: surgical versus conservative treatment. *J. Bone Joint Surg.* 70A:1483, 1988.

19. Czerniecki, J. M., F. Lippert, and J. E. Olerud. A biomechanical evaluation of tibiofemoral rotation in anterior cruciate deficient knees during walking and running. *Am. J. Sports Med.,* 16(4):327–331, 1988.

20. Daniel, D. M., M. L. Stone, B. E. Dobson, D. C. Fithian, D. J. Rossman, and K. R. Kaufman. Fate of the ACL-injured patient: A prospective outcome study. *Am. J. Sports Med.* 22 (5):632, 1994.

21. Draganich, L. F., and T. P. Andriacchi. Three-dimensional moments produced by the knee joint musculature. *Transactions of the 31st Annual Meeting Orthopedic Research Society* 10:137, 1985, vol. 10, p. 137.

22. Feagin, J. A., K. L. Lambert, and R. R. Cunningham. Consideration of the anterior cruciate ligament injury in skiing. *Clin. Orthop.* 216:13–18, 1987.

23. Finsterbush, A., U. Frankl, Y. Matan, and G. Mann. Secondary damage to the knee after isolated injury of the ACL. *Am. J. Sports Med.* 18:475, 1990.

24. Grood, E. S., W. J. Suntay, F. R. Noyes, and D. L. Butler. Biomechanics of the knee-extension exercise: Effect of cutting the anterior cruciate ligament. *J. Bone Joint Surg.* 66A:725, 1984.

25. Jacobsen, K. Osteoarthritis following insufficiency of the cruciate ligament in man: a clinical study. *Acta Orthop. Scand.* 48:520, 1977.

26. Johnson, R. J. The anterior cruciate ligament: a dilemma in sports medicine. *Int. J. Sports Med.* 3:71, 1982.

27. Kålund, S., T. Sinkjaer, L. Arendt-Nielsen, and O. Simonsen. Altered timing of hamstring muscle action in anterior cruciate ligament deficient patients. *Am. J. Sports Med.* 18(3): 245–248, 1990.

28. Kannus, P., and M. Jarvinen. Post-traumatic ACL insufficiency as a cause of osteoarthritis in a knee joint. *Clin. Rheumatol.* 8(2):251, 1989.

29. Laas, P., S. Kaalund, S. LeFebre, L. Arendt-Neilsen, and T. Sinkjær. Muscle coordination following rupture of the anterior cruciate ligament—electromyographic studies of 14 patients. *Acta Orthop. Scand.* 62(1):9–14, 1991.

30. Limbird, T. J., R. Shiavi, M. Frazer, and H. Borra. EMG profilex of knee joint musculature during walking: Changes induced by anterior cruciate ligament deficiency. *J. Orthop. Res.* 6(5):630–638, 1988.

31. Markolf, K. L., A. Kochan, and H.D. Amstutz. Measurement of knee stiffness and laxity inpatients with documented absence of the anterior cruciate ligament. *J. Bone Joint Surg.* 66A:242, 1984.

32. McHugh, M. P., A.L. Spitz, M. P. Lorei, S. J. Nicholas, E. B. Hershman, and G. W. Gleim. Effect of anterior cruciate ligament deficiency on economy of walking and jogging. *J. Orthop. Res.* 12:592–597, 1994.

33. Mikosz, R. P., C. D. Wu, and T. P. Andriacchi. Model interpretation of functional adaptations in the ACL-deficient patient. *Proceedings of the NACOB II, The 2nd North American Congress on Biomechanics* 1992, p. 441.

34. Noyes, F. R., D. S. Matthews, P.A. Mooar, and E.S. Grood. The symptomatic anterior cruciate-deficient knee. Part II. The results of rehabilitation, activity modification and counseling on functional disability. *J. Bone Joint Surg.* 65A:163, 1983.

35. Noyes, F. R., P. A. Mooar, D. S. Matthews, and D. L. Butler. The symptomatic anterior cruciate-deficient knee. Part I. The long-term functional disability in athletically active patients. *J. Bone Joint Surg.* 65A:154, 1983.

36. Noyes, F. R., O. D. Schipplein, T. P. Andriacchi, S. R. Saddemi, and M. Weise. The anterior cruciate ligament-deficient knee with varus alignment: an analysis of gait adaptations and dynamic joint loadings. *Am. J. Sports Med.* 20(6):707, 1992.

37. Prodromos, C. C., T. P. Andriacchi, and J. O. Galante. A relationship between knee joint loads and clinical changes following high tibial osteotomy. *J. Bone Joint. Surg.* 67A(8): 1188–1194, 1985.

38. Renström, P., S. W. Arms, T. S. Stanwyck, R. J. Johnson, and M. H. Pope. Strain within the anterior cruciate ligament during hamstring and quadriceps activity. *Am. J. Sports Med.* 14(1):83–87, 1986.

39. Schipplein, O. D., and T. P. Andriacchi. Interaction between active and passive knee stabilizers during level walking. *J. Orthop. Res.* 9:113, 1991.

40. Shiavi, R., L. Q. Zhang, T. Limbird, and M. A. Edmondstone. Pattern analysis of electromyographic linear envelopes exhibited by subjects with uninjured and injured knees during free and fast speed walking. *J. Orthop. Res.* 10:226–236, 1992.

41. Tibone, J. E., T. J. Antich, G.S. Fanton, D. R. Moynes, and J. Perry. Functional analysis of anterior cruciate ligament instability. *Am. J. Sports Med.* 14:276, 1986.

42. Wang, J. W., K.N. Kuo, T. P. Andriacchi, and J.O. Galante. The influence of walking mechanics and time on the results of proximal tibial osteotomy. *J. Bone Joint Surg.* 72A(6): 905–913, 1990.

43. Wroble, R. R., R. A. Brand. Paradoxes in the history of the ACL. *Clin. Orthop.* 259:183, 1990.

2
Interactions Between Muscle Glycogen and Blood Glucose during Exercise

MARK HARGREAVES, Ph.D.

During prolonged strenuous exercise, muscle glycogen and blood-borne glucose, derived from liver glycogenolysis and gluconeogenesis (and from the gastrointestinal tract when glucose is ingested), are important substrates for contracting skeletal muscle. Fatigue during such exercise is often associated with depletion of these carbohydrate reserves [18, 24, 47, 90]. Increased muscle glycogen availability before exercise and carbohydrate ingestion during exercise have been shown to enhance endurance exercise performance [9, 12, 18, 24], and it is generally believed that this is a result of maintenance of carbohydrate availability and oxidation during the latter stages of exercise. In view of the importance of carbohydrates for exercise performance, interest has focused on the regulation of muscle glycogenolysis and glucose uptake during exercise. This article summarizes the potential interactions between muscle glycogen and blood glucose during exercise (Fig. 2.1). More specifically, the effects of alterations in blood glucose availability on the rate of muscle glycogenolysis and the influence of muscle glycogen availability on muscle glucose uptake will be reviewed.

MUSCLE GLYCOGENOLYSIS AND GLUCOSE UPTAKE DURING EXERCISE

The rate of muscle glycogen breakdown during exercise is primarily dependent on exercise intensity and is most rapid during the early stages of exercise (Fig. 2.2 and refs. 33, 92, and 103). As exercise at a given intensity continues, the rate of muscle glycogen utilization declines (Fig. 2.2), partly as a result of reduced muscle glycogen availability, although a reduction in glycogen phosphorylase activity and increased blood-borne substrate availability may also play a role. The rapid increase in muscle glycogenolysis with the onset of exercise is a result of activation of glycogen phosphorylase, which exists in two forms: a less active b form and a more active a form [56]. Phosphorylase b to a transformation occurs in response to the increased sarcoplasmic [Ca^{2+}] with muscle contractions and hormonal stimulation by epinephrine, mediated via cyclic 3', 5'- adenosine monophosphate (cyclic AMP) [14, 56, 87]. In addition, allosteric modulators such as AMP and inosine monophosphate (IMP), as well as the substrates inorganic phosphate

FIGURE 2.1.

Potential interactions between muscle glycogen and blood glucose during exercise. GLU, glucose; G-6-P, glucose 6-phosphate; GLUT4, glucose transporter isoform 4; GLY, glycogen; HK, hexokinase; LAC, lactate; PYR, pyruvate.

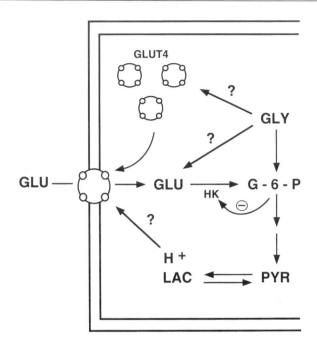

(P_i) and glycogen, influence phosphorylase activity. This complex regulation of glycogen phosphorylase activity ensures that the rate of muscle glycogenolysis is closely coupled to adenosine triphosphate (ATP) demand. As already mentioned, substrate availability plays an important role in the regulation of muscle glycogenolysis. It has been suggested that the increase in muscle [P_i] provides a link between energy demand and glycogen utilization [14], although it is not the sole factor [83]. Increased muscle glycogen availability results in an increased muscle glycogen degradation during exercise [32, 45, 49, 86] as a result of enhanced glycogen phosphorylase activity [49, 56]. This effect of glycogen availability does not appear to operate during high-intensity exercise [6, 96, 101]. During such exercise, the marked increases in ATP turnover, intramuscular Ca^{2+} and Pi levels and plasma epinephrine are likely to result in near maximal activation of glycogen phosphorylase and glycogenolysis, such that increased glycogen availability has no additional effect. There has been much interest in the effect of alterations in blood glucose availability on muscle glycogenolysis, which

FIGURE 2.2.

Muscle glycogen levels and leg glucose uptake during low (○, 30–40% V̇O₂ peak), moderate (●, 60–70% V̇O₂ peak) and high (▲, 90% V̇O₂ peak) intensity exercise. Arrows denote point of fatigue. Redrawn from ref. 91.

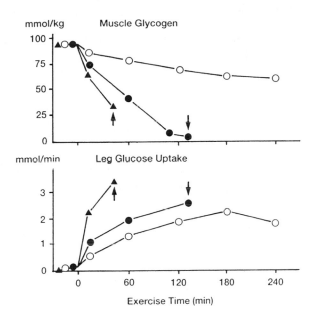

will be discussed in more detail later. Alterations in plasma free fatty acid (FFA) levels have been shown to influence muscle glycogenolysis during exercise. Inhibition of FFA mobilization by nicotinic acid lowers plasma FFA and increases muscle glycogen use during exercise [11]. In contrast, increased plasma FFA availability has been shown to reduce the rate of muscle glycogen utilization during exercise [22, 29, 51, 85, 104] via posttransformational regulation of glycogen phosphorylase activity [29].

Exercise is a powerful stimulus for skeletal muscle glucose uptake, with the increase in glucose uptake by contracting skeletal muscle being greater than that elicited by maximal insulin stimulation [54]. The magnitude of the exercise-induced increase in muscle glucose uptake is related to both the intensity and duration of exercise (Fig. 2.2 and ref. 105). At moderate exercise intensities, the increase in muscle glucose uptake is accompanied by an increase in glucose utilization [58]; however, during intense exercise, an increase in intramuscular glucose suggests that glucose phosphorylation and utilization are inhibited [58]. A potential explanation for this is an increase in muscle glucose-6-phosphate concentration ([G-6-P]), an inhibitor of hexokinase (Fig. 2.1 and ref. 67), as a consequence of increased muscle glycogenolysis. As exercise duration increases at a given exercise intensity, there is an increase in muscle glucose uptake (Fig. 2.2 and refs. 59 and 105). This is because of a progressive increase in sarcolemmal glucose transport [62] and an increase in glucose metabolism, as a result of a lower muscle [G-6-P] as the rate of muscle glycogenolysis declines with continued exercise [59]. During prolonged exercise, glucose delivery to contracting muscle may become a limiting factor as arterial glucose levels decline [2, 3, 59]. Glucose and insulin delivery to contracting skeletal muscle are increased during exercise as a consequence of the increase in muscle blood flow but cannot fully explain the exercise-induced increase in muscle glucose uptake. Thus, local factors within contracting muscle play the major role [112]. These factors include increased membrane transport of glucose and activation of the glycolytic and oxidative enzymes responsible for glucose disposal. Sarcolemmal glucose transport occurs by means of facilitated diffusion, with the GLUT4 glucose transporter isoform being responsible for contraction and insulin-stimulated glucose transport. Numerous studies have demonstrated translocation of GLUT4 from an intracellular site to the plasma membrane with contractions in rat skeletal muscle [31, 34, 68, 88], and this has also been observed in human skeletal muscle [61, 62]. It is less clear whether exercise affects GLUT4 intrinsic activity; however, GLUT4 translocation is generally considered the primary mechanism underlying increased membrane glucose transport with contractions. The intracellular distribution of GLUT1 is unaffected by exercise [34, 61]. The increase in muscle glucose uptake [80, 107] and GLUT4 translocation [35] in response to muscle contraction can occur in the absence of insulin. This is consistent with observations that contractions stimulate muscle glucose uptake via a mechanism different from insulin stimulation [65, 68, 76, 111] and that the effects of insulin and contractions on muscle glucose transport and GLUT4 translocation are additive [31, 76, 106]. Despite these observations, the plasma insulin level remains an important determinant of skeletal muscle glucose uptake during exercise [27, 50, 108]. Substrate availability also influences muscle glucose uptake during exercise. The relationship between muscle glycogen and glucose uptake will be discussed in more detail in a subsequent section. Increased blood glucose availability results in enhanced muscle glucose uptake and disposal during exercise [1, 13, 26, 70], whereas the decline in arterial blood glucose levels during the latter stages of prolonged exercise is likely to limit muscle glucose uptake [2, 3]. There has also been interest in the potential effect of increased plasma FFA on glucose uptake. Conflicting results have been obtained in perfused rat skeletal muscle [8, 84, 87]. Studies in humans have also produced differing results. Increased plasma FFA availability was associated with reduced leg glucose uptake during knee extension exercise [44]; in contrast, other investigators have observed no effect of elevated FFA on leg glucose uptake or the tracer-determined rate of glucose disappearance (glucose Rd), which primarily reflects leg muscle glucose disposal[60], glucose Rd during cycling exercise [89, 97]. Despite the uncertainty regarding the influence of FFA on glucose uptake, it is tempting to speculate that the increase in plasma FFA during prolonged exercise may limit muscle glucose uptake at a time when muscle glycogen and arterial blood glucose levels are low. Under conditions of reduced muscle glycogen availability, inhibition of FFA mobilization by nicotinic acid results in a rapid fall in blood glucose and premature fatigue [32].

ALTERATIONS IN BLOOD GLUCOSE AVAILABILITY: EFFECTS ON MUSCLE GLYCOGEN UTILIZATION

Because a reduction in carbohydrate availability is associated with fatigue during prolonged strenuous exercise, there has been an interest in strategies that enhance exercise performance by increasing or maintaining carbohydrate supply to contracting skeletal muscle. One approach has been to increase blood glucose levels by means of carbohydrate ingestion, which results in increased exercise time to fatigue [18, 24, 25, 95, 100] and the ability to maintain or increase work output [53, 75, 98]. Although it is generally believed that this ergogenic effect of carbohydrate ingestion arises from the maintenance of blood glucose levels and a high rate of carbohydrate oxidation at a time when muscle glycogen and the reliance upon it is low, it is also possible that a reduction in the rate of muscle glycogen utilization may contribute. Increases in glucose and G-6-P have the potential to reduce glycogen phosphorylase activity [56] and carbohydrate ingestion has been shown to increase intramuscular glucose accumulation during prolonged exercise [95], presumably as a consequence of enhanced muscle glucose uptake [1, 13, 70]. Another possibility is an increase in glycogen synthesis as a result of relatively higher blood glucose and insulin levels after carbohydrate ingestion, although this is more likely to occur at lower exercise intensities [64, 81] than during moderate- to high-intensity exercise, during which the stimulus for muscle glycogenolysis is greater. In one of the first investigations on muscle glycogen metabolism during exercise in humans [10], elevation of blood glucose to 13–30 mmol·liter^{-1} by means of intravenous glucose infusion resulted in a 24% reduction in net muscle glycogen use during 1 hr of exercise at 115–150 watts. However, muscle glycogen remained the major fuel source during exercise, and the authors concluded "that sugar supplied via the blood stream is able, only to a minor extent, to replace muscle glycogen as a source of energy during this type of muscular work". In a more recent study [26], elevation of blood glucose to 10–12 mmol·liter^{-1} by glucose infusion had no effect on muscle glycogen use during cycling exercise at 70–75% of peak pulmonary oxygen uptake ($\dot{V}O_2$ peak). Ingestion of carbohydrate during prolonged exercise results in

FIGURE 2.3.

Muscle glycogen levels before, during, and after exercise to fatigue at 71 ± 1% V̇O₂ peak with (CHO) and without (CON) carbohydrate ingestion. Values are means ± SE (n = 7). Redrawn from ref. 24.

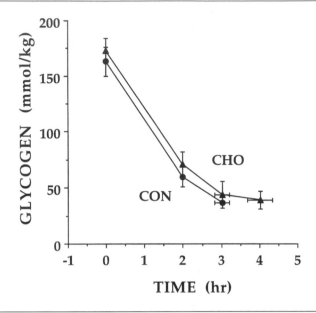

more modest increases in blood glucose, such that it usually remains within normal limits (4–6 mmol·liter⁻¹). Under such conditions, a number of studies have demonstrated that net muscle glycogen utilization during cycling exercise at 70–75% V̇O₂ peak is unaltered [Fig. 2.3 and refs. 13, 24, 40, and 75), despite a tracer-determined glucose uptake increase [13, 70]. In contrast, recent studies during prolonged treadmill running at 70% V̇O₂ peak have demonstrated that carbohydrate ingestion reduces the rate of muscle glycogen utilization and that this effect occurred almost exclusively in Type I muscle fibers [99, 100]. In addition, in those studies that have used an intermittent, variable-intensity cycling exercise protocol, carbohydrate ingestion resulted in a reduction in muscle glycogen use [41, 110]. A possible explanation for these different results may be the relative metabolic demand placed upon vastus lateralis (the muscle sampled) in these various studies. It has been observed previously that muscle glycogen utilization during running is greater in the lower limb muscles (soleus, gastrocnemius) than in vastus lateralis [23]. Despite muscle glycogen being quite low at the point of fatigue during treadmill running [100], it is possible that with a relatively lower rate of muscle glycogenolysis the increased blood glucose and insulin levels after carbohydrate ingestion resulted in a further reduction in muscle glycogen use. A similar mechanism may operate during the intermittent exercise protocols [41, 110], which have included periods of relatively low-intensity cycling exercise, during which muscle glycogen use may be reduced and glycogen synthesis may even be enhanced [64, 81] by higher blood glucose and insulin levels. Thus, during prolonged strenuous cycling exercise in humans, carbohydrate ingestion that results in increased blood glucose availability has no effect on net muscle glycogen utilization. However, whether carbohydrate ingestion can alter muscle glycogen metabolism may depend upon the mode and intensity of exercise. Studies in exercising rats have also observed reductions [5, 109] or no change [36, 94] in muscle glycogen use during exercise with carbohydrate supplementation. Again, differences in exercise intensity and the amount of glucose provided have been proposed as possible reasons for the differing results [36].

To my knowledge, no studies have examined the direct effect of reduced blood glucose availability on muscle glycogen metabolism during exercise. The ingestion of glucose in the hour before exercise results in hyperglycemia and hyperinsulinemia and a rapid fall in blood glucose with the onset of exercise [22, 30, 42, 43], as a result of the combined stimulatory effects of insulin and contractile activity on muscle glucose uptake [27, 69, 108]. This reduction in glucose availability during exercise has been associated with an increase in muscle glycogen utilization in some studies [22, 43], although this may be more related to the blunting of lipolysis that also occurs with pre-exercise hyperglycemia and hyperinsulinemia. In contrast, other studies have observed no effect of pre-exercise hyperinsulinemia, and the subsequent exercise-induced fall in blood glucose, on muscle glycogen use during exercise [30, 42]. Insulin-induced hypoglycemia in exercising rats is associated with a slight increase in muscle glycogen utilization [4]. Again, however, the effects of low blood glucose could not be separated from those resulting from reduced plasma FFA. Whether reduced blood glucose availability will influence muscle glycogen use during exercise is likely to be determined by the magnitude of the reduction in glucose availability and the extent to which blood glucose contributes to energy metabolism during exercise i.e., the proportion of total carbohydrate utilization that must be "replaced" by muscle glycogen degradation. As previously mentioned, however, no studies have directly addressed this question.

INFLUENCE OF MUSCLE GLYCOGEN AVAILABILITY ON MUSCLE GLUCOSE UPTAKE

The interactions between muscle glycogen and glucose uptake depicted in Figure 2.1 suggest a potential role for muscle glycogen in the regulation of muscle glucose uptake. Increases in [G-6-P], derived from muscle glycogenol-

FIGURE 2.4.

*Tracer-determined rate of glucose disappearance (glucose Rd) during 120 min of exercise at 69 ± 1% $\dot{V}O_2$ peak with (GLU) and without (CON) glucose ingestion. Values are means ± SE (n = 6). * denotes difference from CON, P < 0.05. Redrawn from ref. 70.*

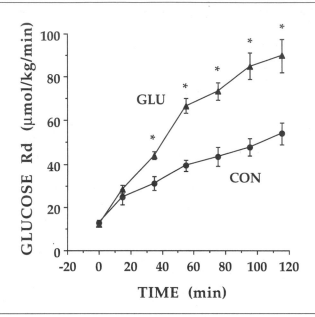

ysis [32], can reduce glucose phosphorylation by inhibiting hexokinase activity [67]. In addition, free glucose may be produced during glycogenolysis, because glucose at branch points in the glycogen molecule is not phosphorylated, although it has been suggested that the majority of free glucose accumulation within contracting skeletal muscle is of extracellular origin [58]. Nevertheless, an increase in the intracellular [glucose] may reduce the gradient for membrane glucose transport. A direct interaction between muscle glycogen and membrane transport/GLUT4 is also possible, but this phenomenon has not been well studied. What, then, is the evidence that muscle glycogen can influence muscle glucose uptake?

Studies in exercising rats [54] and the stimulated, perfused rat hindlimb [80] have suggested that glucose uptake only increases in those muscles that have a decrease in glycogen. In humans, there is a close temporal relationship between the decrease in muscle glycogen and the increase in muscle glucose uptake during cycling [46, 59] and dynamic knee extension [93] exercise. Furthermore, the progressive increase in tracer-determined glucose disposal during prolonged exercise (Fig. 2.4 and refs. 13 and 70), which occurs primarily into contracting muscle [60], may be partly related to the decline in muscle glycogen. It also appears that the relative hyperglycemia after carbohydrate ingestion is more effective in enhancing glucose uptake late in exercise when muscle glycogen is low (Fig. 2.4 and ref. 70). However, these temporal associations may simply reflect independent effects of exercise on muscle glycogenolysis and glucose uptake, rather than a causal relationship. For example, glucose infusion in patients with McArdle's disease improves both dynamic [39] and static [66] exercise performance, presumably as a consequence of increased muscle glucose uptake and oxidation that occurs in the absence of muscle glycogen degradation. Thus, muscle glycogenolysis may not always be a prerequisite for muscle glucose uptake, at least in this patient population. Nevertheless, the strength of the association between muscle glycogenolysis and glucose uptake in the above-mentioned studies suggests a potential link between these processes. This link may not be limited to the exercise situation. An increase in 3-O-methylglucose (3-MG) transport has been observed in nonexercising muscle during exercise [73] and there was a significant relationship between the increment in 3-MG transport and the decrement in glycogen within the nonexercising muscle, although an effect of systemic humoral factors could not be excluded. A 40% reduction in muscle glycogen levels by exposure of rats to epinephrine was associated with an increase in both basal and insulin-stimulated (30 $\mu U \cdot mL^{-1}$) 3-MG transport in incubated epitrochlearis muscles [77]. Finally, overexpression of muscle glycogen phosphorylase in cultured human muscle fibers not only resulted in increased glycogen turnover and reduced basal glycogen levels but also an enhanced capacity for glucose uptake and consumption in the absence of changes in hexokinase activity [7].

The more direct evaluation of the relationship between muscle glycogen and muscle glucose uptake requires the manipulation of muscle glycogen availability and subsequent measurement of glucose uptake during exercise. The difficulty with this approach in humans has been the need to use exercise and dietary interventions to manipulate the pre-exercise muscle glycogen level. Such interventions can produce alterations in other factors (e.g., plasma substrate and hormone levels) that also influence muscle glucose uptake. Gollnick et al. [32] observed a greater glucose extraction during exercise in a limb that commenced exercise with low muscle glycogen levels, compared to that in the contralateral limb with a higher pre-exercise muscle glycogen concentration. Leg glucose uptake during exercise was positively correlated with the percentage of glycogen-empty fibers (determined histochemically) and inversely with the muscle [G-6-P]. In this study, however, the lower muscle glycogen levels were obtained by single-leg exercise on the day before the investigation, which may have resulted in ongoing stimulation of muscle glucose uptake [48] and increased insulin sensitivity [74]. We recently evaluated the influence of muscle glycogen on glucose uptake during exercise using an identical exercise stimulus on the day before the investigation but while varying dietary carbohydrate intake [45]. The increased carbohydrate intake resulted in higher pre-exercise muscle glycogen levels and increased muscle glycogen degradation during exercise at 65–70% $\dot{V}O_2$ peak. In contrast, tracer-determined glucose uptake was not different between the two conditions, implying no effect of muscle glycogen availability. However, plasma insulin and glucose were lower and plasma FFA were higher after the low carbohydrate intake, alterations that would be expected to reduce muscle glucose uptake and oppose the potential stimulatory effect of lower muscle glycogen on glucose uptake. In a recent preliminary report [102], a similar result was obtained during dynamic knee extension. Again, alterations in lipid metabolism within the contracting muscle may have confounded the direct effects of muscle glycogen availability on glucose uptake. Similarly, increases in plasma FFA levels have been used to explain the inability of glycogen-depleted subjects to take and oxidise a greater amount of ingested glucose [82]. These technical problems in human studies are avoided with the use of the perfused rat hindlimb, where perfusate substrate and hormone concentrations can be easily controlled. Under these conditions, an effect of muscle glycogen on muscle glucose uptake [48, 86] and 3-MG transport [48] during contractions has been clearly demonstrated. Increased muscle glycogen resulted in reduced glucose uptake and 3-MG transport, whereas reduced muscle glycogen availability increased both measures (Fig. 2.5). The lower rates of glucose uptake and transport under conditions of muscle glycogen supercompensation were associated with higher intracellular concentrations of G-6-P and glucose [48].

The potential mechanisms linking muscle glycogen and its rate of breakdown with muscle glucose uptake involve effects on both membrane glucose transport and glucose disposal, as summarized in Figure 2.1. It has been suggested that effects on glucose disposal, via alterations in muscle [G-6-P] and hexokinase activity, exert a major influence on muscle glucose uptake during exercise [59]. Indeed, the alterations in muscle glucose uptake with differences in muscle glycogen are related to the muscle [G-6-P] [32, 48]. In addition, the observation that 3-MG transport during muscle contractions is influenced by the muscle glycogen availability [48] indicates that there are also effects on membrane glucose transport. Furthermore, the progressive increase in sarcolemmal vesicle glucose transport and GLUT4 content that has recently been observed during 40 min of exercise at 75% $\dot{V}O_2$ peak [62], may be partly related to the decline in muscle glycogen. The mechanisms underlying effects on membrane glucose transport have been less studied than those related to glucose metabolism. Increases in intracellular glucose have the potential to reduce the gradient for glucose diffusion. In addition, there may be effects on GLUT4 translocation and/or activity. In plasma membrane vesicles from rat skeletal muscle, in-

FIGURE 2.5.

Relationship between muscle glycogen and glucose uptake during contractions in the perfused rat hundlimb (Panel A). Data points represent means ± SE (n = 9–11). Symbols are control (▲), glycogen-depleted (●) and glycogen supercompensated (■) rats. Panel B summarizes glucose transport into contracting muscles with either high (hatched bars) or low (open bars) glycogen levels after 5 and 15 min. Values are means ± SE (n = 8–9). * denotes different from low glycogen, P < 0.05. Reproduced from ref. 48.

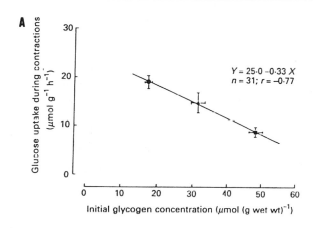

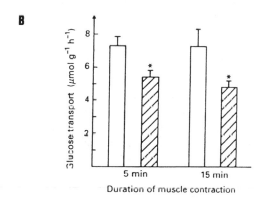

creased [G-6-P] had no effect on GLUT4 intrinsic activity, whereas GLUT4 activity was sensitive to changes in pH [63]. Thus, it is possible that a decrease in muscle pH, as a consequence of increased muscle glycogenolysis associated with higher pre-exercise muscle glycogen concentrations, may modulate membrane glucose transport. Another possibility is a direct effect of glycogen on GLUT4. It has been suggested that "exercise-sensitive" GLUT4 vesicles may be associated with glycogen [16], and a preliminary report provided evidence of binding of skeletal muscle GLUT4 vesicles with immobilized cyclodextrin, a glycogen surrogate that interacts with glycogen-binding proteins [17]. In this proposed scheme, the degradation of muscle glycogen during exercise would release GLUT4 vesicles, thereby making them available for translocation to the plasma membrane. Although this may provide an explanation for the influence of muscle glycogen on membrane glucose transport, further work is required to verify this interesting hypothesis.

ENDURANCE TRAINING

One of the major metabolic adaptations to endurance training is a decrease in the reliance on muscle glycogen [15, 21, 37, 55, 57] and blood glucose [19, 20, 55, 78] as fuel sources during exercise. The potential mechanisms responsible for this blunting of carbohydrate utilization include increased muscle oxidative capacity, tighter metabolic control, alterations in muscle fiber recruitment patterns, and changes in glycogenolytic and glucoregulatory hormone levels and/or action. Is it possible that the blunting of glycogenolysis and glucose utilization after training represents another interaction between muscle glycogen and glucose uptake?

After endurance training, there is a reduction in muscle [G-6-P] during exercise that closely parallels the decrease in muscle glycogen utilization [21]. This suggests a decrease in the rate of G-6-P production from muscle glycogenolysis and/or glucose transport and phosphorylation. A recent study has demonstrated that posttransformational factors, such as reduced P_i and AMP, are responsible for the blunting of muscle glycogenolysis during intense exercise after short-term training [15]. The reduction in muscle AMP and P_i was associated with an increased muscle oxidative capacity. In addition, a reduction in plasma epinephrine levels may contribute during exercise of longer duration [15]. The decrease in muscle glucose uptake during exercise after training occurs despite the fact that skeletal muscle GLUT4 [28, 38, 52, 72, 79] and hexokinase activity [78, 79] are increased and the observation that insulin-stimulated muscle glucose uptake is enhanced by training [28]. Furthermore, we have observed an inverse relationship between tracer-determined glucose uptake during exercise and vastus lateralis GLUT4 and citrate synthase activity in a group of active, but untrained, men [71]. Taken together, these results suggest that GLUT4 translocation and/or activity in response to submaximal exercise is reduced after training in human subjects. It is tempting to speculate that the reduced muscle glycogenolysis and glucose uptake occurs in response to a common signal that is in some way linked to the improved energy status of the muscle after training. An alternative suggestion might be that if GLUT4 vesicles were associated with glycogen [17], and GLUT4 translocation were dependent upon glycogen degradation [16], then the lower muscle glucose uptake was a consequence of the reduced glycogen breakdown. Such suggestions are purely speculative but are worthy of further investigation.

SUMMARY

Muscle glycogen and blood glucose are important substrates for contracting skeletal muscle during exercise. The possibility exists for considerable interaction between muscle glycogen and blood glucose and their effects on muscle glucose uptake and glycogenolysis, respectively. Increases in blood glucose availability have little effect on net muscle glycogen utilization during prolonged, strenuous cycling exercise, but this may be dependent upon the mode and intensity of exercise. No data exist on the direct effect of reduced blood glucose levels on muscle glycogen metabolism. In rats, studies using the perfused hindlimb suggest an inverse relationship between muscle glycogen levels and glucose uptake. A similar conclusion can be drawn from a number of human studies albeit, on occasion, from indirect evidence. The influence of muscle glycogen on glucose uptake involves effects on both membrane glucose transport and intracellular glucose metabolism. Such a relationship would, under conditions of adequate muscle glycogen availability, limit muscle glucose uptake, thereby preserving the relatively small blood glucose supply for the brain, nerves, and blood cells, which are dependent on it for their energy metabolism.

ACKNOWLEDGEMENTS

The collaboration with Associate Professor Joseph Proietto, Professor Erik Richter, Dr. Søren Kristiansen, Dr. Glenn McConell, Dr. Michael McCoy, and Dr. Nelly Marmy-Conus and the excellent technical assistance of Suzanne Fabris have been fundamental to my research activity over the last 4–5 years and are gratefully acknowledged. Financial support for specific projects has been received from the Danish National Science Foundation, Danish Natural Science Research Council, Diabetes Australia Research Trust, Gatorade Sports Science Institute, National Health and Medical Research Council of Australia, and Ross Australia.

REFERENCES

1. Ahlborg, G., and P. Felig. Influence of glucose ingestion on fuel-hormone response during prolonged exercise. *J. Appl. Physiol.* 41:683–688, 1976.
2. Ahlborg, G., and P. Felig. Lactate and glucose exchange across the forearm, legs, and splanchnic bed during and after prolonged leg exercise. *J. Clin. Invest.* 69:45–54, 1982.
3. Ahlborg, G., P. Felig, L. Hagenfeldt, R. Hendler, and J. Wahren. Substrate turnover dur-

ing prolonged exercise in man: splanchnic and leg metabolism of glucose, free fatty acids, and amino acids. *J. Clin. Invest.* 53:1080–1090, 1974.

4. Arogyasami, J., T. L. Sellers, G. I. Wilson, J. P. Jones, C. Duan, and W. W. Winder. Insulin-induced hypoglycemia in fed and fasted exercising rats. *J. Appl. Physiol.* 72:1991–1998, 1992.

5. Bagby, G. J., H. J. Green, S. Katsuta, and P. D. Gollnick. Glycogen depletion in exercising rats infused with glucose, lactate, or pyruvate. *J. Appl. Physiol.* 45:425–429, 1978.

6. Bangsbo, J., T. E. Graham, B. Kiens, and B. Saltin. Elevated muscle glycogen and anaerobic energy production during exhaustive exercise in man. *J. Physiol.* 451:205–227, 1992.

7. Baque, S., J. J. Guinovart, and A. M. Gomez-Foix. Overexpression of muscle glycogen phosphorylase in cultured human muscle fibers causes increased glucose consumption and nonoxidative disposal. *J. Biol. Chem.* 271:2594–2598, 1996.

8. Berger, M., S. A. Hagg, M. N. Goodman, and N. B. Ruderman. Glucose metabolism in perfused skeletal muscle: effects of starvation, diabetes, fatty acids, acetoacetate, insulin and exercise on glucose uptake and disposition. *Biochem. J.* 158:191–202, 1976.

9. Bergstrom, J., L. Hermansen, E. Hultman, and B. Saltin. Diet, muscle glycogen and physical performance. *Acta Physiol. Scand.* 71:140–150, 1967.

10. Bergstrom, J., and E. Hultman. A study of the glycogen metabolism during exercise in man. *Scand. J. Clin. Lab. Invest.* 19:218–228, 1967.

11. Bergstrom, J., E. Hultman, L. Jorfeldt, B. Pernow, and J. Wahren. Effect of nicotinic acid on physical working capacity and on metabolism of muscle glycogen in man. *J. Appl. Physiol.* 26:170–176, 1969.

12. Bosch, A. N., S. C. Dennis, and T. D. Noakes. Influence of carbohydrate loading on fuel substrate turnover and oxidation during prolonged exercise. *J. Appl. Physiol.* 74:1921–1927, 1993.

13. Bosch, A. N., S. C. Dennis, and T. D. Noakes. Influence of carbohydrate ingestion on fuel substrate turnover and oxidation during prolonged exercise. *J. Appl. Physiol.* 76:2364–2372, 1994.

14. Chasiotis, D. Role of cyclic AMP and inorganic phosphate in the regulation of muscle glycogenolysis during exercise. *Med. Sci. Sports Exerc.* 20:545–550, 1988.

15. Chesley, A., G. J. F. Heigenhauser, and L. L. Spriet. Regulation of muscle glycogen phosphorylase activity following short-term endurance training. *Am. J. Physiol.* 270:E328-E335, 1996.

16. Coderre, L., K. V. Kandror, G. Vallega, and P. F. Pilch. Identification and characterization of an exercise-sensitive pool of glucose transporters in skeletal muscle. *J. Biol. Chem.* 270: 27584–27588, 1995.

17. Coderre, L., G. Vallega, and P. F. Pilch. Association of GLUT-4 vesicles with glycogen particles in skeletal muscle: identification of a contraction-sensitive pool (abstract). *Diabetes* 43:159A, 1994.

18. Coggan, A. R., and E. F. Coyle. Reversal of fatigue during prolonged exercise by carbohydrate infusion or ingestion. *J. Appl. Physiol.* 63:2388–2395, 1987.

19. Coggan, A. R., W. M. Kohrt, R. J. Spina, D. M. Bier, and J. O. Holloszy. Endurance training decreases plasma glucose turnover and oxidation during moderate-intensity exercise in men. *J. Appl. Physiol.* 68:990–996, 1990.

20. Coggan, A. R., C. A. Raguso, B. D. Williams, L. S. Sidossis, and A. Gastaldelli. Glucose kinetics during high-intensity exercise in endurance-trained and untrained humans. *J. Appl. Physiol.* 78:1203–1207, 1995.

21. Coggan, A. R., R. J. Spina, W. M. Kohrt, and J. O. Holloszy. Effect of prolonged exercise on muscle citrate concentration before and after endurance training in men. *Am. J. Physiol.* 264:E215-E220, 1993.

22. Costill, D. L., E. Coyle, G. Dalsky, W. Evans, W. Fink, and D. Hoopes. Effects of elevated plasma FFA and insulin on muscle glycogen usage during exercise. *J. Appl. Physiol.* 43: 695–699, 1977.

23. Costill, D. L., E. Jansson, P. D. Gollnick, and B. Saltin. Glycogen utilization in leg muscles of men during level and uphill running. *Acta Physiol. Scand.* 91:475–481, 1974.

24. Coyle, E. F., A. R. Coggan, M. K. Hemmert, and J. L. Ivy. Muscle glycogen utilization during prolonged strenuous exercise when fed carbohydrate. *J. Appl. Physiol.* 61:165–172, 1986.

25. Coyle, E. F., J. M. Hagberg, B. F. Hurley, W. H. Martin, A. A. Ehsani, and J. O. Holloszy. Carbohydrate feeding during prolonged strenuous exercise can delay fatigue. *J. Appl. Physiol.* 55:230–235, 1983.

26. Coyle, E. F., M. T. Hamilton, J. Gonzalez-Alonso, S. J. Montain, and J. L. Ivy. Carbohydrate metabolism during intense exercise when hyperglycemic. *J. Appl. Physiol.* 70:834–840, 1991.

27. DeFronzo, R. A., E. Ferrannini, Y. Sato, P. Felig, and J. Wahren. Synergistic interaction between exercise and insulin on peripheral glucose uptake. *J. Clin. Invest.* 68:1468–1474, 1981.

28. Dela, F., A. Handberg, K. J. Mikines, J. Vinten, and H. Galbo. GLUT4 and insulin receptor binding and kinase activity in trained human muscle. *J. Physiol.* 469:615–624, 1993.

29. Dyck, D. J., S. J. Peters, P. S. Wendling, A. Chesley, E. Hultman, and L. L. Spriet. Regulation of muscle glycogen phosphorylase activity during intense aerobic cycling with elevated FFA *Am J Physiol* E116-E125, 1996.

30. Fielding, R. A., D. L. Costill, W. J. Fink, D.S. King, J. E. Kovaleski, and J. P. Kirwan. Effects of pre-exercise carbohydrate feedings on muscle glycogen use during exercise in well-trained runners. *Eur. J. Appl. Physiol.* 56:225 229, 1987.

31. Gao, J., J. Ren, E. A. Gulve, and J. O. Holloszy. Additive effect of contractions and insulin on GLUT-4 translocation into the sarcolemma. *J. Appl. Physiol.* 77:1597–1601, 1994.

32. Gollnick, P. D., B. Pernow, B. Essen, E. Jansson, and B. Saltin. Availability of glycogen and plasma FFA for substrate utilization in leg muscle of man during exercise. *Clin. Physiol.* 1:27–42, 1981.

33. Gollnick, P. D., K. Piehl, and B. Saltin. Selective glycogen depletion pattern in human muscle fibres after exercise of varying intensity and at varying pedalling rates. *J. Physiol.* 241: 45–57, 1974.

34. Goodyear, L. J., M. F. Hirshman, and E. S. Horton. Exercise-induced translocation of skeletal muscle glucose transporters. *Am. J. Physiol.* 261:E795-E799, 1991.

35. Goodyear, L. J., P. A. King, M. F. Hirshman, C. M. Thompson, E. D. Horton, and E. S. Horton. Contractile activity increases plasma membrane glucose transporters in the absence of insulin. *Am. J. Physiol.* 258:E667-E672, 1990.

36. Gorski, J., M. Zendzian-Piotrowska, M. Gorska, and J. Rutkiewicz. Effect of hyperglycaemia on muscle glycogen mobilization during muscle contractions in the rat. *Eur. J. Appl. Physiol.* 61:408–412, 1990.

37. Green, H. J., S. Jones, M.E. Ball-Burnett, D. Smith, J. Livesey, and B. W. Farrance. Early muscular and metabolic adaptations to prolonged exercise training in humans. *J. Appl. Physiol.* 70:2032–2038, 1991.

38. Gulve, E. A., and R. J. Spina. Effect of 7–10 days of cycle ergometer exercise on skeletal muscle GLUT-4 protein content. *J. Appl. Physiol.* 79:1562–1566, 1995.

39. Haller, R. G., S. F. Lewis, J. D. Cook, and C. G. Blomqvist. Myophosphorylase deficiency impairs muscle oxidative metabolism. *Ann. Neurol.* 17:196–199, 1985.

40. Hargreaves, M., and C. A. Briggs. Effect of carbohydrate ingestion on exercise metabolism. *J. Appl. Physiol.* 65:1553–1555, 1988.

41. Hargreaves, M., D. L. Costill, A. Coggan, W. J. Fink, and I. Nishibata. Effect of carbohydrate feedings on muscle glycogen utilization and exercise performance. *Med. Sci. Sports Exerc.* 16:219–222, 1984.

42. Hargreaves, M., D. L. Costill, W. J. Fink, D. S. King, and R. A. Fielding. Effect of pre-exercise carbohydrate feedings on endurance cycling performance. *Med. Sci. Sports Exerc.* 19: 33–36, 1987.

43. Hargreaves, M., D. L. Costill, A. Katz, and W. J. Fink. Effect of fructose ingestion on muscle glycogen usage during exercise. *Med. Sci. Sports Exerc.* 17:360–363, 1985.

44. Hargreaves, M., B. Kiens, and E. A. Richter. Effect of increased plasma free fatty acid concentrations on muscle metabolism in exercising men. *J. Appl. Physiol.* 70:194–201, 1991.

45. Hargreaves, M., G. McConell, and J. Proietto. Influence of muscle glycogen on glycogenolysis and glucose uptake during exercise. *J. Appl. Physiol.* 78:288–292, 1995.

46. Hargreaves, M., I. Meredith, and G. L. Jennings. Muscle glycogen and glucose uptake during exercise in humans. *Exp. Physiol.* 77:641–644, 1992.

47. Hermansen, L., E. Hultman, and B. Saltin. Muscle glycogen during prolonged severe exercise. *Acta Physiol. Scand.* 71:129–139, 1967.

48. Hespel, P., and E. A. Richter. Glucose uptake and transport in contracting, perfused rat muscle with different pre-contraction glycogen concentrations. *J. Physiol.* 427:347–359, 1990.

49. Hespel, P., and E. A. Richter. Mechanism linking glycogen concentration and glycogenolytic rate in perfused contracting rat skeletal muscle. *Biochem. J.* 284:777–780, 1992.

50. Hespel, P., L. Vergauwen, K. Vandenburghe, and E. A. Richter. Significance of insulin for glucose metabolism in skeletal muscle during contractions. *Diabetes.* 45:S99-S104, 1996.

51. Hickson, R. C., M. J. Rennie, R. K. Conlee, W. W. Winder, and J. O. Holloszy. Effects of increased plasma fatty acids on glycogen utilization and endurance. *J. Appl. Physiol.* 43: 829–833, 1977.

52. Houmard, J. A., M.S. Hickey, G. L. Tyndall, K. E. Gavigan, and G. L. Dohm. Seven days of exercise increase GLUT-4 protein content in human skeletal muscle. *J. Appl. Physiol.* 79: 1936–1938, 1995.

53. Ivy, J. L., D. L. Costill, W. J. Fink, and R. W. Lower. Influence of caffeine and carbohydrate feedings on endurance performance. *Med. Sci. Sports* 11:6–11, 1979.

54. James, D. E., E. W. Kraegen, and D. J. Chisholm. Muscle glucose metabolism in exercising rats: comparison with insulin stimulation. *Am. J. Physiol.* 248:E575-E580, 1985.

55. Jansson, E., and L. Kaijser. Substrate utilization and enzymes in skeletal muscle of extemely endurance-trained men. *J. Appl. Physiol.* 62:999–1005, 1987.

56. Johnson, L. N. Glycogen phosphorylase: control by phosphorylation and allosteric effectors. *FASEB J.* 6:2274–2282, 1992.

57. Karlsson, J., L.- O. Nordesjo, and B. Saltin. Muscle glycogen utilization during exercise after physical training. *Acta Physiol. Scand.* 90:210–217, 1974.

58. Katz, A., S. Broberg, K. Sahlin, and J. Wahren. Leg glucose uptake during maximal dynamic exercise in humans. *Am. J. Physiol.* 251:E65-E70, 1986.

59. Katz, A., K. Sahlin, and S. Broberg. Regulation of glucose utilization in human skeletal muscle during moderate dynamic exercise. *Am. J. Physiol.* 260:E411-E415, 1991.

60. Kjær, M., B. Kiens, M. Hargreaves, and E. A. Richter. Influence of active muscle mass on glucose homeostasis during exercise in humans. *J. Appl. Physiol.* 71:552–557, 1991.

61. Kristiansen, S., M. Hargreaves, and E.A. Richter. Exercise-induced increase in glucose transport, GLUT-4 and VAMP-2 in plasma membrane from human muscle. *Am. J. Physiol.* 270:E197-E201, 1996.

62. Kristiansen, S., M. Hargreaves, and E.A. Richter. Progressive increase in glucose transport and GLUT4 in human sarcolemmal vesicles during moderate dynamic exercise, submitted for publication to *Am. J. Physiol.*, 1996.

63. Kristiansen, S., J. F. Wojtaszewski, C. Juel, and E.A. Richter. Effect of glucose-6-phosphate and pH on glucose transport in skeletal muscle plasma membrane giant vesicles. *Acta Physiol. Scand.* 150:227–233, 1994.

64. Kuipers, H., H. A. Keizer, F. Brouns, and W. H. M. Saris. Carbohydrate feeding and glycogen synthesis during exercise in man. *Pflugers Arch.* 410:652–656, 1987.

65. Lee, A. D., P. A. Hansen, and J. O. Holloszy. Wortmannin inhibits insulin-stimulated but not contraction-stimulated glucose transport activity in skeletal muscle. *FEBS Lett* 361: 51–54, 1995.

66. Lewis, S. F., R. G. Haller, J. D. Cook, and R. L. Nunnally. Muscle fatigue in McArdle's disease studied by ^{31}P-NMR: effect of glucose infusion. *J. Appl. Physiol.* 59:1991–1994, 1985.
67. Lueck, J. D., and H. J. Fromm. Kinetics, mechanism, and regulation of rat skeletal muscle hexokinase. *J. Biol. Chem.* 249:1341–1347, 1974.
68. Lund, S., G. D. Holman, O. Schmitz, and O. Pedersen. Contraction stimulates translocation of glucose transporter GLUT4 in skeletal muscle through a mechanism distinct from that of insulin. *Proc. Natl. Acad. Sci. U. S. A.* 92:5817–5821, 1995.
69. Marmy-Conus, N., S. Fabris, J. Proietto, and M. Hargreaves. Pre-exercise glucose ingestion and glucose kinetics during exercise. *J. Appl. Physiol.* 81:853–857, 1996.
70. McConell, G., S. Fabris, J. Proietto, and M. Hargreaves. Effect of carbohydrate ingestion on glucose kinetics during prolonged exercise. *J. Appl. Physiol.* 77:1537–1541, 1994.
71. McConell, G., M. McCoy, J. Proietto, and M. Hargreaves. Skeletal muscle GLUT-4 and glucose uptake during exercise in humans. *J. Appl. Physiol.* 77:1565–1568, 1994.
72. McCoy, M., J. Proietto, and M. Hargreaves. Effect of detraining on GLUT-4 protein in human skeletal muscle. *J. Appl. Physiol.* 77:1532–1536, 1994.
73. Megeney, L. A., G. C. B. Elder, M. H. Tan, and A. Bonen. Increased glucose transport in nonexercising muscle. *Am. J. Physiol.* 262:E20-E26, 1992.
74. Mikines, K. J., B. Sonne, P. A. Farrell, B. Tronier, and H. Galbo. Effect of physical exercise on sensitivity and responsiveness to insulin in humans. *Am. J. Physiol.* 254:E248-E259, 1988.
75. Mitchell, J. B., D. L. Costill, J. A. Houmard, W. J. Fink, D. D. Pascoe, and D. R. Pearson. Influence of carbohydrate dosage on exercise performance and glycogen metabolism. *J. Appl. Physiol.* 67:1843–1849, 1989.
76. Nesher, R., I. E. Karl, and D. M. Kipnis. Dissociation of effects of insulin and contraction on glucose transport in rat epitrochlearis muscle. *Am. J. Physiol.* 249:C226-C232, 1985.
77. Nolte, L. A., E. A. Gulve, and J. O. Holloszy. Epinephrine-induced in vivo muscle glycogen depletion enhances insulin sensitivity of glucose transport. *J. Appl. Physiol.* 76:2054–2058, 1994.
78. Phillips, S. M., H. J. Green, M. A. Tarnopolsky, and S. M. Grant. Decreased glucose turnover after short-term training is unaccompanied by changes in muscle oxidative capacity. *Am. J. Physiol.* 269:E222-E230, 1995.
79. Phillips, S. M., X.-X. Han, H. J. Green, and A. Bonen. Increments in skeletal muscle GLUT-1 and GLUT-4 after endurance training in humans. *Am. J. Physiol.* 270:E456-E462, 1996.
80. Ploug, T., H. Galbo, and E. A. Richter. Increased muscle glucose uptake during contractions: no need for insulin. *Am. J. Physiol.* 247:E726-E731, 1984.
81. Price, T. B., R. Taylor, G. F. Mason, D. L. Rothman, G. I. Shulman, and R. G. Shulman. Turnover of human muscle glycogen with low-intensity exercise. *Med. Sci. Sports Exerc.* 26: 983–991, 1994.
82. Ravussin, E., P. Pahud, A. Dorner, M. J. Arnaud, and E. Jequier. Substrate utilization during prolonged exercise preceded by the ingestion of ^{13}C-glucose in glycogen depleted and control subjects. *Pflugers Arch.* 382:197–202, 1979.
83. Ren, J. M., and E. Hultman. Regulation of phosphorylase a activity in human skeletal muscle. *J. Appl. Physiol.* 69:919–923, 1990.
84. Rennie, M. J., and J. O. Holloszy. Inhibition of glucose uptake and glycogenolysis by availability of oleate in well-oxygenated perfused skeletal muscle. *Biochem. J.* 168:161–170, 1977.
85. Rennie, M. J., W. W. Winder, and J. O. Holloszy. A sparing effect of increased plasma fatty acids on muscle and liver glycogen content in the exercising rat. *Biochem. J.* 156:647–655, 1976.
86. Richter, E. A., and H. Galbo. High glycogen levels enhance glycogen breakdown in isolated contracting skeletal muscle. *J. Appl. Physiol.* 61:827–831, 1986.
87. Richter, E. A., N. B. Ruderman, H. Gavras, E. R. Belur, and H. Galbo. Muscle glycogenolysis during exercise: dual control by epinephrine and contractions. *Am. J. Physiol.* 242:E25-E32, 1982.

88. Rodnick, K. J., J. W. Slot, D. R. Studelska, D. E. Hanpeter, L. J. Robinson, H. J. Geuze, and D.E. James. Immunocytochemical and biochemical studies of GLUT4 in rat skeletal muscle. *J. Biol. Chem.* 267:6278–6285, 1992.

89. Romijn, J. A., E. F. Coyle, L. S. Sidossis, X.- J. Zhang, and R. R. Wolfe. Relationship between fatty acid delivery and fatty acid oxidation during strenuous exercise. *J. Appl. Physiol.* 79:1939–1945, 1995.

90. Sahlin, K., A. Katz, and S. Broberg. Tricarboxylic acid cycle intermediates in human muscle during prolonged exercise. *Am. J. Physiol.* 259:C834-C841, 1990.

91. Saltin, B., and P. D. Gollnick. Fuel for muscular exercise: role of carbohydrate. E.S. Horton and R. L. Terjung (eds.). *Exercise, Nutrition, and Energy Metabolism.* New York: Macmillan, 1988, pp. 45–71.

92. Saltin, B., and J. Karlsson. Muscle glycogen utilization during work of different intensities. B. Pernow and J. Wahren (eds.). *Muscle Metabolism during Exercise.* New York: Plenum Press, 1971, pp. 289–299.

93. Saltin, B., B. Kiens, and G. Savard. A quantitative approach to the evaluation of skeletal muscle substrate utilization in prolonged exercise. G. Benzi, L. Packer, and N. Siliprandi (eds.). *Biochemical Aspects of Exercise.* Amsterdam: Elsevier Science, 1986, pp. 235–244.

94. Slentz, C. A., J. M. Davis, D. L. Settles, R. R. Pate, and S. J. Settles. Glucose feedings and exercise in rats: glycogen use, hormone responses, and performance. *J. Appl. Physiol.* 69: 989–994, 1990.

95. Spencer, M. K., Z. Yan, and A. Katz. Carbohydrate supplementation attenuates IMP accumulation in human muscle during prolonged exercise. *Am. J. Physiol.* 261:C71-C76, 1991.

96. Spriet, L. L., L. Berardinucci, D. R. Marsh, C. B. Campbell, and T. E. Graham. Glycogen content has no effect on skeletal muscle glycogenolysis during short-term tetanic stimulation. *J. Appl. Physiol.* 68:1883–1888, 1990.

97. Spriet, L. L., L. M. Odland, D. Wong, M.G. Hollidge-Horvat, and G. J. F. Heigenhauser. Effect of elevated [FFA] on glucose uptake and lactate efflux during submaximal exercise in man (abstract). *Med. Sci. Sports Exerc.* 28:S2, 1996.

98. Tsintzas, O. K., R. Liu, C. Williams, I. Campbell, and G. Gaitanos. The effect of carbohydrate ingestion on performance during a 30-km race. *Int. J. Sports Nutr.* 3:127–139, 1993.

99. Tsintzas, O. K., C. Williams, L. Boobis, and P. Greenhaff. Carbohydrate ingestion and glycogen utilization in different muscle fibre types in man. *J. Physiol.* 489:243–250, 1995.

100. Tsintzas, O. K., C. Williams, L. Boobis, and P. Greenhaff. Carbohydrate ingestion and single muscle fibre glycogen metabolism during prolonged running in men. *J. Appl. Physiol.* 81:801–809, 1996.

101. Vandenburghe, K., P.Hespel, B. Vanden Eynde, R. Lysens, and E. A. Richter. No effect of glycogen level on glycogen metabolism during high intensity exercise. *Med. Sci. Sports Exerc.* 27:1278–1283, 1995.

102. Van Hall, G., W. H. M. Saris, B. Saltin, and A. J. M. Wagenmakers. Use of glucose during prolonged exercise in muscle with a normal and low glycogen content (abstract). *Med. Sci. Sports Exerc.* 26:S204, 1994.

103. Vøllestad, N. K.,and P. C. S. Blom. Effect of varying exercise intensity on glycogen depletion in human muscle fibres. *Acta Physiol. Scand.* 125:395–405, 1985.

104. Vukovich, M. D., D. L. Costill, M. S. Hickey, S. W. Trappe, K. J. Cole, and W. J. Fink. Effect of fat emulsion infusion and fat feeding on muscle glycogen utilization during cycle exercise. *J. Appl. Physiol.* 75:1513–1518, 1993.

105. Wahren, J., P. Felig, G. Ahlborg, and L. Jorfeldt. Glucose metabolism during leg exercise in man. *J. Clin. Invest.* 50:2715–2725, 1971.

106. Wallberg-Henriksson, H., S. H. Constable, D. A. Young, and J. O. Holloszy. Glucose transport into rat skeletal muscle: interaction between exercise and insulin. *J. Appl. Physiol.* 65: 909–913, 1988.

107. Wallberg-Henriksson, H., and J. O. Holloszy. Contractile activity increases glucose uptake by muscle in severely diabetic rats. *J. Appl. Physiol.* 57:1045–1049, 1984.

108. Wasserman, D. H., R. J. Geer, D. E. Rice, D. Bracy, P.J . Flakoll, L. L. Brown, J. O. Hill, and N.N. Abumrad. Interaction of exercise and insulin action in humans. *Am. J. Physiol.* 260:E37-E45, 1991.

109. Winder, W. W., J. Arogyasami, H. T. Yang, K. G. Thompson, L. A. Nelson, K. P. Kelly, and D.H. Han. Effects of glucose infusion in exercising rats. *J. Appl. Physiol.* 64:2300–2305, 1988.

110. Yaspelkis, B. B., J. G. Patterson, P. A. Anderla, Z. Ding, and J. L. Ivy. Carbohydrate supplementation spares muscle glycogen during variable-intensity exercise. *J. Appl. Physiol.* 75:1477–1485, 1993.

111. Yeh, J.- I., E. A. Gulve, L. Rameh, and M. J. Birnbaum. The effects of wortmannin on rat skeletal muscle: dissociation of signaling pathways for insulin- and contraction-activated hexose transport. *J. Biol. Chem.* 270:2107–2111, 1995.

112. Zinker, B. A., D. B. Lacy, D. P. Bracy, and D. H. Wasserman. Role of glucose and insulin loads to the exercising limb in increasing glucose uptake and metabolism. *J. Appl. Physiol.* 74:2915–2921, 1993.

3
Thermoregulation at Rest and during Exercise in Healthy Older Adults

W. LARRY KENNEY, PH.D.

This review will focus on the comparative responses of older and younger individuals at rest and during dynamic exercise at environmental extremes, comprising both hot and cold climatic conditions. Several comprehensive reviews have been published in recent years, and the reader is also directed to a pair of exceptional reviews by Pandolf [93] and Young [130], as well as another chapter by this author [58]. For the purpose of this review, "older" will be operationally defined as men and women over the age of 65 years, for the purposes of comparing and contrasting their physiological responses with those of "young" men and women 20–30 yr of age. Furthermore, the focus throughout this paper will be on the apparently healthy adult, excluding the important but complex issue that a disproportionate number of adults over the age of 65 have some underlying disease or disability and/or use prescription medications of varying types. A comprehensive review of human thermoregulation is beyond the scope of this chapter, which will focus on information derived from studies designed specifically to address age or aging comparisons. Where appropriate and where sufficient data exist, additional commentary will address effects of exercise training, acclimation, and genetic influences on purported age-related changes.

As with all age comparisons, there are interpretive caveats to be addressed related to study design, and the initial section of this review will be devoted to a discussion of that important topic. Secondly, although the focus of *Exercise and Sport Science Reviews* is on exercise, it is important to also examine thermoregulation under thermoneutral resting conditions in an attempt to determine what constitutes a normal "baseline" body temperature and hydration state in older individuals. Next, the chapter reviews the impact of age on human physiological responses at rest and during exercise in warm environments. Intervention strategies, notably aerobic fitness, heat acclimation, and hormone replacement therapy in postmenopausal women, are reviewed that may impact the ability of older subjects to regulate body fluids and temperature. Finally, responses to rest and exercise in cold environments are discussed from a similar perspective.

INTERPRETIVE ISSUES

When interpreting comparative aging studies in—but by no means limited to—exercise and environmental physiology, there are several interpretive concerns that must be kept in mind. First, it is essential to remember the inherent error introduced into all cross-sectional aging studies by "selective mortality." That is, the subject pool from which older research subjects are drawn consists of the survivors from a cohort that has already experienced some degree of mortality [24]. Added to this is the difficulty in exercise studies of selecting subjects with physical and physiological characteristics purely reflective of the older population as a whole (i.e., random selection from a large potential pool), simply because of their inability to sustain physical exertion or their lack of interest in such studies.

Secondly, the astute reader of the physiological literature should never lose sight of what question a given study purports to address [58]. Consider for a moment the following three research questions.

Question 1. Are the Elderly at Greater Risk for Hypothermia?

This question is most directly (and most correctly) approached by examining morbidity and mortality data from climatic cold spells in large urban areas. Morbidity and mortality data, coupled with the complex nature of this particular physiological stimulus and effect, tell us little about the effects of chronological age independent of the plethora of other factors that contribute to morbidity and mortality in the elderly. In essence, data are derived from the least healthy few percentiles of the older population. Therefore, although it is common to do so, it is unwarranted to make generalizations about risk of hypothermia from laboratory studies comparing small groups of young and older subjects.

Question 2. Does a Typical 65-yr-Old Man Respond Differently during Cold Exposure Than a Typical 20-yr-Old Man?

The research paradigm that is often used to answer this question selects either a random sample of men from each of two distinct age groups from a large population without regard for effects of concomitant variables or selects "normally active" men. Figure 3.1 depicts the mean population $\dot{V}O_2max$ for four groups of men. Groups A and B are young subjects who are active and inactive (not necessarily sedentary), respectively, and Groups C and D are older men similarly categorized into two activity groups. Question 2 above compares Group B with Group D or, less often, Group A with Group C.

This approach offers the advantage of yielding results that are more applicable to the general aged population, e.g., in making health policy decisions for appropriate room temperatures in facilities which house elderly active men and women. However, one difficulty with this approach is trying

FIGURE 3.1.

*Maximal oxygen uptake (V̇O₂max) as a function of age and exercise habits. This model illustrates the difficulty in isolating age as an independent influence on thermoregulatory responses in cross-sectional studies. Matching 25-year-old and 65-year-old subjects for V̇O₂max (**B** and **C**) results in a comparison of regular exercisers and nonexercisers; matching subjects for activity level (**A** and **C** or **B** and **D**) results in different V̇O₂max levels. Percentiles are based on 1994 data from the Institute for Aerobics Research, Dallas, TX.*

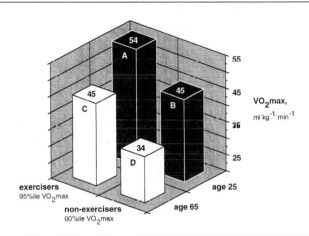

to determine whether notable age differences are truly reflective of chronological age or are more closely related to factors that change in concert with aging — V̇O₂max, activity level, body size and composition, disease presence, etc.

Adding a further degree of complexity to this already complex issue, interpretation of cross-sectional studies that do not match subjects for V̇O₂max becomes even more difficult when exercise is introduced, because it becomes impossible for older and younger subjects who differ in V̇O₂max to exercise at the same absolute *and* relative (i.e., percent V̇O₂max) exercise intensity. A similar absolute intensity imposes a similar metabolic heat production, whereas many heat loss effector responses (sweating rate, for example) are related to relative intensity, i.e., percent V̇O₂max.

Question 3. Does Biological Aging Inevitably Result in Physiological Changes That Impact on Human Responses to Cold Stress?

Like the previous question, this question has most often been addressed by cross-sectional laboratory comparisons. However, in contrast to random subject selection, these studies attempt to match groups of older and younger subjects with respect to as many characteristics as possible, usually such characteristics as $\dot{V}O_2max$, body size, and adiposity. In the illustration shown in Figure 3.1, Groups B and C are compared and contrasted. Additionally, care is taken to control for such factors as hydration and acclimation state. The unstated premise underlying this approach is that, when the healthiest, fittest subset of the older population exhibits responses significantly different from those of their matched younger counterparts, such differences can better be attributed to chronological age. In that way, these experiments come closer to addressing effects attributable to age per se. On the other hand, because such studies test a select subgroup of older adults who are relatively disease- and medication-free, who are highly fit, and who exercise on a regular basis, extrapolation of the results to the general population is unwise.

Unfortunately, there are no comprehensive longitudinal studies of aging and thermoregulation during exercise at extreme ambient temperatures. There are precious few longitudinal case study reports [102], and although these are certainly noteworthy, the results have limited utility because of the low subject numbers (one to a few) and inattention to inherent limitations in this type of design. The cross-sectional approaches previously discussed study differences attributable to age rather than to aging effects. One last approach has been introduced in the literature [36–38] in which a large heterogeneous sample of subjects is tested in a standardized protocol. Dependent variables (e.g., heat storage) are then examined for their relative dependence on the multiple independent variables (e.g., physical size, $\dot{V}O_2max$, age), using multiple regression analyses.

RESTING THERMOREGULATION UNDER THERMONEUTRAL CONDITIONS

Is Baseline Body Temperature "Normal" in Older Individuals?

Before considering the effects of exercise on the body core temperature (T_c) of older men and women, it is important to consider whether there is an inherent difference in their baseline T_c, that is, under resting thermoneutral conditions. There are several published reports that suggest that baseline T_c decreases with advancing age and has greater variability in older populations [47, 100, 108]. The British National Survey [32] reported that as many as 10% of individuals 65 yr of age and older had early morning temperatures $< 35.5°C$. If such an age difference exists, it would have important implications for control of T_c during exercise in the cold (where it would be disadvantageous) and in the heat (where it might provide an advantage [72]).

Keilson et al. [55] investigated the prevalence of low body temperatures in 97 ambulatory elderly (mean age, 74 yr) and 20 younger (mean age, 32 yr) subjects in northern Maine. As in the British National Survey, early morning urine temperatures (T_u) were measured as a proxy measure of T_c. That study detected no T_u < 35.5°C, and average T_u and oral temperatures (T_o) were 0.3 and 0.2°C warmer, respectively, than those in the British study. More importantly, there was no age effect on either T_u or T_o upon waking, which averaged 36.41 ± 0.34 (*SD*) °C and 36.21 ± 0.42°C, respectively, for the older subjects and 36.53 ± 0.36°C and 36.41 ± 0.42°C for the younger subjects.

A careful review of the literature suggests that, rather than being a physiological consequence of aging, lower T_c of older men and women reported in various studies appear to reflect nutritional, disease, and medication effects. The Fox study [32] noted that the subgroup of the elderly with the most reports of low temperatures was the poor. Marion et al. [80] measured the oral and urine temperatures of 93 healthy volunteers (ages 62–96) who were free from a large number of potential confounding factors known to influence T_c. Exclusionary criteria included various diseases (including diabetes and neurological disorders), low body weight and consumption of < 2 meals per day, smoking, lack of self-sufficiency, alcohol intake > 3 oz/wk, and use of various medications. When such factors were excluded, there was no relationship between age and baseline T_u or T_o, which averaged 37.0 and 36.8°C, respectively, across all age groups.

Does the Circadian Temperature Rhythm Change with Age?

The study by Marion et al. [80] also found that the intersubject variability of T_c did not increase with age, with T_c ranging from 36.5 to 37.6°C for each age group studied (64–72, 73–79, and 80–96 yr old). One may ask whether the circadian rhythm, which controls T_c fluctuations independent of activity, changes with age, as has been suggested. T_c is one of the most powerful and stable of all indicators of circadian synchrony, reflecting activity of the so-called "strong oscillator." Several animal studies have found decreased amplitudes and shorter periodicity in older animals [48]. There have been concurring human studies suggesting that aging is associated with flatter and earlier phasing rhythms, even under conditions of self-regulated diurnal activity [123]. However, neither mean 24-hr T_c nor mean T_c during sleep was dependent on age; however, the mean T_c during the time period 2:00–8:00 a.m. was significantly higher in older (69 ± 2 yr) men.

Conversely, a more recent study by Monk et al. [85] showed no evidence that older subjects (in this case, defined as >77 yr old) have different circadian temperature (rectal temperature, T_{re}) rhythm amplitudes than young adults. Possible reasons for this contradiction include the site of T_c measurement (see below) and what appears to be a gender interaction. Older women typically show no alterations in circadian T_c rhythm, when compared with young men or women, whereas more investigations have shown that older men seem to differ more often from their younger counterparts.

Measurement of T_c in Older Individuals

Body T_c refers to the temperature of all tissues located at a depth sufficient so as not to be affected by a temperature gradient through surface tissues [52]. However, thermal gradients occur within the core because of local metabolic rates, tissue mass, and vasomotor influences. Although we know that all of these influences on local T_c change with aging, there is little information available concerning a possible interaction between age and the site of T_c measurement. At rest, T_u, T_o, and T_{re} have most often been used as surrogates of T_c in studies comparing older and young men and women. In general, T_u is systematically lower than T_{re} by 0.2–0.5°C and has a slightly greater time constant [52]. T_o in the elderly is typically lower than T_u [80]. T_o depends on mouth breathing patterns, some medications prevalent in the elderly, environmental conditions that are strong enough to influence face cutaneous temperature, etc. Several other age-related factors, including denture materials and mucosal changes secondary to long-term denture use, may influence the accuracy and reliability of T_o measurements [79].

In laboratory studies involving exercise, T_{re} and esophageal temperature (T_{es}) are the most common sites of T_c measurement, although auditory canal (T_{ac}) and tympanic temperatures (T_{ty}) have also been used. T_{es} most accurately reflects temperature of the blood leaving the heart, and in all probability, the temperature of the blood perfusing the hypothalamus [52]. T_{re} tracks T_{es} well when the rate of heat storage is slow and when exercise involves large muscle groups; otherwise, it lags behind because of the thermal inertia associated with this large tissue mass. Because of aging differences in visceral blood flow during exercise [57, 63, 68], there is the potential for age to affect differentially the T_{re} response to heat storage. However, there have been no studies directly comparing the T_{re} and T_{es} responses in older and young exercising subjects.

What Constitutes "Euhydration" in Older Individuals?

This question is germane because of the close relationship between hydration (acting through both volume and osmolality effects) and thermoregulation. The gerontology literature is replete with reports of altered hydration status in the elderly. Careful reading suggests that most of this information comes from anecdotal evidence and facts extrapolated from clinical and institutionalized older populations. For example, an often-cited clinical survey noted that dehydration was evident in about 25% of nonambulatory geriatric hospital patients [117]. In another, a majority of patients over age 65 from six continuing-care hospital wards were found to have elevated serum osmolalities (>296 mOsmol/kg), and a group of 58 patients randomly selected had a mean plasma osmolality of 304 ± 8 mOsmol/kg at time of hospital admission [92]. Extrapolating such statistics to noninstitutionalized older populations has led to the idea that "healthy, active older [individuals] are hyperosmotic and hypovolemic" [78]. This does not appear to be the case. In fact, despite the statistics cited above for geriatric hospitals, dehydration is evident in only about 1% of older community hospital admissions [116].

When healthy older subjects report for laboratory studies designed to challenge fluid balance, they are typically in a normal state of hydration [12, 66, 98] although a slightly elevated plasma osmolality is often noted in these older subject groups at "baseline" [12, 27, 66, 78, 84]. However, such studies typically require an overnight fast; thus, the "baseline" plasma volumes and tonicity reported really reflect the response to mild dehydration, which selectively renders older subjects slightly hyperosmotic and hypovolemic [58].

Therefore, it is more tenable that hyperosmolar hypohydration [1] accompanies, or results from, various clinical conditions in older individuals, or [2] reflects an age-specific response to mild water deprivation. With respect to baseline conditions, the latter would be important if older men and women, on a day-to-day basis, consumed less fluid than younger men and women.

What dictates spontaneous fluid intake, and do those stimuli change as we age? Under *ad libitum* conditions, in natural environments, neither the amount nor the pattern of fluid intake is regulated physiologically to any great extent [97]. Rather, both are governed by the amount and timing of food intake [16, 17, 97]. Enough fluid is consumed with meals to maintain adequate fluid balance, and under unstressed conditions the kidney response of older persons is sufficient to maintain this balance.

This concept seems to apply to the older adult population as well. When fluids are readily available, independently living healthy older individuals demonstrate daily fluid intakes similar to those of younger individuals. In one study, 262 adults (ages 20–80) were asked to maintain a food and fluid intake diary for 7 consecutive days. There were no notable age differences in total fluid intake (food water content plus fluids drunk), water intake in excess of that required for digestion ("surplus water"), and overall volume of fluid consumed. Nor was there an age effect for thirst, its relationship to fluid intake, or the amount of fluid ingested relative to the amount of solid ingested during a meal [18]. Even those few surveys of community-dwelling older men and women that report slight reductions of fluid intake, their intake is still well within the normal range of 1.6–2.4 liter/day [75].

It seems difficult to reconcile the above discussion with the fact that laboratory studies typically show a deficient thirst sensation and lower fluid intake when older subjects are challenged by water deprivation or heat stress. It appears that problems related to fluid balance in older men and women may only become apparent when homeostasis is challenged. The disturbed fluid and electrolyte homeostasis in older individuals has been linked to both altered renal function [24, 27, 73, 74, 104] and deficiencies in thirst sensation [12, 78, 95, 96, 98].

REST IN COLD ENVIRONMENTS

This section deals with humans exposed to cold under resting conditions and the potential influence age may have on body temperature and effector responses. In general, most cross-sectional studies report that older men and women demonstrate a relative inability to maintain their body temperatures when exposed to cold conditions [10, 32, 45, 76, 132], although there are reports to the contrary showing no age effect [5, 125].

The physiological response to cold involves both decreased heat loss and increased heat production. The former is accomplished by increasing effective tissue insulation, primarily by peripheral vasoconstriction. The latter involves increasing metabolic rate largely by shivering. Arterial (and venous) constriction leads to augmented peripheral thermal resistance equivalent to about 1.4 cm of tissue, which is similar to insulation provided by a similar thickness of cork [13].

In 1977, Collins et al. [10] stated, "People at risk of developing hypothermia also seem to have . . . a nonconstrictor pattern of vasomotor responses to cold." Although this is somewhat of an overgeneralization, advanced age—independent of other factors—does seem to be associated with an attenuated vasoconstrictor response during cold exposure, as shown in Figure 3.2. In separate studies, older (58–67 yr) and young (22–31 yr) subjects were exposed to thermal transients of ambient cooling and heating. In the cooling experiments [60], subjects wore long-sleeved shirts and trousers, and local skin temperature was clamped at 34–35°C. In this way, forearm blood flow (FBF) measured at this site reflected reflex limb responses primarily invoked by whole-body skin cooling to 26°C. The older men decreased FBF more slowly and to a lesser extent than the young men, even though the groups were well matched for $\dot{V}O_2$max and body size and composition. Although T_{es} declined slightly but steadily in the older group and stayed constant in the younger men, T_C differences were not statistically significant. Because these subject groups differed only in age, these data imply that age per se diminishes the peripheral vasoconstrictor response to cold stress.

A similar study confirmed that aerobic fitness has little effect on the T_c drop at rest in the cold [26]. In that study, older (55–66 yr) and young (21–29 yr) subjects sat at 5°C. T_{re} dropped faster in the older men than in the young group, regardless of $\dot{V}O_2$max. Although peripheral blood flow was not measured, estimated heat conductance (by partial calorimetry) suggested diminished peripheral vasoconstriction, in agreement with Kenney and Armstrong [60]. Similarly attenuated vasoconstrictor responses of older subjects have been demonstrated in the skin of the fingertips, using laser Doppler flowmetry [69].

Because both skin and muscle vasoconstriction contribute in series to insulation from cold, the impact of the diminished vasoconstrictor response on thermal balance is exacerbated by sarcopenia—the age-related loss of

FIGURE 3.2.

Mean forearm blood flow (measured as a surrogate for skin blood flow) responses of young and older men (n = 6 per group) sitting at rest during ambient temperature transients. Subjects wore light standard cotton clothing (0.6 clo), and the two age groups were well matched for physical characteristics and $\dot{V}O_2max$. Local forearm skin temperature was clamped at 34–35 °C in order to isolate reflex changes in SkBF as mean body temperature changed. In separate studies, air temperature was systematically raised or lowered to increase or decrease mean body temperature (calculated as $0.8\,T_c + 0.2\,\bar{T}_{sk}$ and $0.67\,T_c + 0.33\,\bar{T}_{sk}$, respectively). Compared to the young subjects, the older men vasoconstricted more slowly and to a lesser extent in the cold, and exhibited an attenuated vasodilation in the heat. Redrawn from data from ref. 2 and 60.

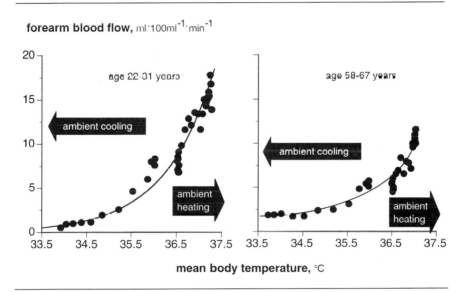

muscle mass. Basal and resting metabolic rates (and, thus, basal and resting heat production) decrease 20% from ages 30 to 70 because of primarily the loss of active muscle mass [99]. This decrement may be associated with a decreased capacity for shivering thermogenesis. As reviewed by Young [130], there is a tendency for cold-induced metabolic heat production to be lower in older adults across studies [5, 44, 70, 126], although reports to the contrary do exist [82, 89, 124]. Again, there is more variability in the responses of older men and women at rest in cold air than in young subject samples [50].

Despite the age difference in vasoconstrictor responses to body cooling, it has been suggested that age may be a secondary factor in determining the overall responses to passive body cooling [61]. There is a notable gender difference when older and younger men and women are exposed to the cold under laboratory conditions. Older women are often able to maintain body temperatures as well as younger women (and better so than older men) during cold exposures [5, 125]. Furthermore, unlike with heat wave statistics, which show increased mortality among women over men in the over-65 age cohort, mortality statistics during cold spells are weighted toward older men [77]. These laboratory and epidemiological data have been interpreted to imply that differences in body size and adiposity (specifically, subcutaneous fat thickness and distribution) may play a larger role than chronological age in determining T_c responses to cold. One study, which matched subject groups for surface area-to-mass ratio [124], reported no age difference in the T_{re} response of men who sat for 30 min at 17°C. No body composition data were reported in that study. However, two studies comparing older and younger women support the above interpretation. Bernstein et al. [5] reported no age difference in the T_{re} response to 3 hr of rest in a cool room (17°C) and Wagner and Horvath [124] reported that women with an average age of 61 yr were able to maintain their baseline T_c during 2 hr at 10°C, whereas the T_c of a group of 21-yr-old women decreased slightly. In both of these studies, the older women had a higher percentage of body fat and a smaller surface area-to-mass ratio than did the young women.

Budd and et al. [8] conducted a study on expedition members (age range, 26–52 yr) at the commencement of the International Biomedical Expedition to the Antarctic in 1991. Twelve men were exposed to 10°C, wearing only nylon shorts, while thermal, metabolic, and cardiovascular responses were monitored. When the relative influences of $\dot{V}O_2$max, adiposity, and age were examined by regression analyses, (1) $\dot{V}O_2$max had no effect on any measured response, (2) increased adiposity was associated with reduced heat loss, whereas age had the opposite effect; and (3) when fatness effects were held constant, the older men had poorer vasoconstrictor responses to the cold. At least in fit, healthy, middle-aged men, these differences in peripheral blood flow distribution do not seem to be accompanied by alterations in atrial natriuretic factor, arginine vasopressin, plasma renin activity, or plasma norepinephrine concentrations [122].

REST IN WARM ENVIRONMENTS

There are several procedures that have been used to raise T_c under resting conditions, as reviewed by Rowell [105]. Rest in hot ambient conditions (natural environments) increases skin temperature ($\bar{T}_{sk}$) but has limited effect on T_c, unless the exposures are extremely prolonged. So-called "indirect heating" usually involves subjects immersing their lower limbs in hot water baths while keeping the upper body warm with blankets. Finally, "direct heating" with water-perfused suits clamps $\bar{T}_{sk}$ at an elevated temperature and allows T_c to systematically increase as that heat is convected to the core. Unfortunately, few if any aging comparisons have used the direct-heating approach to examine responses to a sustained and purely thermoregulatory reflex drive. Studies that have exposed subjects of different ages to hot natural environments have not reported any age differences in the T_c response [22, 113], although this may reflect an inadequate thermal stimulus imposed under such conditions.

Sweat Gland Function

Humans rely to a large degree on the ability to activate eccrine sweat glands and the ability of those glands to secrete sweat to regulate T_c under heat stress conditions. Before examining sweating in response to passive heat stress, a basic question is whether skin aging alters the eccrine gland response to a standardized stimulus. Eccrine glands can be stimulated in vivo by cholinergic analogues [such as methylcholine (MCh) or pilocarpine] injected intradermally or induced via iontophoresis.

Although there is a large variability in the sweat gland responses to such sudorific stimuli, some clear effects of aging are evident. Local sweating rates are lower in older subjects for a given pharmacological stimulus, an effect that can be attributed to a smaller sweat output per activated gland [23, 62, 110, 115]. The density of pharmacologically activated glands appears to be unaffected by age.

When do these changes occur? Sato [109] suggested that "aging has very little effect on the pharmacologically induced maximal sweat rate until the 60s, but glandular function gradually declines in the 70s and 80s." This seems to be an oversimplification for several reasons. In the subjects tested by Ellis and colleagues [23], there was a distinct age difference in MCh-induced sweating in subjects randomly selected from a hospitalized population. However, the authors noted that in the older subjects who exhibited higher sweat outputs, ". . . the texture and appearance of the skin . . . appeared more youthful and elastic and less wrinkled to the naked eye than of those whose sweat response was poor or absent." Lifetime ultraviolet exposure and other environmental factors may have an interactive effect with chronological age in determining sweat gland responsiveness.

When varying concentrations of MCh were injected intradermally into the thighs of three distinct age groups (22–24, 33–40, and 58–67 yr) of men, there were no age differences in active gland density (Fig. 3.3A). All subjects in this study were rigorously heat acclimated, and groups were matched for $\dot{V}O_2$max. Their respective group sweat outputs per active gland at each MCh concentration are shown in Figure 3.3B. Although only the oldest and youngest group responses differed significantly, it is interesting that the 33–40-yr-old group exhibited sweat outputs that were intermediate in each case, suggesting perhaps a continuous decline throughout adulthood. These data also strongly suggest that this decrement is not a function

FIGURE 3.3.

*In vivo comparison of human eccrine sweat gland responses to intradermal injection of various concentrations of acetyl-β-methylcholine chloride, an analogue of the natural sudomotor neurotransmitter, acetylcholine. Panel **A** shows the active sweat gland density resulting from the injection of a 10^{-4}M concentration of methylcholine in 3 distinct age groups (n = 6 men per group) of heat-acclimated men. Maximal activation occurred by 2 min postinjection, and there were no age differences in the density of active glands. On the other hand, the oldest group of men produced significantly less sweat per gland in response to each dose of injected methycholine, compared to that of the youngest group. 50+ heat signifies the injection of this concentration after the subjects exercised in the heat (37°C) for 1 hr. Redrawn from ref. 62.*

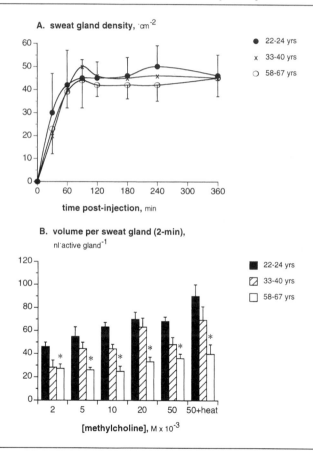

A. sweat gland density, cm^{-2}

time post-injection, min

- ● 22-24 yrs
- x 33-40 yrs
- ○ 58-67 yrs

B. volume per sweat gland (2-min),
nl·active gland^{-1}

[methylcholine], M x 10^{-3}

- ■ 22-24 yrs
- ▨ 33-40 yrs
- □ 58-67 yrs

of decreased V̇O$_2$max or differing body size or composition, as subject groups were matched for these characteristics as well as for acclimation state. Failure to take into account heat acclimation, whether natural or artificial, can obviate any underlying age effects. For example, one study reported that older and young men matched for $\dot{V}O_2$max had similar sweating rates in response to pilocarpine iontophoresis; however, these results were confounded by comparing an older group who were actively training (4 hr of vigorous exercise per week for the previous 23 yr) with a young sedentary group [9]. Sweat glands can even undergo "local training" by means of repeated immersion of the skin in hot water. When such a protocol is performed, older individuals increase local sweat production but to a lesser degree than young men and women [90].

There is also good evidence that there are regional differences in sweat gland function between older and younger persons. Foster et al. [31] demonstrated that forehead and limb sweating was more reduced than trunk sweating by age in response to MCh injection.

Sweating during Passive Heat Exposures

Do older men and women sweat less during passive heat exposure? If so, is it attributable to chronological age or to other factors that change with aging and perhaps are amenable to intervention? Several studies from the 1970s [11, 28, 113] and selected recent papers [51] suggest that the answer to the former question is yes. When men 70–82 and men 16–20 yr old were exposed to warm (30°C) air and placed their hands in hot water, sweating was delayed in the older men [11], confirming an earlier report of an elevated sweating threshold in older men [28]. Shoenfeld et al. [113] reported lower sweating rates in older (46–63 yr) men and women during a short exposure to extreme dry heat of 89–90°C.

The common link among the above cross-sectional comparisons of older and young groups is the lack of control for concomitant influences such as acclimation, body size, or $\dot{V}O_2$max. On the other hand, Drinkwater and colleagues exposed 10 postmenopausal women (mean age, 58 yr) and 10 younger women (mean age, 38 yr) to a 40°C (20% relative humidity (rh)) environment for 2 hr [22]. Subjects were matched for body surface area, but $\dot{V}O_2$max varied within the cohort of women tested. There were no age differences in sweating; rather, sweating rate was correlated with $\dot{V}O_2$max. Similar results were reported in a study examining thermal transients [34]. Forty male and female subjects (ages 8–67 yr) were tested on a Potter bed balance as ambient temperature was systematically raised. Sweating rate was strongly determined by $\dot{V}O_2$max of the subjects, rather than by age. Similar sweating rates and onset thresholds were seen in groups of 21–39-yr-old and 61–73-yr-old men exposed to 40°C (40% rh) for 130 min. The older men in that study were active occupationally as security guards but not as regular endurance exercisers.

The regional pattern of sweating distribution mentioned above was also evident during passive heating (legs and feet in a warm water bath while sitting at 35°C), i.e., an age difference was noted on the thighs but not on the back [49]. In each case, gland output was lower in older men at peripheral sites but not at central locations. A logical hypothesis may be that glandular function declines in a peripheral-to-central direction as skin ages.

Cardiovascular Responses during Passive Heating

Older men sitting at rest in hot environments exhibit attenuated increases in skin blood flow (SkBF), compared to that of younger men [2, 132], even when the young men have similar anthropometry, body composition, and $\dot{V}O_2$max [2]. Data from one such study are included in Figure 3.2. Changes in FBF measured with strain gauges have traditionally been used to assess changes in SkBF, because underlying inactive muscle flow does not change during passive heating [19]. Independent of local effects, reflex skin vasodilation was attenuated in the older men as they sat at rest and as ambient temperature was elevated. In this case, the majority of the reflex drive came from increasing $\bar{T}_{sk}$. When an orthostatic challenge (tilt) is added to passive heating, older (61–73 yr) men respond with a greater tachycardia and a significantly attenuated peripheral blood flow response, compared to those of young men (21–39 yr) [112].

EXERCISE IN WARM ENVIRONMENTS

In an early study, Henschel and colleagues [41] exposed 100 men and women ages 60–93 yr to humid (70% rh) air temperatures of 33°C for 70 min. Subjects performed intermittent exercise at low intensities and heart rate, ventilation rate, and $\dot{V}O_2$ were measured. The authors concluded that "the elderly persons were able to tolerate the work-in-heat stress without evidence of excessive physiological strain." However, the low exercise intensities in this experiment admittedly "did not seriously tax [the subjects'] capacities," so the foregoing conclusion cannot be generalized to more vigorous exercise or to more stressful environments. Since that time, many experiments, using many paradigms, have been conducted, comparing the responses of older and young adults to exercise in hot environments.

Heat Storage and T_c

There are many contradictory papers in the literature about whether or not older subjects increase T_c at a greater rate during exercise, compared to young subjects. Metabolic heat production is a function of the absolute exercise intensity, whereas heat loss mechanisms are closely related to relative intensity. Therefore, heat storage and the resulting increase in T_c are dependent to some degree upon both absolute and relative intensities. It is not surprising then that much of the controversy about exercise T_c responses and aging can be resolved by controlling for the difference in $\dot{V}O_2$max between subject groups.

Much of the older literature documented a relatively larger rise in T_c and a greater physiological strain in general in exercising older men and

FIGURE 3.4.

Published studies present conflicting answers to the question, "Do older exercising subjects show a greater increase in core temperature than young subjects?" When older and young subjects are tested without regard for $\dot{V}O_2$max or chosen as representative of that age group with regard to $\dot{V}O_2$max (A, n = 15 per group), the rise in esophageal temperature during exercise is greater in the older individuals. However, when older and young subjects are healthy and have similar $\dot{V}O_2$max's (B, n = 7 per group), T_c responses are similar as well. These studies illustrate the concept that $\dot{V}O_2$max is more important than chronological age in determining heat storage during exercise and the subsequent T_c response. A was redrawn from ref. 65 and B was redrawn from ref. 66.

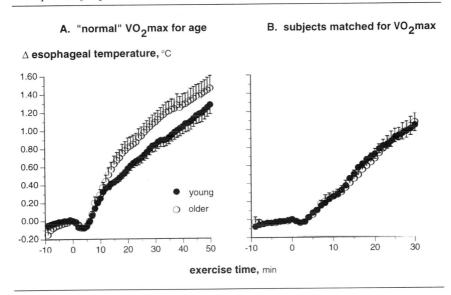

A. "normal" VO₂max for age   B. subjects matched for VO₂max

Δ esophageal temperature, °C

exercise time, min

women [21, 39, 40, 127]. This conclusion is valid for the general population of older men and women, whose lower average $\dot{V}O_2$max predetermines that a given absolute exercise intensity corresponds to a greater percent $\dot{V}O_2$max. However, when older subjects are matched for $\dot{V}O_2$max with young subjects and exercise at the same absolute *and* relative intensity, there are seldom differences in either T_c or calculated heat storage [56, 58, 66, 67, 94, 121]. Figure 3.4 illustrates this concept. When a group of 15 older (ages 60–75 yrs) and 15 young (ages 18–30 yrs) men comprising a fairly wide range of $\dot{V}O_2$max's exercised at 60% $\dot{V}O_2$max in a warm chamber, there was a greater rise in T_{es} (ΔT_{es}) in the older group (Panel A). However, when men from two distinct age groups were matched for $\dot{V}O_2$max in a previous study [66], this difference disappeared (panel B). Another feature noticeable in Figure 3.4 is the larger variability within the older groups, which is typical of aging studies in general.

Havenith et al. [36–38] have used a different approach to determine the relative influences of various individual characteristics on heat strain. Rather than matching subject groups that differ in only one characteristic (such as age), they tested a large number of heterogeneous subjects in a standard heat challenge, then used multiple regression analyses to determine the relative influence of various individual characteristics on a dependent response of interest. This methodology was used in a collaborative project between Penn State University and the TNO Human Factors Institute in the Netherlands to determine the relative influences of several independent variables—age, gender, adiposity and anthropometry, $\dot{V}O_2$max, and regular physical activity level—on dependent variables such as T_{re} and calculated heat storage (S) during 1 hr of low-intensity (60-watt) steady-state cycle exercise in a warm (35°C) environment [37]. Fifty-six subjects were selected such that age (20–73 yr) and $\dot{V}O_2$max (1.86–4.44 liter/min) were not interrelated. Final T_{re} and S were both significantly correlated with $\dot{V}O_2$max. After inclusion of the $\dot{V}O_2$max effect into prediction models, age had no significant influence. The conclusion was that, once natural variation in physical fitness is introduced in a test population, the effect of chronological age per se appears to be negligible.

Cardiovascular Responses during Exercise in the Heat

Rowell [107] has stated, "Probably the greatest stress ever imposed on the human cardiovascular system . . . is the combination of exercise and hyperthermia." When exercise is performed in warm environmental conditions, there is a competition between the need to deliver oxygen to active muscle and the need to increase SkBF for facilitation of heat dissipation. This challenge to blood flow delivery is met by both increasing cardiac output and adjusting vascular resistance in nonactive tissues. Adding to the regulatory challenges are losses of fluid through sweating and losses of intravascular volume as a result of dynamic fluid shifts. Despite these challenges to cardiovascular and thermal homeostasis, *in vivo* regulation is usually accomplished sufficiently so as to minimize heat storage while maintaining blood pressure homeostasis. The following sections address the effects of chronological age on the mechanisms through which the body responds to dynamic exercise in the heat.

CONTROL OF SKIN BLOOD FLOW. During exercise, contracting muscles produce metabolic heat that, if not dissipated to the environment effectively, severely limits the ability to continue exercising. Dissipation of heat in humans is accomplished in series by dramatically increasing SkBF and by producing (and evaporating) sweat. The former (along with the T_c-to-$\bar{T}_{sk}$ gradient) determines the rate at which heat is convected from the core to the skin, whereas the latter primarily accounts for the dissipation of that heat to the environment, although dry heat exchange contributes to heat loss at ambient temperatures appreciably lower than $\bar{T}_{sk}$.

Mechanisms of control of SkBF during exercise have been reviewed recently [53, 64]. SkBF over most of the body during exercise is determined by a competition between vasoconstrictor and vasodilator influences, i.e., dual efferent neural control. The adrenergic vasoconstrictor system is common to all regional circulations; however, the sympathetic vasodilator system is unique to the skin. Activation of this system can fully dilate cutaneous arterioles, increasing whole-body SkBF to levels approaching 8 liters/min [105].

During prolonged upright exercise in warm environments, T_c does not usually reach an equilibrium but continues to increase. Once a threshold (T_c is exceeded, the increase in T_c is accompanied by a parallel steep rise in SkBF. However, SkBF does not increase without bound, and an attenuated rate of increase occurs above a T_c of about 38°C, such that an apparent upper limit to SkBF is reached [7, 67, 86, 105]. When SkBF is plotted as a function of the primary stimulus—T_c or ΔT_c—during exercise, these phases—threshold, steep rise, and attenuated rise—can be appreciated.

Is chronological age associated with an altered SkBF response during exercise in the heat? And, if so, by what mechanism(s) does age exert this effect? A series of studies performed at Penn State University [56, 63, 66, 67] compared the SkBF responses of older fit ($\dot{V}O_2max = 45$–50 ml·kg^{-1}·min^{-1}) healthy men and women (ages 50–75) with a sample of those 20–30-yr-old subjects with similar physical and physiological characteristics. In all cases, older individuals responded to exercise with a lower SkBF at a given T_c, compared to their younger counterparts. Although exercise intensity and ambient conditions differed among the studies, there was a consistent effect of age on the SkBF to T_c relationship, which is shown in Figure 3.5A. In this study [65], 15 men (ages 60–74 yr) and 15 young men (20–25 yr) exercised at 50% $\dot{V}O_2max$ in a 36°C room. Their ΔT_{es} responses are shown in Figure 3.4A. Figure 3.5A depicts the forearm vascular resistance (= FBF divided by mean arterial pressure) as a function of rising T_{es}. Above threshold temperatures, the blood flow response of the older men was greatly attenuated. Although it is not clear from this figure, the threshold T_c for increasing SkBF is typically unchanged by age, but the slope of the relationship is decreased, as is the highest SkBF achieved. A reasonable interpretation of this systematic change would be that age affects SkBF peripherally, rather than altering central hypothalamic control features [88].

Estimated SkBFs for the older exercising subjects range from 25 to 50% lower than those of their matched young counterparts. It is obvious from these data that older men and women increase SkBF to a significantly smaller degree during combined exercise and heat stress than younger men. Although the mean SkBF response across a group of older subjects is lower than that of a fitness-matched group of young subjects, the range of responses within the older group is typically larger. Some individuals over the age of 65 exhibit high levels of SkBF; however, many others demonstrate severe limitations to increasing SkBF during a heat challenge.

FIGURE 3.5.

*During exercise in a warm (36°C) environment, the increase in forearm vascular conductance (= forearm blood flow/mean arterial pressure, reflective of forearm skin vasodilation) is significantly attenuated in older men (**A**) (n = 15 men per group). Because both age groups achieved a similar percentage of the maximal vasodilation possible at a given skin site (**B**), maximal skin vasodilation is decreased with age. Data derived from ref. 65.*

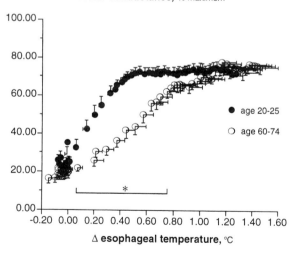

A. forearm vascular conductance, units

B. skin vascular conductance, % maximum

Δ esophageal temperature, °C

What are the mechanisms through which these age differences in the control of SkBF act? The noted age differences are clearly not the result of a lower $\dot{V}O_2max$ in the older subjects, because subject groups were matched for $\dot{V}O_2max$. Thus, the older individuals are actually more active than the young men and women. Nor is the diminished vasodilation caused by the hypovolemia and/or hypertonicity [30] reported as accompaning alterations in hydration in the elderly. In a study that manipulated hydration status in older and young men, then had them exercise in the heat, age and hypohydration independently caused a decreased SkBF, with no interactive effects noted [66].

An alternate hypothesis might be that an increased sympathetic (noradrenergic) vasoconstrictor tone may limit heat-induced skin vasodilation in older individuals. Vasoconstrictor tone in humans is mediated through α-noradrenergic sympathetic pathways. If older individuals have an exaggerated α-receptor-mediated vasoconstriction that limits dilation, blocking the constrictor system should lead to a "normalization" of the SkBF response, i.e., the response should become more like that of younger individuals. When we systemically blocked α-receptors with the selective α¹-antagonist prazosin [67] or blocked the local release of norepinephrine with local administration of bretylium tosylate [65], there was no selective effect of the drug on the SkBF response of older men.

Because structural changes occur in aging skin that are independent of aerobic fitness, the most plausible explanation for the lower skin vasodilation with age results from structural changes within the cutaneous vessels, which limit the degree of active vasodilation. The magnitude of maximal vasodilation, which can be elicited by prolonged local heating of the forearm, appears to be diminished in older men [81, 103], an effect that appears to decline fairly linearly between 12 and 85 yr of age [81]. Figure 3.5 supports this notion. Although the absolute increase in SkBF, shown as forearm vascular conductance in 3.5A, was reduced in the older men, they achieved the same percentage of the site-specific maximal blood flow (3.5B), implying different maximal flows.

Finally, no discussion about age and thermoregulation would be complete without some attention to menopause and postmenopausal hormone status. Surprisingly few studies have been performed on this subject population. Tankersley et al. tested a small group of postmenopausal women before and after 14–23 days of estrogen replacement therapy (ERT) [120]. The daily dosage of E_2 administered was sufficient to signif icantly increase plasma estradiol concentration without significantly affecting progesterone levels. Both at rest and during exercise in a warm environment, T_c was consistently (~0.5°C) lower after ERT. There was no change in resting or exercise $\dot{V}O_2$, but SkBF and local sweating were higher at any given T_c (Fig. 3.6). Furthermore, exercise heart rate (HR) was significantly lower after ERT. Thus, both thermoregulatory and cardiovascular strain experienced during heat and exercise stress seem to be reduced by acute ERT. Whether these are transient effects, or whether continued ERT maintains these advantages is currently under investigation. It may be that the cardiovascular advantages were a consequence of an isotonic hemodilution, because exogenous 17β-estradiol administration has been

FIGURE 3.6.

In postmenopausal women, the acute (approximately 3 weeks) effect of estrogen replacement therapy (ERT) is a shift in the esophageal temperature thresholds for forearm blood flow (A) and local sweating (B) to the left, i.e., to lower temperatures. Data shown are from one representative woman. The result is an increased effector response at any given T_c. Redrawn from ref. 120.

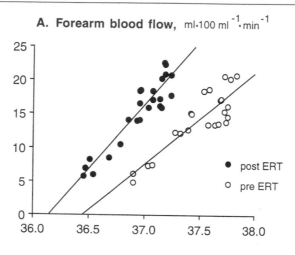

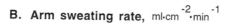

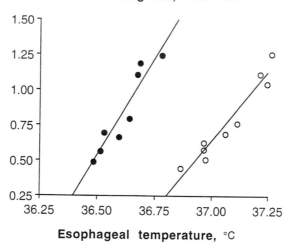

Esophageal temperature, °C

shown to cause the conservation of water and electrolytes in women [1, 6], resulting in a significant hemodilution and expansion of plasma volume [129]. Although estrogen has been shown to increase the firing rate of warm-sensitive neurons in the preoptic anterior hypothalamus in rats

[114], which should stimulate heat loss responses, no similar evidence exists in humans.

CARDIAC OUTPUT. Whether or not exercise cardiac output ($\dot{Q}_c$) declines with age is controversial, and there is abundant contradictory evidence in the literature. The question is confounded by differences in exercise intensity (relative vs. absolute), subject screening for underlying diseases, subject fitness level and training status, and the method used to measure $\dot{Q}_c$. During submaximal exercise in cool or thermoneutral environments, $\dot{Q}_c$ has been reported to be lower [83, 91, 119], the same [29, 35] and, surprisingly, even higher [3, 54] in older subjects than in young subjects.

Examination of the purported mechanisms that account for age-related changes in $\dot{Q}_c$ with advanced age may help clarify this issue. During exercise of moderate-to-high intensity, the mechanisms through which older subjects achieve a high $\dot{Q}_c$ shift from a dependence on a catecholamine-mediated increase in HR and inotropy to a greater reliance on the Frank-Starling mechanism [33, 71, 111]. Left ventricular diastolic filling declines with age, with older men showing lower peak filling rates at rest, at 50% $\dot{V}O_2$max, and at maximal exercise intensities [111], a decline that is not secondary to a lower $\dot{V}O_2$max, but rather to a decreased β-adrenergic responsiveness. Under conditions in which venous return and ventricular filling would be expected to be compromised, one might expect that older subjects to be less able to compensate to lower filling rates by sympathetic means. This would explain why lower stroke volumes and $\dot{Q}_c$s are more often seen in older men during upright, but not supine, exercise [25] and when skin venous pooling is augmented by the imposition of exogenous heat stress [56]. Additionally, there is some evidence that age-related chances in $\dot{Q}_c$ may be gender-specific [46,118], with greater age-related changes seen in men than in women.

Figure 3.7 shows the responses of 8 young and 7 older men to incremental cycle exercise in the heat (36°C). Exercise was progressive but intermittent to allow subjects to reach steady state at each intensity. Subjects were also well matched for peak $\dot{V}O_2$ so that, at each relative intensity, absolute workload was also equal. At intensities at and above 60% $\dot{V}O_2$peak, $\dot{Q}_c$ was significantly lower in the older men, as was HR at rest and at every intensity. Stroke volume was higher in the older men during exercise, albeit not enough to offset the chronotropic age effect.

REGIONAL BLOOD FLOWS. Increasing $\dot{Q}_c$ helps meet the dual demand for increased blood flow to working muscle and to the skin. However, the ability of $\dot{Q}_c$ to increase is limited by attainment of near-maximal heart rates and by an inability to increase stroke volume further in light of a falling central filling pressure. An additional circulatory adjustment during dynamic exercise in the heat is the sympathetically mediated redistribution of blood flow away from splanchnic and renal vascular beds. Diversion of blood from these two regions allows for a redistribution of 1 liter/min or more to the skin circulation [106, 107]. This may be of particular importance for older

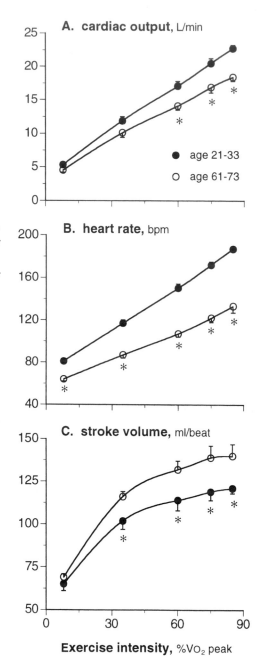

FIGURE 3.7.

*Cardiac output (**A**), heart rate (**B**), and stroke volume (**C**) of V̇O₂max-matched older (n = 7) and young (n = 8) groups of men performing progressive intermittent exercise at 36°C ambient temperature. At rest, only heart rate was different between groups. Stroke volume was significantly higher at every exercise intensity in the older men; however, this increase was not sufficient to offset the lower heart rate response at higher intensities, and cardiac output was significantly lower at and above 60% V̇O₂peak. Because of subject selection criteria (similar V̇O₂max across age groups), each relative intensity also represented the same absolute V̇O₂ for each group. Thus, even in highly trained men over the age of 60, increased inotropism cannot fully compensate for the age-related chronotropic impairment.*

persons with poor left ventricular function and, thus, a limited ability to increase $\dot{Q}_c$, yet few studies have examined the potential effects of age on this integrated response.

A recent study compared the renal blood flow (RBF, measured by clearance of para-amino hippurate) responses of 60–70-yr old and 20–30-yr old men before, during, and after a bout of exercise in a warm (30°C) environment [68]. To better determine the effects of chronological age (i.e., to minimize the effects of confounding variables), the distinct age groups were again matched with respect to body size, adiposity, and $\dot{V}O_2$max. A full day of baseline data were collected, and exercise tests were performed on the 1st and 4th days of a heat acclimation protocol. Age-associated reductions in RBF at rest are well documented [14, 128] and this study was no exception, with baseline RBFs 21% lower in the older group (753 ± 116 vs. 959 ± 104 ml/min). During exercise at 50% $\dot{V}O_2$,max, RBF decreased to a significantly greater extent in the 20–30-yr-old group on each exercise day, decreasing by 508 and 365 ml/min during exercise on Days 1 and 4 (reductions of 45 and 36% from baseline, respectively). For the 60–70-yr-old subjects, RBF decreased only 98 (12%) and 83 (12%) ml/min on each of the 2 days.

Similar RBF results were reported in a follow-up study, which simultaneously measured splanchnic blood flow (SBF by indocyanine green clearance) and FBF [57, 63]. Figure 3.8 shows the reductions in RBF and SBF, along with the increases in FBF, during steady-state exercise at two intensities. Unlike RBF, resting SBF changes little with age. At 35% $\dot{V}O_2$peak, there are little sympathetic activation, relatively minor changes in flow (RBF remained constant and SBF fell by 12–14% in both groups), and no age difference. At 60% $\dot{V}O_2$peak, FBF was significantly lower and SBF decreased to a lesser extent in the older men (e.g., -45 ± 2 vs. -33 ± 3%; p < 0.01). Summing RBF and SBF, the young men redistributed 37% more total blood flow away from these two circulations, compared to that of their older counterparts. It appears that the greater increase in SkBF in young exercising subjects (as compared to that of those older than 60 yr of age) is partially supported by a greater redistribution of blood flow away from splanchnic and renal vascular beds. Regular exercise may alter this pattern of distribution of $\dot{Q}_c$, with fit older men redistributing more flow away from splanchnic and renal circulations than more sedentary men do, but age differences remain [43].

Sweating Responses

The age-related deficit in drug- or heat-activated sweat gland function described above does not necessarily translate into lower sweating rates during exercise in the heat. Sweating rate depends not only on genetic and physiological factors but also is strongly influenced by environmental influences. Table 3.1 provides summary data from 24 papers published since 1956, which compared sweating rates and/or local sweating characteristics

Table 3.1.
Results of Studies Examining the Effects of Age on Sweating Responses, (1956–1994)

Reference (Author and Year)	T_a, rh%	$\dot{V}o_2max$ Similar?	Accli- mated?	Rest or Exercise (%)	Sweating Rate	Onset	Slope
Anderson and Kenney, 1987	48°, 15	Y[a]	Y	E(40)	↓	–	–
Armstrong and Kenney, 1993	46°, 11	Y	Both	R	↓peak	NS	NS
Cable and Green, 1990	22°, 50	N	N	E/R	↓	–	–
Crowe and Moore, 1973	30°[1b]	N	N	R	–	↓	–
Drinkwater and Horvath, 1979	35°, 60	N	N	E (35)	↓	–	–
	48°, 10				↓	–	–
Drinkwater et al., 1982	40°, 40	N	N	R	NS	NS	NS
Fennell and Moore, 1973	27°[1b]	N	N	R	–	–	–
Hellon and Lind, 1956	38°, 60	N	N	R	NS	↓	NS
Hellon et al., 1956	38°, 55	N	N	E/R	NS[2c]	–	–
Inoue et al., 1991	35°[3d]	N	N	R	NS	↓	–
		N	Y		↓	↓	–
Kenney, 1988	37°, 60	Y	N	E (40)	NS	–	–
Kenney and Anderson, 1988	37°, 60	Y	Y	E (40)	NS	–	–
Kenney et al., 1990	48°, 15	Y	N	E (43)	NS	–	–
Lind et al., 1970	various	N	N	E/R	NS[2c]	–	–
Mack et al., 1994	36°, 30	N	N	E (60)	NS	–	–
Miescher and Fortney, 1989	45°, 25	N	N	R	NS	–	–
Pandolf et al., 1988	49°, 20	Y	Both	E (45)	NS	NS	NS
Robinson et al., 1865[e]	40°, 20	N	Both	E	↓	–	–
Sagawa et al.,1988	40°, 40	N	N	R	NS	NS	–
Shoenfeld et al., 1978	90°, 4	N	N	R	↓	–	–
Smolander et al., 1990	30°, 80	Y	N	E (30)	NS	NS	NS
	40°, 20				NS	–	↓
Tankersley et al., 1991	30°, 55	N	N	E (68)	↓	NS	↓
		Y	N		NS	NS	NS
Wagner et al., 1972	49°, 15	N	Both	E	↓	–	–
Yousef et al., 1984	Desert	N	N	E (40)	NS	–	–

[a]Y, yes; E, exercise; R, rest; NS, no significant age difference. ↓ implies a significantly lower response in older subjects.
[b]plus hand in hot water bath.
[c]↓ during work, ↑ during rest.
[d]plus legs in hot water bath.
[e]longitudinal comparison of four men.

FIGURE 3.8.

*During exercise in the heat, blood flow is redistributed away from splanchnic (**A**) and renal (**B**) circulations and to the skin (**C**). At intensities high enough to elicit a substantial sympathetic nervous system activation (60% V̇O₂peak in this study), older men vasoconstricted the splanchnic circulation to a lesser extent than young men did, while also exhibiting less skin vasodilation. Renal blood flow at rest is lower in older individuals, thus the flow redistribution from rest to exercise was likewise less in the older men. In young men (relative to those more than 59 yr of age), a greater skin blood flow is supported by a larger redistribution of the available cardiac output away from splanchnic and renal vascular beds. Redrawn from ref. 63.*

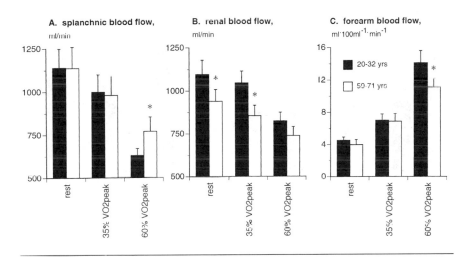

(onset of sweating and/or the slope of the sweating rate to T_c relationship) in subjects differing significantly in age. Most reported no significant age difference in sweating. Upon careful examination of the studies that reported significantly lower sweating rates in older subjects, several conclusions may be drawn.

First, peak sweating rates are usually lower in older men and women and, therefore, sweating differences are more likely to be evident during exercise in hot dry climates, although very large interindividual variability exists. Figure 3.9 depicts the results of a study in which women of two age groups exercised in a warm humid environment (3.9A) and a hot dry environment (3.9B). Differences in regional sweating rates (measured by dew-point hygrometry) existed only in the dry environment, where every skin site tested demonstrated lower sweating rates. In such environments, sweating differences are the result of a lower sweating rate per heat-activated sweat gland and not from fewer active glands (Fig. 3.10). Second, V̇O₂max and heat ac-

FIGURE 3.9.

*Local sweating rates at three skin sites (measured by dew-point hygrometry) for two age groups of women exercising in warm humid (**A**) and a hot dry (**B**) environments. All older women were postmenopausal, and none was on hormone replacement therapy. An age difference was noted at each site (as well as for overall sweating rate) in the drier environment only. Redrawn from ref. 59.*

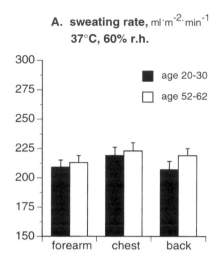
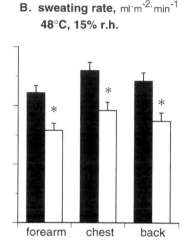

climation are more important in determining sweating rate than is age. Finally, potential age differences in sweating responses may be masked by (among other factors) environmental influences.

Control of Plasma Volume

Resting plasma volume (PV) is influenced by a variety of factors, including body size, lean body mass, various chronic diseases, physical activity and trained state, heat acclimation, and hydration status. Not surprisingly, there is much disagreement in the literature as to whether older men and women have similar or lower PVs than younger persons of the same gender. Tracking changes in PV in older and younger men and women by following changes in hematocrit and hemoglobin concentration [20], as is commonly done, has little utility without one knowing whether substantial baseline differences exist in PV. Three recent studies that used Evan's blue dye dilution to measure absolute PV in older and younger men illustrate the difficulty in drawing irrefutable conclusions in this area. In "healthy active" older and young groups of men, Mack et al. [78] saw significantly lower PVs in subjects >65 yr of age (43 ± 2 ml/kg) vs. the PVs of those <30 years of age (48

FIGURE 3.10.

*The age difference in sweating rate (**A**) in a hot dry environment (48°C, 15% relative humidity (r.h.) is primarily a function of a lower output per gland (**C**), as opposed to fewer active glands (**B**), with the possible exception of early in the exposure. Women (n = 8 per group) were matched for $\dot{V}O_2$max and exercised at 35-40% $\dot{V}O_2$max in each condition. HASG, is heat-activated sweat glands. Redrawn from ref. 59.*

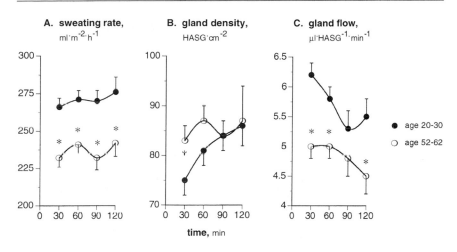

± 3 ml/kg). When Davy and Seals [15] matched men in their 60s with men in their 20s on the basis of regular daily physical activity, a similar difference was noted (50 ± 2 vs. 39 ± 2 ml/kg). A requirement for inclusion in that study was that subjects not be physically active or endurance trained. When Bell, working in the author's laboratory, [4] matched older and younger subjects for $\dot{V}O_2$max rather than for activity, such differences disappear, and a group of older men actually had slightly higher plasma volumes (48 ± 2 vs. 43 ± 3 ml/kg), although this difference was not statistically significant. Standardizing these results for lean body mass rather than for body weight does not account for the differences among studies, although the loss of lean body mass that typically accompanies aging certainly strongly influences PV. It is proposed that, like many other factors that impact on thermoregulation, PV is probably more strongly influenced by physical activity and $\dot{V}O_2$max than by chronological age.

During exercise, fluid is shifted from the vascular space into extravascular compartments. The magnitude of this translocation is determined by Frank-Starling forces (primarily hydrostatic and oncotic pressure gradients), which are, in turn, a function of exercise intensity, ambient conditions, posture, and other factors associated with dynamic exercise. A greater loss of plasma volume is associated with greater increases in T_c, a relative tachycardia, and possible hypotension during exercise in hot environments.

Some authors have also suggested in recent years that PV may be more labile in older exercising subjects. A thorough review of the data in this area makes it difficult to support the contention that age is associated with greater losses of plasma volume (ΔPV) during exercise in hot environments, although this may be true for a given set of conditions. Miescher and Fortney [84] saw larger protein and fluid losses in the older men during 3 hr of passive heating, and that decrement took longer to restore once drinking was initiated. Mack and colleagues [78], on the other hand, noted no age difference in ΔPV during prolonged exercise in the heat. Results from our own studies have been mixed. In one set of studies, we noted that older women demonstrated significantly larger ΔPV during exercise in warm, humid, but not hot dry, conditions [59]. In another, age was associated with a larger loss of PV when subjects were well hydrated, but the age difference disappeared when the subjects were hypohydrated [66]. At present, no conclusions can be drawn about control of intravascular fluid volume during exercise with aging. More systematic investigations, perhaps focusing on age differences in intravascular protein and protein translocation, are necessary before any age effects can be clearly elucidated.

EXERCISE TRAINING AND HEAT ACCLIMATION

Positive homeostatic effects of endurance exercise training and heat acclimation on thermoregulation have been well studied in young subjects. It is, however, difficult to ascribe beneficial aspects purely to training or purely to acclimation effects resulting from inherent difficulties in separating the two intervention strategies. The attainment of a fully heat-acclimated state necessitates performing dynamic exercise in a warm environment. Passive exposure, as in a sauna or steam room, conveys some, but not all, of the benefits of repeated exercise in the heat. Conversely, exercise training involves the regular elevation of body temperature and sweating, which serves to partially acclimate the individual, even when exercise is performed in a cool environment. There is a dearth of exercise training studies in the literature involving men and women over 65 or 70 yr of age, and fewer yet have tested subjects during exercise in the heat before and after a training regimen.

Endurance Training and Exercise in the Heat

One benefit of exercise training is to increase thermoregulatory effector (SkBF and sweating) responses at a given T_c during exercise in the heat. Ten days of high-intensity training, sufficient to increase $\dot{V}O_2$max by 12%, resulted in a higher local sweating rate on the chest and a higher SkBF at a given T_c—the result of lower T_c thresholds for the onset of sweating and skin vasodilation [101]. The slope of the chest sweating rate to T_c response was only slightly increased with training, and that of SkBF to T_c was unaffected. Can older subjects who maintain a high $\dot{V}O_2$max via regular exercise offset the age-related decrements in SkBF and sweating?

Tankersley et al. [121] addressed this question indirectly by recruiting three groups of subjects who differed in age and $\dot{V}O_2$max in the following way. A group of 13 older men (58–74 yr) was recruited, such that 7 were senior athletes with a high $\dot{V}O_2$max relative to their age group (HO). The remaining six older subjects had a normal $\dot{V}O_2$max for their age (NO). Seven young men were tested who were well matched with the HO for $\dot{V}O_2$max and well matched with the NO for training status, i.e., active but not trained. Each subject performed a 20-min exercise bout at 65–70% $\dot{V}O_2$max in a warm (30°C) environment. While significant differences in FBF and sweating rate (SR) were noted only between the young and NO groups, the HO group demonstrated responses that were intermediate—somewhat lower than those of the young men but higher than those of the NO. It follows from these data that regular exercise training in older subjects may help offset the age-related decline in heat loss function.

Although no true longitudinal training studies have been conducted with subjects past 65 yr of age, the work by Havenith et al. [37] supports the conclusions of Tankersley and colleagues. Inclusion of $\dot{V}O_2$max into regression models eliminates age as a significant predictor of T_c. On the other hand, SkBF responses are significantly related to both age and $\dot{V}O_2$max. Weight loss from sweating was a function only of fitness-related variables.

Heat Acclimation and Age

In the 1960s, Robinson et al. [102] published a longitudinal account of sorts on the ability to acclimatize to the heat. Four men (ages 44–60 yr) "acclimatized about as well" during low-intensity exercise (40°C, 25% rh) as they had 21 yr earlier. Others [94, 131] have since confirmed the ability of middle-aged and older men to acclimate to repeated exercise-heat exposures. In a study by Pandolf and associates [94], middle-aged soldiers (mean age, 46 yr) actually responded with less strain than men 25 yr younger during the first several exercise-heat exposures—an advantage apparently conferred by their greater weekly aerobic activity (subjects were matched for $\dot{V}O_2$max). This advantage was negated by the heat acclimation, because the younger men had similar responses after the initial few days.

Similar to training effects, heat acclimation leads to a higher SkBF for a given T_c in young subjects via a change in the T_c threshold for vasodilation [2, 42, 101]. Furthermore, this adaptation can occur without any increase in $\dot{V}O_2$max [101]. This increased SkBF may be independent of the expansion of blood volume that accompanies both exercise training and heat acclimation [30], because an acute hypervolemia fails to alter SkBF significantly [87], but the exact mechanism is unknown.

Rigorous heat acclimation confers similar effects on SkBF and sweating in young and older men during passive heating [2]. After a 9-day active heat acclimation period, both older (61 ± 1 yr) and younger (26 ± 2 yr) men demonstrated similar reductions in baseline rectal and mean body temperatures. There was, in both age groups, a greater effector response at a given T_c, resulting from a leftward shift in the T_c threshold. Although acclimation increased sweating rate in both groups, the older men had significantly lower sweating rates on the chest before and after acclimation.

SUMMARY

Epidemiological evidence of increased mortality among older men and women resulting from hyper- and hypothermia should not be interpreted as implying that aging per se confers an intolerance to environmental extremes. Relatively few studies have attempted to delineate the effects of chronological age from concomitant factors (such as decreases in $\dot{V}O_2$max, lowered habitual activity levels, alterations in body composition, etc.) in determining thermoregulatory responses to rest and exercise in hot environments. When the effects of chronic diseases and sedentary life-style are kept to a minimum, heat tolerance appears to be minimally compromised by age. $\dot{V}O_2$max is more important than age in predicting body temperature during exertion, even though some of the physiological mechanisms associated with heat dissipation (especially control of skin blood flow and distribution of cardiac output) are closely associated with chronological age. Dehydration effects may be magnified in older individuals, and rehydration may be compromised by age-related differences in thirst sensitivity and renal function.

The efficacy of various interventions in improving thermoregulatory responses of older individuals (e.g., aerobic training and heat acclimation) has not been studied adequately. Older men and women are capable of acclimating to hot conditions, but the time course of physiological changes underlying acclimation with age may be different. Another intervention that holds promise is hormone replacement therapy in postmenopausal women, which acutely affects temperature regulation and control of body fluids in a positive direction. The chronic effects of hormone replacement therapy on thermoregulation during exercise and environmental stresses are not known.

Tolerance to cold exposure under resting conditions may be less dependent on age and aerobic fitness than on body composition. Studies of older and younger subjects exercising in cold environments are lacking altogether, including important studies into the possible preventive effects of regular physical activity on physiological responses to cold stress.

ACKNOWLEDGMENTS

The work performed in the author's laboratory was funded primarily by NIH Grants R23 AG05653 and R01 AG07004 and by funding made available by the Penn State Gerontology Center and the College of Health and Human Development. The technical and medical assistance of the Noll Physiological Research Center faculty, staff, and graduate students are thankfully acknowledged.

REFERENCES

1. Aitken, J. M., R. Lindsay, and D. M. Hart. The redistribution of body sodium in women on long term oestrogen therapy. *Clin. Sci. Mol. Med.* 47:179–187, 1974.
2. Armstrong, C. G., and W. L. Kenney. Effects of age and acclimation on responses to passive heat exposure. *J. Appl. Physiol.* 75:2162–2167, 1993.
3. Becklake, M. R., H. Frank, G. R. Dagenais, G. L. Ostiguy, and C. A. Guzman. Influence of age and sex on exercise cardiac output. *J. Appl. Physiol.* 20:938–947, 1965.
4. Bell, G. W. Effect of Age on Control of Plasma Volume During Exercise and Heat Acclimation. [M.S. thesis] University Park, PA: The Pennsylvania State University, 1993.
5. Bernstein, L. M., L. C. Johnston, R. Ryan, T. Inouye, and F.K. Hick. Body composition as related to heat regulation in women. *J. Appl. Physiol.* 9:241–256, 1956.
6. Blahd, W. H., M. A. Lederer, and E. T. Tyler. Effect of oral contraceptives on body water and electrolytes. *J. Reprod. Med.* 13:223–225, 1974.
7. Brengelmann, G. L., J. M. Johnson, L. Hermansen, and L. B. Rowell. Altered control of skin blood flow during exercise at high internal temperatures. *J. Appl. Physiol.* 43:790–794, 1977.
8. Budd, G. M., J. R. Brotherhood, A. L. Hendrie, and S. E. Jeffery. Effects of fitness, fatness, and age on men's responses to whole body cooling in air. *J. Appl. Physiol.* 71:2387–2393, 1991.
9. Buono, M. J., B. K. McKenzie, and F. W. Kasch. Effects of ageing and physical training on the peripheral sweat production of the human eccrine sweat gland. *Age Ageing* 20:439–441, 1991.
10. Collins, K. J., C. Dore, A. N. Exton-Smith, R. H. Fox, I. C. Macdonald, and P. M. Woodward. Accidental hypothermia and impaired temperature homeostasis in the elderly. *Br. Med. J.* 1:353–356, 1977.
11. Crowe, J. P., and R. E. Moore. Physiological and behavioral responses of aged men to passive heating. *J. Physiol. (Lond.)* 236:1973.
12. Crowe, M. J., M. L. Forsling, B. J. Rolls, P.A. Phillips, J. G. G. Ledingham, and R. F. Smith. Altered water excretion in healthy elderly men. *Age Ageing* 16:285–293, 1987.
13. Daniels, F. Physiologic factors in the skin's reaction to heat and cold. T. B. Fitzpatrick (ed.). *Dermatology in General Medicine.* New York: McGraw-Hill, 1987, pp. 1412–1424.
14. Davies, D. F., and N. W. Shock. Age changes in glomerular filtration rate, effective renal plasma flow and tubular excretory capacity in adult males. *J. Clin. Invest.* 29:496–507, 1950.
15. Davy, K. P., and D. R. Seals. Total blood volume in healthy young and older men. *J. Appl. Physiol.* 76:2059–2062, 1994.
16. de Castro, J. M. A microregulatory analysis of spontaneous fluid intake by humans: evidence that the amount of fluid ingestion and its timing is governed by feeding. *Physiol. Behav.* 43:705–714, 1988.
17. de Castro, J. M. The relationship of spontaneous macronutrient and sodium intake with fluid ingestion and thirst in humans. *Physiol. Behav.* 49:513–519, 1991.
18. de Castro, J.M. Age-related changes in natural spontaneous fluid ingestion and thirst in humans. *J. Gerontol.* 47:P321-P330, 1992.

19. Detry, J. R., G. L. Brengelmann, L. B. Rowell, and C. Wyss. Skin and muscle components of forearm blood flow in directly heated resting man. *J. Appl. Physiol.* 32:506–511, 1972.

20. Dill, D. B., and D. L. Costill. Calculation of percentage changes in volume of blood, plasma, and red cell in dehydration. *J. Appl. Physiol.* 37:247–248, 1974.

21. Drinkwater, B. A., and S. M. Horvath. Heat tolerance in aging. *Med. Sci. Sports Exerc.* 11:49–55, 1979.

22. Drinkwater, B. L., J. F. Bedi, A. B. Louks, S. Roche, and S. M. Horvath. Sweating sensitivity and capacity of women in relation to age. *J. Appl. Physiol.* 53:671–676, 1982.

23. Ellis, F. P., A. N. Exton-Smith, K. G. Foster, and J. S. Weiner. Eccrine sweating and mortality during heat waves in very young and very old persons *Isr. J. Med. Sci.* 12:815–817, 1976.

24. Epstein, M. Effects of aging on the kidney. *Fed. Proc.* 38:168–172, 1979.

25. Fagard, R., and J. Staessen. Relation of cardiac output at rest and during exercise in essential hypertension. *Am. J. Cardiol.* 67:585–589, 1991.

26. Falk, B., O. Bar-Or, J. Smolander, and G. Frost. Response to rest and exercise in the cold: effects of age and aerobic fitness. *J. Appl. Physiol.* 76:72–78, 1994.

27. Faull, C. M., C. Holmes, and P. H. Baylis. Water balance in elderly people: is there a deficiency of vasopressin? *Age Ageing* 22:114–120, 1993.

28. Fennell, W. H., and R. E. Moore. Responses of aged men to passive heating. *J. Physiol. (Lond.)* 231:118P, 1973.

29. Fleg, J. L. Alterations in cardiovascular structure and function with advancing age. *Am. J. Cardiol.* 57:33C–44C, 1986.

30. Fortney, S. M., E. R. Nadel, C. B. Wenger, and J. R. Bove. Effect of acute alterations of blood volume on circulatory performance in humans. *J. Appl. Physiol.* 50:292–298, 1981.

31. Foster, K. G., F. P. Ellis, C. Dore, A. N. Exton-Smith, and J. S. Weiner. Sweat responses in the aged. *Age Ageing* 5:91–101, 1976.

32. Fox, A., P. M. Woodward, and A. N. Exton-Smith. Body temperature in the elderly: a national study of physiological, social and environmental conditions. *Br. Med. J.* 1:200–206, 1973.

33. Gerstenblith, G., D. G. Renlund, and E. G. Lakatta. Cardiovascular response to exercise in younger and older men. *Fed. Proc.* 46:1834–1839, 1987.

34. Gonzalez, R. R., L. G. Berglund, and J. A. J. Stolwijk. Thermoregulation in humans of different ages during thermal transients. Z. Szelenyi and M. Szekely (eds.). *Proceedings of the Satellite of 28th International Congress of Physiological Sciences.* Pecs, Hungary: Pergamon Press, 1980, pp. 357–361.

35. Hagberg, J.M., W. K. Allen, D. R. Seals, B. F. Hurley, A. A. Ehsani, and J. O. Holloszy. A hemodynamic comparison of young and older endurance athletes during exercise. *J. Appl. Physiol.* 58:2041–2046, 1985.

36. Havenith, G., Y. Inoue, V. Luttikholt, and W. L. Kenney. Combined effect of age and V̇o₂max on body temperature during work in a warm humid climate in a heterogenous subject population. A. S. Milton (ed.). *Thermal Physiology 1993.* Aberdeen, Scotland: IUPS Thermal Physiology Commission, 1993, p. 44.

37. Havenith, G., Y. Inoue, V. Luttikholt, and W. L. Kenney. Age predicts cardiovascular, but not thermoregulatory responses to humid heat stress. *Eur. J. Appl. Physiol.* 70:88–96, 1995.

38. Havenith, G., and H. van Middendorp. The relative influence of physical fitness, acclimation state, anthropometric measures and gender on individual reactions to heat stress. *Eur. J. Appl. Physiol.* 61:419–427, 1990.

39. Hellon, R. F., and A. R. Lind. Observations on the activity of sweat glands with special reference to the influence of ageing. *J. Physiol. (Lond.)* 133:132–144, 1956.

40. Hellon, R. F., A. R. Lind, and J. S. Weiner. The physiological reactions of men of two age groups to a hot environment. *J. Physiol. (Lond.)* 133:118–131, 1956.

41. Henschel, A., M. B. Cole, and O. Lyczkowskyj. Heat tolerance of elderly persons living in a subtropical climate. *J. Gerontol.* 23:17–22, 1968.

42. Hessemer, V., A. Zeh, and K. Bruck. Effects of passive heat adaptation and moderate sweatless conditioning on responses to heat and cold. *Eur. J. Appl. Physiol.* 55:281–289, 1986.

43. Ho, C.- W., J. L. Beard, P. A. Farrell, and W. L. Kenney. Distribution of cardiac output during exercise/heat stress: influence of age and fitness level (abstract). *FASEB J.* 10:118, 1996.

44. Horvath, S. M., C. E. Radcliffe, B. K. Hutt, and G. B. Spurr. Metabolic responses of older people to a cold environment. *J. Appl. Physiol.* 8:145–148, 1955.

45. Horvath, S. M., and R. D. Rochelle. Hypothermia in the aged. *Environ. Health Perspect.* 20:127–130, 1977.

46. Hossack, K. F., and R. A. Bruce. Maximal cardiac function in sedentary normal men and women: comparison of age-related changes. *J. Appl. Physiol.* 53:799–804, 1982.

47. Howell, T. H. Normal temperature in old age. *Lancet* i:517–518, 1948.

48. Ingram, D. K., E. D. London, and M. A. Reynolds. Circadian rhythmicity and sleep: effects of aging in laboratory animals. *Neurobiol. Aging* 3:287–297, 1982.

49. Inoue, Y., M. Nakao, T. Araki, and H. Murakami. Regional differences in the sweating responses of older and younger men. *J. Appl. Physiol.* 71:2453–2459, 1991.

50. Inoue, Y., M. Nakao, T. Araki, and H. Yeda. Thermoregulatory responses of young and older men to cold exposure. *Eur. J. Appl. Physiol.* 65:492–498, 1992.

51. Inoue, Y., M. Nakao, S. Okudaira, H. Ueda, and T. Araki. Seasonal variation in sweating responses of older and younger men. *Eur. J. Appl. Physiol.* 70:6–12, 1995.

52. International Organization for Standardization (ISO). Ergonomics—Evaluation of thermal strain by physiological measurements. International Organization for Standardization Draft Standard 9886, 1989, pp. 1–13.

53. Johnson, J. M. Exercise and the cutaneous circulation, J. O. Holloszy (ed.). *Exercise and Sport Science Reviews.* Baltimore: Williams & Wilkins, 1992, pp. 59–97.

54. Kanstrup, I.- L., and B. Ekblom. Influence of age and physical activity on central hemodynamics and lung function in active adults. *J. Appl. Physiol.* 45:709–717, 1978.

55. Keilson, L., D. Lambert, D. Fabian, et al. Screening for hypothermia in the ambulatory elderly. *J. Am. Med. Assoc.* 254:1781–1784, 1985.

56. Kenney, W. L. Control of heat-induced vasodilation in relation to age. *Eur. J. Appl. Physiol.* 57:120–125, 1988.

57. Kenney, W. L. Age and control of visceral blood flow during work. *Environ. Ergon.* 6:204–205, 1994.

58. Kenney, W. L. Body fluid and temperature regulation as a function of age. C. V. Gisolfi E. R. Nadel, D. R. Lamb (eds.). *Exercise in Older Adults: Perspectives in Exercise Science and Sports Medicine.* Carmel, IN: Cooper Publishing Group, 1995, vol.8, pp. 305–351.

59. Kenney, W. L., and R. K. Anderson. Responses of older and younger women to exercise in dry and humid heat without fluid replacement. *Med. Sci. Sports Exerc.* 20:155–160, 1988.

60. Kenney, W. L., and C. G. Armstrong. Reflex peripheral vasoconstriction is diminished in older men. *J. Appl. Physiol.* 80:512–515, 1996.

61. Kenney, W. L., and E. R. Buskirk. Functional consequences of sarcopenia: effects on thermoregulation. *J. Gerontol.* 20A:78–85, 1995.

62. Kenney, W. L., and S. R. Fowler. Methylcholine activated eccrine sweat gland density and output as a function of age. *J. Appl. Physiol.* 65:1082–1088, 1988.

63. Kenney, W. L., and C.- W. Ho. Age alters regional distribution of blood flow during moderate-intensity exercise. *J. Appl. Physiol.* 79:1112–1119, 1995.

64. Kenney, W. L., and J. M. Johnson. Control of skin blood flow during exercise. *Med. Sci. Sports Exerc.* 24:303–312, 1992.

65. Kenney, W. L., A. L. Morgan, W. B. Farquhar, E. M. Brooks, and J. M. Pierzga. Mechanism underlying the attenuated cutaneous vasodilation of older subjects exercising in the heat (abstract). *FASEB J.* 10:118, 1996.

66. Kenney, W. L., C. G. Tankersley, D. L. Newswanger, D. E. Hyde, and S. M. Puhl. Age and hypohydration independently influence the peripheral vascular response to heat stress. *J. Appl. Physiol.* 68:1902–1908, 1990.

67. Kenney, W. L., C. G. Tankersley, D. L. Newswanger, and S. M. Puhl. α1-Adrenergic blockade does not alter control of skin blood flow during exercise. *Am J Physiol.* 260:H855-H861, 1991.

68. Kenney, W. L., and D. H. Zappe. Effect of age on renal blood flow during exercise. *Aging Clin. Exp. Res* 6:293–302, 1994.

69. Khan, F., V. A. Spence, and J. J. F. Belch. Cutaneous vascular responses and thermoregulation in relation to age. *Clin. Sci.* 82:521–528, 1992.

70. Krag, C. L., and W. B. Koontz. Stability of body function in the aged. I. Effect of exposure of the body to cold. *J. Gerontol.* 5:227–235, 1950.

71. Lakatta, E. G. Hemodynamic adaptations to stress with advancing age. *Acta Med. Scand. Suppl.* 711:39–52, 1986.

72. Lee, D. T., and E. M. Haymes. Exercise duration and thermoregulatory responses after whole body precooling. *J. Appl. Physiol.* 79:1971–1976, 1995.

73. Lindeman, R. D., and R. Goldman. Anatomic and physiologic age changes in the kidney. *Exp. Gerontol.* 21:379–406, 1986.

74. Lindeman, R. D., H. C. Van Buren, and L. G. Raisz. Osmolar renal concentrating ability in healthy young men and hospitalized patients without renal disease. *N. Engl. J. Med.* 262:1306–1314, 1960.

75. Löwik, M. R. H., S. Westenbrink, K. F. A. M. Hulshof, C. Kistemaker, and R. J. J. Hermus. Nutrition and aging: dietary intake of apparently healthy elderly. *J. Am. Coll. Nutr.* 8:347–356, 1989.

76. Lybarger, J. A., and E. M. Kilbourne. Hyperthermia and hypothermia in the elderly: an epidemiology review. B. B. Davis and W. G. Wood (eds.) *Homeostatic Function and Aging.* New York: Raven Press, 1985, pp. 149–156.

77. Macey, S. M., and D. F. Schneider. Deaths from excessive heat and excessive cold among the elderly. *Gerontologist* 33:497–500, 1993.

78. Mack, G. W., C. A. Weseman, G. W. Langhans, H. Scherzer, C. M. Gillen, and E. R. Nadel. Body fluid balance in dehydrated healthy older men: thirst and renal osmoregulation. *J. Appl. Physiol.* 76:1615–1623, 1994.

79. Maeda, T., K. Stoltz, A. User, H. Kroone, and N. Brill. Oral temperature in young and old people. *J. Oral Rehabil.* 6:159–166, 1979.

80. Marion, G. S., K. P. McGann, and D. L. Camp. Core body temperature in the elderly and factors which influence its measurement. *Gerontology* 37:225–232, 1991.

81. Martin, H. L., J. L. Loomis, and W. L. Kenney. Maximal skin vascular conductance in subjects aged 5 to 85 yr. *J. Appl. Physiol.* 79:297–301, 1995.

82. Mathew, L., S. S. Purkayastha, R. Singh, and J. Sen Gupta. Influence of aging in the thermoregulatory efficiency of man. *Int. J. Biometeorol.* 30:137, 1986.

83. McElvaney, G. N., S. P. Blackie, N. J. Morrison, M. S. Fairbarn, P. G. Wilcox, and R. L. Pardy. Cardiac output at rest and in exercise in elderly subjects. *Med. Sci. Sports Exerc.* 21:293–298, 1989.

84. Miescher, E., and S. M. Fortney. Responses to dehydration and rehydration during heat exposure in young and older men. *Am. J. Physiol.* 257:R1050-R1056, 1989.

85. Monk, T. H., D. J. Buysse, C. F. Reynolds, D. J. Kupfer, and P. R. Houck. Circadian temperature rhythms of older people. *Exp. Gerontol.* 30:455–474, 1995.

86. Nadel, E. R., E. Cafarelli, M. F. Roberts, and C. B. Wenger. Circulatory regulation during exercise in different ambient temperatures. *J. Appl. Physiol.* 46:430–437, 1979.

87. Nadel, E. R., S. M. Fortney, and C. B. Wenger. Effect of hydration state on circulatory and thermal regulations. *J. Appl. Physiol.* 49:715–721, 1980.

88. Nadel, E. R., J. W. Mitchell, B. Saltin, and J. A. J. Stolwijk. Peripheral modifications to the central drive for sweating. *J. Appl. Physiol.* 31:828–833, 1971.

89. O'Hanlon, J. F., and S. M. Horvath. Changing physiological relationships in men under acute cold stress. *Can. J. Physiol. Pharmacol.* 48:1–10, 1970.

90. Ogawa, T., and N. Ohnishi. Trainability of sweat glands in the aged. M. K. Yousef (ed.). *Milestones in Environmental Physiology.* The Hague: SPB Academic Publishing, 1989, pp. 63–71.

91. Ogawa, T., R. J. Spina, W. H. Martin, W. M. Kohrt, K. B. Schechtman, J. O. Holloszy, and

A. A. Ehsani. Effects of aging, sex, and physical training on cardiovascular responses to exercise. *Circulation* 86:494–503, 1992.

92. O'Neill, P. A., E. B. Faragher, I. Davies, R. Wears, K. A. McLean, and D. S. Fairweather. Reduced survival with increasing plasma osmolality in elderly continuing care patients. *Age Ageing* 19:68–71, 1990.

93. Pandolf, K. B. Aging and heat tolerance at rest or during work. *Exp. Aging Res* 17:189–204, 1991.

94. Pandolf, K. B., B. S. Cadarette, M. N. Sawka, A. J. Young, R. P. Francesconi, and R. R. Gonzalez. Thermoregulatory responses of middle-aged and young men during dry-heat acclimation. *J. Appl. Physiol.* 65:65–71, 1988.

95. Phillips, P.A., M. Bretherton, J. Risvanis, D. Casley, C. Johnston, and L. Gray. Effects of drinking on thirst and vasopressin in dehydrated elderly men. *Am. J. Physiol.* 264:R877-R881, 1993.

96. Phillips, P. A., C.I. Johnston, and L. Gray. Thirst and fluid intake in the elderly. D. J. Ramsay and D.A. Booth (eds.). *Thirst: Physiological and Psychological Aspects.* London: Springer-Verlag 1991, pp. 403–411.

97. Phillips, P. A., B. J. Rolls, J. G. G. Ledingham, and J. J. Morton. Body fluid changes, thirst and drinking in man during free access to water. *Physiol. Behav.* 33:357–363, 1984.

98. Phillips, P. A., B. J. Rolls, M. L. Ledingham, M. L. Forsling, J. J. Morton, M. J. Crowe, and L. Wollner. Reduced thirst after water deprivation in healthy elderly men. *N. Engl. J. Med.* 311:753–759, 1984.

99. Poehlman, E. Endurance exercise in aging humans: effects on energy metabolism. J. O. Holloszy (ed.) *Exercise and Sports Science Reviews.* Baltimore: Williams and Wilkins, 1994, pp. 251–284.

100. Primrose, W. R., and L. R. N. Smith. Oral and environmental temperatures in a Scottish urban geriatric population. *J. Clin. Exp. Gerontol.* 42:151–165, 1982.

101. Roberts, M. F., C. B. Wenger, J. A. J. Stolwijk, and E. R. Nadel. Skin blood flow and sweating changes following exercise training and heat acclimation. *J. Appl. Physiol.* 43:133–137, 1977.

102. Robinson, S., H. S. Belding, F. C. Consolazio, S. M. Horvath, and E. S. Turrell. Acclimatization of older men to work in the heat. *J. Appl. Physiol.* 20:583–586, 1965.

103. Rooke, G. A., M. V. Savage, and G. L. Brengelmann. Maximal skin blood flow is decreased in elderly men. *J. Appl. Physiol.* 77:11–14, 1994.

104. Rowe, J. W., N. W. Shock, and R. A. DeFronzo. The influence of age on the renal response to water deprivation in man. *Nephron* 17:270–278, 1976.

105. Rowell, L. B. Human cardiovascular adjustments to exercise and thermal stress. *Physiol. Rev.* 54:75–159, 1974.

106. Rowell, L. B. Measurement of hepatic-splanchnic blood flow in man by dye techniques. D. A. Bloomfield (ed.). *Dye Curves: The Theory and Practice of Indicator Dilution.* Baltimore: University Park Press, 1974, pp. 209–229.

107. Rowell, L. B. *Human Circulation: Regulation During Physical Stress.* New York: Oxford University Press, 1986.

108. Salvosa, C. B., P. R. Payne, and E. F. Wheeler. Environmental conditions and body temperatures of elderly women living alone or in local authority homes. *Br. Med. J.* 2:656–659, 1971.

109. Sato, K. The mechanism of eccrine sweat secretion. C. V. Gisolfi, D. R. Lamb, E. R. Nadel (eds.). *Exercise, Heat, and Thermoregulation: Perspectives in Exercise Science and Sports Medicine.* Dubuque, IA: Brown & Benchmark, 1993, pp. 85–117.

110. Sato, K., and D. Timm. Effect of aging on pharmacological sweating in man. A. M. Klingman and Y. Takase (eds.). *Cutaneous Aging.* Tokyo: University of Tokyo Press, 1988, pp. 127–134.

111. Schulman, S. P., E. G. Lakatta, J. L. Fleg, L. Lakatta, L. C. Becker, and G. Gerstenblith. Age-related decline in left ventricular filling at rest and exercise. *Am. J. Physiol.* 263:H1932-H1938, 1992.

112. Shiraki, K., S. Sagawa, M. K. Yousef, N. Konda, and K. Miki. Physiological responses of aged men to head-up tilt during heat exposure. *J. Appl. Physiol* 63:576–581, 1987.
113. Shoenfeld, Y., R. Udassin, Y. Shapiro, A. Ohri, and E. Sohar. Age and sex differences in response to short exposure to extreme dry heat. *J. Appl. Physiol.* 44:1–4, 1978.114.
114. Silva, N. L., and J. A. Boulant. Effects of testosterone, estradiol, and temperature on neurons in preoptic tissue slices. *Am. J. Physiol.* 250:R625-R632, 1986.
115. Silver, A., W. Montagna, and I. Karaean. Age and sex differences in spontaneous, adrenergic, and cholinergic human sweating. *J. Invest. Dermatol.* 43:255–256, 1964.
116. Snyder, M. A., D. W. Feigal, and A. L. Arieff. Hypernatraemia in elderly patients: a heterogenous, morbid and iatrogenic entity. *Ann. Intern. Med.* 107:309–319, 1987.
117. Spangler, P. F., T. R. Risley, and D. D. Bilyew. The management of dehydration and incontinence in non-ambulatory geriatric patients. *J. Appl. Behav. Anal.* 17:397–401, 1984.
118. Spina, R. J., T. Ogawa, W. M. Kohrt, W. H. Martin, J. O. Holloszy, and A. A. Ehsani. Differences in cardiovascular adaptations to endurance exercise training between older men and women. *J. Appl. Physiol.* 75:849–855, 1993.
119. Strandell, T. Circulatory studies on healthy older men. *Acta Med. Scand.* 175:1–44, 1964.
120. Tankersley, C. G., D. J. Mikita, W. C. Nicholas, and W. L. Kenney. Estrogen replacement in middle-aged women: thermoregulatory, cardiovascular, and body fluid responses to exercise in the heat. *J. Appl. Physiol.* 73:1238–1245, 1992.
121. Tankersley, C. G., J. Smolander, W. L. Kenney, and S. M. Fortney. Sweating and skin blood flow during exercise: effects of age and maximal oxygen uptake. *J. Appl. Physiol.* 71:236–242, 1991.
122. Therminarias, A., P. Flore, M. F. Oddou-Chirpaz, C. Gharib, and G. Gauquelin. Hormonal responses to exercise during moderate cold exposure in young vs. middle-aged subjects. *J. Appl. Physiol.* 73:1564–1571, 1992.
123. Vitiello, M.V., R.G. Smallwood, D. H. Avery, R. A. Pascualy, D. C. Martin, and P. A. Prinz. Circadian temperature rhythms in young adult and aged men. *Neurobiol. Aging* 7:97–100, 1986.
124. Wagner, J. A., and S. M. Horvath. Influences of age and gender on human thermoregulatory responses to cold exposures. *J. Appl. Physiol.* 58:180–186, 1985.
125. Wagner, J. A., and S. M. Horvath. Cardiovascular reactions to cold exposures differ with age and gender. *J. Appl. Physiol.* 58:187–192, 1985.
126. Wagner, J. A., S. Robinson, and R. Marino P. Age and temperature regulation of humans in neutral and cold environments. *J. Appl. Physiol.* 37:562–565, 1974.
127. Wagner, J. A., S. Robinson, S. P. Tzankoff, and R. P. Marino. Heat tolerance and acclimatization to work in the heat in relation to age. *J. Appl. Physiol.* 33:616–622, 1972.
128. Watkin, D. M., and N. W. Shock. Agewise standards for CIN, CPAH, and TmPAH in adult males. *J. Clin. Invest.* 34:969, 1955.
129. Whitten, C. L., and J. T. Bradbury. Hemodilution as a result of estrogen therapy. Estrogenic effects in the human female. *Proc. Soc. Exp. Biol. Med.* 78:626–629, 1951.
130. Young, A. J. Effects of aging on human cold tolerance. *Exp. Aging Res.* 17:205–213, 1991.
131. Yousef, M. K., D. B. Dill, T. F. Vitez, S. D. Hillyard, and A. S. Goldman. Thermoregulatory responses to desert heat: age, race and sex. *J. Gerontol.* 39:406–414, 1984.
132. Yousef, M. K., and L. A. Golding. Thermal homeostasis and aging. M. K. Yousef (ed.). *Milestones in Environmental Physiology*. The Hague: SPB Academic Publ., 1989, pp. 53–61.

4
Effects of Endurance Exercise on Adipose Tissue Metabolism

BARBARA J. NICKLAS, Ph.D.

Adipose tissue, once considered an inert connective tissue, is an essential storage site for key substrates used as sources of energy. Adipocytes have numerous metabolic functions (see ref. 10), the most important of which are the hydrolysis (lipolysis) and synthesis (lipogenesis) of triacylglycerol (TG) for the release and storage of nonesterified free fatty acids (FFA) and glycerol (Fig. 4.1). The regulation of adipocyte lipid metabolism during periods of excess energy expenditure is critical for the maintenance of fuel homeostasis. For example, adipocytes adapt to acute and long-term increases in physical activity by enhancing their capacity to mobilize and replenish lipid that is used for energy by exercising muscle.

The exercise-induced adaptations in muscle metabolism are widely recognized [49]; however, adaptations in adipose tissue metabolism are less familiar. The purpose of this review is to summarize the effects of endurance exercise on the metabolic functions of adipose tissue. The information will focus on studies performed in humans, unless the only available data are from other species. The effects of both a single exercise bout and endurance exercise training on lipolysis and lipogenesis, the two principal metabolic properties of adipose tissue, are summarized. Additionally, the limited data regarding the effects of endurance exercise on FFA reesterification and blood flow to adipose tissue are discussed. Evolving research examining the role of exercise in the modification of adipocyte size and regional pattern of fat distribution is also reviewed. Collectively, this review gives the reader insight into the significance of these adaptations in adipose tissue metabolism for the supply of lipid substrate during endurance exercise.

REGULATION OF LIPOLYSIS IN HUMAN ADIPOSE TISSUE

Dole [31] showed that one of the principal metabolic functions of adipose tissue is to hydrolyze stored TG into FFA and glycerol. Today, the complex steps leading to this reaction in the adipocyte are well known (Fig. 4.2). Lipolysis is regulated through a chain of events that involve hormone binding and the coupling of the hormone-receptor complex to the membrane-bound enzyme, adenylate cyclase. Lipolytic hormones bind to their receptors and activate the stimulatory guanine nucleotide protein (G_s), while

FIGURE 4.1.

Major pathways of nonesterified FFA storage and mobilization in adipocytes by the enzymes LPL and HSL.

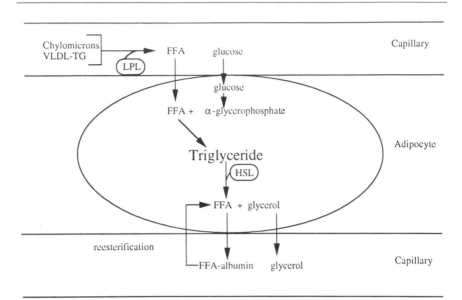

antilipolytic hormones bind to their receptors and activate the inhibitory guanine nucleotide protein (G_i). The balance between these opposing pathways determines the magnitude of cyclic adenosine monophosphate (cAMP) production by adenylate cyclase. The concentration of cAMP controls the activity of cAMP-dependent protein kinase, which ultimately controls the phosphorylation and activation state of hormone-sensitive lipase (HSL), the rate-limiting enzyme that catalyzes the hydrolysis of TG [37]. Thus, the regulation of HSL activity is the most important factor in the mobilization of lipid from adipocytes.

The FFA hydrolyzed from TG are either reesterified by the adipocyte or released to the plasma, where they bind to albumin and are transported to other tissues for oxidation and/or TG synthesis. The glycerol released during lipolysis is not reutilized by the adipocyte but is transported to the liver or kidney, where it is converted to glucose via glycerol kinase and other gluconeogenic enzymes [36]. Cyclic AMP is degraded to 5'-AMP via a phosphodiesterase-catalyzed reaction. Intracellular phosphatases dephosphorylate and inactivate protein kinase and HSL. Through these series of reactions, FFAs, stored as TG in adipocytes, are made readily available as a source of energy substrate for other body tissues.

FIGURE 4.2.

Adrenergic regulation of the lipolytic cascade in adipocytes. GTP, guanosine triphosphate; GDP, guanosine diphosphate; ATP, adenosine triphosphate; ADP, adenosine diphosphate; TAG, triacylglycerol.

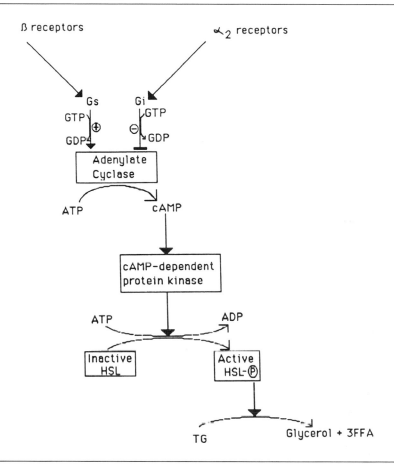

The release of FFA from adipose tissue is regulated by hormones acting on the adipocyte. In humans, insulin and the catecholamines are the most physiologically important hormones regulating adipocyte lipolysis. Insulin is a potent antilipolytic hormone whose effects are mediated through receptor and postreceptor mechanisms [10, 69]. Norepinephrine secreted from nerve endings in adipose tissue, or epinephrine and norepinephrine released from the adrenal medulla, are the main stimulatory hormones of lipolysis [1]. Catecholamines exert a dual effect in humans, either stimulating lipolysis via β-adrenergic receptors or inhibiting lipolysis via α2-adrenergic receptors. Under normal conditions, the lipolytic β-effect dominates, but the balance in the density and affinity of these receptors can change so that catecholamines have a net inhibitory effect on lipolysis [1].

Adipose tissue metabolism is measured in vitro in samples of subcutaneous adipose tissue obtained by means of a needle biopsy [44]. The biopsy can be conducted in any subcutaneous adipose tissue site, although the lower abdomen and upper gluteal regions are most frequently used. After the adipose tissue is removed, experiments are performed on whole pieces of the tissue or on isolated cells obtained by treating the tissue with collagenase to separate the adipocytes [89]. Adipocyte lipolytic sensitivity and maximal responsiveness to stimulatory or inhibitory agonists are measured in vitro, using a double-radioisotope technique [65], or by measuring the concentration of the end products, FFA and glycerol, as indices of the lipolytic rate. Because FFA can be esterified into new TG for reutilization by adipocytes, the release of glycerol is a more accurate index of lipolysis. Glycerol is not reutilized by human adipocytes because of their lack of glycerol kinase, the enzyme necessary for metabolizing glycerol [111].

Although in vitro techniques are useful for studying adipose tissue lipolysis under controlled conditions, the results may not directly reflect actual FFA release from intact adipose tissue [67]. For this reason, in vivo methods are also used to measure the rate of lipid mobilization from adipose tissue. Microdialysis is one such technique that was recently applied to the study of adipose tissue metabolism [3]. This method allows measurement of small water-soluble metabolites, such as glycerol in the interstitial space of a specific adipose tissue region. A hollow permeable tube is inserted, and the tissue is perfused with a dialysis solvent. Measurements of the concentration of metabolites in the outgoing solvent are combined with xenon washout measurements of local blood flow to quantify the rate of lipolysis [60].

Another method for assessing adipose tissue lipolysis in vivo uses the measurement of arteriovenous concentration differences across subcutaneous adipose tissue depots [39]. For abdominal adipose tissue, the superficial epigastric vein is used for venous sampling, whereas a heated dorsal hand vein (arterialized) or a radial artery is used for arterial sampling. This method also relies on accurate measurement of local blood flow to adipose tissue. Finally, the constant-infusion isotope-dilution method, using either radioactive or stable isotopes, is used to measure rates of glycerol and FFA release into circulation [54]. However, because this technique measures whole-body lipolysis and does not distinguish FFA mobilization from adipose tissue only, studies using this methodology are not included in this review. The reader is referred to a recent review of these studies that examines the effects of endurance exercise on whole-body lipolysis [71].

EFFECTS OF ENDURANCE EXERCISE ON
ADIPOSE TISSUE LIPOLYSIS

Effects of acute endurance exercise

The oxidation of lipid is important for meeting the body's excess energy demands during exercise, especially exercise of a low-to-moderate-intensity [92]. Up to 90% of the total energy expended during this type of exercise may be supplied by oxidation of FFA [81]. The FFA used for this enhanced fat oxidation is derived from circulating TG-rich lipoproteins in plasma, intramuscular TG stores, and circulating albumin-bound FFA mobilized from adipose tissue. Adipose tissue is the most important source of FFA during prolonged bouts of endurance exercise [15]. Consequently, physiological changes occur during exercise to enhance the lipid mobilization from adipose tissue. Specifically, sympathetic nervous system activity increases, resulting in elevated catecholamine levels that stimulate adipocyte lipolysis [41]. In addition, insulin concentration decreases during a prolonged exercise bout, reducing the inhibitory effects of insulin on lipolysis. These hormonal changes raise circulating levels of FFA and glycerol during continuous exercise, which is indicative of an increase in FFA mobilization from adipose tissue. During higher-intensity exercise, the accumulation of lactate inhibits HSL activity and reduces lipid mobilization from adipose tissue, allowing muscles to utilize glycogen as an energy source [11]. Furthermore, both in vitro and in vivo studies examining the effects of acute exercise on adipose tissue lipolysis suggest that these hormonal changes are complemented by changes in adipocytes themselves to further enhance FFA mobilization during exercise.

IN VITRO STUDIES. Studies using in vitro techniques show that adipocytes become more responsive to catecholamine stimulation during endurance exercise. This phenomenon was first documented in rat [7, 98] and later in human [97, 120, 121] adipocytes taken immediately after an exercise bout. In one study, basal lipolysis in abdominal adipocytes was unchanged in lean, young males after 90 min of cycling exercise at 88% of maximal heart rate, but maximal catecholamine-stimulated lipolysis increased by 23% [97]. Similar results were seen in gluteal fat cells from a mixed group of young men and women after 30 min of cycling exercise at 67% of maximal aerobic capacity ($\dot{V}O_2$max) [121]. The latter study demonstrated that the cellular mechanism responsible for the exercise-induced increase in catecholamine-stimulated lipolysis was an increase in β-adrenergic receptor responsiveness, rather than changes in either β- or α_2-adrenergic receptor sensitivity. Moreover, radioligand binding experiments showed that the increase in β-adrenergic receptor responsiveness was not caused by a change in the availability of β-adrenergic receptor binding sites. These findings indicate that the exercise-induced increase in catecholamine-stimulated lipolysis is a re-

FIGURE 4.3.

Lipolytic effects of norepinephrine in adipocytes from gluteal (A) and abdominal (B) regions in 10 men and 9 women before (open symbols) and after (closed symbols) exercise. Values are means ± SE. Reproduced from ref. 120.

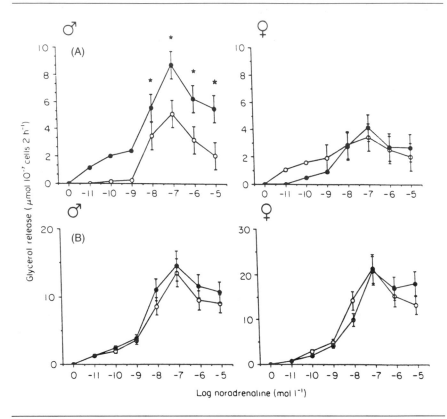

sult of enhancement of a step in the β-adrenergic pathway that is distal to receptor binding.

Not all studies demonstrate an increase in catecholamine-stimulated lipolysis with acute endurance exercise [21, 120]. However, discrepant results among studies are most likely due to differences in the gender of the subjects or the site of the adipose tissue sampling. In an attempt to clarify the effects of gender and fat location on adipocyte changes in lipolysis induced by acute exercise, both abdominal and gluteal adipocyte lipolysis were examined in separate groups of men and women before and after 30 minutes of cycling exercise at 67% of V̇O₂max [120]. As with previous findings, exercise did not affect basal lipolysis in either abdominal or gluteal adipose tissue in men or women. In abdominal adipocytes, exercise did not change catecholamine-stimulated lipolysis in either the men or women (Fig. 4.3). However, in gluteal adipocytes, exercise increased catecholamine-stimulated lipolysis in men but not in women. Furthermore, exercise increased postreceptor-stimulated lipolysis by 30% in gluteal adipocytes in men but not in women. The lack of an increase in catecholamine-stimulated lipolysis after exercise in women was caused by greater α_2-adrenergic antilipolytic responsiveness in gluteal cells, because the β-adrenergic responsiveness was equally enhanced in both men and women (Fig. 4.3). The lack of an increase in lipolytic responsiveness in abdominal adipocytes in men contradicts an earlier finding [95], but the discrepency may be the result of differences in the length of the exercise stimulus (i.e., 90 vs. 30 min).

These in vitro data indicate that there is an increase in catecholamine-stimulated lipolytic responsiveness of adipocytes after acute cycling exercise in men but not in women (Table 4.1). This effect may be more pronounced in gluteal, compared to abdominal, adipocytes, because an increase in lipolysis of abdominal adipose tissue was only seen after a longer exercise bout. The mechanism for this exercise-induced increase in catecholamine-stimulated lipolysis is not caused by changes in adrenergic receptors but is the result of enhancement of a step in the β-adrenergic pathway that is distal to receptor binding.

IN VIVO STUDIES. Studies using in vivo measures of adipose tissue lipolysis yield results that differ from those of in vitro studies. Findings of microdialysis and arteriovenous difference studies show that acute, cycling exercise increases FFA mobilization from gluteal as well as abdominal sites in both men and women. For example, one study demonstrated a progressive increase in glycerol and FFA release from subcutaneous abdominal adipose tissue of both men and women during 60 min of cycling exercise at 50–70% of $\dot{V}O_2$max [48]. In another study, the glycerol concentration in the mi-

TABLE 4.1.
Summary of the Effects of Endurance Exercise on Abdominal and Gluteal Adipose Tissue Lipolysis in Men and Women

	Acute Exercise	Exercise Training	
		Cross-sectional	Longitudinal
Lipolysis (in vitro)			
Abdominal	↑ (M[a] only)	↑ (M and W)	↑ (M > W)
Gluteal	↑↑ (M only)	—	—
Lipolysis (in vivo)			
Abdominal	↑↑ (M and W)	↔	—
Gluteal	↑ (M and W)	—	—

[a]Dash, not studied; M, men; W, women.

crodialysis effluent of both abdominal and gluteal adipose tissue increased significantly during 30 min of cycling exercise at 67% of $\dot{V}O_2$max in young lean men and women [4]. Moreover, in women, gluteal adipose tissue was three times less responsive to exercise than abdominal adipose tissue. In men, gluteal adipose tissue was 50% less responsive than abdominal adipose tissue. After exercise, the glycerol concentration gradually decreased and reached the resting concentration within 30 min. These results indicate that during acute exercise, FFA are mobilized more readily from intact abdominal than gluteal adipose tissue for up to approximately 30 min after the cessation of exercise. This preferential mobilization of FFA from abdominal adipose tissue occurs despite the exercise-induced increase in lipolytic responsiveness of gluteal adipocytes to catecholamine-stimulation (Table 4.1). Thus, other mechanisms, such as an enhanced blood flow to abdominal adipose tissue, may account for the preferential mobilization of FFA from intact abdominal, as compared to gluteal, sites during cycling exercise.

In summary, adipose tissue lipolysis is increased during and immediately after exercise because of changes in concentrations of regulatory hormones, as well as changes in the lipolytic capacity of adipose tissue itself (Table 4.1). However, this effect varies, depending on the methodology used in the study, the length of the exercise session, the location of adipose tissue studied, and the gender of the subjects. Measured in vitro, 30 min of acute exercise increases lipolytic responsiveness in gluteal, but not abdominal, adipocytes of men, but no effect is seen in adipocytes of female subjects. However, measured in intact adipose tissue, FFA are mobilized during 30 min of exercise to a greater extent from abdominal adipose tissue in both men and women, suggesting that blood flow and other factors affect the net release of FFA from adipocytes during exercise. This exercise-induced increase in adipose tissue lipolysis provides a continuous flow of FFA that is used as a substrate for energy production by working muscles during prolonged exercise of a low-to-moderate-intensity.

Effects of Endurance Exercise Training

Physiological adaptations occur after a period of endurance exercise training to improve the transport of oxygen to muscle and to change the relative resting substrate oxidation rate toward a greater reliance on lipid for energy production [43, 49]. In muscle, this shift in substrate utilization results from an increased capacity for lipid oxidation [72] and greater hydrolysis of intramuscular TG [51]. In addition, results from both cross-sectional and exercise training studies show that there is a concurrent training-induced adaptation in adipose tissue to increase its capacity for FFA mobilization [20–22, 28, 88].

CROSS-SECTIONAL STUDIES. Parizkova and Stankova were the first to report a greater lipolytic responsiveness to catecholamine stimulation in adipocytes of exercise-trained rats [80]. Subsequently, studies in humans confirmed and extended this finding. When abdominal adipocytes from male endurance athletes and sedentary men were compared, the basal rate of lipolysis was similar, but lipolytic responsiveness and sensitivity to catecholamine-stimulation were greater in athletes because of an increase in the efficiency of the β-adrenergic pathway [20, 22, 119]. Similar results were seen in female runners, as compared to those in sedentary women, except that the increase in catecholamine-stimulated lipolysis in the runners was caused by a greater β-adrenergic stimulation, as well as a reduction in α2-adrenergic inhibition of lipolysis [21, 22, 88]. Furthermore, two of these studies [21, 88] showed that dibutyryl cAMP-stimulated lipolysis (an analogue of cAMP that diffuses into the cell and activates protein kinase) was also higher in women runners. This indicates that the greater responsiveness of the β-adrenergic pathway in abdominal adipocytes of trained athletes results from an adaptation distal to adenylate cyclase in the lipolytic cascade.

The results of a study using microdialysis to compare intact abdominal adipose tissue lipolysis in trained and sedentary men differ from these in vitro data. This study showed rates of lipolysis were similar in trained and untrained young men in the basal state and during epinephrine infusion [109]. The discrepancy between these findings and the results of in vitro experiments may be a result of the substantially higher concentration of epinephrine used in vitro (10^{-7} to 10^{-6} M), compared to the more physiological concentration used in vivo (5×10^{-9} M). Thus, a higher concentration of epinephrine may be necessary to observe differences in lipolysis between trained and untrained subjects, using the technique of microdialysis.

LONGITUDINAL STUDIES. There are only a few longitudinal studies in humans that examined the effects of endurance exercise training on adipose tissue lipolysis. In one study [28], 20 wk of exercise that increased $\dot{V}O_2$max by 29% in young, lean men and 33% in young, lean women did not change the basal rate of abdominal adipocyte lipolysis, but increased catecholamine-stimulated lipolysis by 66% in men and 46% in women (Fig. 4.4). In a similar study, 20 wk of endurance exercise training increased abdominal adipocyte catecholamine-stimulated lipolysis in men but not in women [26]. These results demonstrate a gender difference in the magnitude of the response of adipose tissue lipolysis to exercise training. Another study showed basal and catecholamine-stimulated lipolysis were significantly higher in marathon runners and men who had exercise-trained for 20 wk than in sedentary men [27]. However, lipolytic responsiveness did not differ between the recently trained men and the marathon runners, indicating that the lipolytic capacity of adipose tissue does not progressively increase with the duration of exercise training. It is also likely that genetic factors influence the effects of exercise training on adipose tissue lipolysis, because the magnitude of the increase in catecholamine-stimulated lipolysis after exercise training was more similar within than between pairs of twins [25].

FIGURE 4.4.

Effects of a 20-wk endurance training program on basal and epinephrine-stimulated lipolysis in 11 women and 11 men. Values are means ± SE. Reproduced from ref. 28.

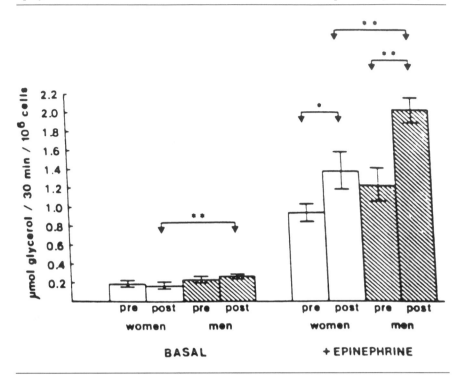

Cumulatively, these findings suggest that abdominal adipocyte responsiveness and sensitivity to catecholamine stimulation are enhanced with endurance exercise training, mostly because of changes in the stimulatory β-adrenergic pathway of the lipolytic cascade (Table 4.1). This lipolytic adaptation occurs within 20 wk of training and may be greater in men than in women. Because previous studies examined the effects of exercise training in abdominal adipose tissue only, it is unknown whether there are regional differences in the response of adipose tissue to endurance exercise training.

Cellular Mechanisms for Enhanced Adipose Tissue Lipolysis with Exercise Training

The results of the studies mentioned above suggest that endurance exercise training enhances the capacity of adipose tissue to mobilize FFA. However, the cellular mechanisms for this adaptation are unknown, especially in humans. Results of one study in rats suggest that differences in adipocyte size between trained and untrained rats could account for the increased adipocyte lipolysis after exercise training [13]. However, other results dispute this idea, because increased adipocyte lipolysis did not relate to variations in adipocyte size after exercise training [28, 79], nor did expressing lipolytic activity per cell size affect the magnitude of the increase in lipolysis observed between trained and sedentary subjects [22, 88]. Thus, there is an effect of exercise training per se on adipocyte lipolysis that is independent of differences in adipocyte size.

This exercise training-induced adaptation in adipocytes could potentially occur at any or all of the biochemical steps in the lipolytic cascade (see Fig. 4.2). Because each of these steps has been studied more thoroughly in rats than in humans, data from both models are reviewed here. First, lipolysis may be enhanced with exercise training by an increase in receptor number or binding affinity. However, in rats, exercise training had no effect on hormone binding to fat cell membranes taken from epididymal fat pads [13, 124]. This finding suggests that the lipolytic capacity of rat adipocytes increases with training through a step distal to receptor binding. At present, there are no studies in humans examining the effects of exercise training on adrenergic receptor number or binding affinity.

Endurance exercise training also may influence the adenylate cyclase activation/cAMP formation step of lipolysis. However, studies in rats show adenylate cyclase activity was both lower [105], as well as higher [52, 124] in exercise-trained, as compared to untrained, rats. The latter two studies suggest that, in rats, exercise training could enhance lipolysis by increasing receptor-cyclase coupling [52, 124]. These conflicting results may be a result of differences in the gender of the rats studied or methodological differences in the measurement of adenylate cyclase activity. Studies examining the effects of exercise training on hormone-stimulated cAMP formation show that, at every concentration of lipolytic agonist, trained rats accumulate less cAMP than untrained littermates [5, 104]. Additionally, cAMP accumulation was lower after fat cell stimulation with isoproteronol (a β-adrenergic agonist) in trained rats, even though their lipolytic rate was elevated [5, 104]. The finding of an elevated level of phosphodiesterase, the enzyme responsible for the breakdown of cAMP, in both of these studies suggests that exercise training enhances lipolysis by some other mechanism besides increasing cAMP levels, possibly by increasing the activity of protein kinase or HSL. Likewise, in humans, adipocytes from exercise-trained subjects show a greater lipolytic response to dibutyryl cAMP (dcAMP) stimulation than adipocytes from untrained subjects [22, 88]. This also points to an adaptation in the protein kinase/HSL steps of the lipolytic cascade with endurance exercise training.

In a study of the final steps of the lipolytic process (i.e., protein kinase and HSL), endurance exercise training did not change protein kinase activity of adipose tissue from female rats [105]. However, in another study, exercise training reduced the activity of protein kinase, suggesting a decreased capacity to activate HSL [76]. Similarly, HSL activity was lower in exercise-trained, compared to control rats [104], and higher in rats after 13 wk of treadmill running [6]. In humans, there are no data regarding the effects of endurance exercise training on protein kinase or HSL activity or expression in adipocytes.

It is also important to note a study that reported elevated activities of mitochondrial enzymes in white adipose tissue of swim-trained rats [110]. Because lipolysis requires ATP, this enhanced ability to synthesize ATP may contribute to the increase in adipocyte lipolysis with exercise training. Thus, to date there is no definitive mechanism known to explain the enhanced rate of adipocyte lipolysis after endurance exercise training in rats or humans. The most feasible mechanism for greater epinephrine-stimulated lipolysis after exercise training is based on the data showing a training-induced increase in lipolysis after dcAMP stimulation [21, 88]. This suggests that exercise training alters adipocyte lipolytic responsiveness at a step distal to adenylate cyclase, probably by increasing expression and/or phosphorylation of HSL.

REGULATION OF LIPOGENESIS IN HUMAN ADIPOSE TISSUE

The synthesis of TG (from FFA and α-glycerophosphate) is the other important metabolic function of adipose tissue (Fig. 4.1). The glycerol moiety is derived from glucose transported across the adipocyte membrane. The FFAs for TG synthesis are derived principally from the hydrolysis of circulating TG-rich chylomicrons and very low-density lipoproteins (VLDL) by the enzyme lipoprotein lipase (LPL) at the surface of the capillary endothelium. A minor source of FFA for TG synthesis is de novo synthesis of lipid from glucose by the adipocyte [10]. Lastly, FFA derived from hydrolyzed TG can be reesterified without leaving the cell. Insulin is the key hormone regulating lipogenesis through its ability to enhance glucose uptake, TG formation, and conversion of glucose into FFA [23, 46]. Numerous other factors, including exercise, can influence the availability of FFA and glucose, and thus the rate of lipogenesis, by altering LPL activity, glucose uptake, and glucose incorporation into TG.

Advances in biochemistry and molecular biology have led to identification and measurement of the steps in the lipogenic process [34, 94]. Radioactive substrate is used to measure LPL activity in pieces of adipose tissue after the enzyme is released from the capillary endothelium by heparin. Heparin-releasable LPL activity is considered the most physiologically active fraction [113]. Glucose transport is directly measured in isolated adipocytes, using a radioactive glucose analogue [2]. Glucose incorporation into TG is determined by adding radioactive glucose to the incubation medium with subsequent detection of radioactivity in extracted lipid [38]. A number of studies have used these methods to examine the effects of acute and chronic endurance exercise on factors affecting the lipogenic process, including LPL activity, glucose uptake, and glucose incorporation into TG.

Endurance Exercise on LPL Activity

Lipoprotein lipase is synthesized within the adipocyte and then transported to the luminal surface of the capillary endothelium [33], where it is the rate-limiting enzyme for the hydrolysis of circulating TG-rich chylomicrons and VLDL. This extracellular source of lipid is the predominant source of FFA for synthesis of TG in adipocytes and indicates the importance of LPL in the lipogenic process [32]. Both acute exercise and endurance exercise training increase LPL activity and expression in muscle and in postheparin plasma in rats and humans [58, 59, 73, 77, 84]. On the other hand, acute and chronic endurance exercise decreases LPL activity in rat adipose tissue but seems to increase adipose tissue LPL activity in humans. Although the reason for these species differences remains unclear from the available data, there are differences in the hormonal regulation of LPL between rats and humans that may cause a differential response of LPL activity to endurance exercise [12].

ACUTE EXERCISE STUDIES. All studies show an exercise-induced increase (ranging from 20 to 44%) in adipose tissue LPL activity in humans after an acute exercise bout [68, 97, 113]. However, there were large interindividual differences in the response of adipose tissue LPL to prolonged endurance exercise in monozygotic and dizygotic pairs of male twins [93]. These changes in LPL activity with exercise appeared to be genotype dependent, suggesting there may be a hereditary component involved in the effects of exercise on adipose tissue LPL activity. Although the cellular and hormonal mechanisms responsible for this increase in adipose tissue LPL activity with acute exercise are unknown, the physiological implication is that an enhanced adipose tissue LPL activity raises FFA concentrations in blood, which are a critical energy source for skeletal muscular contraction during exercise. On the other hand, studies in rats show a decrease in adipose tissue LPL activity after a single exercise session [7, 58, 75, 82], which can last for up to 24 hr postexercise [7]. This decreased enzyme activity is not a result of suppression of LPL by elevated serum levels of FFA [82] but is caused by pretranslational regulation by the LPL gene [58].

EXERCISE TRAINING STUDIES. There is also evidence for changes in adipose tissue LPL activity as a result of endurance exercise training. However, again data from human and animal studies (see ref. 73 for review) are contradictory. Most animal studies show decreases in adipose tissue LPL activity with exercise training, whereas in normal-weight humans, endurance training increases adipose tissue LPL activity. Cross-sectional studies in humans show physically active males have higher adipose tissue LPL activity than sedentary men [70, 74, 95]. In one of these studies, a similar trend was also observed in female runners [74]. Furthermore, a significant positive correlation exists between adipose tissue LPL activity and the average amount of weekly physical activity, with the most active men exhibiting a 70% higher LPL activity than untrained subjects [70, 74].

Although the data from cross-sectional studies clearly show a training-induced increase in LPL activity, results from longitudinal training studies are less consistent. In previously sedentary subjects, endurance exercise training either increased [84], decreased [59], or did not change [85, 103] adipose tissue LPL activity. Furthermore, in young runners, 2 wk of detraining increased adipose tissue LPL activity through posttranslational changes in LPL immunoreactive mass [107]. Disparities in these results may result from differences in the length of the exercise training, the timing of the adipose tissue biopsy relative to the last bout of exercise, the subject's degree of obesity, or to the site of the adipose tissue studied. A relatively long (15-wk) training period increased adipose tissue LPL activity in the abdominal region of normal-weight men [84]. On the other hand, both studies that showed no changes in adipose tissue LPL activity were of a short duration (1–3 wk) with small increases in $\dot{V}O_2$max [85, 103]. In obese young women, 6 mo of endurance exercise decreased both abdominal and gluteal adipose tissue LPL activity [59]. However, obese subjects have higher adipose tissue LPL activity, compared to that of lean individuals [32], suggesting the response of obese subjects to exercise training may differ from that of a lean person. Since there are regional differences in LPL activity at rest [40, 86, 87], the effects of endurance exercise on LPL activity could differ by region of adipose tissue studied. To date, only the study in obese women compared the response of LPL activity in two different adipose tissue sites, and there was no difference in the magnitude of the decline in LPL activity between the abdominal and gluteal regions [59].

In summary, these studies show adipose tissue LPL activity is greater in endurance-trained compared to untrained lean individuals (Table 4.2). However, in obese subjects, with higher initial adipose tissue LPL activity, endurance exercise training decreased both abdominal and gluteal adipose tissue LPL activity. Because adipose tissue LPL activity correlates positively with plasma high-density lipoprotein cholesterol (HDL-C) concentrations [74] and negatively with TG concentrations [84], the increase in LPL with exercise may explain the low VLDL and high HDL-C levels typically seen in endurance-trained individuals. Furthermore, the increase in adipose tissue LPL in response to endurance exercise training would enhance the lipogenic capacity of adipose tissue and is consistent with studies showing a training-induced increase in glucose uptake and TG formation in adipose tissue.

TABLE 4.2.
Summary of the Effects of Endurance Exercise on Factors Regulating Abdominal Adipose Tissue Lipogenesis[a] (LPL Activity, Glucose Uptake, and Glucose Conversion into TG) in Men and Women.

	Acute Exercise	Exercise Training	
		Cross-sectional:	Longitudinal:
LPL Activity	↑ (lean M)	↑ (M > W)	↑ (lean M) and ↓ (obese W)
Glucose uptake	—	↑ (in rats—no human studies)	
Glucose into TG	↓ (lean M)	↑ (lean M)	↑ (M > W)

[a]LPL, lipoprotein lipase; TG, triglyceride; M, men; W, women; dash, not studied.

Endurance Exercise and Adipocyte Glucose Metabolism

The adipocyte's capacity for lipogenesis is dependent on the availability of α-glycerophosphate and, thus, on insulin-mediated glucose transport across the adipocyte plasma membrane [23]. Presently, the effects of an acute exercise bout on adipocyte glucose transport are not known. However, numerous studies in rats show endurance exercise training increases basal and insulin-stimulated glucose uptake, as well as glucose oxidation, in adipose tissue [17–19, 47, 56, 79, 116, 117, 122]. In two of these studies [47, 117], the increase in glucose uptake was supported by an increase (67 and 42%, respectively) in the number of adipocyte glucose transporters in exercise-trained rats. After cessation of exercise training, the enhanced glucose uptake by adipose tissue is rapidly lost [19], suggesting that the increased adipocyte glucose uptake after exercise training may be a transient effect of glucose transporters.

Inside the adipocyte, glucose is either incorporated into the glycerol backbone of TG or converted to FFA and esterified into TG. In humans, glucose conversion into FFA (de novo lipogenesis) is minimal, and most glucose is incorporated into the glycerol fraction of TG [46]. Both a single endurance exercise bout, as well as long-term endurance exercise training, affect the adipocyte's capacity for glucose incorporation into TG. For example, 90 min of cycling exercise inhibited basal and insulin-stimulated glucose incorporation into TG in abdominal adipocytes by 25 and 16%, respectively [97], in young males. These results are similar to those reported in rats after an acute exercise bout [6]. On the other hand, endurance exercise training increases adipocyte glucose incorporation into TG in both rats [18, 117] and humans [95, 96, 119]. In a cross-sectional study, abdominal adipocyte basal and insulin-stimulated glucose incorporation into TG were greater in male marathon runners compared to sedentary controls,

FIGURE 4.5.

Pre- and posttraining values for fat cell maximal insulin-stimulated glucose conversion into triglyceride in 13 women and 10 men. Reproduced from ref. 96.

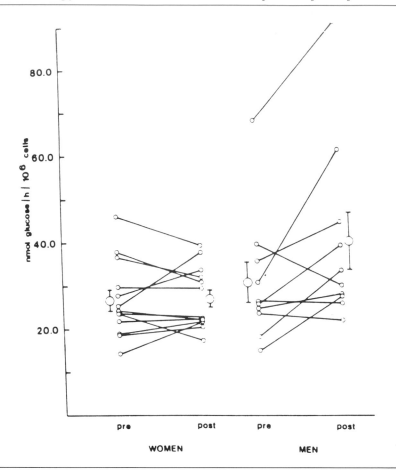

even when subjects were matched for fat cell size [95]. Similarly, basal and insulin-stimulated rates of glucose incorporation into TG in abdominal adipocytes were approximately 2-fold higher in male recreational athletes, compared to those in sedentary men [119]. In response to endurance exercise training, basal and insulin-stimulated glucose incorporation into TG increased 15–20% in previously sedentary male, but not female, subjects (Fig. 4.5) [96]. This suggests that there are gender differences in the effects of exercise training on lipogenesis. The effects of exercise training on the rate of adipocyte TG synthesis from glucose also may be influenced by the length of the training, because no adaptation was seen after a short-term period (22 days) of exercise training [85]. Thus, glucose incorporation into TG is enhanced after endurance exercise training but is inhibited after an acute exercise bout, especially in men (Table 4.2).

OTHER EXERCISE-INDUCED ADAPTATIONS IN ADIPOSE TISSUE

In addition to adaptations in adipocyte lipolysis and lipogenesis, there are other factors involved in the net release and uptake of FFA from adipose tissue that are altered with exercise. These factors include: FFA transport across the adipocyte plasma membrane, reesterification of FFA hydrolyzed during lipolysis, and blood flow to adipose tissue. Presently, there is little information regarding the effects of either an acute exercise bout or of endurance exercise training on these factors.

Effects of Endurance Exercise on Adipocyte FFA Transport

Unlike glucose, whose uptake into adipocytes has been well characterized [23], the mechanism for cellular uptake of FFA is unclear. FFA may diffuse freely through the adipocyte plasma membrane, or its transport may be facilitated by a transport protein. Recently, such a protein was cloned and shown to be localized to plasma membranes of cultured adipocytes [99]. This transport protein is expressed at high levels in skeletal, cardiac, and adipose tissues, sites of importance for FFA metabolism and storage. This study also showed that an isoform of long-chain fatty acyl CoA synthetase is involved in the uptake of FFA, suggesting that the transport protein may work with this enzyme to facilitate diffusion of FFA. It would be of interest to examine whether expression of this fatty acid transport protein and enzyme adapt to changes in the need for FFA uptake in adipose tissue. However, there are no studies examining the effects of acute or chronic endurance exercise on FFA uptake by the adipocyte.

Effects of Endurance Exercise on Adipocyte FFA Reesterification

Two studies demonstrate that reesterification of FFA decreases during an acute exercise bout. The first measured whole-body FFA reesterification but calculated rates of intracellular (adipose tissue) and extracellular (liver) FFA reesterification [125], and the other directly measured arteriovenous differences in FFA and glycerol release from subcutaneous abdominal adipose tissue [48]. In both studies, approximately 20% of FFA released from TG was reesterified by adipose tissue at rest, and this percentage gradually declined during exercise, to the point where no FFAs were reesterified after 70 min of exercise [48]. A decrease in FFA reesterification by adipose tissue during exercise would increase release of hydrolyzed FFA into circulation for use as substrate by working skeletal muscles.

Effects of Endurance Exercise on Blood Flow to Adipose Tissue

Adipocytes are surrounded by an extensive network of capillaries (see ref. 91 for a review of adipose tissue vascularity). To date, only one study examined the effects of acute endurance exercise on adipose tissue blood flow [14]. This study demonstrated a progressive increase in abdominal subcutaneous adipose tissue blood flow (up to 3-fold higher) during four 50-min bouts of exercise in the upright position [14]. It is logical that capillary density in adipose tissue would be increased after endurance exercise training to facilitate the transport of substrates. However, the effects of endurance exercise training on the vascularity of adipose tissue have not been examined.

EFFECTS OF ENDURANCE EXERCISE ON ADIPOCYTE SIZE

The morphological characteristics of the adipocyte are unique in that the cytoplasm constitutes only a small part of the total cell volume, whereas more than 95% of the cell consists of TG. Adipocytes are capable of large changes in their TG volume and, thus in their diameter, to accommodate alterations in energy balance within the body. There is a continuous cycle of lipogenesis and lipolysis within adipocytes, with subsequent storage or release of FFA [36]. Integration of the rates of synthesis and hydrolysis determines the amount of TG stored and, thus, the adipocyte volume. Therefore, exercise-induced alterations in the rates of lipogenesis and lipolysis can have considerable effects on adipocyte size.

There is substantial evidence to suggest that adipose tissue mass is controlled by the size of individual adipocytes, rather than by the number of cells in a specific adipose tissue region. The absolute and relative amounts of body fat correlate positively with adipocyte volume in young lean men and women [16, 28, 119] and in obese, older men and women (B. J. Nicklas unpublished data). Furthermore, weight loss by caloric restriction decreases adipocyte size, rather than adipocyte number [45]. Consequently, it is likely that the effects of exercise training on adipose tissue mass are related to changes in adipocyte size. Presently, because of its high degree of reliability [16, 62], the direct microscopic measurement of isolated adipocyte diameter is the most widely used technique for determining adipocyte size [30].

Most data show that adipocyte size is significantly lower in exercise-trained than in sedentary subjects in all adipose tissue sites studied [9, 22, 27, 88, 95, 115]. Furthermore, exercise-trained men have a similar adipocyte size, regardless of age, suggesting that the age-related increase in adipocyte size is partly the result of a lack of physical activity [9]. Similarly, exercise training studies that result in loss of body fat demonstrate decreases in fat cell size [28, 90, 96]. However, adipocyte size is not reduced in subjects who do not lose weight with exercise training [28, 59]. These findings suggest that the loss of adipose tissue mass with exercise training is caused by reductions in the amount of TG stored in adipocytes.

EFFECTS OF ENDURANCE EXERCISE ON ADIPOSE TISSUE DISTRIBUTION

Recent studies provide evidence that the anatomical distribution of adipose tissue is more important than total adiposity in the assessment of risk for cardiovascular disease (CVD) [8, 83]. A predominantly abdominal distribution of adipose tissue (android or upper body obesity), as opposed to a lower body fat distribution (gynoid obesity), is independently associated with several CVD risk factors (dyslipidemia, hypertension, hyerpinsulinemia and insulin resistance) and with increased mortality from CVD [42, 53, 61, 83]. Exercise training improves these same metabolic risk factors, possibly in part by favorably altering body fat distribution towards lower body sites [29, 55].

The TG storage and mobilization capacity of adipose tissue varies, depending on its anatomical location [35, 64, 122]. In general, adipocytes in the abdominal region, particularly the omental cells, show a greater sensitivity and responsiveness to the lipolytic effect of catecholamines, compared to adipocytes from the gluteal-femoral region [78, 122]. In one study, abdominal adipose tissue was preferentially mobilized for energy needs during exercise in both men and women [4]. Thus, endurance exercise training could cause a consistent preferential release of lipid from abdominal, as opposed to gluteofemoral fat stores, which would favor a lower-body fat distribution. In this regard, numerous studies suggest that exercise training changes body fat distribution, despite little or no change in body weight.

Epidemiological studies show an inverse relationship between amount of physical activity and the degree of upper body obesity, especially in young men [102, 108, 114] This relationship is significant even after adjustment for smoking and body mass index (BMI) [102]. Furthermore, when physical fitness is measured by a $\dot{V}O_2$max test, the most aerobically fit male and female subjects have the lowest waist to hip ratio (WHR) [114]. Data also show a significant inverse relationship between physical activity and WHR in older men, which is independent of both age and BMI [63, 116]. However, regular exercise is not independently associated with a lower WHR in older women [63], suggesting that gender may affect the relationship of endurance exercise training to body fat distribution in older individuals.

There are a few longitudinal studies examining the influence of an exercise training intervention on body fat distribution. One study showed a significant reduction in WHR after 14 wk of endurance exercise training in middle-aged, obese men [50]. Likewise, after 20 wk of endurance training the sum of the trunk skinfolds was reduced by 22% in young males, whereas the sum of the extremity skinfolds was decreased by only 12.5% [24]. However, the reduction in each skinfold measurement, except the calf and bicep, was related to the initial size of the skinfold, implying that regional differences in fat mobilization with exercise training could be accounted for by the initial skinfold size. The same authors studied obese premenopausal women after 14 mo of exercise training and found, using computed tomography, that the ratio of abdominal to femoral subcutaneous fat area decreased after training [29]. This finding indicates that exercise training resulted in a comparatively greater fat loss from the abdominal region than the femoral-gluteal region in these women. Similarly, there was a significant decrease in WHR after 6 mo of exercise training in obese, young women who lost weight, as well as in those who did not lose weight, as a result of the exercise [57].

Older individuals typically have an upper body fat distribution caused by increases in abdominal fat storage with aging and changes in hormonal status [66, 100, 106]. For this reason, two studies investigated the effects of endurance exercise training on body fat distribution in older subjects [55, 101]. To determine whether there are age-related differences in regional fat mobilization with exercise, a 6-mo endurance exercise training study was conducted in both younger and older men [101]. $\dot{V}O_2$max increased by 18 and 22% in the younger and older men, respectively. Body weight, percent fat, and fat mass declined significantly in the older men but not in the younger men. Likewise, WHR decreased significantly only in the older men, but this change was related to the size of the fat depot at the start of the study. In the second study, the effects of 9–12 mo of endurance exercise training on fat distribution were studied in 60- to 70-yr old men and women [55]. Although total weight loss during the training was greater for men, relative changes in weight were similar between men and women. However, the relative changes in skinfold thickness were larger at central sites than at peripheral sites in both men and women. Likewise, relative changes in circumferences of the chest, waist, umbilicus and hips were larger than in the arm and thigh in both genders. The results of these studies suggest a preferential mobilization of subcutaneous abdominal, compared to peripheral, fat stores during exercise training in both young and old individuals. This reduction in abdominal fat accumulation may be one mechanism by which exercise improves risk factors for CVD.

SUMMARY AND FUTURE RESEARCH

The physiological purposes of the exercise-induced adaptations in adipose tissue metabolism are to increase its capacity to release lipid substrate during exercise and to enhance its capacity for lipid replenishment for use during future muscular activity. A number of adipocyte functions are able to adapt for these purposes. Most importantly, adipocyte responsiveness to catecholamine stimulation increases during a single bout of exercise and after a period of endurance exercise training. Exercise training also improves the lipogenic capacity of adipose tissue by increasing the number of glucose transporters, the incorporation of glucose into TG, and the activity of LPL. Additional research is needed to elucidate the cellular mechanisms for these adaptive changes in adipocyte metabolism, as well as the type of exercise and the time course and duration of the exercise stimulus necessary to elicit them. It also will be important to determine whether the interaction of other factors, such as age, gender, genotype, body composition, body fat distribution, and dietary habits, alters the response of adipose tissue metabolism to endurance exercise.

Studies using more precise measurement techniques, such as computed tomography or magnetic resonance imaging, are needed to establish whether intra-abdominal fat is preferentially mobilized during exercise training, compared to subcutaneous abdominal fat. Further research is also needed to determine whether exercise-induced changes in lipolysis or lipogenesis differ between adipose tissue sites and whether these regional adaptations in adipocyte metabolism provide a mechanism for alterations in body fat distribution with exercise training. Elucidation of these details will provide information regarding the most effective exercise prescription for reducing abdominal obesity and CVD risk factors in overweight, sedentary populations.

ACKNOWLEDGMENTS

The author thanks Dr. Andrew Goldberg for his invaluable input during the preparation of this review, and Dr. Ellen Rogus and Dr. Alice Ryan for their insightful comments. Dr. Nicklas was supported by a National Institutes of Aging training grant (T32 AG 00219), a NIH Geriatric Leadership Academic Award (K07 AG-00608) to Dr. Andrew Goldberg, and a NIH research grant (R01 NR-03514–01) to Dr. Karen Dennis and Dr. Andrew Goldberg.

REFERENCES

1. Arner, P. Control of lipolysis and its relevance to development of obesity in man. *Diabetes Metab. Rev.* 4:507–515, 1988.
2. Arner, P. Techniques for the measurement of white adipose tissue metabolism: a practical guide. *Int. J. Obes.* 19:435–442, 1995.
3. Arner, P., and J. Bulow. Assessment of adipose tissue metabolism in man: comparison of Fick and microdialysis techniques. *Clin. Sci.* 85:247–256, 1993.
4. Arner, P., E. Kriegholm, P. Engfeldt, and J. Bolinder. Adrenergic regulation of lipolysis in situ at rest and during exercise. *J. Clin. Invest.* 85:893–898, 1990.
5. Askew, E. W., A. L. Hecker, V. G. Coppes, and F. B. Stifel. Cylic AMP metabolism in adipose tissue of exercise-trained rats. *J. Lipid Res.* 19:729–736, 1978.

6. Askew, E. W., R. L. Huston, C. G. Plopper, and A. L. Hecker. Adipose tissue cellularity and lipolysis. *J. Clin. Invest.* 56:521–529, 1975.

7. Barakat, H., D. S. Kerr, E. B. Tapscott, and G. L. Dohm. Changes in plasma lipids and lipolytic activity during recovery from exercise of untrained rats. *Proc. Soc. Exp. Biol. Med.* 166:162–166, 1981.

8. Bjorntorp, P. The associations between obesity, adipose tissue distribution and disease. *Acta Med. Scand.* 723S:121–134, 1988.

9. Bjorntorp, P., G. Grimby, H. Sanne, L. Sjostrom, G. Tibblin, and L. Wilhelmsen. Adipose tissue fat cell size in relation to metabolism in weight-stabile, physically active men. *Horm. Metab. Res.* 4:178–182, 1972.

10. Bjorntorp, P., and J. Ostman. Human adipose tissue dynamics and regulation. *Adv. Metab. Disord.* 5:277–327, 1971.

11. Boyd, A. E., S. R. Giamber, M. Mager, and H. E. Lebovitz. Lactate inhibition of lipolysis in exercising man. *Metabolism* 23:531–542, 1974.

12. Brunzell, J. D., and A. P. Goldberg. Hormonal regulation of human adipose tissue lipoprotein lipase. G. Schettler, Y. Goto, Y. Hata, and G. Klose (eds.). *Atherosclerosis IV: Proceedings of the Fourth International Symposium,* Berlin: Springer-Verlag, 1977, pp. 336–341.

13. Bukowiecki, L., J. Lupien, N. Follea, A. Paradis, D. Richard, and J. LeBlanc. Mechanism of enhanced lipolysis in adipose tissue of exercise-trained rats. *Am. J. Physiol.* 239:E422-E429, 1980.

14. Bulow, J. Adipose tissue blood flow during exercise. *Danish Med. Bull.* 30:85–100, 1983.

15. Bulow, J., and J. Madsen. Regulation of fatty acid mobilization from adipose tissue during exercise. *Scand. J. Sports Sci.* 8:19–26, 1986.

16. Clarkson, P. M., F. I. Katch, W. Kroll, R. Lane, and G. Kamen. Regional adipose cellularity and reliability of adipose cell size determination. *Am. J. Clin. Nutr.* 33:2245–2252, 1980.

17. Craig, B.W., and P.J. Folley. Effects of cell size and exercise on glucose uptake and metabolism in adipocytes of female rats. *J. Appl. Physiol.* 57:1120–1125, 1984.

18. Craig, B. W., G. T. Hammons, S. M. Garthwaite, L. Jarett, and J. O. Holloszy. Adaptations of fat cells to exercise: response of glucose uptake and oxidation to insulin. *J. Appl. Physiol.: Respir. Environ. Exerc. Physiol.* 51:1500–1506, 1981.

19. Craig, B. W., K. Thompson, and J. O. Holloszy. Effects of stopping training on size and response to insulin of fat cells in female rats. *J. Appl. Physiol. Respir. Environ. Exerc. Physiol.* 54:571–575, 1983.

20. Crampes, F., M. Beauville, D. Riviere, and M. Garrigues. Effect of physical training in humans on the response of isolated fat cells to epinephrine. *J. Appl. Physiol.* 61:25–29, 1986.

21. Crampes, F., M. Beauville, D. Riviere, M. Garrigues, and M. Lafontan. Lack of desensitization of catecholamine-induced lipolysis in fat cells from trained and sedentary women after physical exercise. *J. Clin. Endocrinol. Metab.* 67:1011–1017, 1988.

22. Crampes, F., D. Riviere, M. Beauville, M. Marceron, and M. Garrigues. Lipolytic response of adipocytes to epinephrine in sedentary and exercise-trained subjects: sex-related differences. *Eur. J. Appl. Physiol.* 59:249–255, 1989.

23. Cushman, S. W., and L. J. Wardzala. Potential mechanism of insulin action on glucose transport in the isolated rat adipose cell. *J. Biol. Chem.* 255:4758–4762, 1980.

24. Despres, J. P., C. Allard, A. Tremblay, J. Talbot, and C. Bouchard. Evidence for a regional component of body fatness in the association with serum lipids in men and women. *Metabolism* 34:967–973, 1985.

25. Despres, J. P., C. Bouchard, R. Savard, D. Prud'homme, L. Bukowiecki, and G. Theriault. Adaptive changes to training in adipose tissue lipolysis are genotype dependent. *Int. J. Obes.* 8:87–95, 1984.

26. Despres, J. P., C. Bouchard, R. Savard, A. Tremblay, M. Marcotte, and G. Theriault. Effects of exercise-training and detraining on fat cell lipolysis in men and women. *Eur. J. Appl. Physiol.* 53:25–30, 1984.

27. Despres, J. P., C. Bouchard, R. Savard, A. Tremblay, M. Marcotte, and G. Theriault. Level

of physical fitness and adipocyte lipolysis in humans. *J. Appl. Physiol. Respir. Environ. Exercise Physiol.* 56:1157–1161, 1984.

28. Despres, J. P., C. Bouchard, R. Savard, A. Tremblay, M. Marcotte, and G. Theriault. The effect of a 20-week endurance training program on adipose-tissue morphology and lipolysis in men and women. *Metabolism* 33:235–239, 1984.
29. Despres, J. P., M. C. Pouliot, S. Moorjani, et al. Loss of abdominal fat and metabolic response to exercise training in obese women. *Am. J. Physiol.* 261:E159-E167, 1991.
30. Di Girolamo, M., S. Mendlinger, and J. W. Fertig. A simple method to determine fat cell size and number in four mammalian species. *Am. J. Physiol.* 221:850–858, 1971.
31. Dole, V. P. A relation between non-esterified faty acids in plasma and the metabolism of glucose. *J. Clin. Invest.* 35:150–154, 1956.
32. Eckel, R. H. Adipose tissue lipoprotein lipase. J. Borenszytajn (ed.). *Lipoprotein Lipase,* Chicago: Evener, 1987, pp. 79–132.
33. Eckel, R. H. Lipoprotein lipase. A multifunctional enzyme relevant to common metabolic diseases. *N. Engl. J. Med.* 320:1060–1068, 1989.
34. Eckel, R. H., P. A. Kern, C. N. Sadur, and T. J. Yost. Methods for studying lipoprotein lipase in human adipose tissue. W. L. Clarke, J. Larner, and S. L. Pohl (eds.). *Methods in Diabetes Research.* New York: John Wiley & Sons, 1986, pp. 259–274.
35. Englfeldt, P., and P. Arner. Lipolysis in human adipocytes, effects of cell size, age and regional differences. *Horm. Metab. Res. Suppl.* 19:26–29, 1988.
36. Fain, J. N. Hormonal regulation of lipid mobilization from adipose tissue. *Biochemical Actions of Hormones.* New York: Academic Press, 1980.
37. Fain, J. N., and J. A. Garcia-Sainz. Adrenergic regulation of adipocyte metabolism. *J. Lipid Res.* 24:945–966, 1983.
38. Foley, J. Measurement of *in vitro* glucose transport and metabolism in isolated human adipocytes. W.C. Clarke, J. Larner, and S.L. Pohl (eds.). *Methods in Diabetes Research.* New York: John Wiley & Sons, 1986, pp. 211–232.
39. Frayn, K. N., S. W. Coppack, S. M. Humphreys, and P. L. Whyte. Metabolic characteristics of human adipose tissue in vivo. *Clin. Sci. Lond.* 76:509–516, 1989.
40. Fried, S. K., and J. G. Kral. Sex differences in regional distribution of fat cell size and lipoprotein lipase activity in morbidly obese patients. *Int. J. Obes.* 11:129–140, 1987.
41. Galbo, H. *Hormonal and Metabolic Adaptations to Exercise.* Stuttgart, Germany: Georg Thieme Verlag, 1983.
42. Gillum, R. F. The association of body fat distribution with hypertension, hypertensive heart disease, coronary heart disease, diabetes and cardiovascular risk factors in men and women aged 18–79 years. *J. Chron. Dis.* 40:421–428, 1987.
43. Henriksson, J. Training induced adaptation of skeletal muscle and metabolism during submaximal exercise. *J. Physiol.* 270:661–675, 1977.
44. Hirsch, J., J.W. Farquhar, E. H. Ahrens, M. L. Peterson, and W. Stoffel. Studies of adipose tissue in man—a microtechnic for sampling and analysis. *Am. J. Clin. Nutr.* 8:499–512, 1960.
45. Hirsch, J., S. K. Fried, N. K. Edens, and R. L. Leibel. The fat cell. *Med. Clin. North Am.* 73: 83–96, 1989.
46. Hirsch, J., and R. B. Goldrick. Serial studies on the metabolism of human adipose tissue. I. Lipogenesis and free fatty acid uptake and release in small aspirated samples of subcutaneous fat. *J. Clin. Invest.* 43:1776–1780, 1964.
47. Hirshman, M. F., L. J. Wardzala, L. J. Goodyear, S. P. Fuller, E. D. Horton, and E. S. Horton. Exercise training increases the number of glucose transporters in rat adipose cells. *Am. J. Physiol.* 257:E520-E530, 1989.
48. Hodgetts, V., S. W. Coppack, K. N. Frayn, and T. D. R. Hockaday. Factors controlling fat mobilization from human subcutaneous adipose tissue during exercise. *J. Appl. Physiol.* 71: 445–451, 1991.
49. Holloszy, J. O., and E. F. Coyle. Adaptations of skeletal muscle to endurance exercise and

their metabolic consequences. *J. Appl. Physiol.: Respir. Environ. Exerc. Physiol.* 56:831–838, 1984.

50. Houmard, J. A., C. McCulley, L. K. Roy, R. K. Bruner, M. R. McCammon, and R. G. Israel. Effects of exercise training on absolute and relative measurements of regional adiposity. *Int. J. Obes.* 18:243–248, 1994.

51. Hurley, B. F., P. M. Nemeth, I. W. H. Martin, J. M. Hagberg, G. D. Dalsky, and J. O. Holloszy. Muscle triglyceride utilization during exercise: effect of training. *J. Appl. Physiol.* 60:562–567, 1986.

52. Izawa, T., T. Komabayashi, M. Tsuboi, E. Koshimizu, and K. Suda. Augmentation of catecholamine-stimulated [^{3}H] GDP release in adipocyte membranes from exercise-trained rats. *Jpn. J. Physiol.* 36:1039–1045, 1986.

53. Kissebah, A. H., N. Vydelingum, R. Murray, et al. Relation of body fat distribution to metabolic complications of obesity. *J. Clin. Endocrinol. Metab* 54:254–260, 1982.

54. Klein, S., and R. R. Wolfe. The use of isotopic tracers in studying lipid metabolism in human subjects. *Baillieres Clin. Endocrinol. Metab.* 4:797–816, 1987.

55. Kohrt, W. M., K. A. Obert, and J. O. Holloszy. Exercise training improves fat distribution patterns in 60- to 70-year old men and women. *J. Gerontol. Med. Sci.* 47:M99-M105, 1992.

56. Kral, G. J., B. Jacobsson, U. Smith, and P. Bjorntorp. The effects of physical exercise on fat cell metabolism in the rat. *Acta Physiol. Scand.* 90:664–672, 1974.

57. Krotkiewski, M. Can body fat patterning be changed? *Acta Med. Scand.* Suppl. 723:213–223, 1988.

58. Ladu, M. J., H. Kapsas, and W. K. Palmer. Regulation of lipoprotein lipase in muscle and adipose tissue during exercise. *J. Appl. Physiol.* 71:404–409, 1991.

59. Lamarche, B., J.- P. Despres, S. Moorjani, et al. Evidence for a role of insulin in the regulation of abdominal adipose tissue lipoprotein lipase response to exercise training in obese women. *Int. J. Obes.* 17:255–261, 1993.

60. Larsen, O. A., N. A. Lassen, and F. Quaade. Blood flow through human adipose tissue determined with radioactive xenon. *Acta Physiol. Scand.* 66:337–345, 1966.

61. Larsson, B., K. Svardsudd, L. Welin, L. Wilhelmsen, P. Bjorntorp, and G. Tibblin. Abdominal adipose tissue distribution, obesity, and risk of cardiovascular disease and death: 13 year follow up of participants in the study of men born in 1913. *Br. Med. J.* 288:1401–1404, 1984.

62. Lavau, M., C. Susini, J. Knittle, S. Blanchet-Hirst, and M. R. C. Greenwood. A reliable photomicrographic method for determining fat cell size and number: application to dietary obesity. *Proc. Soc. Exp. Biol. Med.* 156:251–256, 1977.

63. Laws, A., R. B. Terry, and E. Barrett-Connor. Behavioral covariates of waist-to-hip ratio in Rancho Bernardo. *Am. J. Public Health* 80:1358–1362, 1990.

64. Leibel, R. L., and J. Hirsch. Site- and sex-related differences in adrenoceptor status in human adipose tissue. *J. Clin. Endocrinol. Metab.* 64:1205–1210, 1987.

65. Leibel, R. L., J. Hirsch, E. M. Berry, and R. K. Gruen. Radioisotopic method for the measurement of lipolysis in small samples of human adipose tissue. *J. Lipid Res.* 25:49–54, 1984.

66. Ley, C. J., B. Lees, and J. C. Stevenson. Sex- and menopause-associated changes in body-fat distribution. *Am. J. Clin. Nutr.* 55:950–954, 1992.

67. Lillioja, S., J. Foley, C. Bogardus, D. Mott, and B. Howard. Free fatty acid metabolism and obesity in man: in vivo in vitro comparisons. *Metabolism* 35:505–514, 1986.

68. Lithell, H., K. Hellsing, G. Lundqvist, and P. Malmberg. Lipoprotein-lipase activity of human skeletal-muscle and adipose tissue after intensive physical exercise. *Acta Physiol. Scand.* 105:312–315, 1979.

69. Lonnroth, P., and U. Smith. The antilipolytic effect of insulin in human adipocytes requires activation of the phophodiesterase. *Biochem. Biophys. Res. Commun.* 141:1157–1161, 1986.

70. Marniemi, J., P. Peltonen, I. Vuori, and E. Hietanen. Lipoprotein lipase of human postheparin plasma and adipose tissue in relation to physical training. *Acta Physiol. Scand.* 110:131–135, 1980.

71. Martin, W. H. I. Effects of acute and chronic exercise on fat metabolism. J. O. Holloszy (ed.). *Exercise and Sports Science Reviews.* Baltimore: Williams & Wilkins, 1996, pp. 203–231.

72. Mole, P. A., L. B. Oscai, and J. O. Holloszy. Adaptation of muscle to exercise. Increase in levels of palmityl CoA synthetase, carnitine palmityltransferase, and palmityl CoA dehydrogenase, and in the capacity to oxidize fatty acids. *J. Clin. Invest.* 50:2323–2330, 1971.

73. Nikkila, E. A. Role of lipoprotein lipase in metabolic adaptation to exercise and training. J. Borensztajn (ed). *Lipoprotein Lipase.* Chicago: Evener, 1987, pp. 187–199.

74. Nikkila, E. A., M.- R. Taskinen, S. Rehunen, and M. Harkonen. Lipoprotein lipase activity in adipose tissue and skeletal muscle of runners: relation to serum lipoproteins. *Metabolism* 27:1661–1671, 1978.

75. Nikkila, E. A., P. Torsti, and O. Penttila. The effect of exercise on lipoprotein lipase activity of rat heart, adipose tissue and skeletal muscle. *Metab. Clin. Exp.* 12:863–865, 1963.

76. Oscai, L. B., R. A. Caruso, A. C. Wergeles, and W. K. Palmer. Exercise and the cAMP system in rat adipose tissue. I. Lipid mobilization. *J. Appl. Physiol.* 50:250–254, 1981.

77. Oscai, L. B., D. A. Essig, and W. K. Palmer. Lipase regulation of muscle triglyceride hydrolysis. *J. Appl. Physiol.* 69:1571–1577, 1990.

78. Ostman, J., P. Arner, P. Engfeldt, and L. Kager. Regional differences in the control of lipolysis in human adipose tissue. *Metabolism* 28:1198–1204, 1979.

79. Owens, J. L., E. O. Fuller, D. O. Nutter, and M. DiGirolama. Influence of moderate exercise on adipocyte metabolism and hormonal responsiveness. *J. Appl. Physiol. Respir. Environ. Exerc. Physiol.* 43:425–430, 1977.

80. Parizkova, J., and L. Stankova. Influence of physical activity on a treadmill on the metabolism of adipose tissue in rats. *Br. J. Nutr.* 18:325–332, 1964.

81. Paul, P. Effects of long lasting physical exercise and training on lipid metabolism. H. H. and J. R. Poortsmans (eds.). *Metabolic Adaptation to Prolonged Physical Exercise.* Basel, Switzerland: Birkhauser Verlag, 1975, pp. 186–193.

82. Paulin, A., and Y. Deshaies. Serum free fatty acids are not involved in acute exercise-induced reduction of LPL in rat tissues. *Am. J. Physiol.* 262:E377-E382, 1992.

83. Peiris, A. N., J. I. Stagner, R. L. Vogel, A. Nakagawa, and E. Samols. Body fat distribution and peripheral insulin sensitivity in healthy men: role of insulin pulsatility. *J. Clin. Endocrinol. Metab.* 75:290–294, 1992.

84. Peltonen, P., J. Marniemi, E. Hietanen, I. Vuori, and C. Ehnholm. Changes in serum lipids, lipoproteins, and heparin releasable lipolytic enzymes during moderate physical training in man: a longitudinal study. *Metabolism* 30:518–526, 1981.

85. Poehlman, E. T. Heredity and changes in body composition and adipose tissue metabolism after short-term exercise-training. *Eur. J. Appl. Physiol.* 56:398–402, 1987.

86. Rainson, J., A. Basdevant, Y. Sitt, and B. Guy Grand. Regional differences in adipose tissue lipoprotein lipase activity in relation to body fat distribution and menopausal status in obese women. *Int. J. Obes.* 12:465–479, 1988.

87. Rebuffe-Scrive, M., L. Enk, N. Crona, et al. Fat cell metabolism in different regions in women. Effect of menstrual cycle, pregnancy, and lactation. *J. Clin. Invest.* 75:1973–1976, 1985.

88. Riviere, D., F. Crampes, M. Beauville, and M. Garrigues. Lipolytic response of fat cells to catecholamines in sedentary and exercise-trained women. *J. Appl. Physiol.* 66:330–335, 1989.

89. Rodbell, M. Metabolism of isolated fat cells, I. Effects of hormones on glucose metabolism and lipolysis. *J. Biol. Chem.* 239:375–380, 1964.

90. Rognum, T. O., K. Rodahl, and P. K. Opstad. Regional differences in the lipolytic response of the subcutaneous fat depots to prolonged exercise and severe energy deficiency. *Eur. J. Appl. Physiol.* 49:401–408, 1982.

91. Rosell, S., and E. Belfrage. Blood circulation in adipose tissue. *Physiol. Rev.* 59:1078–1104, 1979.

92. Saltin, B., and P. O. Astrand. Free fatty acids and exercise. *Am. J. Clin. Nutr.* 57:752S-758S, 1993.

93. Savard, R., and C. Bouchard. Genetic effects in the response of adipose tissue lipoprotein lipase activity to prolonged exercise: a twin study. *Int. J. Obes.* 14:771–777, 1990.

94. Savard, R., Y. Deshaies, J.-P. Despres, et al. Lipogenesis and lipoprotein lipase in human adipose tissue: reproducibility of measurements and relationships with fat cell size. *Can. J. Physiol. Pharmacol.* 62:1448–1452, 1984.

95. Savard, R., J. P. Despres, Y. Deshaies, M. Marcotte, and C. Bouchard. Adipose tissue lipid accumulation pathways in marathon runners. *Int. J. Sports Med.* 6:287–291, 1985.

96. Savard, R., J.-P. Despres, M. Marcotte, and C. Bouchard. Endurance training and glucose conversion into triglycerides in human fat cells. *J. Appl. Physiol.* 58:230–235, 1985.

97. Savard, R., J. P. Despres, M. Marcotte, G. Theriault, A. Tremblay, and C. Bouchard. Acute effects of endurance exercise on human adipose tissue metabolism. *Metabolism* 36: 480–485, 1987.

98. Savard, R., L. J. Smith, J. E. Palmer, and M. R. C. Greenwood. Site specific effects of acute exercise on muscle and adipose tissue metabolism in sedentary female rats. *Physiol. Behav.* 43:65–71, 1988.

99. Schaffer, J. E., and H. F. Lodish. Expression cloning and characterization of a novel adipocyte long chain fatty acid transport protein. *Cell* 79:427–436, 1994.

100. Schwartz, R. S., W. P. Shuman, V.L. Bradbury, et al. Body fat distribution in healthy young and older men. *J. Gerontol.* 45:M181-M185, 1990.

101. Schwartz, R. S., W. P. Shuman, V. Larson, et al. The effect of intensive endurance exercise training on body fat distribution in young and older men. *Metabolism* 40:545–551, 1991.

102. Seidell, J. C., M. Cigolini, J. Deslypere, J. Charzewska, B. Ellsinger, and A. Cruz. Body fat distribution in relation to physical activity and smoking habits in 38-year-old European men. *Am. J. Epidemiol.* 133:257–265, 1991.

103. Seip, R. L., T. J. Angelopoulos, and C. F. Semenkovich. Exercise induces human lipoprotein lipase gene expression in skeletal muscle but not adipose tissue. *Am. J. Physiol.* 268: E229-E236, 1995.

104. Shepherd, R. E., E. G. Noble, G. A. Klug, and P. D. Gollnick. Lipolysis and cAMP accumulation in adipocytes in response to physical training. *J. Appl. Physiol. Respir. Environ. Exerc. Physiol.* 50:143–148, 1981.

105. Shepherd, R. E., W. L. Sembrowich, H. E. Green, and P. D. Gollnick. Effect of physical training on control mechanisms of lipolysis in rat fat cell ghosts. *J. Appl. Physiol.* 42: 884–888, 1977.

106. Shimokata, H., R. Andres, P. Coon, D. Elahi, D. Muller, and J. Tobin. Studies in the distribution of body fat. II. Longitudinal effects of change in weight. *Int. J. Obes.* 13:455–464, 1989.

107. Simisolo, R. B., J. M. Ong, and P. A. Kern. The regulation of adipose tissue and muscle lipoprotein lipase in runners by detraining. *J. Clin. Invest.* 92:2124–2130, 1993.

108. Slattery, M. L., A. McDonald, D. E. Bild, et al. Associations of body fat and its distribution with dietary intake, physical activity, alcohol, and smoking in blacks and whites. *Am. J. Clin. Nutr.* 55:943–949, 1992.

109. Stallknecht, B., L. Simonsen, J. Bulow, J. Vinten, and H. Galbo. Effect of training on epinephrine-stimulated lipolysis determined by microdialysis in human adipose tissue. *Am. J. Physiol.* 269:E1059–E1066, 1995.

110. Stallknecht, B., J. Vinten, T. Ploug, and H. Galbo. Increased activities of mitochondrial enzymes in white adipose tissue in trained rats. *Am. J. Physiol.* 261:E410–E414, 1991.

111. Steinberg, D., M. Vaughan, and S. Margolis. Studies of triglyceride biosynthesis in homogenates of adipose tissue. *J. Biol. Chem.* 236:1631–1635, 1961.

112. Taskinen, M., and E. A. Nikkila. Effect of acute vigorous exercise on lipoprotein lipase activity of adipose tissue and skeletal muscle in physically active men. *Artery* 6:471–483, 1980.

113. Taskinen, M. R., E. A. Nikkila, J. K. Huttunen, and H. Hilden. A micromethod for assay of lipoprotein lipase activity in needle biopsy samples of human adipose tissue and skeletal muscle. *Clin. Chim. Acta* 104:107–117, 1980.

114. Tremblay, A., J. Despres, C. Leblanc, et al. Effect of intensity of physical activity on body fatness and fat distribution. *Am. J. Clin. Nutr.* 51:153–157, 1990.

115. Tremblay, A., J. P. Despres, and C. Bouchard. Adipose tissue characteristics of ex-obese long-distance runners. *Int. J. Obes.* 8:641–648, 1984.

116. Troisi, R. J., J. W. Heinold, P.S. Vokonas, and S.T. Weiss. Cigarette smoking, dietary intake, and physical activity: effects on body fat distribution—the Normative Aging Study. *Am. J. Clin. Nutr.* 53:1104–1111, 1991.

117. Vinten, J., and H. Galbo. Effect of physical training on transport and metabolism of glucose in adipocytes. *Am. J. Physiol.* 244:E129–E134, 1983.

118. Vinten, J., L. N. Petersen, B. Sonne, and H. Galbo. Effect of physical training on glucose transporters in fat cell fractions. *Biochim. Biophys. Acta* 841:223–227, 1985.

119. Viru, A., K. Toode, and A. Eller. Adipocyte responses to adrenaline and insulin in active and former sportsmen. *Eur. J. Appl. Physiol.* 64:345–349, 1992.

120. Wahrenberg, H., J. Bolinder, and P. Arner. Adrenergic regulation of lipolysis in human fat cells during exercise. *Eur. J. Clin. Invest.* 21:534–541, 1991.

121. Wahrenberg, H., P. Engfeldt, J. Bolinder, and P. Arner. Acute adaptation in adrenergic control of lipolysis during physical exercise in humans. *Am. J. Physiol.* 253:E383–E390, 1987.

122. Wahrenberg, H., F. Lonnfqvist, and P. Arner. Mechanisms underlying regional differences in lipolysis in human adipose tissue. *J. Clin. Invest.* 84:458–467, 1989.

123. Wardzala, L. J., M. Crettaz, E. D. Horton, B. Jeanrenaud, and E. S. Horton. Physical training of lean and genetically obese Zucker rats: effect on fat cell metabolism. *Am. J. Physiol.* 243:E418–E426, 1982.

124. Williams, R. S., and T. Bishop. Enhanced receptor-cyclase coupling and augmented catecholamine-stimulated lipolysis in exercising rats. *Am. J. Physiol.* 243:E345–E351, 1982.

125. Wolfe, R. R., S. Klein, F. Carraro, and J. M. Weber. Role of triglyceride-fatty acid cycling in controlling fat metabolism in humans during and after exercise. *Am. J. Physiol.* 258:E382–E389, 1990.

5
The Cellular Stress Response to Exercise: Role of Stress Proteins

MARIUS LOCKE, Ph.D.

A feature common to all concepts of "stress" is the disruption of home-ostasis. Although this concept is easily applied to whole organisms, it can also be applied at the cellular level. Indeed, the initial focus of many stressors begins at the cellular level, and it is not until certain organs or systems become sufficiently impaired that homeostatic disruption becomes evident and intervention is required. Furthermore, during episodes of stress, a decreased ability of cells from vital organs to maintain homeostasis may compromise the survival of the entire organism. Conversely and consequently, minimizing disruptions and maintaining cellular homeostasis may contribute to an increased ability of the whole organism to withstand various forms of stress.

At the cellular level, proteins play an important role in maintaining cellular homeostasis. Damage or impairment to either existing proteins or newly synthesized polypeptides often results in the disruption of cellular homeostasis. To combat protein-related homeostatic disruptions, cells respond by rapidly synthesizing a group of highly conserved proteins, termed "stress proteins" (SPs). This universal biological response has been termed the "cellular stress response" and occurs in all cells examined thus far. Although the exact function for many of the SPs remains unclear, what is clear is that cells demonstrating elevated levels of certain SPs are capable of withstanding normally lethal stresses.

Some of the conditions known to induce the cellular stress response include increased temperature, ischemia, reactive oxygen species, generation of abnormal proteins, uncoupling of oxidative phosphorylation, alterations in pH, alterations in calcium, and glucose deprivation. Because the conditions experienced by cells of an exercising animal are often physiologically and/or biochemically similar to the conditions known to elicit the cellular stress response, it is not surprising that exercise scientists have become interested in the cellular stress response and SPs. Therefore, understanding the role and expression of SPs will aid researchers in understanding how exercise may provide protection to cells and tissues and may have important health implications. In addition, for the athlete, an increased content of certain SPs may provide an advantage when he or she is exercising in certain environments. Consequently, the general objective of this chapter is to introduce SPs and the cellular stress response, as well as to discuss the relevant information on SPs as it pertains to exercise. This chapter is not intended to be a comprehensive review on SPs or the stress response. For those interested in more detailed information, I would refer them to two excellent books [119, 122] and other reviews [96, 120, 121, 155, 169, 185]. It is hoped that this chapter will familiarize initiates to the terms, concepts, and importance of SPs as they pertain to exercise.

HISTORY AND NOMENCLATURE

The heat shock response was first identified in *Drosophila busckii* by Ritossa [143]. Exposure to elevated temperatures or heat shock, as it was termed, was reported to cause puffing of polytene chromosomes in the salivary glands of *Drosophila* larvae. This report received little attention, and it was not until Tissières et al. [173] demonstrated the synthesis of new proteins in *Drosophila* during heat shock that the "new field" was started. Because exposure to an elevated temperature or "heat shock" was the first stressor used, the newly synthesized proteins were initially termed "heat shock proteins" (HSPs). The first report of mammalian HSPs showed that in addition to heat, other stressors also induced the synthesis of HSPs [74]. As the list of stressors capable of inducing HSPs and the "heat shock response" grew, the terms "cellular stress response" and SP were introduced to reflect accurately the universal nature of the response and the myriad of agents known to induce these new proteins of unknown function [61].

After further investigation, it was discovered that two homologous but differentially regulated sets of stress genes exist [84, 140, 180]. SPs could be divided into at least two specific groups: the HSPs, which were induced by heat shock and other stressors, and a second, different set of proteins, termed glucose-regulated proteins (GRPs). GRPs were induced in cells by subjecting them to glucose starvation, anoxia, calcium ionophores, glucose analogues, and other agents that perturb the N-linked glycosylation of nascent proteins but were not induced by heat shock [136, 180]. Thus, it should be emphasized that although HSPs and GRPs are both considered SPs, GRPs and HSPs refer to distinctly different sets of proteins that exhibit different sensitivities to stresses. Some of the differences between HSPs and GRPs are presented in Figure 5.1.

As investigation into SPs progressed, it became apparent that the term "stress protein" was somewhat of a misnomer, because many SPs were shown to be involved in normal cellular processes during unstressed conditions. Indeed, SPs may comprise up to 5% of cell protein [43] and have been shown to be involved in a wide variety of cellular processes. In view of their involvement with cellular proteins, the term "molecular chaperones" originated. The term "molecular chaperones" describes proteins that facilitate the correct folding of polypeptides or assembly of oligomeric struc-

FIGURE 5.1.
Differences between HSPs and GRPs.

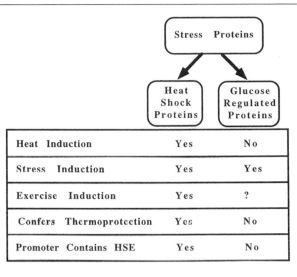

	Heat Shock Proteins	Glucose Regulated Proteins
Heat Induction	Yes	No
Stress Induction	Yes	Yes
Exercise Induction	Yes	?
Confers Thermoprotection	Yes	No
Promoter Contains HSE	Yes	No

tures but are not part of the complex themselves [41]. Some, but not all, of the HSPs and GRPs can be considered molecular chaperones. For the purpose this review, the term HSP will be used to identify genes that contain a heat shock element (HSE) within their promoter region. Genes that do not contain an HSE but are nevertheless induced by stress, such as the GRPs, will be identified as precisely as possible. The term SPs will be used to describe both HSPs and GRPs.

CLASSIFICATION OF SPS

In general, SPs are usually referred to by their molecular weight, as determined by migration on gels or from nucleic acid sequence analysis. Although this might seem straightforward, it should be noted that protein families consisting of various isoforms exist. In addition, because many SPs have been identified in many different species and by many different methods, exact classification and comparisons are often difficult and confusing. For example, HSP 70 and HSP 68 refer to the same protein families in humans and mice, respectively [63, 102]. In addition, the term, HSP 70, is often used to refer to one or more of the 70,000 dalton family of HSPs. In this review, specific isoforms will be identified where possible. The term HSP 70 will be used to refer to the whole family of proteins, or where a specific isoform could not be identified.

TABLE 5.1.
Some of the SPs Identified in Mammalian Cells/Tissues

SP	Cell/Tissue	Exercise Induction	Reference
CPN 10	Rat Tibialis anterior	?	134
Ubiquitin	Human biceps	Yes	172
HSP 27	Mouse heart	?	170
HSP 32	Rat heart	?	73
HSP 47	Fibroblasts	?	154
HSP 60	Rat soleus	Possibly	134
HSP 72	Rat Soleus	Yes	94
HSP 73	Rat soleus	Yes	94
GRP 75	Rat tibialis anterior	?	134
GRP 78	Rabbit adductor	?	177
HSP 90	Rat Soleus	Yes	93
GRP 94	HeLa cells	?	70
HSP 100	Rat soleus	Possibly	93
HSP 110	Mouse 3T3 cells	?	85

Many SPs have been identified in mammalian cells (see Table 5.1). However, information regarding the role and expression of many of these SPs in most cells/tissues is limited. Investigations involving exercise are fewer still. Thus, although certain SPs (HSP 90, HSP 27, HSP 60, and the GRPs) will be introduced and discussed briefly, the vast majority of space is devoted to the HSP 70 family of SPs, because a greater number of exercise related investigations have focused on the expression of these particular SPs.

THE 70-KD FAMILY OF SPS

The most highly conserved SPs, both within and between species, are members of the HSP 70 family [63]. All HSP 70 family members are capable of binding both adenosine triphosphate (ATP) [182] and polypeptides [10, 20, 80]. The N-terminal domain of the protein contains an ATP binding site [113], whereas regions in the C-terminal domain are responsible for polypeptide binding [62] and nuclear localization [113]. In mammalian cells, four main isoforms of the HSP 70 family have been identified [10, 185], although other tissue-specific HSP 70-like proteins also exist [37, 188, 190]. The main HSP 70 isoforms are localized to specific cellular compartments, where they mediate specific events involving proteins [10]. A cognate isoform, termed the heat shock cognate (HSC 73) is constitutively (present under control or unstressed conditions) synthesized in most cells and is only slightly stress inducible [93, 136, 166, 175]. A second isoform, HSP 72, is closely related to HSC 73 and often referred to as the inducible

TABLE 5.2.
Location of the Major HSP 70 Isoforms during Stressed and Unstressed Conditions.

	Cellular Location		
HSP 70 Isoform	Unstressed	Stressed	Reference
HSC 73	Cytoplasm	Nucleus	181
HSP 72	Cytoplasm	Nucleus	181
GRP 75	Mitochondrion	Mitochondrion	116
GRP 78	Endoplasmic/ sarcoplasmic reticulum	Endoplasmic/ sarcoplasmic reticulum	127

isoform of the HSP 70 family [20, 93, 136]. Two other HSP 70 isoforms, GRP 78 and GRP 75, are located in the sarcoplasmic/endoplasmic reticulum and mitochondria, respectively [116, 136, 166, 177]. As their name suggests, these isoforms are GRPs and are not heat inducible. Table 5.2 describes the major HSP 70 isoforms and their cellular location(s).

HSC 73 and HSP 72

In most cells, both a cognate isoform, HSC 73, and an inducible isoform, HSP 72, can be detected after exposure to a variety of stresses, including exercise [93, 94]. These proteins have been shown to be involved in protein synthesis [10, 80], folding [10], transport [25, 26, 36, 174], disassembly [23, 175], degradation [25], preventing protein aggregation, and denaturation, as well as in restoring the function of proteins that are damaged during stress [164, 192].

At present, it remains unclear as to why cells require both a cognate and an inducible isoform that are so closely related in both sequence and putative function [20]. However, one distinguishing feature between HSC 73 and HSP 72 is the presence of intervening sequences in the HSC 73 gene and the lack of intervening sequences in the HSP 72 gene [53, 63, 111, 166]. Because mRNA processing is highly sensitive to stresses, such as heat [107, 190], it may help explain why the cognate isoform is only slightly stress inducible [20, 166]. In contrast, the lack of intervening sequences in the HSP 72 gene may facilitate its rapid transcription during episodes of stress [63]. Differences in the 5' promoter regions of HSP 72 and HSC 73 may also contribute to the observed differences in stress inducibility [111, 166].

When mammalian cells are challenged with stress, both isoforms migrate from the cytoplasm to the nucleus and become associated with preribosomal-containing granular region of nucleoli [181, 184]. During the recovery from stress, they return to the cytoplasm and become associated with proteins and polyribosomes [183, 184]. Both isoforms may form a stable association with each other during stress and associate with nascent polypeptides and newly synthesized proteins [10, 20]. In muscle, the association of HSC 73/HSP 72 with the nascent polypeptides may mediate the speed of nascent polypeptide elongation, and this process may be affected, at least in part, by the level of ATP [80]. However, although ATP hydrolysis accelerates the dissociation of HSP 70 from nascent polypeptides, it is not required for it [156]. HSP 70 associates with polypeptides substrates in the presence of adenosine diphosphate (ADP); ATP binding causes release of the polypeptides [62]. Although the ability to bind and hydrolyze ATP may seem of critical importance, even in the absence of its ATP binding domain, the peptide-binding domain of HSP 72 can still bind to certain critical cellular proteins and prevent denaturation and/or aggregation, thereby preventing cell death at elevated temperatures [89, 90].

Another function of HSP 70 appears to be the restoration of damaged proteins. In agreement with this, DNAK, the prokaryotic homologue of HSP 70, has been shown to reactivate heat-damaged RNA polymerase [164], as well as to protect lactate dehydrogenase from heat inactivation [192]. During or after episodes of stress, the restoration of damaged proteins that are crucial for normal cell functioning would undoubtedly contribute to the restoration of cellular homeostasis, and this may be one of the mechanisms by which HSP 70 members confer protection to cells.

As previously mentioned, HSC 73 is present under control or unstressed conditions (constitutively expressed) in most cells and is only slightly heat inducible [93, 136, 166, 175]. Despite having a slightly higher molecular weight than HSP 72, the mRNA for HSC 73 is shorter [53, 111]. HSC 73 has been shown to play a role in the transport of proteins into the nucleus [160], peroxisome [178], as well as the mitochondrion and endoplasmic reticulum [26, 36]. In contrast to other HSP members, only HSC 73 has been shown to bind to proteins containing a specific peptide motif that targets proteins for lysosomal import and degradation [25]. A fraction of intracellular HSC 73 also appears to reside within the lysosome and may be an essential component of the proteolytic machinery [171].

HSC 73 has also been shown to be an "uncoating ATPase" [23], in that it catalyzes the dissociation of clathrin triskelion from clathrin-coated vesicles. The energy from ATP hydrolysis is used to disrupt or depolymerize the coated vesicles into clathrin triskelions. In the process, HSC 73 is released from the clathrin triskelions [23, 175]. Thus, HSC 73 may play an important role in the degradation of specific cellular proteins.

At present, it remains unclear as to whether HSP 72 and HSC 73 are repair proteins involved in the renaturation of aggregated/denatured proteins or protectors against damage, or both. Whatever the case may be, a vast amount of evidence suggests that cells with an elevated HSP 72 content (and, to a lesser extent, HSC 73) are more resistant to protein-damaging stresses, including heat and ischemia. Thus, the relevance of an elevated

HSP 72/HSC 73 content to the cells/tissues of an exercising organism is obvious: an elevation in cellular HSP 72/HSC 73 content may allow the cells/tissues of an exercising animal to more easily withstand the biochemical and physiological stresses that often accompany exercise.

GRP 75 and GRP 78

Both GRP 75 and GRP 78 are constitutively synthesized soluble proteins that share sequence homology with the HSP 72 and HSC 73 [53]. Both proteins are not induced by heat stress and remain compartmentalized after stress [127, 182]. GRP 78, also known as the immunoglobulin heavy-chain binding protein, or BIP, contains a cleavable signal peptide that is cleaved once it is inside the lumen of the endoplasmic reticulum [127]. GRP 78 appears to have a role in the assembly of secretory proteins and has been shown to bind to incomplete immunoglobulin G proteins until the light chains are attached [136]. GRP 78 has been identified in the sarcoplasmic reticulum (SR) of fast and slow skeletal muscle and localizes with an even distribution within the longitudinal SR and the terminal cisternae [177]. Its role in muscle is less clear than in other cells but may be related to its Ca^{2+} binding ability.

GRP 75, the mitochondrial HSP 70 isoform, is also synthesized in precursor form in the cytoplasm, whereas the mature form of GRP 75 is located in the mitochondrion [116]. GRP 75 facilitates the translocation of precursor proteins across the mitochondrial membrane and is involved with the subsequent stabilization and folding of proteins once they are in the mitochondrion [71, 117, 187]. In rat striated muscle, GRP 75 is expressed in proportion to mitochondrial content and has been shown to increase in the rat tibialis anterior muscle after chronic electrical stimulation [134]. In the rat myocardium, GRP 75 content parallels adaptive growth during hypertrophy and atrophy induced by pressure overload and hypothyroidism, respectively [131]. GRP induction after exercise remains to be examined.

OTHER SPS

The 90-kd HSP Family

The HSP 90 family is comprised of three proteins: two closely related cytoplasmic isoforms, termed HSP 90α and HSP 90β, as well as a glucose-regulated protein (GRP 94), located in the endoplasmic reticulum [71, 108]. In mouse, HSP 90α and 90β proteins are 86% homologous, and both proteins are present to some extent in unstressed cells [118]. HSP 90 has been shown to bind to a number of proteins, including actin [77, 78], tubulin [149], tyrosine kinases [133, 189], serine-threonine kinases [145], as well as other HSPs [150]. However, HSP 90 is best known for binding to unoccupied steroid hormone receptors [141]. These receptors include estrogen, progesterone, glucocorticoid, progesterone, and androgen receptors [21, 34, 141]. The exact role of HSP 90 in steroid hormone receptor binding is still somewhat unclear, but it seems to be that of a chaperone. HSP 90 appears to work in conjunction with HSP 70, as well as other HSPs and non-HSPs in the receptor maturation process [141]. In the absence of the hormone, HSP 90 is thought to bind to the receptor and maintain it in an inactive form [21, 34]. On hormone presentation, the receptor-HSP 90 complex dissociates, and the receptor is rendered capable of binding to DNA. The synthesis of HSP 90 has been shown to increase in lymphocytes, spleen cells, and soleus muscles from untrained rats after an acute bout of exercise [93]. Interestingly, an increased synthesis of HSP 90 was observed in some cells/tissues after only 20 min of exercise and before the increased synthesis of other SPs.

HSP 60

HSP 60 is synthesized in precursor form in the cytoplasm but functions in mitochondria after being processed into its mature form [116]. HSP 60 facilitates the folding and assembly of proteins as they enter the mitochondria and has been shown to stabilize preexisting proteins under stress conditions [24, 104]. This folding has been shown to occur in an ATP-dependent manner, followed by the release of the bound proteins [116]. Newly synthesized mitochondrial proteins have been shown to interact and coprecipitate with HSP 60 [117]. As a result of this "chaperone-like" activity, HSP 60 has been termed a molecular chaperone, or chaperonin [40].

Similar to GRP 75, HSP 60 is also constitutively expressed in muscle in proportion to mitochondrial content and increases after chronic electrical stimulation [134]. Myocardial HSP 60 content has been shown to parallel the cellular adaptive growth that accompanies hypertrophy and atrophy induced after pressure overload and hypothyroidism, respectively [131]. A single bout of exercise induced the synthesis of a 65-kd protein in rat lymphocytes, spleen cells, and soleus muscles [93]. However, it was not confirmed to be HSP 60.

HSP 27

HSP 27 or HSP 25, as it is referred to in rodents, is less universally conserved than other HSPs but contains a conserved domain similar to a domain in the lens protein, α-crystallin [65]. Another important difference from other HSPs is that HSP 27 accumulates with slower kinetics and is synthesized for a longer time after stress [5, 82]. In unstressed mammalian cells, HSP 27 is localized to the cytoplasm, but during stress it localizes to inside or around the nucleus [5, 176]. Although the exact function of HSP 27 remains unknown, it has been shown to be involved in signal transduction, growth, and differentiation, as well as the transformation process [6]. HSP 27 can be activated through the P38 kinase pathway and appears to be a necessary component of a signaling pathway between mitogens and actin polymerization at the cell membrane [6].

An elevated HSP 27 content has been associated with cell thermoresistance [81]. Cell lines expressing elevated levels of HSP 27 were found to be extremely thermoresistant, compared to parental cell lines. A good correlation between the amount of HSP 27 and its thermoresistance was also established. In addition, it was observed that the amount of HSP 27 in the cell before stress may be more important than the level attained after stress induction [81]. Although the exact mechanism for thermoresistance remains unknown, it may involve stabilizing the microfilament network.

In mammals, HSP 27 stems from a single gene, but up to four isoelectric variants can be generated by phosphorylation [81, 83]. A number of agents that activate signal transduction pathways, such as cytokines and growth factors, have been shown to cause a rapid phosphorylation of HSP 27 [6]. Constitutive and stress-induced expression of HSP 27 in mammalian cells appears to be complex, as considerable tissue-specific expression exists [170]. However, an induction of more than 10-fold after stress is not uncommon [6]. HSP 27 is known to exist in very large aggregates (500,000 daltons) in the native state [5], and although HSP 27 has been reported to be constitutively expressed in mammalian muscle [48, 170], its role and expression, pertaining to exercise, remain to be investigated.

Similar to all HSPs, HSP 27 contains several heat shock elements within its promoter region that confer stress inducibility [60]. However, the promoter regions of both the human and rodent HSP 27 genes also contain an estrogen-response element [46]. Thus, in addition to stress induction, HSP 27 may be elevated after estrogen treatment. In agreement with this, HSP 27 is one of the major products synthesized by certain mammalian cells after estrogen treatment [45]. This may have important implications regarding the protective effects conferred to striated muscle after estrogen administration.

GRPs

In higher organisms, GRPs are not induced by heat shock, although coinduction with HSPs and GRPs can result from treating cells with amino acid analogues [185]. The regulation of GRPs is distinct from HSPs, yet they share considerable homology [53, 108, 127]. Interestingly, GRP 78 is more highly conserved between species than between HSP 70 isoforms of the same species [55]. As previously mentioned, GRPs are induced in cells by subjecting them to glucose deprivation [116, 140], calcium ionophores [22, 116, 180], low extracellular pH [186], glucose analogues [116, 140], and other agents that perturb the N-linked glycosylation of nascent proteins [127, 140] but are not induced by heat shock [136]. Induction of GRPs does not confer thermotolerance [158, 167]. However, induction of the GRPs does confer resistance to certain drugs [17, 28]. Although HSPs have been extensively studied, less attention has been paid to the GRPs. Certain GRPs have been reported to be constitutively expressed in mammalian muscle [131, 134, 177]. However, exercise induction of GRPs has not been investigated.

Additional SPs

In addition to the SPs mentioned previously, a number of other SPs have been identified. HSP 110 is a normal constituent of mammalian cells and is induced by heat shock [168]. Its expression correlates with thermotolerance and is associated with the nucleus [168, 180]. The hamster HSP 110 has been cloned and demonstrates a sequence similar to that of the ATP-binding region of HSP 70-related proteins [85]. Another lesser known SP, HSP 100, is a glycoprotein located in the endoplasmic reticulum and golgi membranes. HSP 100 synthesis can be induced by the calcium ionophore A23187 [66], elevated temperature [180], and amino acid analogues [66]. Despite similarities to other stress proteins, the physiological function of HSP 100 and HSP 110 remains unknown. Interestingly, protein of 100 kd demonstrates an increased synthesis in rat cells and tissues after an acute bout of exercise [93].

A 47-kd collagen binding protein has also been shown to be induced by heat shock [129]. HSP 47 is located in the endoplasmic reticulum and has been shown to bind to various types of collagen. The function of HSP 47 is presumed to be similar to that of GRP 78, in that it binds to incomplete pro-collagen polypeptides in the endoplasmic reticulum [114]. A number of other proteins are known to contain heat shock elements within their pro-motor regions, thereby making them HSPs. Some of these proteins include heme oxygenase [161], ubiquitin [16], and α-crystallin [76]. All of these proteins have been identified in muscle, although the exact reason for these proteins possessing a heat-inducible expression remains unclear. However, it has been suggested that they may also be involved in the stress response and, possibly, induced by exercise.

INDUCTION OF HSPs

The promoter regions for many of the HSPs from several organisms have been sequenced and shown to contain a highly conserved *cis*-acting element, termed the HSE [13, 135]. The HSE consists of a 5'-nGAAn-3' sequence and often exists in multiple copies [2, 13]. The HSE is the binding site for the heat shock transcription factors (HSFs) and, as alluded to earlier, the presence of one or more functional HSEs is the identifying feature of an HSP gene.

At least two different mammalian HSF genes, HSF1 and HSF2, have been identified [151]. The identity between mouse HSF1 and HSF2 is only 38%

at the nucleic acid level and only the DNA binding and trimerization domains appear to be similar [151]. HSF1 is activated by heat, heavy metals, oxidative stress, and denatured proteins, whereas HSF2 is activated by hemin, a protoporphyrin ring structure used in the heme-binding groups of myoglobin and catalase. HSF2 appears to regulate HSP expression during differentiation and development [153]. Two isoforms for both HSF1 and HSF2 have been identified [50, 51]. These isoforms, termed α and β, are generated by alternative spicing and are regulated in a tissue-dependent manner. The existence of these isoforms suggests additional ways in which the expression of HSPs can be regulated.

Stress-induced regulation of the HSPs is mediated by HSF1 binding to the HSE [152]. In mammals, the expression of HSF1 is constitutive and not stress inducible [152]. HSF1 contains a regulatory domain consisting of 20 amino acids that confers heat responsiveness [130]. HSF1 exists in the cytoplasm of unstressed cells as a non-DNA-binding monomer, but after exposure to protein-damaging stresses, HSF1 undergoes a conversion to a trimeric state and acquires DNA-binding activity [8, 29, 152]. The process of trimerization and DNA binding is termed HSF activation. The various steps for stress-induced activation of HSPs are diagrammed in Figure 5.2. HSF1 activation has been shown to occur in cells within minutes after exposure to heat-shock [75, 97, 124, 125], hypoxia [11, 49], ATP depletion [12], changes in pH [138], metabolic inhibitors [12], and exercise [96].

HSF activation (presumably, HSF1) has been detected in the hearts of exercising rats [96]. Rats were exercised on a treadmill for 0, 20, 40, 60 min or to exhaustion at 24 m/min. Eighty percent of the hearts from animals that ran for at least 40 min demonstrated a detectable HSF activation. In addition, some of the animals that ran for only 20 min also demonstrated HSF activation. The HSF activation observed in hearts from exercised animals was similar, if not identical, to HSF activation observed in hearts from heat-shocked animals, suggesting that exercise and heat shock may induce HSPs by the same general mechanism. However, it should be noted that in some cases, the rectal temperatures obtained by the exercising animals were well below the temperatures required for HSF activation by heat shock. Thus, factors other than heat per se may also contribute to the exercise-induced HSF activation.

Exactly how HSF activation and inactivation is regulated in cells remains unclear. However, HSPs, and HSP 70 members in particular, have been suggested as being involved in the regulation of HSF1 activation [1, 7, 126]. During unstressed conditions, HSF1 exists in the cytoplasm, possibly complexed with HSP 70 members (Fig. 5.2). A common component of the stressors shown to induce HSPs is that they are proteotoxic or protein damaging. Thus, during episodes of stress, the accumulation of damaged and/or malfolded proteins is thought to compete HSP 70 away from HSF1, allowing the non-DNA-binding HSF1 monomers to form DNA-binding trimers.

FIGURE 5.2.

Induction of HSP 70 following activation of the heat shock transcription factor and possible mechanisms of protein protection.

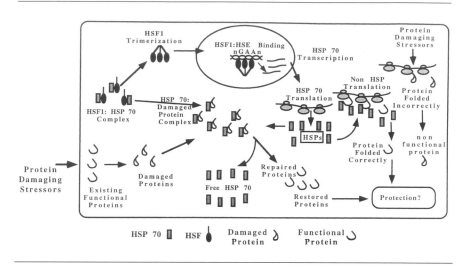

It has suggested that when ATP levels are reduced to a "critical" level, HSP 70 remains complexed to unfolded proteins and cannot be recycled [12]. This reduces the pool of free HSP 70 and increases its demand, creating a competition between unfolded proteins and the HSF for HSP 70. Eventually, as the affinity for HSP 70 by unfolded proteins exceeds the affinity for HSP 70 by the HSF, HSP 70 will be depleted to a level at which it releases HSF for trimerization and DNA binding. After activation of the HSP 70 gene, HSP 70 eventually accumulates to a level at which "free" HSP 70 forms a complex with the activated HSF and, through some yet to be determined mechanism, inhibits further activation. Thus, the competition for HSP 70 by newly damaged proteins may alter the equilibrium between "free" and "substrate-bound" forms of HSP 70. Altering this equilibrium has been suggested as the signal that leads to activation of the HSF and the stress response [7].

Although HSPs are primarily regulated at the level of transcription, other steps have also been shown to be important. HSP 70 mRNA appears very unstable when expressed at normal temperatures [137] and is virtually undetectable in unstressed muscle, using Northern blot analyses [32, 97]. After a 15-min, 42°C whole-animal heat shock, myocardial HSP 70 mRNA rapidly accumulates, peaks 2–4 hr post-heat shock and returns to control levels by 6 hr [32, 97]. A similar pattern of HSP 70 mRNA accumulation and decay has been observed after exercise [97, 147].

The rapid degradation of HSP 70 mRNA may be the result of adenine, uracil-rich sequences in the 3′ untranslated region (3′-UTR) that targets mRNAs for rapid turnover [159]. The 3′-UTR of HSP 70 has been shown to influence HSP 70 production [123]. Heat-shocked COS-1 cells transfected with the HSP 70 3′-UTR linked to a reporter gene demonstrated an increase in reporter gene activity relative to heat-shocked COS-1 cells transfected with a β-globin 3′-UTR reporter gene construct, suggesting a mechanism of posttranscriptional control for HSP 70 [123].

SP RESPONSE TO ACUTE EXERCISE

The first attempt using exercise as a stimulus to induce SPs was made by Hammond et al. [57]. However, no HSP 70 was detected in the translation products from mRNAs present in rat heart muscles directly after exhaustive swimming. In contrast, several investigators have shown that the physiological stress created by treadmill running can induce SPs in a variety of tissues [93, 98, 147, 163]. In one study demonstrating SP induction after exercise, rats were run at 24 m/min for 20, 40, or 60 min or to exhaustion. An increased incorporation of ^{35}S-methionine into SPs with molecular weights of 65, 72, 73, 90, and 100 kd was detected in lymphocytes, spleen cells, and soleus muscle [93]. In the soleus, an increased synthesis of HSP 72, HSC 73, and HSP 90 was detected after only 20 min of exercise. Although in spleen cells and lymphocytes the enhanced synthesis of the 72 kd SP occurred only at, or near, exhaustion.

Salo et al. [147] ran rats to exhaustion (mean time, 64.9 ± 8 min at 26.8 m/min on a 10% grade) and examined proteins from the liver, heart, and hindlimb muscles immediately after exercise. Significant increases in at least 15 protein bands, ranging in molecular weight from 20 to 190 kd were detected. In addition, HSP 70 mRNA was shown to accumulate in the plantaris, extensor digitorum longus, and soleus muscles after exercise. HSP 70 mRNA levels increased 6-fold, peaked 30–60 min after exercise, and declined to control levels by 6 hr postexercise. It was proposed that heat generated by muscle contraction may cause mitochondrial uncoupling, elevating ubisemiquinone concentrations, and increasing superoxide ion generation.

Although the exact component of exercise responsible for the induction of SPs remains unknown, increased temperature might seem to be a major component. Indeed, Blake et al. [14] reported that in vivo temperature increases of only 1–1.5°C are capable of increasing HSP 70 content in certain rat tissues. To examine the role of internal temperature on HSP 70 accumulation, Skidmore et al. [163] exercised rats (17 m/min on a 0% grade, for approximately 60 min) in a cool environment so that colonic temperature did not differ from baseline. The soleus, extensor digitorum longus, and gastrocnemius muscles, as well as the left ventricle, were collected 30 min after exercise and analyzed for HSP 70 content. After exercise, an accumulation of HSP 70 was detected in the soleus, gastrocnemius, and the left ventricle but not in extensor digitorum longus. These increases in HSP 70 content, independent of body temperature, suggest that factors other than the heat generated during exercise contribute to the accumulation of HSP 70 during exercise. Thus, although the increased temperature generated during exercise may contribute to HSP induction, it may not be the only factor.

Additional evidence for factors other than an exercise-induced elevation in temperature, as HSPs inducers, can be obtained from cold stress studies. Matz et al. [106] examined HSP expression in the brown adipose tissue of mice during cold stress. When animals are challenged with a cold environment, shivering takes place, and heat is generated by the activation of the mitochondrial uncoupling protein (UCP). After cold stress exposure, it was observed that HSPs were induced in brown adipose tissue but not in heart or skeletal muscle. Because both the core body temperature and the local temperature of brown adipose tissue decline during cold stress, it appears unlikely that the increased HSP expression resulted from the heat generated by UCP activity. Furthermore, the induction of HSPs in brown adipose tissue was shown to be mediated through adrenergic receptors. This suggests that factors other than heat are capable of inducing HSPs and emphasizes the importance of other physiological factors in inducing the HSP response.

Surprisingly, only a few studies have investigated SP induction in humans. Ryan et al. [146] investigated whether exercise can induce the synthesis of SPs in leukocytes obtained from exercising humans who maintained a rectal temperature greater than 40°C for 75 min. Although no differences were detected in the profile of proteins synthesized in leukocytes obtained before and after exercise, leukocytes obtained after exercise and incubated at 41°C demonstrated a decreased HSP 72 synthesis. Thus, it was concluded that a cell's thermal history might be evaluated based on its ability to synthesize HSP 72 [146]. Another study examined SP accumulation after high-force eccentric arm exercise [16]. Muscle proteins obtained from biopsies taken 48 hr postexercise were assessed for ubiquitin by immunoblotting. Both free and conjugated ubiquitin levels were increased in biceps muscles subjected to eccentrically biased exercise. Unfortunately, other SPs were not examined. However, because ubiquitin is a heat shock protein [16], it suggests that exercise-induced muscle damage may activate the heat shock response in human muscle.

The exact perturbations caused by exercise that are responsible for HSP induction remain to be determined. However, because HSPs have been shown to be induced in a synergistic manner [144], it remains plausible that two or more factors may be acting together. The common feature of the inducers of the stress response is thought to be damaged or denatured proteins [121]. Indeed, abnormal proteins have been shown to activate the heat shock response [3]. Thus, any process that damages or denatures proteins may activate the heat shock response.

SP RESPONSE TO CHRONIC EXERCISE

At present, little is known regarding the expression of HSPs in tissues after exercise training. A number of preliminary reports have suggested that certain HSPs may be elevated with exercise training [19, 148, 162]. These findings have important implications regarding the mechanism(s) by which exercise may provide protection to cells/tissues from stress and disease. Although all of these studies provide useful information, in all cases, either the speed or duration was progressively increased. Thus, any increased HSP content may simply reflect the relative change in exercise intensity or duration from the previous exercise level. Because the HSP response is generally regarded as a transient response required by cells to allow them cope or adapt to a new level of stress, it remains unknown what happens to HSP content after exercise at the same intensity and duration for several weeks. Does an adaptation occur? Does HSP content (and protection) decline to preexercise values? Or, alternatively, is the daily stress of exercise the stimulus that continually induces HSPs and maintains them at elevated levels? These questions warrant further investigation.

PROTECTIVE EFFECTS AFTER SP EXPRESSION

An elevated level of certain HSPs has been associated with a phenomenon termed acquired thermotolerance, which may be defined as a transient resistance to the cytotoxic effects from a subsequent lethal heat shock induced by a short exposure to a nonlethal heat treatment [115, 155]. The concept of acquired thermotolerance may have important implications for the protection conferred to cells and tissues after exercise induction of SPs.

Although both HSP 27 [81] and, to a lesser extent, HSP 90 [9] have been associated with cellular protection, the vast majority of evidence implicates HSP 70 members, particularly HSP 72, as the cytoprotective proteins responsible for conferring protection to cells. Although the first evidence for HSP 70 as a cytoprotection protein was correlative in nature and largely based on an association with protection, more recent studies involving the transfection of constructs into cultured cells, as well as transgenic mice models, have provided direct evidence for HSP 72 as a cytoprotective protein [4, 18, 69, 88, 103, 139, 142].

Cell Culture Studies

An elevated HSP 70 content has been shown to confer thermotolerance to mammalian cells, such that cells expressing a high HSP 72 content become capable of surviving normally lethal temperatures [88]. In addition, when HSPs are induced by stressors other than heat, thermotolerance is still conferred [86]. Li [87] examined the relationship between heat sensitivity and the concentration of the various HSPs in Chinese hamster HA-1 cells and found that the best predictor of survival during heat stress was the content of HSP 70. A good correlation was also observed between HSP 70 synthesis and the logarithm of cell survival. Examination of the HSP 70 isoforms demonstrated no difference between HSC 73 and HSP 72 isoforms in conferring thermotolerance. Thus, Li [87] concluded that together these isoforms may confer heat resistance to cells. Angelidis et al. [4] elevated the constitutive expression of HSP 70 in CV1 monkey cells by transfecting the cells with a plasmid construct consisting of the human HSP 70 gene under the control of the β-actin promotor. Cell lines expressing high amounts of HSP 70 were resistant to elevated temperatures, whereas cells that expressed little or no HSP 70 were not resistant to elevated temperatures. Taken together, these results suggest that HSP 70 protects cells against a lethal heat treatment and may be responsible for thermotolerance.

In another series of experiments, Li et al. [88] transfected a constitutively expressed recombinant human HSP 72-encoding gene into rat fibroblasts and examined the relationship between levels of human HSP 72 and thermal resistance of transfected rat cells. When individual cloned lines were exposed to 45°C (a normally lethal temperature) and their thermal survival was determined by colony formation assay, the expression of human HSP 72 was found to confer a heat resistance to rat cells. These results reinforce the hypothesis that HSP 72 has a protective function against thermal stress.

Additional experiments have shown that expression of the human HSP 72 gene in rat cells confers heat resistance and translational thermotolerance, as well as enhances the ability of cells to recover from heat-induced inhibition of RNA and protein synthesis [90]. Similar experiments have demonstrated protection to muscle cells. Heads et al. [58] used a rat myocyte cell line transfected with the human HSP 70 gene under control of the β-actin promoter. Compared to controls, the transfected cells were significantly protected against lethal heat stress (47°C for 2 hr). In addition to protecting cells from heat stress, an elevated HSP 70 expression has been shown to protect muscle cells against ischemic stress [67, 112]. Thus, a large amount of evidence suggests that an increased HSP 70 expression provides protection to cells from stress.

Animal Studies

Evidence for protection conferred by HSPs can also be obtained from investigations using whole animals. Most of these studies have used the idea of "cross-tolerance." This concept suggests that when HSPs are induced by heat, protection against a different stress, such as ischemia, will be conferred. Thus, most of these studies involved heating anesthetized animals, thereby elevating core temperature to approximately 42°C for 10–20 min, followed by a recovery period (usually 24 hr) and evaluating protection after ischemic stress. The theory behind these studies is that after the heat shock, HSPs will accumulate during recovery, thus conferring protection to a subsequent stress. This allows HSP content and the extent of protection to be evaluated.

The first studies of this type evaluated myocardial function, using either Langendorff isolated heart technique or myocardial infarct size using the triphenyl-tetrazolium staining method. After whole-animal heat shock, an increased myocardial HSP 72 content has been associated with an improved postischemic functional recovery [30, 31, 72] and a reduction in infarct size [33, 39, 64]. Furthermore, a direct correlation between the amount of HSP 72 and reduction in infarct size has been demonstrated [64]. Currie et al. [33] heat stressed rabbits 24 or 40 hr before a 30-min coronary artery occlusion, followed by 3 hr of reperfusion. Although an elevated HSP 72 content was also detected in both groups, myocardial infarct size was reduced only in rabbits heat stressed 24 hr before, not 40 hr before. The exact reasons for the lack of protection at 40 hr remains unclear, but it suggests that the protection conferred to the heart by HSPs may be transient.

Studies employing transgenic mice overexpressing either the rat [103] or human [18, 139] HSP 72 transgene product in their myocardium also provide evidence for an HSP 72-mediated myocardial protection from ischemia. When hearts from mice were subjected to ischemia, the hearts from HSP 72 transgenic mice demonstrated a reduction in infarct size [103]. Similarly, Plumier et al. [139] showed an enhanced postischemic recovery in the hearts of HSP 72 transgenic mice subjected to global ischemia. Bradford et al. [18] demonstrated an enhanced recovery of high-energy phosphates and correction of metabolic acidosis after global ischemia in HSP 72 transgenic mice, compared to those in nontransgenic controls. Taken together, these studies strongly suggest that the accumulation of HSPs, HSP 72 in particular, can provide direct protection to the myocardium during episodes of ischemic stress.

Little is known regarding the protective functions of HSPs in skeletal muscle. At present, only one study has investigated the protective role of heat shock to skeletal muscle [47]. This study found that prior heat shock treatment conferred significant biochemical protection against ischemic injury to rat muscle. After 20 min of ischemia, muscles from heat-shocked rats demonstrated a lesser reduction in creatine phosphate levels. However, CP content was so severely reduced in both cases that it is unclear what protection, if any, may have been conferred.

Exercise Studies

The concept of "cross-tolerance" has tremendous implications for exercise induction of HSPs and disease prevention. If induction of HSPs by heat stress provides protection to the heart from ischemic stress, it follows then that induction of HSPs by exercise might also provide protection. This cross-tolerance concept, using exercise as the initial stressor, has been examined [98]. In this study, rats were subjected to either exercise or heat shock, allowed to recover for 24 hr, and myocardial function was examined after ischemic stress. Exercise consisted of either one or three consecutive daily bouts of treadmill running at 30 m/min (0% grade for 60 min), whereas heat shock consisted of elevating rectal temperature to 42°C for 15 min. Twenty-four hr after exercise or heat shock, the hearts were removed, and cardiac function was assessed before and after 30 min of global ischemia, using the Langendorff isolated heart technique. During reperfusion, animals that were previously heat shocked or subjected to three bouts of exercise demonstrated a significant recovery in left ventricular-developed pressure (LVDP) and rates of contraction and relaxation ($\pm dP/dt$), compared to nonexercise animals (Fig. 5.3). Animals that exercised only once demonstrated no difference in recovery of LVDP and $\pm dP/dt$ from nonexercised controls. Western blot analyses for HSP 72 showed a significantly elevated myocardial HSP content in the hearts from both heat-shocked animals and animals exposed to three bouts of exercise, compared to those of either nonexercised controls or animals subjected to only one bout of exercise. One bout of exercise did not significantly elevate myocardial HSP 72 content above that of nonexercised controls. When myocardial HSP 60, HSP 90β, or GRP 75 content was examined, no differences were observed between those of exercised, heat-shocked, and nonrunning animals [M. Locke, unpublished observations]. The results from this study suggest that exercise induction of HSPs, particularly HSP 72, can also confer protection to cells and tissues from stress.

Although no studies have investigated the protective effects of SPs in skeletal muscle, their involvement in muscle protection is strongly implicated. For example, it has been known for some time that a single bout of eccentric exercise can provide protection against future injury [157]. Exercise of a similar intensity and duration has been shown to increase HSP synthesis in muscle [93, 147]. Thus, considering the repair- and protection-related functions of certain SPs, it is conceivable that induction of SPs by exercise may provide protection against injury from future exercise bouts. This concept is similar, if not identical, to that of "acquired thermotolerance" discussed earlier.

SPs may also be involved in protecting specific fiber types. It has been shown that predominantly slow or Type I muscles, such as the soleus, constitutively express a greater content of HSP 72, HSC 73, and perhaps other SPs, than predominantly fast/Type IIB muscles, such as the white gastroc-

FIGURE 5.3.

Recovery of left ventricular pressure following 30 min of global ischemia. Modified from ref. 97.

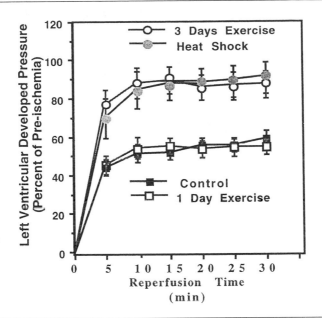

nemius [94, 100]. Assuming that the various fiber types also express similar differences, slow/Type I muscle fibers may be less vulnerable to certain stresses because of their elevated SP content. Although there is evidence to support this concept, the susceptibility of the various fiber types to damage remains equivocal [91, 179]. Interestingly, it has been suggested that vulnerability to eccentric contraction-induced injury is related more to the recent contractile and loading history of a muscle than to fiber-type composition [179]. Thus, the expression of SPs may play a role in the susceptibility of the various muscle fiber types to specific types of injury.

TISSUE-SPECIFIC EXPRESSION OF SPs

Certain SPs are readily detectable in unstressed tissues, and tissue-specific stress responses have been reported [44, 100, 170]. In unstressed striated muscle, the constitutive expression of several SPs has been reported [52, 54, 94, 99, 131, 134, 177]. Although generally considered to be primarily an inducible protein, HSP 72 is constitutively expressed in rat skeletal muscle in proportion to the number of Type I or slow oxidative fibers [94]. Because two members of the yeast HSP 70 family have been implicated in facilitating the transport of proteins into mitochondria [26, 36] and HSP 60/GRP 75 are both known to assist with mitochondrial protein transport, it might be assumed that HSP 72 content is also related to the oxidative capacity or mitochondrial content of a muscle or tissue. In agreement with this idea, the mitochondrial generation of reactive oxygen species, such as hydrogen peroxide, might appear to necessitate an elevated content of specific SPs [38]. However, a number of facts suggest this explanation may not be so simple. First, while HSP 72 is constitutively expressed at high levels in predominantly slow/Type I muscles, such as the rat soleus, it is at very low levels in rat heart, a very highly oxidative and mitochondrial rich tissue. In addition, muscles rich in the highly oxidative Type IIA and IIX fibers, such as the plantaris, express much lower amounts of HSP 72 than the soleus [94]. Second, when the Type I and Type IIB fiber composition of rat muscles was manipulated by compensatory hypertrophy or by thyroid hormone administration, changes in HSP 72 content did not parallel the changes in oxidative capacity of the muscle [95]. In the case of thyroid hormone treatment, the oxidative capacity of the soleus muscle increased as did the number of Type IIB fibers; yet, HSP 72 content decreased. After compensatory hypertrophy of the plantaris muscle, although there was an increase in HSP 72 content, the change appeared unrelated to oxidative capacity. Thus, unlike GRP 75 and HSP 60, the constitutive expression of HSP 72 in rat skeletal muscle does not appear to be strictly related to muscle oxidative capacity or mitochondrial content.

A constitutive expression of HSP 72 has also been observed in the hearts of large mammals, including humans [109, 110] and swine [99]. In the latter study, the constitutive expression HSP 72 was detected at equal levels in all chambers of the swine heart. No HSF activation was observed in protein extracts, suggesting that the constitutive expression of HSP 72 in these hearts may not be the result of an HSF-HSE interaction. Thus, the constitutive expression of HSP 72 might be a result of other transcription factors acting on other parts of the HSP 72 promoter.

Although the reason for the constitutive expression of HSP 72 within the swine and human heart remains unknown, insight into the reason for its high expression may be obtained by examining the biochemical and physiological differences between the hearts from swine and rodents. First, because the rat heart has a greater oxidative capacity than the swine heart, it suggests that HSP 72 is not related to the oxidative capacity of a tissue. Second, because the rat heart exhibits a higher heart rate and rate pressure product than the swine heart, it suggests that the higher content of HSP 72 is not an indicator of the amount of hemodynamic work imposed on the myocardium. Third, the basal expression of HSP 72 may not be related to calcium cycling, because these parameters are also higher in the rat myocardium [56]. Lastly, since the right and left sides of the swine heart differ 4 to 5-fold in systolic pressure, yet demonstrated a similar HSP 72 content, it is suggested that the basal expression of HSP 72 is not directly related to systolic pressure.

One known difference between the heart of large and small mammals is the type of myosin heavy-chain protein (MHC) expressed [56, 128]. Hearts from small mammals, such as the rat, are comprised of primarily the fast α-MHC in both atria and ventricles, whereas hearts from large mammals express the Type I or β-MHC in their ventricles but the fast α-MHC in their atria. In agreement with this idea, the constitutive expression of HSP 72 in rat skeletal muscles appears related to the proportion of Type I/β-MHC muscle fibers [94], and the switch in MHC gene expression in the rat heart after pressure overload is accompanied by induction of HSP 70 [35, 68, 165].

To clarify the relationship between the pattern of expression for HSP 72 and Type I MHC, the content of the two proteins in the hearts from small (rat) and large (swine) mammals was compared [99]. All chambers of the rat heart expressed little, if any, HSP 72, whereas all chambers of the swine heart expressed relatively high levels of HSP 72. Because the atria of the swine express the α-MHC and the ventricles express the β-MHC yet both had similar levels of HSP 72, it may be that HSP 72 is not strictly related to the expression of the Type I MHC. The reason why certain muscles constitutively express a relatively high HSP 72 content remains unknown, but some interesting questions can be raised about the necessity for such proteins, as well as about their possible roles in providing protection. In addition, because HSP 70 has been suggested to be a negative regulator of HSF activation, its constitutive expression has important implications regarding induction of the HSP response.

SPs AND AGING

The heat shock response of aged cells has been examined [15, 27, 42, 59, 92, 132]. In the unstressed state, aged and adult cells appear to demonstrate similar levels of HSPs, at least for the ones examined thus far [59, 101, 132]. However, when subjected to stress, cells from aged animals demonstrate a diminished stress response [59, 132]. More specifically, a reduced accumulation of HSP 72 in aged cells after stress has been reported for rat heart [79, 101, 132] and liver [59], as well as for certain human cell lines [27, 92]. These studies suggest that aged cells demonstrate a reduced ability to mount a stress response.

A diminished stress response in vital organs of an aged animal may compromise the ability of the entire animal to survive during episodes of stress [79, 101, 132]. Aged rats (> 18 mo old) given a 10-min 41°C heat shock and allowed to recover for various amounts of time demonstrated a 47% reduction in HSF activation, a reduction in HSP 72 mRNA, and a 35% reduction in HSP 72 protein content, compared to hearts from adults (6 mo old)[101]. Interestingly, myocardial HSF (monomer) protein content was similar between aged and adult animals, suggesting that the reduced HSF activation observed in the aged rats' hearts was not a result of decreased content of the HSF monomer protein. In addition, the hearts from previously heat-shocked, aged animals (24 hr earlier) did not demonstrate myocardial protection, as indicated by recovery of left ventricular pressure and rate of contraction. In contrast, the hearts from previously heat-shocked adult animals demonstrated significantly enhanced postischemic recovery. These results suggest that aging is associated with an impaired ability to translate stress signals into the biochemical steps necessary for induction of the stress response. Thus, the diminished ability of aged cells to mount a stress response and synthesize HSPs may render an aged organism more susceptible to certain stresses.

At this time, the only known method of retarding or reversing the age-related decline in HSP induction is caloric restriction [59]. Heat stressed hepatocytes from aged rats fed a calorie restricted diet demonstrated a greater induction of HSP 72 synthesis, mRNA levels, transcription and HSF1 activation than hepatocytes from aged rats fed ad libitum [59]. In addition, the level of HSP 72 induction in heat-stressed hepatocytes from aged rats fed a calorie-restricted diet was similar to that of young rats fed ad libitum. Interestingly, caloric restriction is also the only experimental manipulation shown to consistently prolong the longevity of mammals [105]. Whether exercise can also retard the age-related decline in the HSP response remains unknown.

CONCLUSIONS AND FUTURE DIRECTIONS

The induction of SPs by exercise has provided a new and exciting area of research for exercise science and has only recently been addressed. It is clear that in animals, exercise is a stimulus capable of inducing the stress response and increasing expression of certain SPs in certain cells and tissues. Preliminary evidence suggests that although the exercise-induced SP induction may occur by the same mechanism as heat shock, it may not be simply the consequence of heat liberated during muscular contraction. More importantly, the exercise induction of SPs has been associated with providing protection to tissues during episodes of stress. Although one can only speculate regarding transfer of these studies to humans, it remains conceivable that exercise induction of certain SPs may also provide a similar protection to humans. That exercise is capable of increasing cellular SP content provides a mechanism for explaining how it may protect vital organs and tissues from stress and disease.

By linking environmental stress(es) and gene expression, SPs may allow exercise scientists studying exercise in environmentally stressful conditions to define limiting or critical factors more precisely. Also, with the advancement of molecular biological techniques, such as polymerase chain reaction, coupled with an increasing ability to analyze smaller tissue samples, questions regarding SPs and exercise may link previously separated areas. These mergers will hopefully allow investigators to address important exercise-related questions. Is the exercise induction of SPs in the heart a mechanism by which exercise may directly protect the heart? Can exercise induce a stress/heat shock response in humans? Do elevated levels of SPs provide an advantage to an exercising organism? If so, how? How does exercise training influence SP expression? What protective benefits can be derived from exercise induction of SPs? Can HSPs be used as markers of cellular damage? What role(s) do SPs play in skeletal muscle adaptation? Undoubtedly, these and many other exciting questions will be addressed in the near future.

REFERENCES

1. Abravaya, K., M. P. Myers, S. P. Murphy, and R. I. Morimoto. The human heat shock protein hsp70 interacts with hsf, the transcription factor that regulates heat shock gene expression. *Genes. Dev.* 6:1153–1164, 1992.
2. Amin, J., J. Ananthan, and R. Voellmy. Key features of heat shock regulatory elements. *Mol. Cell. Biol.* 8:3761–3769, 1988.
3. Ananthan, J., A. L. Goldberg, and R. Voellmy. Abnormal proteins serve as eukaryotic stress signals and trigger the activation of the heat shock genes. *Science* 232:522–524, 1986.
4. Angelidis, C. E., I. Lazaridis and G. N. Pagoulatos. Constitutive expression of heat-shock protein-70 in mammalian cells confers thermoresistance. *Eur. J. Biochem.* 199:35–39, 1991.
5. Arrigo, A.-P., and W. J. Welch. Characterization and purification of the small 28,000-dalton mammalian heat shock protein. *J. Biol. Chem.* 262:15359–15369, 1987.
6. Arrigo, A.-P., and J. Landry. Expression and function of the low-molecular-weight heat shock proteins. R. I. Morimoto, A. Tissières, and C. Georgopoulos (eds.). *The Biology of Heat Shock Proteins and Molecular Chaperones.* Cold Spring Harbor, NY: Cold Spring Harbor Laboratory Press, 1994, pp. 335–373.
7. Baler, R., W. J. Welch, and R. Voellmy. Heat-shock gene regulation by nascent polypeptides and denatured proteins: hsp70 as a potential autoregulatory factor. *J. Cell. Biol.* 117:1151–1159, 1992.
8. Baler, R., G. Dahl, and R. Voellmy. Activation of heat shock genes is accompanied by oligomerization, modification, and rapid translocation of heat shock factor HSF1. *Mol. Cell. Biol.* 13:2486–2496, 1993.
9. Bansal, G. S., P. M. Norton, and D. S. Latchman. The 90-kDa heat shock protein protects mammalian cells from thermal stress but not from viral infection. *Exp. Cell Res.* 195:303–306, 1991.
10. Beckmann, R. P., L. A. Mizzen, and W. J. Welch. Interaction of hsp 70 with newly synthesized proteins: implications for protein folding and assembly. *Science* 248:850–854, 1990.
11. Benjamin, I. J., B. Kroger, and R. S. Williams. Activation of the heat shock transcription factor by hypoxia in mammalian cells. *Proc. Natl. Acad. Sci. U. S. A.* 87:6263–6267, 1990.
12. Benjamin, I. J., S. Horie, M. L. Greenberg, R. J. Alpern, and R. S. Williams. Induction of stress proteins in cultured myogenic cells. *J. Clin. Invest.* 89:1685–1689, 1992.
13. Bienz, M., and H. R. B. Pelham. Heat shock regulatory elements function as an inducible enhancer in the Xenopus hsp70 gene when linked to a heterologous promoter. *Cell* 45:753–760, 1986.

14. Blake, M. J., D. Gershon, J. Fargnoli, and N. J. Holbrook. Discordant expression of heat shock protein mRNAs in tissues of heat-stressed rats. *J. Biol. Chem.* 265:15275–15279, 1990.

15. Blake, M. J., J. Fargnoli, D. Gershon, and N. J. Holbrook. Concomitant decline in heat-induced hyperthermia and HSP70 messenger RNA expression in aged rats. *Am. J. Physiol.* 260:R663-R667, 1991.

16. Bond, U., and M. J. Schlesinger. The chicken ubiquitin gene contains a heat shock promotor and expresses an unstable mRNA in heat-shocked cells. *Mol. Cell Biol.* 6:4602–4610, 1986.

17. Born, R., and H. Eichholtz-Wirth. Effects of different physiological conditions on the action of adriamycin on Chinese hamster cells in vitro. *Br. J. Cancer* 44:1981.

18. Bradford, N. B., M. Fina, I. J. Benjamin, R. W. Moreadith, K. H. Graves, P. Zhao, S. Gavva, A. Wiethoff, A. D. Sherry, C. R. Malloy, and R. S. Williams. Cardioprotective effects of 70-kDa heat shock protein in transgenic mice. *Proc. Natl. Acad. Sci. U. S. A.* 93:2339–2342, 1996.

19. Brickman, T. M., M. G. Flynn, E. Sanchez, W. A. Braun, C. P. Lambert, F. F. Andres, and J. Hu. Stress protein synthesis and content following acute and chronic exercise. *Med. Sci. Sports Exerc.* 28:S100, 1996.

20. Brown, C. R., R. L. Martin, W. J. Hansen, R. P. Beckmann, and W. J. Welch. The constitutive and stress inducible form of hsp 70 exhibit functional similarities and interact with one another in an ATP dependent fashion. *J. Cell. Biol.* 120:1101–1112, 1993.

21. Catelli, M. G., N. Binart, I. Jung-Testas, J. M. Renoir, E. E. Baulieu, J. R. Feramisco, and W. J. Welch. The common 90-kd protein component of non-transformed '8S' steroid receptors is a heat-shock protein. *E M B O J.* 4:3131–3135., 1985.

22. Chao, C. C.-K., W.-C. Yam, and S. Lin-Chao. Coordinated induction of two unrelated glucose-regulated protein genes by a calcium ionophore: human Bip/GRP78 and GAPDH. *Biochem. Biophys. Res. Commun.* 171:431–438, 1990.

23. Chappell, T., W. J. Welch, D. M. Schlossman, K. B. Palter, M. J. Schlesinger, and J. E. Rothman. Uncoating ATPase is a member of the 70 kilodalton family of stress proteins. *Cell* 45: 3–13, 1986.

24. Cheng, M. Y., F. U. Hartl, J. Martin, R. A. Pollock, F. Kalousek, W. Neupert, E. M. Hallberg, R. L. Hallberg, and A. L. Horwich. Mitochondrial heat-shock protein hsp60 is essential for assembly of proteins imported into yeast. *Science* 337:620–625, 1989.

25. Chiang, H.-L., S. R. Terlecky, C. P. Plant, and J. F. Dice. A role for a 70-kilodalton heat shock protein in lysosomal degradation of intracellular proteins. *Science* 246:382–385, 1989.

26. Chirico, W. J., M. G. Waters, and G. Blobel. 70K heat shock related proteins stimulate protein translocation into microsomes. *Nature* 332:805–810, 1988.

27. Choi, H.-S., Z. Lin, B. Li, and A. Y.-C. Liu. Age-dependent decrease in the heat-inducible DNA sequence-specific binding activity in human diploid fibroblasts. *J. Biol. Chem.* 265: 18005–18011, 1990.

28. Colofiore, J. R., G. Ara, D. Berry, and J. A. Belli. Enhanced survival of adriamycin-treated Chinese hamster cells by 2-deoxy-D-glucose and 2, 4-dinitrophenol. *Cancer Res.* 42: 3934–3940, 1982.

29. Cunniff, N. F. A., J. Wagner, and W. D. Morgan. Modular recognition of 5-base-pair DNA sequence motifs by human heat shock transcription factor. *Mol. Cell Biol.* 11:3504–3514, 1991.

30. Currie, R. W., M. Karmazyn, M. Kloc, and M. K. Heat-shock response is associated with enhanced postischemic ventricular recovery. *Circ. Res.* 63:543–549, 1988.

31. Currie, R. W., and M. Karmazyn. Improved post-ischemic ventricular recovery in the absence of changes in energy metabolism in working rat hearts following heat shock. *J. Mol. Cell. Cardiol.* 22:631–636, 1990.

32. Currie, R. W., and R. M. Tanguay. Analysis of rat heart RNA for transcripts for catalase and SP 71 after in vivo hyperthermia. *Biochem. Cell. Biol.* 67:375–382, 1991.

33. Currie, R. W., R. M. Tanguay, and J. G. Kingma, Jr. Heat-shock response and limitation of tissue necrosis during occlusion/reperfusion in rabbit hearts. *Circulation* 87:963–971, 1993.

34. Dalman, F. C., L. C. Scherrer, L. P. Taylor, H. Akil, and W. B. Pratt. Localization of the 90-kDa heat shock protein-binding site within the hormone-binding domain of the glucocorticoid receptor by peptide competition. *J. Biol. Chem.* 266:3482–3490, 1991.

35. Delcayre, C., J. L. Samuel, F. Marotte, M. Best-Belpomme, J. J. Mercadier, and L. Rappaport. Synthesis of stress proteins in rat cardiac myocytes 2–4 days after imposition of hemodynamic overload. *J. Clin. Invest.* 82:460–468, 1988.

36. Deshaies, R. J., B. D. Koch, M. Werner-Washburne, E. A. Craig, and R. Schekman. A subfamily of stress proteins facilitates translocation of secretory and mitochondrial precursor polypeptides. *Nature* 332:800–805, 1988.

37. Domanico, S. Z., D. C. DeNagel, J. N. Dahlseid, J. M. Green, and S. K. Pierce. Cloning of the gene encoding peptide-binding protein 74 shows that it is a new member of the heat shock protein 70 family. *Mol. Cell. Biol.* 13:3598–3610, 1993.

38. Donati, Y. R. A., D. O. Slosman, and B. S. Polla. Oxidative injury and the heat shock response. *Biochem. Pharmacol.* 40:2571–2577, 1990.

39. Donnelly, T. J., R. E. Sievers, F. L. J. Vissern, W. J. Welch, and C. L. Wolfe. Heat shock protein induction in rat hearts. A role for improved myocardial salvage after ischemia and reperfusion? *Circulation* 85:769–778, 1992.

40. Ellis, J. Proteins as molecular chaperones. *Nature* 328:378–379, 1987.

41. Ellis, R. J., and S. M. van der Vies. Molecular chaperones. *Annu. Rev. Biochem.* 60:321–347, 1991.

42. Fargnoli, J., T. Kunisada, A. J. Fornace, Jr., E. L. Schneider, and N. J. Holbrook. Decreased expression of heat shock protein 70 mRNA and protein after heat treatment in cells of aged rats. *Proc. Natl. Acad. Sci. U. S. A.* 87:846–850, 1990.

43. Feige, U., and B. S. Polla. Heat shock proteins; the hsp70 family. *Experientia* 50:979–986, 1994.

44. Flanagan, S. W., A. J. Ryan, C. V. Gisolfi, and P. L. Moseley. Tissue-specific HSP70 response in animals undergoing heat stress. *Am. J. Physiol.* 268:R28–R32, 1995.

45. Fuqua, S. A., M. Blum-Salingaros, and W. L. McGuire. Induction of the estrogen-regulated "24K" protein by heat shock. *Cancer Res.* 49:4126–4129, 1989.

46. Gaestel, M., R. Gotthardt, and T. Muller. Structure and organization of a murine gene encoding small heat-shock protein Hsp25. *Gene* 128:279–283, 1993.

47. Garramone, R. R., R. M. Winters, D. Das, and P. J. Deckers. Reduction of skeletal muscle injury through stress conditioning using the heat shock response. *Plast. Reconstr. Surg.* 93: 1242–1247, 1994.

48. Gernold, M., U. Knauf, M. Gaestel, J. Stahl and P.-M. Kloetzel. Development and tissue-specific distribution of mouse small heat shock protein hsp25. *Dev. Genet.* 14:103–111, 1993.

49. Giaccia, A. J., F. A. Auger, A. Koong, D. J. Terris, A. I. Minchinton, G. H. Hahn, and J. M. Brown. Activation of the heat shock transcription factor by hypoxia in normal and tumer cell lines in vivo and in vitro. *Int. J. Radiat. Oncol. Biol. Phys.* 23:891–897, 1992.

50. Goodson, M. L., O.-K. Park-Sarge, and K. D. Sarge. Tissue-dependent expression of heat shock factor 2 isoforms with distinct transcriptional activities. *Mol. Cell Biol.* 15:5288–5293, 1995.

51. Goodson, M. L., and K. D. Sarge. Regulated expression of heat shock factor 1 isoforms with distinct leucine zipper arrays via tissue-dependent alternative splicing. *Biochem. Biophys. Res. Commun.* 211:943–949, 1995.

52. Guerriero, V., Jr., D. A. Raynes, and J. A. Gutierrez. Hsp70-related proteins in bovine skeletal muscle. *J. Cell Physiol.* 140:471–477, 1989.

53. Gunther, E., and L. Walter. Genetic aspects of the hsp70 multigene family in vertebrates. *Experientia* 50:987–1000, 1994.

54. Gutierrez, J. A., and V. Guerriero. Quantitation of hsp70 in tissues using a competitive enzyme-linked immunosorbent assay. *J. Immunol. Methods* 143:81–88, 1991.
55. Haas, I. G. Bip (GRP78), and essential hsp70 resident protein in the endoplasmic reticulum. *Experientia* 50:1012–1020, 1994.
56. Hamilton, N., and C. D. Ianuzzo. Contractile and calcium regulating capacities of myocardia of different sized mammals scale with resting heart rate. *Mol. Cell. Biochem.* 106: 133–141, 1991.
57. Hammond, G. L., Y.-K. Lai, and C. L. Markert. Diverse forms of stress lead to new patterns of gene expression through a common and essential pathway. *Proc. Natl. Acad. Sci. U. S. A.* 79:3485–3488, 1982.
58. Heads, R. J., D. S. Latchman, and D. M. Yellon. Stable high level expression of a transfected human hsp70 gene protects a heart-derived muscle cell line against thermal stress. *J. Mol. Cell. Biol.* 26:1994.
59. Heydari, A. R., B. Wu, R. Takahashi, R. Strong, and A. Richardson. Expression of heat shock protein 70 is altered by age and diet at the level of transcription. *Mol. Cell. Biol.* 13: 2909–2918, 1993.
60. Hickey, E., S. E. Brandon, R. Potter, G. Stein, J. Stein, and L. A. Weber. Sequence and organization of genes encoding the human 27 kDa heat shock protein. *Nucleic Acids Res.* 14: 4127–4145, 1986.
61. Hightower, L. E., and F. P. White. Cellular response to stress: comparison of a family of 71–73 kilodalton proteins rapidly synthesized in rat tissue slices and canavanine-treated cells in culture. *J. Cell. Physiol.* 108:261–275, 1981.
62. Hightower, L. E., S. E. Sadis, and I. M. Takenaka. Interaction of vertebrate hsc70 and hsp70 with unfolded proteins and peptides. R. I. Morimoto, A. Tissières, and C. Georgopoulos (eds.). *The Biology of Heat Shock Proteins and Molecular Chaperones.* Cold Spring Harbor, NY: Cold Spring Harbor Laboratory Press, 1994, pp 179–207.
63. Hunt, C., and R. I. Morimoto. Conserved features of eukaryotic HSP70 genes revealed by comparison with the nucleotide sequence of human HSP70. *Proc. Natl. Acad. Sci. U. S. A.* 82:6455–6459, 1985.
64. Hutter, M. M., R. E. Sievers, V. Barbosa, and C. L. Wolfe. Heat-shock protein induction in rat hearts. A direct correlation between the amount of heat-shock protein and the degree of myocardial protection. *Circulation* 89:355–360, 1994.
65. Ingolia, T. D., and E. A. Craig. Four small *Drosophila* heat shock proteins are related to each other and to mammalian alpha-crystallin. *Proc. Natl. Acad. Sci. U. S. A.* 79:2360–2364, 1982.
66. Itoh, H., Kobayashi, R., and Y. Tashima. Isolation and some properties of bovine brain 100 kDa heat shock protein. *Int. J. Biochem.* 22:1445–1452, 1990
67. Iwaki, K., S.-H. Chi, W. H. Dillmann, and R. Mestril. Induction of HSP 70 in cultured neonatal cardiomyocytes by hypoxia and metabolic stress. *Circulation* 87:2023–2032, 1993.
68. Izumo, S., B. Nadal-Ginard, and V. Mahdavi. Protooncogene induction and reprogramming of cardiac gene expression produced by pressure overload. *Proc. Natl. Acad. Sci. U. S. A.* 85:339–343, 1988.
69. Johnston, R. N., and B. L. Kucey. Competitive inhibition of *hsp70* gene expression causes thermosensitivity. *Science* 242:1551–1554, 1988.
70. Kang, H. S., and W. J. Welch. Characterization and purification of the 94-kDa glucose-regulated protein. *J. Biol. Chem.* 266:5643–5649, 1991.
71. Kang, P.-J., J. Ostermann, J. Shilling, W. Neupert, E. Craig, and N. Pfanner. Requirement for hsp70 in the mitochondrial matrix for translocation and folding of precursor proteins. *Nature* 348:137–142, 1990.
72. Karmazyn, M., K. Mailer, and W. R. Currie. Acquisition and decay of heat-shock-enhanced postischemic ventricular recovery. *Am. J. Physiol.* 259:H424–H431, 1990.
73. Katayose, D., S. Isoyama, H. Fujita, and S. Shibahara. Separate regulation of heme oxygenase and heat shock protein 70 mRNA expression in the rat heart by hemodynamic stress. *Biochem. Biophys. Res. Commun.* 191:587–594, 1993.

74. Kelley, P. M., and M. J. Schlesinger. The effect of amino acid analogues and heat-shock on gene expression in chicken embryo fibroblasts. *Cell* 15:1277–1286, 1978.

75. Kim, D., H. Ouyang, and G. C. Li. Heat shock protein hsp70 accelerates the recovery of heat-shocked mammalian cells through its modulation of heat shock transcription factor HSF1. *Proc. Natl. Acad. Sci. U. S. A.* 92:2126–2130, 1995.

76. Klemenz, R., E. Froehli, R. H. Steiger, R. Schasfer, and A. Aoyama. Alpha-crystallin is a small heat shock protein. *Proc. Natl. Acad. Sci. U. S. A.* 88:3652–3656, 1991.

77. Koyasu, S., E. Nishida, T. Kadowaki, F. Matsuzaki, K. Iida, F. Harada, M. Kasuga, H. Sakai, and I. Yahara. Two mammalian heat shock proteins, HSP90 and HSP100 are actin-binding proteins. *Proc. Natl. Acad. Sci. U. S. A.* 83:8054–8058, 1986.

78. Koyasu, S., E. Nishida, Y. Miyata, H. Sakai, and I. Yahara. HSP100, a 100-kDa heat shock protein, is a Ca^{2+}-calmodulin-regulated actin-binding protein. *J. Biol. Chem.* 264:15083–15087, 1989

79. Kregal, K. C., P. L. Moseley, R. Skidmore, J. A. Gutierrez, and J. Guerriero V. HSP70 accumulation in tissues of heat-stressed rats is blunted with advancing age. *J. Appl. Physiol.* 97:1673–1678, 1995.

80. Ku, Z., J. Yang, V. Menon, and D. B. Thomason. Decreased polysomal HSP-70 may slow polypeptide elongation during skeletal muscle atrophy. *Am. J. Physiol.* 268:C1369-C1374, 1995.

81. Landry, J., P. Chretien, H. Lambert, E. Hickey, and L. Weber. Heat shock resistance conferred by expression of the human HSP 27 gene in rodent cells. *J. Cell Biol.* 109:7–15, 1989.

82. Landry, J., P. Chretien, A. Laszlo, and H. Lambert. Phosphorylation of HSP27 during development and decay of thermotolerance in Chinese hamster cells. *J. Cell. Phsyiol.* 147:93–101, 1991.

83. Landry, J., H. Lambert, M. Zhou, J. N. Lavoie, E. Hickey, L. A. Weber, and C. W. Anderson. Human hsp27 is phosphorylated at serines-78 and serines-82 by heat shock and mitogen-activated kinases that recognize the same amino acid motif as S6 kinase-II. *J. Biol. Chem.* 267:794–803, 1992.

84. Lee, A.S. The accumulation of three specific proteins related to glucose-regulated protein in a temperature-sensitive hamster mutant cell line K12. *J. Cell. Physiol.* 106:119–125, 1981.

85. Lee-Yoon, D., D. Easton, M. Murawski, R. Burd, and J. R. Subjeck. Identification of a major subfamily of large hsp70-like proteins through cloning of the mammalian 110-kDa heat shock protein. *J. Biol. Chem.* 270:15725–15733, 1995.

86. Li, G. C. Induction of thermotolerance and enhanced heat shock protein synthesis in Chinese hamster fibroblasts by sodium arsenite and by ethanol. *J. Cell. Physiol.* 115:116–122, 1983.

87. Li, G. C. Elevated levels of 70,000 dalton heat shock protein in transiently thermotolerant Chinese hamster fibroblasts and in their heat resistant variants. *Int. J. Radiat. Oncol. Biol. Phys.* 11:165–177, 1985.

88. Li, G. C., L. G. Li, Y. K. Liu, J. Y. Mak, L. L. Chen, and W. M. F. Lee. Thermal response of rat fibroblasts stably transfected with the human 70-kDa heat shock protein-encoding gene. *Proc. Natl. Acad. Sci. U. S. A.* 88:1681–1685, 1991.

89. Li, G. C., L. Li, R. Y. Liu, M. Rehman, and W. M. Lee. Heat shock protein hsp70 protects cells from thermal stress even after deletion of its ATP-binding domain. *Proc. Natl. Acad. Sci. U. S. A.* 89:2036–2040, 1992.

90. Li, L., G. Shen, and G. C. Li. Effects of expression human Hsp70 and its deletion derivatives on heat killing and RNA and protein synthesis. *Exp. Cell. Res.* 217:460–468, 1995.

91. Lieber, R. L., and J. Friden. Selective damage of fast glycolytic muscle fibre with eccentric contraction of the rabbit tibialis anterior. *Acta Physiol. Scand.* 133:587–588, 1988.

92. Liu, A. Y.-C., Z. Lin, H.-S. Choi, F. Sorhage, and B. Li. Attenuated induction of heat shock gene expression in aging diploid fibroblasts. *J. Biol. Chem.* 264:12037–12045, 1989.

93. Locke, M., E. G. Noble, and B. G. Atkinson. Exercising mammals synthesize stress proteins. *Am. J. Physiol.* 258:C723-C729, 1990.

94. Locke, M., E. G. Noble, and B. G. Atkinson. Inducible isoform of HSP70 is constitutively expressed in a muscle fiber type specific pattern. *Am. J. Physiol.* 261:C774-C779, 1991.

95. Locke, M., B. G. Atkinson, R. M. Tanguay, and E. G. Noble. Shifts in type I fiber proportion in rat hindlimb muscle are accompanied by changes in HSP 72 content. *Am. J. Physiol.* 266:C1240–1246, 1994.

96. Locke, M., and E. G. Noble. Review. Stress proteins: the exercise response. *Can. J. Physiol.* 20:p156–168, 1995.

97. Locke, M., E. G. Noble, R. M. Tanguay, M. R. Feild, S. E. Ianuzzo, and C. D. Ianuzzo. Activation of heat-shock transcription factor in rat heart after heat shock and exercise. *Am. J. Physiol.* 268:C1387- C1394, 1995.

98. Locke, M., R. M. Tanguay, K. R. E., and C. D. Ianuzzo. Enhanced post-ischemic myocardial recovery following exercise induction of HSP 72. *Am. J. Physiol.* H320-H325, 1995.

99. Locke, M., R. M. Tanguay, and C. D. Ianuzzo. Constitutive expression of HSP 72 in swine heart. *J. Mol. Cell. Cardiol.* 28:467–474, 1996.

100. Locke, M., and R. M. Tanguay. Increased HSF activation in muscles with a high constitutive HSP 70 expression. *Cell Stress Chaperones* 1:189–196, 1996.

101. Locke, M., and R. M. Tanguay. Diminished heat shock response of the aged myocardium. *Cell Stress Chaperones,* in press, 1996.

102. Lowe, D. G., and L. A. Moran. Molecular cloning and analysis of DNA complementary to three mouse M_r=68,000 heat shock protein mRNAs. *J. Biol. Chem.* 261:2102–2112, 1986.

103. Marber, M. S., R. Mestril, S.-H. Chi, M. R. Sayen, D. M. Yellon, and W. H. Dillmann. Overexpression of the rat inducible 70-kD heat stress protein in a transgenic mouse increases the resistance of the heart to ischemic injury. *J. Clin. Invest.* 95:1446–1456, 1995.

104. Martin, J., A. L. Horwich, and F. U. Hartl. Prevention of protein denaturation under heat stress by the chaperonin Hsp60. *Science* 258:995–998, 1992.

105. Masoro, E. J. Nutrition and aging: a current assessment. *J. Nutr.* 115:842–848, 1985.

106. Matz, J. M., M. J. Blake, H. M. Tatelman, K. P. Lavoi, and N. J. Holbrook. Characterization and regulation of cold-induced heat shock expression in mouse adipose tissue. *Am. J. Physiol.* 269:R38-R47, 1995.

107. Mayrand, S., and T. Pederson. Heat shock alters ribonucleoprotein assembly in Drosophila cells. *Mol. Cell. Biol.* 3:161–171, 1983.

108. Mazzarella, R. A., and M. Green. ERp99, an abundant conserved glycoprotein of the endoplasmic reticulum, is homologous to the 90kDa heat shock protein (hsp90) and the 94kDa glucose regulated protein (grp94). *J. Biol. Chem.* 262:8875–8883, 1987.

109. McGrath, L. B., and M. Locke. Myocardial self preservation: absence of heat shock factor activation and HSP 70 mRNA accumulation in the human heart during cardiac surgery. *J. Card. Surg.* 10:400–405, 1995.

110. McGrath, L. B., M. Locke, M. Cane, C. Chen, and C. D. Ianuzzo. Heat shock protein (HSP 72) expression in patients undergoing cardiac surgery. *J. Thorac. Cardiovasc. Surg.* 109: 370–376, 1995.

111. Mestril, R., S.-H. Chi, M. R. Sayen, and W. H. Dillmann. Isolation of a novel inducible rat heat shock protein (HSP70) gene and its expression during ischemia/hypoxia and heat shock. *Biochem. J.* 298:561–569, 1994.

112. Mestril, R., S.-H. Chi, M. R. Sayen, K. O'Reilly, and W. H. Dillman. Expression of inducible stress protein 70 in rat heart myogenic cells confers protection against simulated ischemia-induced injury. *J. Clin. Invest.* 93:759–767, 1994.

113. Milarski, K. L., and R. I. Morimoto. Mutational analysis of the human HSP70 protein: distinct domains for nucleolar localization and adenosine triphosphate binding. *J. Cell Biol.* 109:1947–1962,1989.

114. Miyaishi, O., K. Kozaki, S. Saga, T. Sato, and Y. Hashizume. Age-related alteration of proline hydroxlyase and collagen-binding heat shock protein (HSP47) expression in human fibroblasts. *Mech. Ageing Dev.* 85:25–36, 1995.

115. Mizzen, L. A., and W. J. Welch. Characterization of the thermotolerant cell. I. Effects on

protein synthesis activity and the regulation of heat-shock protein 70 expression. *J. Cell Biol.* 106:1105–1116, 1988.

116. Mizzen, L. A., C. Chang, J. I. Garrels, and W. J. Welch. Identification, characterization, and purification of two mammalian stress proteins present in mitochondria, grp 75, a member of the hsp 70 family and hsp 58, a homolog of the bacterial groEL protein. *J. Biol. Chem.* 264:20664–20675, 1989.

117. Mizzen, L. A., A. N. Kabiling, and W. J. Welch. The 2 mammalian mitochondrial stress proteins, grp-75 and hsp-58, transiently interact with newly synthesized mitochondrial proteins. *Cell Regul.* 2:165–179, 1991.

118. Moore, S. K., C. Kozak, E. A. Robinson, S. J. Ullrich, and E. Appella. Murine 86- and 84-kDa heat shock proteins, cDNA sequences, chromosome assignments, and evolutionary origins. *J. Biol. Chem.* 264:5343–5351, 1987.

119. Morimoto, R. I., A. Tissières, and C. Georgopoulos (eds.). *Stress Proteins in Biology and Medicine.* Cold Spring Harbor, NY: Cold Spring Harbor Laboratory Press, 1990.

120. Morimoto, R. I., K. D. Sarge, and K. Abravaya. Transcriptional regulation of heat shock genes. *J. Biol. Chem.* 267:21987–21990, 1992.

121. Morimoto, R. I. Cells in stress: transcriptional activation of heat shock genes. *Science* 259: 1409–1410, 1993.

122. Morimoto, R. I., A. Tissières, and C. Georgopoulos (eds.). *The Biology of Heat Shock Proteins and Molecular Chaperones.* Cold Spring Harbor, NY: Cold Spring Harbor Laboratory Press, 1994.

123. Moseley, P. L., E. S. Wallen, J. D. MaCafferty, S. Flanagan, and J. A. Kern. Heat stress regulates the human 70-kDa heat shock gene through the 3′-untranslated region. *Am. J. Physiol.* 264:L533-L537, 1993.

124. Mosser, D. D., G. Theodorakis, and R. I. Morimoto. Coordinate changes in heat shock element-binding activity and HSP70 transcription rates in human cells. *Mol. Cell. Biol.* 8: 4736–4744, 1988.

125. Mosser, D. D., P. T. Kotzbauer, K. D. Sarge, and R. I. Morimoto. *In vitro* activation of heat shock transcription factor DNA-binding by calcium and biochemical conditions that affect protein conformation. *Proc. Natl. Acad. Sci. U. S. A.* 87, 3748–3752, 1990.

126. Mosser D.D., J. Duchaine and B. Massie. The DNA-binding activity of the human heat shock transcription factor is regulated *in vivo* by Hsp70. *Mol. Cell. Biol.* 13, 5427–5438, 1993.

127. Munro, S., and H. R. B. Pelham. An HSP70-like protein in the ER: identity with the 78 kd glucose-regulated protein and immunoglobulin heavy chain binding protein. *Cell* 46: 291–300, 1986.

128. Nadal-Ginard, B., and V. Mahdavi. Basic mechanisms of cardiac gene expression. *Eur. Heart J.* 14:2–11, 1993.

129. Nagata, K., S. Saga, and K. M. Yamada. A major collagen-binding protein of chick embryo fibroblasts is a novel heat shock protein. *J. Cell Biol.* 103:223–229, 1986.

130. Newton, E. M., U. Knauf, M. Green, and R. E. Kingston. The regulatory domain of the human heat shock factor 1 is sufficient to sense heat stress. *Mol. Cell Biol.* 16:839–846, 1996.

131. Nishio, M. L., O. I. Ornatsky, and D. A. Hood. Effects of hypothyroidism and aortic constriction on mitochondria during cardiac hypertrophy. *Med. Sci. Sports Exerc.* 27:1500–1508, 1995.

132. Nitta, Y., K. Abe, M. Aoki, I. Ohno, and S. Isoyama. Diminished heat shock protein 70 mRNA induction in aged rat hearts after ischemia. *Am. J. Physiol.* 267:H1795-H1803, 1994.

133. Oppermann, H., W. Levinson, and J. M. Bishop. A cellular protein that associates with the transforming protein of Rous sarcoma virus is also a heat-shock protein. *Proc. Natl. Acad. Sci. U. S. A.* 78:1067–1071, 1981.

134. Ornatsky, O. L., M. K. Connor, and D. A. Hood. Expression of stress proteins and mito-

chondrial chaperonins in chronically stimulated skeletal muscle. *Biochem. J.* 311:119–123, 1995.

135. Pelham, H. R. B. A regulatory upstream promotor element in *Drosophila* hsp 70 heat shock gene. *Cell* 30:517–528, 1982.

136. Pelham, H. R. B. Speculations of the functions of the major heat shock and glucose regulated proteins. *Cell* 46:959–961, 1986.

137. Petersen, R. B., and S. Lindquist. Regulation of HSP70 synthesis by messenger RNA degradation. *Cell Regul.* 1:135–149, 1989.

138. Petronini, P. G., R. Alfieri, C. Campanini, and A. F. Borghetti. Effect of an alkaline shift on induction of the heat shock response in human fibroblasts. *J. Cell. Physiol.* 162:322–329, 1995.

139. Plumier, J.-C. L., B. M. Ross, R. W. Currie, C. E. Angelidis, H. Kazlaris, G. Kollias, and G. N. Pagoulatos. Transgenic mice expressing the human heat shock protein 70 have improved post-ischemic myocardial recovery. *J. Clin. Invest.* 95:1854–1860, 1995.

140. Pouyssegur, J., R. P. C. Shiu, and I. Pastan. Induction of two transformation-sensitive membrane polypeptides in normal fibroblasts by a block in glycoprotein synthesis or glucose deprivation. *Cell* 11:941–947, 1977.

141. Pratt, W. B. Transformation of glucocorticoid and progesterone receptors to the DNA-binding state. *J. Cell. Biochem.* 35:51–68, 1987.

142. Riabowol, K. T., L. A. Mizzen, and W. J. Welch. Heat shock is lethal to fibroblasts microinjected with antibodies against hsp70. *Science* 242:433–436, 1988.

143. Ritossa, F. A new puffing pattern induced by temperature shock and DNP in Drosophila. *Experientia* 15:571–573, 1962.

144. Rodenhiser, D. I., J. H. Jung, and B. G. Atkinson. The synergistic effect of hyperthermia and ethanol of changing gene expression of mouse lymphocytes. *Can. J. Cytol.* 28:1986.

145. Rose, D. W., R. E. H. Wettenhall, W. Kudlicki, G. Kramer, and B. Hardesty. The 90-kilodalton peptide of the heme-regulated eIF-2a kinase has sequence similarity with the 90-kilodalton heat shock protein. *Biochemistry* 26:6583–6587, 1987.

146. Ryan, A. J., C. V. Gisolfi, and P. L. Moseley. Synthesis of 70K stress protein by human leukocytes—effect of exercise in the heat. *J. Appl. Physiol.* 70:466–471, 1991.

147. Salo, D. C., C. M. Donovan, and K. J. A. Davies. HSP70 and other possible heat shock or oxidative stress proteins are induced in skeletal muscle, heart, and liver during exercise. *Free Radic. Biol. Med.* 11:239–246, 1991.

148. Samelman, T. R., and S. E. Alway. Heat shock protein expression after training in the plantaris muscle of Fischer 344 rats. *Med. Sci. Sports. Exerc.* 28:S115, 1996.

149. Sanchez, E. R., T. Redmond, L. C. Scherrer, E. H. Bresnick, M. J. Welsh, and W. B. Pratt. Evidence that the 90-kilodalton heat shock protein is associated with tubulin-containing complexes in L cell cytosol and intact PtK cells. *Mol. Endocrinol.* 2:756–760, 1988.

150. Sanchez, E. R., L. E. Faber, W. J. Henzel, and W. B. Pratt. The 56–59-kilodalton protein identified in untransformed steroid receptor complexes is a unique protein that exists in cytosol in a complex with both the 70- and 90-kilodalton heat shock proteins. *Biochemistry* 29:5145–5152, 1990.

151. Sarge, K. D., V. Zimarino, K. Holm, C. Wu, and R. I. Morimoto. Cloning and characterization of two mouse heat shock factors with distinct inducible and constitutive DNA-binding ability. *Genes Dev.* 5:1902–1911, 1991.

152. Sarge, K. D., S. P. Murphy, and R. I. Morimoto. Activation of heat shock gene transcription by heat shock factor 1 involves oligomerization, acquisition of DNA-binding activity, and nuclear localization and can occur in the absence of stress. *Mol. Cell Biol.* 13:1392–1407, 1993.

153. Sarge, K. D., O.-K. Park-Sarge, J. D. Kirby, K. E. Mayo, and R. I. Morimoto. Expression of heat shock factor 2 in mouse testis: potential role as a regulator of heat-shock gene expression during spermatogenesis. *Biol. Reprod.* 50:1334–1343, 1994.

154. Sauk, J. J., C. L. Van Kampen, K. Norris, R. Foster, and M. J. Somerman. Expression of

constitutive and inducible hsp70 and hsp47 is enhanced in cells persistently spread on OPN1 or collagen. *Biochem. Biophys. Res. Commun.* 172:135–142, 1990.

155. Schlesinger, M. J. Heat shock proteins. *J. Biol. Chem.* 265:12111–12114, 1990.

156. Schmid, D., A. Baici, H. Gehring, and P. Christen. Kinetics of molecular chaperone action. *Science* 263:971–973, 1994.

157. Schwane, J. A., and R. B. Armstrong. Effect of training on skeletal muscle injury from downhill running in rats. *J. Appl. Physiol.* 55:969–975, 1983.

158. Sciandra, J. J., and J. R. Subjeck. The effects of glucose on protein synthesis and thermosensitivity in Chinese hamster ovary cells. *J. Biol. Chem.* 258:12091–12093, 1983.

159. Shaw, G., and R. A. Karmen. Conserved AU sequence from the 3′ untranslated region of GM-CSF mRNA mediates selective mRNA degradation. *Cell* 46:659–667, 1986.

160. Shi, Y., and J. O. Thomas. The transport of proteins into the nucleus requires the 70-kilodalton heat shock protein or its cytosolic cognate. *J. Mol. Cell. Biol.* 12:2186–2192, 1992.

161. Shibahara, S. Muller, R. M., and H. Taguchi. Transcriptional control of rat heme oxygenase by heat shock. *J. Biol. Chem.* 262:12889–12892, 1987.

162. Sim, J. D., M. Locke, and E.G. Noble. Increased heat shock protein 72 content in rat skeletal muscle after short term exercise training. *Med. Sci. Sports Exerc.* 23:S3, 1991.

163. Skidmore, R., J. A. Gutierrez, V. Guerriero, and K. Kregel. HSP70 induction during exercise and heat stress in rats: role of internal temperature. *Am. J. Physiol.* 268:R92-R97, 1995.

164. Skowyra, D., C. Georgopoulos, and M. Zylicz. The E.coli dnaK gene product, the hsp 70 homologue, can reactivate heat inactivated RNA polymerase in an ATP hydrolysis dependent manner. *Cell* 62:939–944, 1990.

165. Snoeckx, L. H. E. H., F. Contard, J. L. Samuel, F. Marotte, and L. Rappaport. Expression and cellular distribution of heat-shock and nuclear oncogene proteins in rat hearts. *Am. J. Physiol.* 261:H1443-H1451, 1991.

166. Sorger, P. K. and H. R. B. Pelham. Cloning and expression of a gene encoding hsc 73, the major hsp70-like protein in unstressed rat cells. *EMBO J.* 6:993–998, 1987.

167. Stevenson, M. A., S. K. Calderwood, and G. M. Hahn. Effect of hyperthermia (45°C) on calcium flux in Chinese hamster ovary HS-1 fibroblasts and its potential role in cytotoxicity and heat resistance. *Cancer Res.* 47:3712–3717, 1987.

168. Subjeck, J., Shyy, T., Shen, J., and R. J. Johnson. Association between the mammalian 110,000-dalton heat-shock protein and nucleoli. *J. Cell. Biol.* 97:1389–1395, 1983.

169. Subject, J. R., and T.-T. Shyy. Stress protein systems of mammalian cells. *Am J. Physiol.* 250:C1-C17, 1986.

170. Tanguay, R. M., Y. Wu, and E. W. Khandjian. Tissue-specific expression of heat shock proteins of the mouse in the absence of stress. *Dev. Genet.* 14:112–188, 1993.

171. Terlecky, S. R. Hsp70s and lysosomal proteolysis. *Experientia* 50:1021–1025, 1994.

172. Thompson, H. S., and S. P. Scordilis. Ubiquitin changes in human biceps muscle following exercise-induced damage. *Biochem. Biophys. Res. Commun.* 204:1193–1198, 1994.

173. Tissières, A., H. K. Mitchell, and U. M. Tracy. Protein synthesis in salivary glands of *Drosophila melanogaster*: relation to chromosome puffs. *J. Mol. Biol.* 84:389–398, 1974.

174. Ungermann, C., W. Neupert, and D. M. Cry. The role of Hsp70 in conferring unidirectionality on protein translocation into mitochondria. *Science* 266:1250–1253, 1994.

175. Ungewickell, E. The 70-kd mammalian heat shock proteins are structurally and functionally related to the uncoating protein that releases clathrin triskelia from coated vesicles. *EMBO J.* 4:3385–3391, 1985.

176. Vincent, M., and R. M. Tanguay. Heat shock induced proteins present in the cell nucleus of Chironomus tentans salivary gland. *Nature* 281:501 503, 1979.

177. Volpe, P., A. Villa, P. Podini, A. Martini, A. Nori, M. C. Panzeri, and J. Meldolesi. The endoplasmic reticulum-sarcoplasmic reticulum connection: distribution of endoplasmic reticulum markers in the sarcoplasmic reticulum of skeletal muscle fibres. *Proc. Natl. Acad. Sci. U. S. A.* 89:6142–6146, 1992.

178. Walton, P. A., J. P. Morello, and W. J. Welch. Inhibition of the peroxisomal import of a microinjected protein by coinjection of antibodies to members of the 70 kD heat shock protein family. *J. Cell Biochem.* 17C suppl. 22, 1993.

179. Warren, G. L., D. A. Hayes, D. A. Lowe, J. H. Williams, and R. B. Armstrong. Eccentric contraction-induced injury in normal and hindlimb-suspended mouse soleus and EDL muscles. *J. Appl. Physiol.* 77:1421–1430, 1994.

180. Welch, W. J., J. I. Garrels, G. P. Thomas, J. J. Lin, and J. R. Feramisco. Biochemical characterization of the mammalian stress proteins and identification of two stress proteins as glucose and Ca^{2+}-ionophore-regulated proteins. *J. Biol. Chem.* 258:7102–7111, 1983.

181. Welch, W. J., and J. R. Feramisco. Nuclear and nucleolar localization of the 72,000-dalton heat shock protein in heat-shocked mammalian cells. *J. Biol. Chem.* 259: 4501–4513, 1984.

182. Welch, W. J., and J. R. Feramisco. Rapid purification of mammalian 70,000-dalton stress proteins: affinity of the proteins for nucleotides. *Mol. Cell Biol.* 5:1229–1237, 1985.

183. Welch, W. J., and J. P. Suhan. Cellular and biochemical events in mammalian cells during and after recovery from physiological stress. *J. Cell Biol.* 103:2035–2053, 1986.

184. Welch, W. J., and L. A. Mizzen. Characterization of the thermotolerant cell. II. Effects on the intracellular distribution of heat-shock protein 70, intermediate filaments, and small nuclear ribonucloprotein complexes. *J. Cell Biol.* 106:1117–1130, 1988.

185. Welch, W. J., L. A. Mizzen, and A.-P. Arrigo. Structure and function of mammalian stress proteins. *Stress-Induced Proteins.* New York: Alan R. Liss, 1989, pp 187–202.

186. Whelan, S. A., and L. E. Hightower. Differential induction of glucose-regulated and heat shock proteins: effects of pH and sulfhydryl-reducing agents on chicken embryo cells. *J. Cell. Physiol.* 125:251–258, 1985.

187. Wienhues, U., and W. Neupert. Protein translocation across mitochondrial membranes. *Bioessays* 14:17–23, 1992.

188. Wisniewski, J., T. Kordula, and Z. Krawczyk. Isolation and nucleotide sequence analysis of the rat testis-specific major heat-shock protein (HSP70)-related gene. *Biochim. Biophys. Acta* 1048:93–99, 1990.

189. Xu, Y., and S. Lindquist. Heat-shock protein hsp 90 governs the activity of pp60v-src kinase. *Proc. Natl. Acad. Sci. U. S. A.* 90:7074–7078, 1993.

190. Yost, H. J., and S. Lindquist. Heat shock proteins affect RNA processing during the heat shock response of *Saccharomyces-Cerevisiae. Mol. Cell. Biol.* 11:1062–1068, 1991.

191. Zakeri, Z. F., D. J. Wolgemuth, and C. R. Hunt. Identification and sequence analysis of a new member of the mouse HSP70 gene family and characterization of its unique cellular and developmental pattern of expression in the male germ line. *Mol. Cell Biol.* 8: 2925–2932, 1988.

192. Zietara, M. S., and E. F. Skorkowski. Thermostability of lactate dehydrogenase LDH-A4 isoenzyme: effect of heat shock protein DnaK on the enzyme activity. *Int. J. Biochem. Cell Biol.* 27:1169–1174, 1995.

6

High-Protein Diets, "Damaged Hearts," and Rowing Men: Antecedents of Modern Sports Medicine and Exercise Science, 1867–1928

ROBERTA J. PARK, Ph.D.

Arriving at agreement about *beginnings* is always problematic. Does "democracy" begin with the 5th century B.C. Athenian Assembly, John Locke's *Two Treatises on Civil Government* (1688), or the Declaration of Independence in 1776? The same is true for "sports medicine" and "exercise science." Should the establishment of the Association Internationale Médico-Sportive (renamed Fédération Internationale de Médicine Sportive in 1934) at the time of the 1928 St. Moritz Winter Olympics be the acknowledged origin of *modern* sports medicine? The formation in 1912 of the Deutsche Reichskomitee für die Wissenschaftliche Erforschung des Sportes und der Leibesübungen? Or some other event? Did "exercise science" begin in the 1960s when that term was increasingly applied to a range of research specialties? In the 1920s, with the rapid growth of monographs and books such as F. A. Bainbridge's *The Physiology of Muscular Exercise* (1919) and the establishment of the Deutsche Hochschule für Leibesübungen (1920), the Harvard Fatigue Laboratory (1927), and other venues in which the scientific study of the exercising body as an important focus? Or did it begin at some earlier date?

In this chapter, I argue that the *antecedents* of modern "sports medicine" and "exercise science" are to be found in the mid-1800s. The major—but by no means exclusive—catalyst was new concepts of "sport" that emerged at schools such as Eton, Harrow, and Rugby and the two great English universities, Oxford and Cambridge [63, 106]. This was wholly distinct (in both form and *ethos*) from the exercises provided for working class children in government schools after the passage of the Education Act of 1876 [31, 100, 148]. By 1914, this new games-playing had spread to other countries where it was shaped by national traditions. Yet, ideologies encapsulated in the Victorian notion of "the gentleman-amateur" [94, 107, 108] remained remarkably consistent throughout the first 5 decades of the present century.

Important, too, was the proliferation of the biomedical sciences. By 1850, experimental physiology was rapidly replacing comparative anatomy as the preferred mode of "investigative enterprise"—a term that is especially appropriate for this chapter. The eight chapters that comprise *The Investigative Enterprise: Experimental Physiology in 19th Century Medicine* (1988) illustrate the complexities of the "thoughts, actions, and conditions" that affect the questions scientists ask, how they carry out their investigations, etc. These chapters also draw attention to the need for diverse studies, ranging from "the single scientist engaged in . . . day-by-day thoughts and operations" [33] to large intellectual, institutional, and cultural networks within which events take place.

Equally broad perspectives will be needed to arrive at a full appreciation of the history of "sports medicine" and "exercise science." *Sportsmedizin: Gestern-Heute-Morgen* (1993), which emanated from a symposium celebrating 80 years of sports medicine in Germany, in one example of recent studies that may help extend our understanding [75, 157]. Jack Berryman's *Out of Many, One* (1995) provides a detailed analysis of the evolution of a major organization—the American College of Sports Medicine [17]. The December 1995 edition of *The Sport Psychologist* is devoted to an as yet underresearched subject—the historical development of sports psychology. The insightful "Exercise Physiology: Roots and Historical Perspectives," which introduces the 4th edition of McArdle, Katch and Katch's *Exercise Physiology: Energy, Nutrition, and Human Performance,* is a much-needed innovation [97]. Written by specialists in biomechanics, sports and exercise psychology, exercise physiology, and related disciplines, the chapters that comprise *The History of Exercise and Sport Science* also should be a useful addition [111].

The contributions of professional groups—e.g., the British Medical Society; the American Physical Education Association (APEA)[1]; Deutscher Ärztebund zur Förderung der Leibesübungen (Association of German Physicians for the Promotion of Physical Exercises); and Ligue Girondine d'Éducation Physique—need to be examined, as must the role of specialist colleges and universities. In English-speaking countries, educational institutions have played a particularly powerful role in shaping athletic sports. The rise of the German research institute in the mid-1800s fostered the growth of biomedical research and, in so doing, laid the foundations for various "sciences" of exercise. International congresses—and certainly the modern Olympics movement—also have had a significant role in promoting "sports medicine" and "exercise science" during the 20th century.

SETTING THE CONTEXT

Athletes from 197 countries participated at the 1996 Atlanta Olympics. When the first modern Olympic Games were held at Athens a century ago,

---

[1]There have been several names for the professional organization that is now known as the American Alliance for Health, Physical Education, Recreation, and Dance: Association for the Advancement of Physical Education (1885), American Association for the Advancement of Physical Education (1886–1902), American Physical Education Association (1903–1937), etc.

few clubs devoted to sports existed outside of English-speaking countries. Fussball-Club Hannover was founded in 1878—shortly thereafter clubs in tennis, cycling, and other sports developed [159]. *Sport im Bild (Sport in Pictures)* and other early German sporting journals owe their origins to Anglo-Saxons living in Berlin. Englishmen also were instrumental in fostering various early sports clubs in Germany [50, 59]. In the early 1900s, sports began to attract important allies like physician and athlete Arthur Mallwitz (an early contributor to the emerging field of sports medicine) and Carl Diem (the leading figure in German sports during the first several decades of the 20th century). However, before World War I, gymnastics remained the preferred form of organized exercise for German-speaking peoples. By 1914, the Deutsche Turnerschaft (German Turner Federation), with 1.4 million members, was the largest such organization in the world [48, 83]. Turnen was both an exercise form and a political movement. The English word "gymnastics" cannot adequately convey its complex meanings.

Spanish expatriate Francisco Amaros had opened a Paris gymnasium in 1817; however, few gymnastic societies existed in France before 1870. By the 1890s, an array of competing groups (some established by physicians) had been organized around domestic and imported systems of exercise. Athletics were not widely embraced. Historian Eugene Weber has observed that in 19th century France, the term "sportsman" usually referred to "a man who owned, or betted on horses" [162, 163]. Early groups such as the Havre Athletic Club (which dominated French football until 1914) owe their origins largely to English businessmen and students. Historian Hippolyte Taine's *Notes sur l'Angleterre* (1871) had brought English public school virtues to a French readership—including the young Pierre de Coubertin, who would become an ardent and unswerving supporter of the "character-building" ethos of Victorian sports [95]. Although some important personages (e.g., former minister of education and premier Jules Simon) endorsed their educational value [145], most of Coubertin's countrymen were highly skeptical of any attempt to introduce English games into the lycées [87, 153, 165].

Nineteenth century medical practice also differed from country to country, as did the status of physicians and their active association with physical education societies. In 1870, it was generally acknowledged that German-speaking universities offered the most advanced medical education available [21, 29, 55]. After the Franco-Prussian War (1870–71) and the consolidation of power in a unified German Reich, the length of medical education increased, and the field became more crowded. In France, the clinic, rather than the laboratory, remained "the core and purpose of . . . medical teaching" (22). In 1871, efforts were begun in the United States to reorganize the medical curriculum along modern lines. However, most American physicians continued to be educated in 2- or 3-year programs until the reforms called for in the Flexner Report (1910) were enacted [22, 52].

In Britain, some 20 licensing boards had existed before the Medical Act of 1858. Of the three traditional groups (physicians, surgeons, and apothecaries), physicians enjoyed the greatest prestige. The Royal College of Physicians was dominated by graduates of Oxford and Cambridge—institutions in which a humanistic and classical emphasis took precedence [130]. A strong national resistance to vivisection impeded biomedical experimentation. David Ferrier, a leading contributor to research on localization of motor and sensory functions, was prosecuted under the 1876 Anti-Vivisection Act. The famous biologist, Thomas Huxley, an outspoken proponent of the new physiology, could not bear to watch animal experiments, much less perform them [56, 58].

Nonetheless, physiological science in Britain advanced along several fronts. From 1870 to 1903, Michael Foster and his students at Cambridge University made important contributions to the problem of heartbeat. At preparatory school, Foster had pursued classical studies and captained his cricket team; at University College Medical School, he excelled in science. Gerald Geison has observed that Foster's student career: "evokes the image of a well-rounded young man of impressive attainments in a variety of pursuits" [58]. This was the vaunted Victorian ideal that found expression in the public school "muscular Christian" ethos and the Ox-Bridge conception of "the gentleman-amateur" [63, 106]. *Ideal*, in fact, was often reality. Several of Foster's students who went on to outstanding research careers had been athletes. Charles Sherrington, a specialist in nerve physiology, was a rugby player; Walter Morely Fletcher's participation in track may have contributed to his interest in studying the chemistry of muscle. Similarly, A. V. Hill, 1922 Nobel award-winning physiologist, was an accomplished track athlete. Roger Bannister, an outstanding Oxford trackman, was a student at St. Mary's Hospital when he became the first man to break the 4-min mile [8, 58].

Physicians closely allied to amateur sports were instrumental in launching the British Association for Sports Medicine in 1952. Adolphe Abrahams (brother of Olympian Harold Abrahams, author of books on training and physician to the British Olympic team) and Arthur Porritt (New Zealand Olympian and Rhodes Scholar) announced the establishment of an association "open to medical representatives nominated by all national sporting bodies and to any interested medical men and women with a qualification registerable in the United Kingdom" [2]. Yet, in 1995, the editor of the *British Journal of Sports Medicine* lamented the failure of sports medicine to attain "academic, institutional and government recognition," citing, as one reason, reluctance on the part of the Royal Colleges to lay down "stringent criteria" (as they did for other medical specialties) for those who worked with athletes [149]. Control of prestige and authority within medicine were surely one reason; but the persistence of views reflected in Sir Stanley Rous's Foreword to *Fitness and Injury in Sport* (1950), a work intended to bring together "in simple language" relevant information for the use of trainers, cannot be discounted:

> For a people to whom sport is a serious matter, the British, com-
> pared with many other nations, usually go about their games in
> a surprisingly un-serious way. . . . Who cares about what effect
> [sport] has on the chemical structure of a certain muscle, or
> what it does to the parasympathetic nervous system? [137]

(This attitude, it should be noted, was quite different from those that in-fused Eastern European sports in the 1950s.) Perhaps it was time, Rous contended, for the British to pay a little more attention to "the scientific approach."

Thomas N. Bonner's *Becoming a Physician: Medical Education in Great Britain, France, Germany, and the United States, 1750–1945* (1995) and W. F. Bynum's *Science and the Practice of Medicine in the 19th Century* (1994) demonstrate the merits of examining developments from more than one national perspective [22, 29]. A comparative approach also may be useful for tracing the antecedents of modern "sports medicine" and "exercise science." Although several countries made significant contributions, the emphasis in this chapter is directed to Britain and the United States—with some attention paid to the contributions of France and Germany.

There were numerous contacts between North America and Europe during the late 19th and early 20th centuries. The bicycle ergometer that Wilbur Atwater and Francis Gano Benedict used in their metabolic studies—as well as apparatus from various American gymnasia—were displayed at the 1911 Dresdan International Hygiene Exhibition [133]. A contingent headed by Carl Diem visited the United States in 1913 to gather information regarding American successes at the 1908 London and 1912 Stockholm Olympic Games. Both Austria and Germany engaged American coaches (Alexander Copland and Alvin Kraeanzlein) to help prepare their country's athletes for the Berlin games in 1916. The "Olympic Lectures" that Carl Diem organized as part of German preparations for the forthcoming Games served as the bases for the diploma course that was initiated at the Deutsch Hochschule für Leibesübungen (German College of Physical Education) after World War I [84].

Many Americans (women as well as men) had gone abroad for training in medicine and the physiological sciences—first, to France (where Claude Bernard was a powerful magnate), and after 1870, to German-speaking universities and research institutes. Henry Pickering Bowditch, author of several late 19th century growth studies [23] and an Honorary member of the A.P.E.A., studied at Carl Ludwig's laboratory in Leipzig. After his 1871 appointment as Dean of the Harvard Medical School, Bowditch initiated America's first successful efforts to make experimental science a part of the medical curriculum [21, 57, 127]. Edward M. Hartwell (Ph.D. in biology, Johns Hopkins University; M.D., Miami Medical School; twice President of the APEA) spent most of 1889 in Germany, Austria, and Sweden, investigating medicine and physical training [124].

Wilbur Atwater, considered by many "the founder of the science of nutrition in the United States," spent 2 years in Leipzig and Berlin. America's first professor of physiological chemistry, Yale's Russell Chittenden, also studied in Germany. As Atwater had done for his dietary studies, Chittenden engaged athletes as subjects for studies of nitrogen balance [30, 32]. R. Tait McKenzie, M.D. (Director of Physical Education at the University of Pennsylvania; President of the APEA; President of the American Academy of Physical Education, etc.) was a delegate to the 1907 International Congress of School Hygiene and other European meetings [92]. The multitalented McKenzie had a significant influence on cardiologist Joseph Wolffe and several of those physical educators who founded the American College of Sports Medicine in 1954 [17].

Three themes run through the following sections of this chapter. The first, and in some ways most important, is that of *organized exercise* (i.e., gymnastics and athletics). The second involves *physiological* and *biomedical* concerns, especially (a) those that coalesced in the phenomenon that came to be known as *athlete's heart* and (b) matters pertaining to *nutrition* and *metabolism*. The third theme involves a look at institutions, professional organizations, and international gatherings in which exercise and sport in relation to medicine and/or science were discussed.

HIGH-PROTEIN DIETS, "DAMAGED HEARTS," AND ROWING MEN: BRITAIN AT MIDCENTURY

When Georgian (1714–1830) writers referred to "sport," they meant something quite different from the athletic competitions that rose to prominence in Victorian England. Riding, hunting, or an occasional leisurely game of cricket were typical pastimes of the gentry. Pugilists, pedestrians, and rowers (who earned their livings as watermen) were drawn from the laboring classes. As one contemporary noted, gentlemen had not yet "attained a taste for [engaging in] vigorous exercise" [4]. Training methods drew from classical sources (especially the Roman physician Claudius Galen) and practices used in preparing racehorses and gamecocks. These were set down in the extensive section on "Athletic Training" that John Sinclair included in *Code of Health and Longevity; or Concise View of the Principles Calculated for the Preservation of Health and the Attainment of Long Life* in 1807 [146].

Before training began, a strong purgative—usually, Glauber's salt (sodium sulfate)—was administered. Classical beliefs regarding alimentation prevailed; reasoning by analogy suggested that underdone beef and mutton (which resembled muscle) were the best food for a man "in training." The athlete might have a little dry bread; vegetables—including potatoes— were eschewed. Water (thought to swell the belly and affect "the wind") was withheld: but several pints of beer a day might be consumed. Flannel clothing and concoctions made of such things as caraway seed, coriander, root liquorice, and sugar candy, boiled together with two bottles of cider, were used to induce "sweating" [125, 146].

Around midcentury, new attitudes began to emerge. The catalyst was the Oxford-Cambridge Boat Race, which became an *annual* affair in 1856. By the 1860s, it attracted more than 100,000 spectators [5]. As more young gentlemen took up rowing they turned to the only source available for information about training—the professionals, whose regimens reflected practices set down in Sinclair's 1807 treatise. In 1846, T. S. Egan had objected to the "extravagance . . . enveloped in a proportionate degree of mystery" that was so often imparted to amateur crews by professional watermen [49]. However, it would be several decades before new ideas slowly began to gain acceptance.

It is tempting—but not accurate—to conclude that discoveries in the physiological sciences initiated the debates over athletic training that began in England during the 1860s. These, at least initially, were prompted by the growth of "amateur" athletics, and the manly games-playing sentiments reflected in Thomas Hughes's immensely popular 1857 fictionalized account of life at Rugby School (*Tom Brown's Schooldays*), as well as *Tom Brown at Oxford* (1861) [63, 106]. The "training systems" then in vogue at the two universities called for little more than an hour's exertion each day. In an effort to prepare for rowing, some men took up running. Oxford and Cambridge held their first "inter-varsity" *athletics* (i.e., track and field) meeting on former's Christ Church Cricket Ground in 1864. The Amateur Athletic Club (AAC) was founded in 1866. The following year the AAC added the *mechanics* clause to its definition of an amateur, effectively excluding those who were by "trade or employment a mechanic, artisan, or laborer" [125]. Although competitions for professionals in rowing and running did continue, it was "amateur" sports (and the "gentleman-amateur" ethos) that predominated.

Baily's Magazine of Sports and Pastimes for 1870 reflects the new developments. Still heavily devoted to the horse and the turf, it now included accounts of the annual boat race and *athletics* meeting. Whereas formerly training for track competitions had been "irrational," one writer noted, athletes now had begun to use methods based upon "knowledge of the human frame and hygienic laws" [6]. It is not quite clear to what the author was referring, but in 1865 Adolf Fick and Johannes Wislicenus had undertaken a practical test of the question: "Does the amount of body substance broken down, and converted in part to urea, always provide enough energy to account for the energy expended in muscular exertion"? Taking along tea laced with sugar and cakes made from starch paste fried in fat, they climbed the 1956-m Faulhorn, collected and analyzed their urine, calculated the energy expended, and concluded that they had disproved the famous chemist Justis von Liebig's assertion that "muscle substance" provided the needed energy [30]. However, the debate over the exact source of energy for muscular contraction would remain unresolved for several decades.

A more likely influence on the training habits of young English gentlemen was Archibald Maclaren's *Training in Theory and Practice* (1866). In the 1850s, the respected Director of the Oxford Gymnasium had spent time in Paris studying fencing, gymnastics, and medicine where, perhaps, he became acquainted with Claude Bernard's work on digestion. Maclaren found fault with every training "system" currently in vogue. Athletes should *not* be dosed with tartar emetic, subjected to forced sweating, and stuffed with underdone beefsteaks. Rather, their diets should include vegetables and water sufficient to replace fluids lost in perspiration and exhalation. He also stipulated that crews in training needed 3 hours of exercise a day—more than twice as much as the Oxford and Cambridge "systems" recommended [101].

An even more intense debate arose over the phenomenon that came to be known as "athlete's heart." This would be waged with particular vigor in English-speaking countries. After the 1867 Oxford-Cambridge Boat Race, London surgeon F. C. Skey submitted a long article to the *Times* criticizing such events and warning that overexertion could lead to permanent injury [147]. The *British Medical Journal* reported that Dr. Thomas Allbutt's clinical report on "Over Strain of the Heart and Aorta" had been a major topic at the Clinical Society's 1873 meetings [3]. Finding the medical literature to be "barren" of scientific works dealing with "training for the guidance of athletes," Dr. Robert J. Lee assembled what he could locate of "scattered physiological and pathological truths" and published these as *Exercise and Training: Their Effects upon Health* 1873. Studies of the effects of training on the musculocardiac and pneumocardiac functions—and the whole "vexed question of diet"—Lee concluded, were virtually nonexistent [91].

Reacting to Skey's assertions, John Morgan (physician to the Manchester Royal Infirmary and former captain of crew at Oxford University) initiated what would become a long series of similar investigations. Publishing his results in 1873 as *University Oars, Being a Critical Enquiry into the After Health of Men Who Rowed in the Oxford and Cambridge Boat-Race from the Year 1829 to 1869*, Morgan concluded from the responses of 251 former oarsmen that they had lived approximately 2 years longer than other men of their cohort [113, 114]. The extensive review of *University Oars* that Maclaren prepared for the prestigious journal *Nature* ended on a precautionary note. Although rowing could be a healthful activity, no man should take up racing "until his chest ha[d] the girth of 30 in" [102].

Given the limited understanding of the heart that was possible before the invention of instruments such as the x-ray in 1895 and the electrocardiograph in 1893, Maclaren's admonition may not seem surprising. Judgments were inferred from percussion, auscultation, and pulse rate, and when such instruments did become available, many clinicians continued to prefer "the trained finger" [89]. Heart size was a matter of much concern and debate. Enlargement might be explained by hypertrophy (increase in thickness of the walls) or dilatation (enlargement of the cavities and thinning of the walls). Some athletes did have undiagnosed heart disease. Should an individual die while engaged in strenuous feats, and the autopsy reveal an enlarged heart, it was all too easy to conclude that activity had *caused* the pathological condition.

As James Whorton [168] observed in his study of the debate over "athlete's heart" between 1870 and 1920, much of the discussion was conditioned by whether the commentator was a proponent or a critic of athletics. Benjamin Ward Richardson, a physician especially concerned with public health issues, maintained that in England there was not an "athlete of the age of thirty-five, who has been ten years at his calling, who is not disabled" [136]. By contrast, Walter Bradford Woodgate, a recognized rowing authority and author of training manuals addressed to "gentlemen," insisted that more men had been injured by overindulgence after competition "than by all the severities [sic] of training" [171].

Drawing upon a wide range of contemporary and classical sources, Philadelphia physician J. William White concluded that competitive athletics were "far less dangerous and much more beneficial than is usually supposed" [167].

The debate was taken up in other countries. In the early 1880s, the German physician George Kolb, conducted various studies on members of the Berlin Ruder-Club. His *Beiträge zur Physiologie Maximaler Muskelarbeit Besonders des Modernen Sports* (1888), almost certainly the first truly *modern* exercise physiology text, reflects a dedication to careful collection and recording of data. The English edition, which appeared in 1893 as *Physiology of Sport,* contains extensive sphygmographic tracings of pulse rates and measures of fatigue, respiration, energy consumption, weight loss in training, etc. In a short chapter entitled "Alkaloids," Kolb stated that he had found that camphor, digitalis, morphine, and cocaine all decreased maximum efficiency. His observation that athletes were not interested in discoveries of physiologists (who, they believed, approached men in training as they would laboratory specimens) probably accurately reflects attitudes then current [81, 88]. How different things would be a century later!

Across the Atlantic, Dr. Edward H. Bradford inquired into the health of men who had rowed in the Harvard-Yale races between 1852 and 1870. As had Morgan, Bradford relied upon information supplied by respondents [25]. A more comprehensive study of Harvard oarsmen between 1852 and 1892 was made by George Meylan, M.D. (Director of the Gymnasium at Columbia University and APEA President), who included pulse rates, urine analysis, and other data. The average athlete, he concluded, lived considerably longer than "the normal expectation." Reflecting a concern that appeared repeatedly in several countries as part of turn-of-the-century anxieties about a decline in the "general vitality" of the educated classes, Meylan reported that oarsmen had "a higher percentage of marriage and of size of family than all other graduates together" [112, 113].

Pedestrianism (professional long-distance walking) enjoyed a brief resurgence during the 1870s. This enabled Dr. Austin Flint, Jr. (Professor of Physiology at New York's Bellevue Hospital Medical College) to make detailed analyses of the food and liquid consumed by Edward Payson Weston during a 400-mile walk, as well as other long distance walks. Flint had studied with Claude Bernard and was well acquainted with current work on metabolism (e.g., Fick and Wislicenus, Liebig, Carl Voit). Flint reported his initial findings in 1871, and he extended these in *On the Source of Muscular Power* (1878) [53, 54]. Dr. F. W. Pavy, a Fellow of the Royal College of Physicians, disputed Flint's hypothesis that food contained force in a "latent state" that was "liberated" in muscular (or nervous) action, and Pavy made his own investigations when Weston competed in Britain [129]. Rejecting Pavy's conclusions, Flint pointed out that the question of whether food is used for repairing muscular tissue consumed in work "or in the direct production of work itself" remained unresolved [54].

By the beginning of the 20th century, a growing number of scientists and physicians had turned to athletes in an effort to gain a better understanding of bodily functions. French physiologist Etienne-Jules Marey conducted a range of locomotor and physiological investigations [109, 172]. German physiologist Nathan Zuntz was interested in the energy efficiency of "the marching soldier, the alpinist, the high-altitude balloonist, and the (sportive) cyclist" [73]. Leo Zuntz used the cyclist to study oxygen consumption; Philippe Tissié did likewise to study fatigue [155]. Wilbur Atwater carried out detailed analyses of the Harvard and Yale crews in 1898 as part of nutrition investigations for the United States Department of Agriculture. Among those who assisted him were Dr. William Anderson (Director of the Gymnasium at Yale and a founding member of the APEA) and Dr. George Wells Fitz, editor of the *American Physical Education Review* and former head of Harvard's short-lived B.S. degree program (1892–1896) in Anatomy, Physiology, and Physical Training [10, 127].

Among his many contributions, Fitz conducted experiments on the effects of exercise on lung ventilation, muscular fatigue, and reaction time—all before 1900 [51, 82]. He also expressed interest in emerging theories of the educational value of "play" [127]. Developments in neurophysiology, as well as the formulation of an experimental approach to psychology (Wilhelm Wundt established the first laboratory in 1878 at the University of Leipzig), suggested that long-standing beliefs about intimate relationships between mind and body might be amenable to scientific verification. Having reviewed contemporary research relating to "the motor ability of children" for G. Stanley Hall's new *Pedagogical Seminary* (today's *Journal of Genetic Education*), John Hancock pointed out that the close relation between muscle, nerve, and mind made "it impossible for exercise to affect one alone." Psychologist Edward Scripture's studies at the Elmira, New York Reformatory found "improvements in self-control and general behavior in those individuals who had participated in a program of athletics, calisthenics, and manual training" [39]—a conclusion similar to that which Dr. Hamilton Wey came to among Elmira inmates in the 1880s [166]. According to Davis et al., it was Norman Triplett's 1898 paper (pacemakers and competition improved bicycle racing performance) that "cut to the heart of the [early American] interface between sport and psychology" [39].

Formulating paradigms to investigate psychological phenomena has been a difficult task, and the science of neurophysiology is still in its infancy. Early forays into "sports medicine" and "exercise science" were directed largely to cardiovascular (subsequently respiratory) and metabolic issues. Atwater's decision to set "the protein standard for physically active men at 125g/day," Kenneth Carpenter has suggested, may have been influenced by both Nathan Zuntz's contention that intense work over a short period "resulted in increased metabolism of protein" and his own personal observations that athletes consumed large quantities of beef [30]. (Indeed, the persistence of practices that had been in vogue with early 19th century pugilists continued to enjoy popularity among coaches and athletes long after science had confirmed the merits of other regimens.) Yale's Russell Chittenden doubted that the body needed such high levels of protein and conducted studies on soldiers and student-athletes during the early 1900s. He found that those individuals who consumed only one-half of Atwater's and Voit's recommended standard remained healthy and vigorous [32]. At the invitation of the Harvard Athletic Committee Dr. Eugene Darling took metabolic and cardiac measures of the crew and football team in an effort to shed light on the much-debated question of "overtraining" [38]. *The Boston Medical and Surgical Journal* spoke approvingly of these efforts to establish "a science instead of a theory of physical training" [7]; yet, in their 1913 monograph on "the efficiency of the human body as a machine," Benedict and Cathcart would state: "Our knowledge of training . . . is woefully deficient" [14].

Ancient legend was turned into concrete reality when the Baron de Coubertin and Michel Bréal created a race from the city of Marathon to the Athens stadium as part of the first modern Olympic program. That same year, the Boston Athletic Association (which had sent competitors to the 1896 Games) organized an annual race [94]. Harold Williams and Horace Arnold (Professors at Tufts College Medical School) and other physicians took blood count, urinary, and other measures of contestants at the 1899

Boston Marathon. Sphygmographic tracings, as well as percussion and auscultation, were used to judge the condition of the heart. "One of the most interesting conclusions," Williams observed, was "evidence of the preparatory enlargement that the heart undergoes." This, he suggested, confirmed the accuracy of noted physician William Osler's contention that "no man becomes a great runner or oarsman who has not naturally a capable if not a large heart" [169]. Drs. J. B. Blake and R. C. Larrabee studied participants in the 1900, 1901, and 1902 Boston Marathons, and found no evidence of "permanent injury" [20].

Although it is not recorded in official sources (probably a concession to Coubertin's aversion to a "scientific" approach to sports), physicians had made brief examinations of men who participated in the 1896 Olympic marathon. Thomas Hicks (winner of the 1904 Olympic marathon) was given sulphate of strychnine, white of egg, and brandy in an effort to allay exhaustion. After the race, pulse rate, heart size, and anthropometric measures were taken of Hicks and other competitors by Drs. R. Tait McKenzie, Joseph Raycroft, and other American physical educators [152].[2]

Upon entering the London stadium, Italy's Dorando Pietri (who was leading the 1908 Olympic marathon) fell repeatedly and was assisted by officials. The rules required his disqualification; and victory was awarded to Irish-American John Hayes. Interest in distance running promptly increased in the United States. The 1909 Pittsburgh Marathon was organized in a manner that would enable Dr. Watson Savage (APEA President) and other investigators to gather extensive data (e.g., pulse rate, temperature, and urine samples) from 55 competitors [140]. That same year, the noted British cardiologist Sir James Mackenzie published *Diseases of the Heart,* and the British Medical Association's annual meeting devoted considerable attention to "the athlete's heart" and the problem of crippling injuries sustained in rugby and soccer. Discussant James Barr observed: "The opinions of medical men var[ied] enormously as to the amount of strain required to damage the heart" [44, 144].

Four papers directed to exercise and physical training were read at Section K (Physiology and Experimental Medicine) during the 1908 meeting of the American Association for the Advancement of Science. Frederic S. Lee (Professor of Physiology at Columbia University) summarized Dr. James H. McCurdy's studies of increased blood flow during exercise, and the work of Chittenden, Zuntz, Tissié, and other contributors to "exercise physiology" [90]. Dr. Thomas A. Storey (soon to become Superintendent of Physical Education for the State of New York) discussed relationships between hygiene and physical training and declared that unless physical education became a

---

[2]Karl Lennartz: "Sportmedical Care of Marathon Runners in the Early Modern Olympic Games." Paper presented at the Olympic Scientific Congress, Dallas, July 10–14, 1996.

more "academic" field, it would not gain the respect that its potential warranted [151]. The other speakers were University of Virginia physiologist Theodore Hough and R. Tait McKenzie, whose *Exercise in Education and Medicine* (1909) [103] was arguably the most comprehensive pre-World War I American text devoted to medicine, physiology, and therapeutic exercise. At the Physiology of Exercise section of the 1912 International Congress of Hygiene and Demography, McKenzie reported the results of tests he had made on 266 University of Pennsylvania students and concluded that the presence of "murmur" was not necessarily an indication of heart lesion. The time had come, he stated, "for a complete reconsideration of the whole question of exercise in relation to the heart" [104].

The assassination of Francis Ferdinand, Archduke of Austria, and 4 years of devastating trench warfare, brought about a reconsideration of many medical problems. In 1915, the British War Office set up a special hospital to study and treat men suffering from "soldier's heart" and "effort syndrome" [77]. The foundations upon which the profession of physical therapy would be established were laid down when physicians, surgeons, and physical educators (especially those well-versed in exercise forms based on the Swedish "system") combined their efforts to care for incapacitated servicemen. As a major in the Royal Medical Corps, McKenzie organized a large recuperative facility and developed an extensive program of rehabilitative exercises, publishing *Reclaiming the Maimed* in 1918.

"FROM CHILDREN'S GAMES" TO VARSITY SPORT: AMERICAN PERSPECTIVES

Before the Civil War, Americans had exhibited little interest in the types of sports that were coming to prominence in England. In 1869, baseball would be called "the national game." However, a decade earlier most had considered it "a child's pastime that no dignified gentleman should pursue" [80]. When she visited the United States in 1867, the pioneering British physician, Sophia Jex-Blake, had expressed surprise at the absence of "athletic sports or exercise." Things would rapidly change! In 1869, Rutgers and Princeton played America's first "intercollegiate" football (soccer) game, and Harvard rowed against Oxford in the first *international* intercollegiate contest. When they first met in 1874, Harvard and Montreal's McGill University played rugby. By 1894, a unique form of American "football" was entrenched. That same year, a protracted debate erupted in the medical press over crippling injuries and deaths in football that foreshadowed the 1905 outcry that led to the formation of the National Collegiate Athletic Association in 1906.

During the 1870s, the *British Medical Journal* and the *Lancet* had begun to report deaths and injuries (e.g., fractured skulls, ruptured spleens) sustained by rugby and soccer players. As football in America became more popular, injury rates escalated.[3] With few antiseptics available, even small wounds might lead to death; internal injuries were frequently fatal. Dr. Edward Nichols, physician to the Harvard team, noted that the knee-joint was "extremely susceptible to bacterial infection." The detailed statistics of injuries sustained by Ivy League football players for the seasons 1905 through 1908, which Nichols published in the *Boston Medical and Surgical Journal* [119], bear striking resemblances to those that *The Physician and Sportsmedicine* would report in the 1970s.

Whereas intercollegiate athletics were the product of student initiative, physical education had its origins in antebellum "health reform" movements in which educators and physicians often shared a common cause. The first issue of the *American Journal of Education* (1826) had urged all educational institutions to "provide proper means of healthful exercise and innocent recreation." Before 1861, both established medical publications (e.g., *Boston Medical Intelligencer; Boston Medical and Surgical Journal*—today's *New England Journal of Medicine*) and short-lived publications directed to "health" (e.g., *Health Journal and Advocate of Physiological Reform*) frequently discussed exercise, hygiene, and physical education [16, 123]. During the 1880s and 1890s, improved health and proper neuromuscular development were the paramount reasons advanced for making physical education part of the curriculum. The goals of physical training, as set forth by Dr. W. M. Conant (Instructor in Anatomy at the Harvard Medical School) at the 1894 meeting of the Boston Society for Medical Improvement were: *hygienic* (health, as well as "fitness" of the muscular, circulatory, and digestive systems) and *educational* (neuromotor and psychosocial development) [126].

Histories of physical education tend to neglect the many and often cordial connections that existed between medicine and physical training before World War I. Of the 49 individuals present at the 1885 founding of the American Association for the Advancement of Physical Education (AAAPE), 11 were physicians. The only AAAPE/APEA President before 1920 who did not hold a medical degree was New York lawyer William Blaikie, a former Harvard athlete who had helped train his *alma mater* for the 1869 Boat Race with Oxford. From the outset, the APEA attracted a broad membership—one reflective of the American Physiological Society that William Andrus Alcott, M.D., and Sylvester Graham had established in 1837 [27]. In this earlier period, "physiology" frequently was used to connote "living according to the laws of life" (i.e., proper diet, rest, exercise)—goals that have their roots in classical conceptions of preventative medicine. By contrast, the American Physiological society that was founded in 1887, like most other turn-of-the-

---

[3]Roberta J. Park: "A Tolerance for Football Injuries in Britain and America, 1873–1914." Paper presented at the 24th Convention of the North American Society for Sport History, Auburn University, May 24–27, 1996.

century professional organizations, attracted a much more restricted membership [57].

The diversity of interests among the APEA's membership—initially a source of strength–became a liability during the last third of the 20th century, as divergent aspirations—indeed wholly different "world views"—increasingly divided the membership. (The American College of Sports Medicine (ACSM) recently expressed concerns about similar centrifugal tendencies.) In the 1970s and early 1980s, growing numbers of researchers—disenchanted that the American Alliance for Health, Physical Education, and Recreation was unwilling to make greater commitments to science and scholarship—transferred their allegiances to the ACSM and other specialized groups (e.g., North American Society for the Psychology of Sport and Physical Activity.)

A century earlier, however, supporters of the APEA had envisioned possibilities not unlike those that ACSM President Joseph Wolffe set forth when he addressed the College Physical Education Association in 1956. Teamwork among the psychologist, sociologist, nutritionist, physiologist, physical educator, and medical specialists, Wolffe declared, was "the aim of the American College of Sports Medicine" [170]. The Massachusetts Medical Society, especially active in seeking to advance the cause of physical education, created a Special Committee in 1887 to investigate Physical Culture in Schools. The *Boston Medical and Surgical Journal* then noted that physical training recently had been "organized into a profession of considerable importance, involving and implying study, training, thought and research." Addressing colleagues at the 1890 AAAPE meeting, Dr. Luther Halsey Gulick enumerated opportunities for scientific work (e.g., effects on the heart of short- and long-distance running; effects of complicated movements on the brain and nerve centers; relation of blood flow to psychical activities). The possibility exists, Gulick observed more than a century ago, to shape "the profession of physical education as it will never be possible again" [62].

The 1899 APEA annual meeting is illustrative of the breadth of turn-of-the-century interest in the new field. Among the speakers was William Townsend Porter, a graduate of St. Louis Medical College and founder of the *American Journal of Physiology* (which he financed from 1897 to 1914). Before joining the Harvard Medical School in 1893, Porter had completed comprehensive growth studies of 33,500 St. Louis children [132]. William James spoke of the importance of understanding the child from the social, psychological, *and* physical perspectives. Noting that the "effect of exercise on mood" was now generally recognized, he speculated that the causes of "mental disease" were chemical [135].

Dr. Jay W. Seaver (Medical Examiner, formerly Head of the Department of Physical Training, at Yale) discussed "The Athletic Trainer." Despite important discoveries, he noted, outmoded ideas "derived largely from English pugilistic practices" were still widespread. It was imperative, Seaver maintained, that trainers who gave digitalis to runners in the belief that increased heart beat would improve performance be replaced by those who had had "a course of study in a Medical School" combined with practical knowledge of exercise [135]. Harvard's President Charles William Eliot, an advocate of healthful exercise, albeit an implacable critic of highly organized college athletics, closed the meeting. He complemented the AAAPE on what it had achieved; but he cautioned that constant vigilance would be needed to shape a mature profession.

At the beginning of the 20th century, APEA membership exceeded 600 women and men, nearly 15% of whom were physicians. Anthropologist Franz Boas, surgeon Henry G. Beyer (a cofounder of the American Physiological Society), psychologist G. Stanley Hall (President of Clark University), and Boston neurologist D. F. Lincoln were among those who presented papers based on original work [18, 126]. The *American Physical Education Review,* founded in 1896, published research reports, professional articles, and reviews of foreign and domestic books dealing with medicine, pedagogy, and relevant sciences. In size, diversity of membership, possession of a comprehensive journal and ties to medical societies as well as universities, the APEA was unique among turn-of-the-century physical education organizations.

By contrast, in Britain there were several small groups. The National Society of Physical Education (1897) and the Gymnastic Teachers Institute (1897) drew their members largely from commercial establishments and teachers in government schools [31, 128]. The Earl of Heath was the nominal president of the National Union of Physical Training Teachers (1891). The Ling Association, founded in 1899, was open to women who had completed the two-year course at either Dartford Physical Education Training College or Stockholm's Royal Central Gymnastic Institute [116]. These organizations had virtually no connection with Oxbridge or "public" school sport. By 1954, there were seven specialist physical education colleges for women. With the exception of Scotland's Dunfermline College (which enrolled both women and men), it was 1930 (when Carnegie College began a 1-yr course) before a permanent program for men was established. The University of Birmingham first offered physical education as part of the Bachelor of Arts degree in 1946. British and Commonwealth students who desired higher degrees in physical education typically sought them in North America [131].

ACROSS "LA MANCHE"

How did things differ across the Channel? Jean Jacques Rousseau's *Emile, ou de l'Éducation* (1762) may be the best-known 18th commentary on the role of exercise and play in human development (of males); but French physicians were equally ardent supporters. Recommendations in Nicholas Andry's *L'Orthopédie ou l'Art de Prévenir et Corriger dans les Enfants les Déformités du Corps* (1741) anticipates ideas that would be advocated a century and a half later. Jean Charles Desessartz (Professor of Surgery and Pharmacy) was not alone in insisting that females—no less than males—require adequate exercise [121]. The concepts set down in army surgeon Clement-Joseph Tissot's comprehensive *Gymnastique Médicinale et Chirurgicale; ou Essai Sur L'Utilité du Mouvement, ou des Différens Exercises du Corps, et du Repos dans la Cure des Maladies* (1780) as palliative for rickets, digestive disorders, rheumatism, and other ailments [93] are remarkably similar to those that appear in early 20th century texts.

Political developments ignited an interest in exercise and physical education in late 19th century France. Humiliating defeats in the Franco-Prussion War prompted a search for "regeneration" that was frequently debated in terms of medical and hygienic problems [120]. Physical exercises of one form or another were seen as integral to France's quest for "national revival." Such sentiments were encapsulated in "Patrie—Courage—Moralité," the motto of the Union des Sociétés de Gymnastique de France, founded in 1873. Bataillons Scolaires (which emphasized military drilling) were established in 1882 but declined within the decade. The Republican-inspired Ligue d'Enseignement advocated gymnastics and games of French derivation. The Swedish, the German, and other systems of gymnastics all had adherents [9, 153, 172]. Both France and Belgium established separate societies for their large Catholic populations in the 1890s and, as was the case elsewhere on the Continent, workers' gymnastic and sports societies were organized [15, 48, 158].

Any possibility of a "French physical education movement," John MacAloon maintains, was rendered impossible as competing organizations proliferated. In June 1888, Coubertin founded le Comité pour la Propagation des Exercises Physiques dans l'Éducation. The Ligue Nationale de l'Éducation Physique, created 5 months later by Paschal Grousset, listed among its members microbiologist Louis Pasteur, physiologist Etienne-Jules Marey, and physician Fernand Lagrange. In December, physician Philippe Tissié founded la Ligue Girondine d'Éducation Physique. Shortly thereafter, Coubertin seized upon the occasion of the 1889 Paris Universal International Exposition to organize athletic competitions and cofound the Union des Sociétés Françaises de Sport Athlétique (USFSA) as part of his efforts to create the modern Olympic Games [9, 153, 160]. Over the next half century, various local and national groups continued to emerge [172].

Four contending schools of thought have been identified [95]. The "hygienists" were committed more to health than to some particular form of exercise. In addition to teachers, this group included physicians like Lagrange, whose *Physiologie des Exercises du Corps* (1889) was published in several English editions as part of the International Scientific Series [86], and Marey, whose interest in applying the laws of physics and chemistry to the body's functions [109] placed him squarely in the tradition of his celebrated countrymen Antoine Lavoisier and Claude Bernard. The second group (also committed to health) consisted of proponents of a particular form of gymnastics. Some, like Tissié, advocated the "rational movements" of the Swedish system [156] developed by Per Hendrick Ling and son Hjalmar Ling (who had attended Claude Bernard's lectures in 1854). Others favored exercises based on the more vigorous movements set down in Friedrich Ludwig Jahn's *Die Deutsche Turnkunst* (1816). The third group supported exercises directed to military needs. The smallest group, led by Coubertin, favored English athletic games, with their emphasis on character development and "manly" virtues [95].

In 1887, the same year that Coubertin initiated his efforts to revive the Olympic Games, Marey was named head of a Commission (members included Lagrange and Georges Demény) charged with reviewing the teaching of gymnastics in schools. In the final report, Marey stated that assertions regarding which were the best types of exercise needed to be subjected to the type of careful physiological and mechanical studies that he and his Assistant Demēny had been conducting [110]. An active gymnast, Demēny had studied medicine. At the Paris Physiological Station, he collaborated with Marey in locomotor and physiological experiments using chronophotography, the odograph, and other apparatus. When their association ended in 1894, Demeny became professor of physiology at the École Militaire de Joinville, then director of the Cours Supérieur d'Éducation Physique in Paris [134, 153, 172]. He authored *Bases Scientifiques de l'Éducation Physique* (1903) [41] and other texts and served as Secretary for various congresses directed to physical education. The *Scientific American,* in 1914, credited Demēny, Marey, and Italian physiologist Angelo Mosso with valuable contributions to the scientific study of respiration, circulation, and muscular action and commented favorably on investigations currently under way at Joinville [24].

The appearance of George Hébert's "natural method" and other systems of exercise in the 1900s added further complexity to a landscape already crowded with competing programs. Before World War II, the École Normale de Gymnastique et d'Escrime, which had emerged from a 1872 reorganization of the military school of gymnastics, was the major venue for preparing teachers for schools and the army. Its curriculum (which drew, in part, from Hébert's work) has been described as "eclectic" [172]. The consequences of all this was reflected in the preface to *Traité d'Éducation Physique* (1930), wherein Dr. Marcel Labbé observed that R. Tait McKenzie had accurately characterized France as a "battleground" of ideas regarding exercise [85].

In *The Anthropology of World's Fairs* (1983), Burton Benedict makes the intriguing observation that the Olympic Games came to fulfill several of the functions that international expositions once had performed. Between

1851 and 1915, 12 major International Universal Expositions were held in Europe and the United States. Beginning with the second (Paris in 1855), "Education, Health, and Social Life" (physical education and sports were often included) was a major division [13]. At the session dedicated to "Gymnastics Considered from a Hygienic Point of View" (organized as part of a Hygiene Congress held during the 1878 Paris International Exposition), physicians discussed the need to improve physical education in their respective countries [37].

The 1900 (Paris) and 1904 (St. Louis) Olympic Games were held during (and largely submerged within) international expositions [105]. Each exposition also hosted meetings devoted to sports and physical culture. At the 1900 Paris International Congress of Physical Education both gymnastics and sports were discussed by French and foreign delegates. A Commission Internationale pour l'Éducation Physique (with Mosso as President and Demény as one of the Secretaries) was founded, and slow motion studies were made of athletes. The 1904 Louisiana Purchase Exposition included within its Department of Physical Culture annual conventions of the APEA and Young Men's Christian Association (YMCA) and an "Olympic Lecture Course." Physician Ferdinand A. Schmidt, who accompanied the German team, spoke on the "Physiology of Exercise." The title of New York physician and APEA member C. Ward Crampton's lecture was "Some Recent Advances in the Sciences of Physical Training" [152].[4]

Polarizations created by the establishment in 1989 of the International Olympic Committee (IOC) World Congresses of Sport Sciences (dominated by medicine and the physiological sciences) vis-à-vis the more traditional, broadly based Olympic Scientific Congresses have been discussed by John MacAloon [96]. Two congresses held in Belgium during the summer of 1905 reflect similar, although not identical, contending "world views." At Liége delegates from 20 countries attended the Second International Congress on Physical Education of Youth organized by Commission Internationale pour L'Éducation Physique. The program included reports on national statistics and the training of teachers, as well as discussions of what was purported to be "the scientific basis of physical education" [35]. Two months earlier, an International Congress of Sport and Physical Education organized under the auspices of the IOC (and carefully orchestrated by IOC President Coubertin) had been held at Brussels. Although gymnastics was discussed, attention was directed to rowing, rugby, golf, fencing, and yachting. In his Introduction to the Report of the Brussels Congress, Coubertin criticized what he called that "group of tenacious and noisy young doctors . . . worshipers of theoretical science and perfectly disdainful of practical knowledge" [34]. The Baron might claim, when it suited his pur-

---

[4]Karl Lennartz: "Sportmedical Care of Marathon Runners in Early Modern Olympic Games." Paper presented at the Olympic Scientific Congress, Dallas, July 10–14, 1996.

pose, that he had been "urging specialists" study questions relating to sport. His commitment, however, was to "soaring ideals," not objective science. Although the theme of the 1913 IOC Congress was "Psychology and Physiology of Sport," the report suggests that discussions were speculative, not scientific [117].

ACROSS THE RHINE

The distinction of establishing the first organization specifically directed to "sports medicine" belongs to German physicians. Many things had brought this about. In the 18th century, physicians as well as educators endorsed the merits of exercise. Johann Christoph Guts Muths, author of influential treatises like *Gymnastik für die Jugend* (1793), referred to medical works[5] and chose for his title the Greek word *gymnastik*. Rapid advances in experimental science and clinical medicine were a factor, as was a desire on the part of physicians to create a niche in a crowded profession.[6] Unification after the Franco-Prussian War made Germany the chief power on the European Continent.

In the 1790s, when French legislative assemblies were attempting to establish a *national* scheme of education, the political entity that came to be known as Germany had consisted of some 300 free cities and independent states, the largest of which was Prussia. Defeat by Napoleon's armies resulted in a growing sense of patriotism and a striving for national unity that found expression in the Turnen movement, initiated by Friedrich Ludwig Jahn in 1811. The tone of Guts Muths's 1817 *Turnbuch für die Söhne des Vaterlands (Book of Gymnastics for the Sons of the Nation)* reflects these reactions to a foreign invader. Commitment to preserving the purity of German traditions remained a fundamental tenant of German gymnastics despite differences that resulted in the formation of various confederations (e.g., Demokratischer-Turnerbund, Arbeiter-Turnerbund) and other developments [15, 45, 48, 159].

When Major Hugo Rothstein introduced the Swedish gymnastic system at Berlin's Zentralturnanstalt, what came to be known as the *Barrenstreit* (parallel bars dispute) erupted. The Minister of Education appointed members of the University of Berlin's Royal Medical Department (e.g., pathologist Rudolph Virchow, nerve physiologist Emil DuBois-Reymond) to adjudicate the matter. Drawing upon his experiences in Ernst Eislen's gymnasium, as well as on his laboratory research, Bois-Reymond denounced the so-called "physiological theories" on which the Swedish system was based [47]. Al-

---

[5]Michael Krüger: "Sport, Health, and Military Fitness." Paper presented at the Olympic Scientific Congress, Dallas, June 10–14, 1996.
[6]Gertrud Pfister: "Between Performance and Health." Paper presented at the IOC Scientific Congress, Dallas, July 10–14, 1996.

though most Turners rejected Anglo-Saxon sports (and refused to participate in early Olympic Games), Ferdinand A. Schmidt, an active Turner, as
well as a physician, endorsed the value of both traditional games and English sports [64]. His comprehensive *Unser Körper* (1899) brought together
relevant turn-of-the-century information regarding the effects of exercise on
the body [141]. Together with Schmidt, the English sportsman Eustis Miles
published a considerably modified version in 1901 as *The Training of the Body
for Games, Athletics, Gymnastics, and Other Forms of Exercise* [142].

By the early 1900s, the scientific interest in sport that George Kolb had
already exhibited had begun to attract the attention of other German physicians. Arthur Mallwitz, a participant at the 1908 London Olympics, reported that he and other medical men were beginning to see sportsmen
who exhibited cardiovascular problems [74]. The 1911 Dresden Internationale Hygiene Ausstellung (International Hygiene Exhibition) marked
an important turning point [75]. German-born United States Naval Surgeon Henry G. Beyer wrote a lengthy article for *Popular Science Monthly*, in
which he praised the exhibits devoted to sanitation, the rapidly developing
field of bacteriology, and sports. The Sports Division, organized by Mallwitz,
included a special laboratory at which effects of exhausting exercise were
studied [18, 75]. To accompany the Exhibition's offerings, an extensive bibliography and two volumes containing chapters written by physicians on
medical, scientific, and pedagogical aspects of exercise and sports were
edited by Berlin doctor Siegfried Weissbein [164, 165]. The United States,
Beyer lamented, lagged considerably behind what Germany had achieved
with regard to the scientific study of hygiene and physical education [19].

Building on the Dresden success, an institute for the "scientific study of
sport and physical training" was initiated in Berlin's Charlottenburg district, and the term "Sportartz" (sports physician) was used for the first time.
A laboratory was designed for the Grunewald stadium in anticipation of the
1916 Berlin Olympics. Physicians meeting at the Golfhotel at Oberhof,
Thuringia on September 21, 1912 established the Deutsche Reichskomitee
für die Wissenschaftliche Erforschung des Sportes und der Leibesübungen
(German Imperial Committee for Scientific Research of Sport and Physical
Training) with Dr. Kraus (Professor of Internal Medicine at the University
of Berlin) as chairman [75]. Whereas the fields of medicine (especially cardiology), physiology, and physical education all contributed to the formation and growth of the ACSM, German sports medicine was established and
controlled by members of the medical profession.

DEVELOPMENTS AFTER WORLD WAR I

The decade of the 1920s witnessed an acceleration in development pertaining to various "sciences" of human performance. When Sir Arthur

Keith (Fellow of the Royal College of Surgeons and formerly Fullerian Professor of Physiology) prepared a second (1925) edition of *The Engines of the Body: Being the Substance of Christmas Lectures Given at the Royal Institution of Great Britain, Christmas 1916–17)*, he chose to discuss new discoveries in a series of appendices. After a short dedication, Keith turned to "Muscles as Combustion Engines and How They Serve the Needs of Athletes"—which focused largely on "the Oxygen Debt" and the work of Fletcher, Hill, and Meyerhoff. He also devoted attention to exercise at altitude (e.g., the work of Haldane and Barcroft), to McCollum and Davis's discovery of fat-soluble Vitamin A, to the discovery of insulin (1922), and to other recent discoveries [79].

The sciences were changing, and so were sports! Hundreds of thousands of servicemen had received their first introductions to organized physical activity through military preparedness programs. Six months after the November 11, 1918 Armistice, 1500 athletes from 18 countries met at Pershing Stadium, Joinville-le-Pont for the Inter-Allied Games of 1919. Conceived of by Elwood S. Brown (a YMCA official serving as Director of Athletics for the American Expeditionary Forces), these games were intended as a friendly assemblage of cooperating nations [78] and a positive diversion for troops awaiting demobilization. In Germany, a bill for compulsory physical education was presented in 1919, and athletic clubs began to emerge in increasing numbers. Spared the devastation of occupying armies and enjoying comparatively good economic times, Americans invested large sums of time and money in college and professional sports, prompting a journalist to write in 1922: A new Golden Age of sport and outdoor amusements is admittedly with us" [94].

Escalating college enrollments contributed to the rapid growth of undergraduate majors in physical education in the United States. By 1927, 135 institutions offered bachelor's degree programs, and 4 offered the master's degree. A doctorate could be obtained at Teachers College. Columbia University, and New York University's School of Education. That same year, the APEA urged its membership to undertake more anatomical, chemical, physiological, and psychological studies of physical activity and recommended the establishment of a *Research Quarterly* to stimulate such investigations [122]. The *Journal of Health and Physical Education* (1930) began a column by physiologist Arthur Steinhaus (George Williams College) entitled "Physiology at the Service of Physical Education." With his considerable knowledge of developments in German and his facility with the language, Steinhaus was able to bring to the American reader insightful reports of the work of Herxheimer, Zuntz, Thörner, and other researchers [150].

A small number of individuals (e.g., Thomas K. Cureton at the University of Illinois, Franklin M. Henry at the University of California) headed extensive research programs between the wars. More typical of leaders in the field of physical education was the multifaceted career of James H. Mc-

Curdy at the International YMCA Training School at Springfield, Massachusetts. McCurdy (who held both the master's and a medical degree) had studied experimental physiology at the Harvard Medical School with William T. Porter. He served as editor of the *American Physical Education Review* (1906–1929) and, during the War, as Director of the Division of Athletics for the YMCA in France [92]. The 369-page work, *Bibliography of Physical Training* (that included numerous foreign as well as domestic medical and scientific references), which he published in 1905 made available to the American reader what Weissbein's *Bibliographie des Gesamten Sports* (1911) would do for the German reader [98, 165]. McCurdy's *Physiology of Exercise: A Text-book for Students of Physical Education* (1924) provided a synthesis of major English-language studies: And may be considered a prototype for subsequent works [99]. A 1927 translation of the work of Drs. Felix Deutsch (University of Vienna) and Emil Kauf (Vienna Heart Station), *Heart and Athletics: Critical Researches upon the Influence of Athletics upon the Heart* (1927), brought to the attention of American readers important European research bearing on this topic [42].

During the 1920s, exercise and high-performance sport became the focus of a growing number of investigators in physiology, psychology, and other disciplines. A comparison of the bibliographies in the 1919 edition of Bainbridge's *The Physiology of Muscular Exercise* [11] and the revised 1931 edition (by Bock and Dill) [12] is illustrative of the changes—as is Edward C. Schneider's *Physiology of Muscular Action* (1933) [143]. During the late 1800s, Paul Bert and Angelo Mosso produced pioneering studies of exercise at high altitude [115, 161]. Before World War I, Schneider and Yale's Yandell Henderson (who would perform respiratory studies on Yale's 1924 gold medal Olympic crew) participated in studies at Pike's Peak. During the War, both were engaged to study the ability of aviators to withstand altitude [66, 67]. Archibald Vivian Hill (1922 Nobel Prize in Physiology and Medicine with German physiologist Otto Meyerhoff) was a proponent of using sport to elucidate physiological questions. In his inaugural address as Joddrell Professor of Physiology at University College, London, he stated: "Athletics, physical training, flying, working, submarines or coal-mines, all require a knowledge of man. . . . The observation of sick men in hospitals is not the best training for the study of normal man at work" [43].

Possessed of the ability to write both exemplary scientific papers [72] and informative syntheses for the general reader [69], Hill once observed that as a youth he had shared with other boys the most ridiculous notions about training: "Drink as little as possible, don't eat potatoes or pastry" [70]. Because he could hear it beating, he had been anxious about his heart. Of his mentor Walter Morley Fletcher, Hill observed: his "chief pride"—despite all that Fletcher had achieved in medical research—was that during his student days he had represented Cambridge against the American universities

[70]. Speaking of his own athletic experiences, Hill noted that "the stiffness and exhaustion" that so often followed a race had stimulated his interest in the dynamics of muscular activity. A comment in his preface to *Muscular Movement in Man: The Factors Governing Speed and Recovery from Fatigue* (1927) underscores different contemporary attitudes: "in America . . . people are more inclined to treat the subject of athletics scientifically. . . . there are, I fear, many athletes and sportsmen in England who would be shocked by such an idea" [71].

According to D. B. Dill, Hill's suggestion that he and Arlie Bock prepare a 3rd edition of Bainbridge's text significantly influenced the research programs that emerged at the Harvard Fatigue Laboratory [43]. Opened in 1927 under the direction of Lawrence Henderson, the Harvard Fatigue Laboratory (subsequently directed by Dill) was, according to Horvath and Horvath, "a unique concept in biological research [in that it] recognized that the systems and organs which comprise a biological organism are interrelated; and they need to be studied in an interrelated context if the biological and social functioning of human beings is to be fully understood" [76]. The laboratory attracted a wide range of domestic and foreign investigators: physiologists, biochemists, psychologists, biologists, physicians, sociologists, anthropologists, and it is generally agreed that it made signal contributions to research on metabolic and respiratory adaptations to exercise, blood changes, renal function, fatigue, training, and other physiological parameters of performance [76, 118].

Between 1925 and 1931 Coleman Griffith (University of Illinois) headed the first research laboratory directed to the study of psychological parameters of sports in the United States [60, 61]. Both psychological and physiological research was conducted at the Deutsch Hochschule für Leibesübungen after its founding in 1920. Ernst Kretschmer's theory of "constitutional types" (asthenic, athletic, pyknic—suggestive of later ecto-, meso-, and endomorphic classifications) was expounded in *Physique and Character* (1921). German physician Wolfgang Kohlrauschs's anthropometric survey of athletes who had competed in the 1922 Deutsche Kampfspiele [74] drew on a lengthy history of interest in body typology and might be considered—at least in part—as in the same genre as Dr. Dudley Allen Sargent's late 19th century anthropometric studies of college athletes [139].

August Bier, professor surgery at the University of Berlin (Director at the Deutsche Hochschule until 1932) and other Berlin physicians were instrumental in forming the German Medical Society for the Advancement of Physical Training (Deutscher Ärztebund zur Förderung der Leibesübungen (DÄB)) in 1924. Ferdinand A. Schmidt and Arthur Mallwitz were named, respectively, Chairman and Vice-Chairman [75]. Regular membership in the DÄB was restricted to registered doctors; honorary membership might be conferred, on appropriate recommendation, to others. The Prussian Ministry of Health and Welfare was persuaded to support the effects of the DÄB, and membership grew from 64 in 1924 to 2289 in 1927.[7] The reasons for such an increase need to be investigated. It is quite possible that the growing surplus of physicians that occurred during the Weimar Republic made this new specialty particularly attractive.

The 1928 Olympic year witnessed a number of events that were especially significant in the history of sports medicine and exercise science. The universities of Hamburg and Leipzig created full-time sports medicine positions. For his Arris and Gale Lecture before the Royal College of Surgeons, Adolphe Abrahams selected "Physiology of Violent Exercise in Relation to the Possibility of Strain." The literature dealing with "physiological and pathological" aspects of exercise, he stated, was "a great deal more voluminous than is generally recognized." Having summarized recent work on oxygen consumption, efficiency of the heart, metabolism, and "effort syndrome," Abrahams noted the thoroughness of "Teutonic discipline" and opportunities that Americans had for "research upon the athlete in their numerous colleges and universities [1]. At the 1928 St. Moritz Winter Olympics, physicians representing 11 countries established the organization that would be renamed Fédération Internationale de Médicine Sportive (FIMS) in 1934 [138, 157].

The first congress of the Association Internationale Médico-Sportive was held in conjunction with the 1928 Amsterdam Olympic Games. Under the direction of Professor F. J. J. Buytendijk and the Netherlands Olympic Committee, teams of physicians, physiologists, and psychologists undertook cardiovascular, electrocardiographic, neuromuscular, blood chemistry, reaction time, anthropometric, and other tests on some 260 male and female competitors [28]. The results of these investigations were published as *Ergebnisse der Sportärztlichen Untersuchungen bei den IX. Olympische Spielen in Amsterdam 1928 (Results of the Sportsmedicine Examinations at the IX Olympic Games in Amsterdam)* and in journals such as *Klinische Wochenschrift* and *Arbeitsphysiologie: Zeitschrift für die Physiologie des Menschen bei Arbeit und Sport (Journal of Human Work and Sport Physiology)*, which was founded in 1928 [26, 68, 154]. It is interesting to note that a Congress of the genre inspired by Coubertin was also held during the Amsterdam Olympics. This attracted several hundred physical educators, physicians, and other individuals [35]. Few data-based papers appear to have been presented, however.

It was John Morgan's inquiry into "the after life" of men who had rowed in the Oxford-Cambridge Boat Race from 1829 to 1869 that initiated medical inquiries into effects of strenuous activity on health and longevity. It seems fitting, therefore, to end this short excursion through early "sports medicine/exercise science" with a similar—but much more extensive—study that was published in *Harper's Monthly Magazine* in 1928. Having re-

---

[7]Gertrud Pfister: "Between Performance and Health." Paper presented in the IOC Scientific Congress, Dallas, July 10–14, 1996.

viewed the records of 4976 men who had participated in baseball, football, crew, track, and "minor sports" at 10 eastern colleges, Louis Dublin concluded that although it was "not easy to draw final conclusions . . . the group of college athletes studied presented a favorable picture." Nevertheless, he cautioned, a great deal still needed to be learned about causal relationships among health, longevity, and participation in athletics [46]. This issue [65], as with other questions concerning the limits and effects of human performance, would receive ever-increasing attention in the second half of the 20th century.

SUMMARY

There are many criteria by which advances in "sports medicine" and "exercise science" may be assessed. Historical developments in the basic and applied sciences—and in clinical practices, as well—may best be explored by those who are experts in particular fields. It is encouraging that more studies of this type have begun to appear. Studies of the evolution of organizations that have fostered various aspects of physical training, exercise science, and sports medicine may provide another useful approach. Whereas 910 individuals participated in the 1976 ACSM Annual Meeting, in 1992, attendance reached 3661. In 1954 (the year the American College of Sports Medicine was organized), *Index Medicus* listed approximately 250 items under the headings Athletics, Exercise, and Physical Education. In 1993, some 4000 citations were reported as being about Athletics, Exercise, Physical Fitness, Exercise-Related Physical Therapy, and Sports Medicine. According to the *Congress Proceedings of the Third IOC World Congress on Sport Sciences* (September 16–22, 1995), 225 individuals made presentations. More than 1650 women and men representing a vast array of contributing fields participated in symposia, lectures, and poster sessions during "Physical Activity, Sport, and Health"—The 1996 International Pre-Olympic Scientific Congress (July 10th—14th). What advances await in the 21st century?

ACKNOWLEDGMENTS

I am especially indebted to the following individuals for their generosity in sending relevant materials: Wildor Hollmann, Hans Langenfeld, Arnd Krüger, Gertrud Pfister, and Horst UEberhorst.

REFERENCES

1. Abrahams, A. On the physiology of violent exercise in relation to the possibility of strain. *Lancet* 214:429–435, 1928.
2. Abrahams, A., and A. Porritt. Sport and medicine. *Br. Med. J.* 2:98, 1952.
3. Allbutt, T. C. On overwork and strain of the heart and aorta. *Clinical Society of London.* London: Longmans, Green, 1873.

4. Anonymous: Athletics. *Contemp. Rev.* 3:374, 1866.
5. Anonymous: The Oxford and Cambridge university boat race. *Illust. London News*, March 31, 1866.
6. Anonymous: The present aspect of athletics. *Baily's Mag. Sport and Pastimes* 18:197–204, 1870.
7. Anonymous: Scientific study of physical training. *Bost. Med. Surg. J.* 140:272, 1899.
8. Anonymous: A great runner. *Br. Med. J.* 1:1143, 1954.
9. Arnaud, P. (ed.). *Les Athlètes de la République: Gymnastique, Sport et Idéologie Republicaine, 1870–1914.* Toulouse: Bibliothèque Historique Privat, 1987.
10. Atwater, W. O., and A. P. Bryant. *Dietary Studies of University Boat Crews.* Bulletin No. 75, U. S. Department of Agriculture, Office of Experiment Stations. Washington, DC: Government Printing Office, 1900.
11. Bainbridge, F. A. *The Physiology of Muscular Exercise.* London: Longmans, Green, 1919.
12. Bainbridge, F. A. *The Physiology of Muscular Exercise.* 3rd rev. ed. by A. V. Bock and D. B. Dill. London: Longmans, Green and Co., 1931.
13. Benedict, B. *The Anthropology of World's Fairs: San Francisco's Panama Pacific International Exposition of 1915.* Berkeley, CA: Scholar Press, 1983.
14. Benedict, F. G., and E. P. Cathcart. *Muscular Work: A Metabolic Study with Special Reference to the Efficiency of the Human Body as a Machine.* Washington, DC: Carnegie Institution of Washington, 1913, p. 3.
15. Beier, W., G. Erbach, W. Schröder, H. Schuster, L. Skorning, G. Wieczisk, and B. Wilk. *Bilder und Dokumente aus der Deutschen Turn- und Sportgeschichte.* Berlin: Staatliches Komitee für Körperkultur und Sport, 1956.
16. Berryman, J. W. Exercise and the medical tradition from Hippocrates through antebellum America: a review essay. J. W. Berryman and R. J. Park (eds.). *Sport and Exercise Science: Essays in the History of Sports Medicine.* Urbana, IL: University of Illinois Press, 1992, pp. 1–56.
17. Berryman, J. W. *Out of Many—One: A History of the American College of Sports Medicine.* Urbana, IL: Human Kinetics Publishers, 1995.
18. Beyer, H. G. The influence of exercise on growth. *J. Exp. Med.* 1:546–558, 1896.
19. Beyer, H. G. The international hygiene exhibition at Dresden. *Pop. Sci. Mo.* 80:105–128, 1912.
20. Blake, J. B., and R. C. Larabee. Observations upon long distance runners. *Bost. Med. Surg. J.* 148:195–206, 1903.
21. Bonner, T. N. *American Doctors and German Universities: A Chapter in International Intellectual Relations, 1870–1914.* Lincoln, NE: University of Nebraska Press, 1963.
22. Bonner, T. N. *Becoming a Physician: Medical Education in Great Britain, France, Germany and the United States, 1750–1945.* New York: Oxford University Press, 1995, p. 258.
23. Bowditch, H. P. The growth rate of children studied by Galton's percentile grades. *22nd Annual Report of the State Board of Health of Massachusetts.* Boston: Wright & Potter, 1891, pp. 479–525.
24. Boyer, J. The scientist and the athlete: The physiology laboratory of the French military school at Joinville. *Sci. Am.* 23:480–481, 1914.
25. Bradford, E. H. Health of rowing men. *Sanitarian* 5:529–536, 1877.
26. Bramwell, C., and R. Ellis. Clinical observations on Olympic athletes. *Arbeitsphysiologie* 1:51–60, 1928.
27. Brobeck, J. R., O. E. Reynolds, and T. A. Appel (eds.). *History of the American Physiological Society: The First Century, 1887–1987.* Bethesda, MD: The American Physiological Society, 1987.
28. Buytendijk, F. J. J. (ed). *Ergebnisse der Sportärztlichen Untersuchungen bei den IX. Olympischen Spielen in Amsterdam 1928.* Berlin: Verlag von Julius Springer, 1929.
29. Bynum, W. F. *Science and the Practice of Medicine in the 19th Century.* Cambridge, England: Cambridge University Press, 1994.
30. Carpenter, K. J. *Protein and Energy: A Study of Changing Ideas in Nutrition.* Cambridge, England: Cambridge University Press, 1994.

31. Chesterton, T. *The Theory of Physical Education in Elementary Schools.* rev. ed. London: Gale & Polden, Ltd., 1897.

32. Chittenden, R. H. *The Nutrition of Man.* New York: Frederick A. Stokes Co., 1907.

33. Coleman, W., and F. L. Holmes (eds.). *The Investigative Enterprise: Experimental Physiology in 19th Century Medicine.* Berkeley, CA: University of California Press, 1988, pp. 1 and 2.

34. Comité International Olympique. *Congrès International de Sport et d'Éducation Physique. Bruxelles, 9–14 Juin 1905.* Paris: Auxerre, 1905, p. 5.

35. *Compte Rendu du Deuxième Congrès International de l'Éducation Physique de la Jeunesse. Liége, 28 Août au 1 Septembre 1905.* Nivelles: Imprimerie Lanneau et Despert.

36. *Compte Rendu du Congrès International d'Éducation Physique et du Sport. Amsterdam, Août 1–4, 1928.* Amsterdam: D'Oliveira.

37. Dally, E. De l'éducation corporelle en France: Son état présent, ses lacunes, son programme. *Congrès International d'Hygiène.* Paris: Imprimerie Nationale, 1880.

38. Darling, E. The effects of training: a study of the Harvard university crew. *Bost. Med. Surg. J.* 141:205–290; 229–233, 1899.

39. Davis, D. F., M. T. Huss, and A. H. Becker. Norman Tripplett and the dawning of sport psychology. *Sport Psychologist* 9:366–375, 1995.

40. Demēny, G. Address of M. Georges Demēny. *Am. Phys. Educ. Rev.* 5:291–300, 1900.

41. Demēny, G. *Les Bases Scientifiques de l'Éducation Physique.* Paris: F. Alcan, 1903.

42. Deutsch, F., and E. Kauf. *Heart and Athletics: Clinical Researches upon the Influence of Athletics upon the Heart.* L. M. Warfield (trans.). St. Louis: C. V. Mosby, 1927.

43. Dill, D. B. Historical review of exercise physiology science. W. R. Johnson and E. R. Buskirk (eds.). *Science and Medicine of Sport and Exercise.* 2nd ed. New York: Harper & Row, 1974, pp. 37–41.

44. Discussion on medical aspects of athleticism. *Br. Med. J.* 2:829–838, 1909.

45. Dixon, J. G. Prussia, politics and physical education. J. G. Dixon, P. C. McIntosh, A. D. Munrow, and R. F. Willetts (eds.). *Landmarks in the History of Physical Education.* London: Routledge & Kegan Paul, 1954, pp. 107–148.

46. Dublin, L. I. Longevity of college athletes. *Harper's Monthly* 157:229–238, 1928.

47. DuBois-Reymond, E. Swedish gymnastics and German gymnastics from a physiological point of view. *Essays Concerning the German System of Gymnastics.* Milwaukee, WI: Freuekner Publishing Co.

48. Eichel, W. *Illustrierte Geschichte der Körperkultur.* Berlin: Sportverlag Berlin, 1983, 2 vols.

49. Egen, T. S. *Principles of Rowing by an Oarsman.* London: F. C. Westley, 1846.

50. Eisenberg, C. Football in Germany: beginnings, 1890–1914. *Int. J. Hist. Sport.* 8:205–220, 1991.

51. Fitz, G. W. A study of types of respiratory movements. *J. Exp. Med.* 1:677–694, 1896.

52. Flexner, A. *Medical Education in the United States and Canada.* Bulletin No. 4. New York: Carnegie Foundation for the Advancement of Teaching, 1910.

53. Flint, A. *On the Physiological Effects of Severe and Protracted Muscular Exercise; with Special Reference to its Influence upon the Excretion of Nitrogen.* New York: D. Appleton & Co., 1871.

54. Flint, A. *On the Source of Muscular Power: Arguments and Conclusions Drawn from Observations upon the Human Subject, under Conditions of Rest and of Muscular Exercise.* New York: D. Appleton & Co., 1878.

55. Frank, R. G. American physiologists in German laboratories, 1865–1914, G. L. Geison (ed.). *Physiology in the American Context, 1850–1940.* Bethesda, MD: American Physiological Society, 1987, pp. 11–46.

56. French, R. D. *Antivivisection and Medical Science in Victorian Society.* Princeton, NJ: Princeton University Press, 1975.

57. Fye, W. B. *The Development of American Physiology: Scientific Medicine in the 19th Century.* Baltimore: Johns Hopkins University Press, 1987.

58. Geison, G. L. *Michael Foster and the Cambridge School of Physiology: the Scientific Enterprise in Late Victorian Society.* Princeton, NJ: Princeton University Press, 1978, pp. 50–66.

59. Gillmeister, H. English editors of German sporting journals at the turn of the century. *Sports Historian* 13:38–65, 1995.
60. Gould, D., and S. Pick. Sport psychology: the Griffith era, 1920–1940. *Sport Psychologist* 9:391–405, 1995.
61. Griffith, C. R. *Psychology and Athletics.* New York: Charles Scribner's Sons, 1928.
62. Gulick, L. H. Physical education: a new profession. *Proceedings of the 5th Annual Meeting of the American Association for the Advancement of Physical Education.* Ithaca, NY: Andrus & Church, 1890, pp. 59–66.
63. Haley, B. *The Healthy Body and Victorian Culture.* Cambridge, MA: Harvard University Press, 1987.
64. Hamer, E. U., and W. Hollmann. *Zwei Medizin-Professoren als Turnreformer: F. A. Schmidt und F. Hueppes*—Kreuzzug für Hygiene und Körperpflege. Eine Dokumentation in Form ihrer Biographien und Bibliographien. Köln, Germany: Bundesinstitut für Sportwissenschaft, 1992.
65. Hartley, P. H., and G. F. Llewellyn. The longevity of oarsmen: a study of those who rowed in the Oxford and Cambridge boat race from 1829 to 1928. *Br. Med. J.* 1:657–662, 1939.
66. Henderson, Y. The physiology of the aviator. *Science* 49:431–441, 1919.
67. Henderson, Y., and H. W. Haggard. The maximum of human power and its fuel. *Am J. Physiol.* 72:264–282, 1925.
68. Herxheimer, H. Die Herzgrösse der Amsterdamer Olympiadeteilnehmer. *Klin. Woch.* 8:402–404, 1929.
69. Hill, A. V. The scientific study of athletics. *Sci. Am.* April: 224–225, 1926.
70. Hill, A. V. *Living Machinery.* New York: Harcourt, Brace & Co., 1927, p. ix.
71. Hill, A. V. *Muscular Movement in Man: The Factors Governing Speed and Recovery from Fatigue.* New York: McGraw-Hill Book Co., 1927, pp 1–4.
72. Hill, A. V. *Trails and Trials in Physiology.* Baltimore: Williams & Wilkins, 1965.
73. Hobermann, J. M. The early development of sports medicine in Germany. J. W. Berryman and R. J. Park (eds.). *Sport and Exercise Science: Essays in the History of Sports Medicine.* Urbana, IL: University of Illinois Press, 1992, pp. 233–282.
74. Hobermann, J. M. *Mortal Engines: The Science of Performance and the Dehumanization of Sport.* New York: The Free Press, 1992.
75. Hollmann, W. Entwicklung der sportmedizin in Deutschland. K. Tittel, K. H. Arndt, and W. Hollmann (eds.). *Sportmedizin: Gestern-Heute-Morgen. Bericht von Jubiläum-symposium des Deutschen Sportärztebundes, Oberhof, 25. bis 27. September 1992.* Leipzig/Berlin/Heidelberg, Germany: 1993, pp. 22–31.
76. Horvath, S. M. and E. C. Horvath. *The Harvard Fatigue Laboratory: Its History and Contributions.* Englewood Cliffs, NJ: Prentice-Hall, 1973, p. 3.
77. Howell, J. D. "Soldier's heart": the redefinition of heart disease and specialty formation in early 20th-century Great Britain. W. F. Bynum, C. Lawrence, and V. Nutton (eds.). *The Emergence of Modern Cardiology.* London: The Wellcome Institute for the History of Medicine, 1985, pp. 34–52.
78. *Inter-Allied Games, Paris 22nd June to 6th July 1919* Published by the Games Committee. Paris: Sté Ane de Publications Périodiques, 1919.
79. Keith, A. *The Engines of the Human Body.* London: Williams & Norgate, Ltd., 1926.
80. Kirsch, G. B. *The Creation of American Team Sports: Baseball and Cricket, 1838–72.* Urbana, IL: University of Illinois Press, 1989, p. 70.
81. Kolb, G. *Physiology of Sport: Contributions toward the Physiology of Maximum Muscular Exertion, Especially in Modern Sports.* London: Krohne & Sesemann, 1893.
82. Kroll W. P. *Graduate Study and Research in Physical Education.* Champaign, IL: Human Kinetics, 1982, pp. 51–59.
83. Krüger, A. *Sieg heil* to the most glorious era of German sport: Continuity and change in the modern German sports movement. *Int. J. Hist. Sport.* 4:5–20, 1987.

84. Krüger, A. "We are sure to have found the true reasons for the American superiority in sports": the reciprocal relationship between the United States and Germany in physical culture and sport. R. Naul (ed.). *Turnen and Sport: the Cross-Cultural Exchange.* Munster, Germany: Waxmann Verlag, 1991, pp. 51–80.

85. Labbé, M. *Traité d'Éducation Physique.* Paris: Gaston, Doin & Co., 1930.

86. Lagrange, F. *Physiology of Bodily Exercise.* London: Kegan Paul, Trench & Co., 1887.

87. Lagrange, F. La reforme de l'éducation physique. *Rev. Deux Mondes* 112:338–374.

88. Langenfeld, H. Auf dem wege zur sportwissenschaft: mediziner und leibesübungen im 19 jahrhundert. *Stadion* 14:125–148, 1988.

89. Lawrence, C. Moderns and ancients: the "new cardiology" in Britain, 1880–1930. W. F. Bynum, C. Lawrence, and V. Nutton (eds.). *The Emergence of Modern Cardiology.* London: Wellcome Institute for the History of Medicine, 1985, pp. 1–33.

90. Lee, F. S. Physical exercise from the standpoint of physiology. *Science* 29:521–527, 1909.

91. Lee, R. J. *Exercise and Training: Their Effects upon Health.* London: Smith, Elder & Co., 1873.

92. Leonard, F. E. *A Guide to the History of Physical Education.* Philadelphia: Lea & Febiger, 1947.

93. Licht, E., and S. Licht. *A Translation of Joseph Clément Tissot's Gymnastique Médicinale et Chirurgicale.* Baltimore: Williams & Wilkins, 1964.

94. Lucas, J. A., and R. A. Smith. *Saga of American Sport.* Philadelphia: Lea Febiger, 1978, p. 305.

95. MacAloon, J. J. *This Great Symbol: Pierre de Coubertin and the Origins of the Modern Olympic Games.* Chicago: University of Chicago Press, 1981.

96. MacAloon, J. J. Sport, science, and intercultural relations: reflections on recent trends in Olympic scientific meetings. *Olympika* 1:1–28, 1994.

97. McArdle, W. D., F. I. Katch, and V. L. Katch. *Exercise Physiology: Energy, Nutrition and Human Performance,* 4th ed. Baltimore: Williams & Wilkins, 1996.

98. McCurdy, J. H. *A Bibliography of Physical Training.* Springfield, MA: Physical Directors' Society of the Young Men's Christian Association, 1905.

99. McCurdy, J. H. *The Physiology of Exercise: a Text-Book for Students of Physical Education.* Philadelphia: Lea & Febiger, 1924.

100. McIntosh, P. C. Games and gymnastics for two nations in one. J. G. Dixon, P. C. McIntosh, A. D. Munrow, and R. F. Willetts (eds.). *Landmarks in the History of Physical Education.* London: Routledge & Kegan Paul, 1957, pp. 177–207.

101. Maclaren, A. *Training in Theory and Practice.* London: Macmillan & Co., 1866.

102. Maclaren, A. University oars. *Nature.* 17 April: 458–460, 1873.

103. McKenzie, R. T. *Exercise in Education and Medicine.* Philadelphia: W. B. Saunders, 1909.

104. McKenzie, R. T. The influence of exercise on the heart. *Am. J. Med. Sci.* 145:69–74, 1913.

105. Mandell, R. D. *Paris 1900: the Great World's Fair.* Toronto: University of Toronto Press, 1967.

106. Mangan, J. A. *Athleticism in the Victorian and Edwardian Public School: the Emergence and Consolidation of an Educational Ideology.* Cambridge, England: Cambridge University Press, 1981.

107. Mangan, J. A. *The Games Ethic and Imperialism: Aspects of the Diffusion of an Ideal.* New York: Viking, 1986.

108. Mangan, J. A. (ed.) *The Cultural Bond: Sport, Empire, Society.* London: Frank Cass, 1993.

109. Marey, E-J. *La Machine Animale: Locomotion Terrestre et Aérienne.* Paris: Librairie G. Baillière, 1878.

110. Marey, E. J. Rapport présenté à M. le Ministre au nom de la Commission de Gymnastique. *Travaux de la Commission de Gymnastique: Ministère de l'Instruction Publique et des Beaux-Arts.* Paris: Imprimerie Nationale, 1889.

111. Massengale, J. D., and R. A. Swanson (eds.). *The History of Exercise and Sport Science.* Champaign, IL: Human Kinetics, 1996.

112. Meylan, G. L. Harvard university oarsmen. *Am. Phys. Educ. Rev.* 9:115–124;362–376, 1904.

113. Montoye, H. J. Health and longevity of former athletes. W. R. Johnson and E. R. Buskirk (eds.). *Science and Medicine of Sport and Exercise,* 2nd ed. New York: Harper & Row, 1974, pp. 366–376.

114. Morgan, J. E. *University Oars, Being a Critical Enquiry into the After Health of Men Who Rowed in the Oxford and Cambridge Boat Race from the Year 1829 to 1869, Based on the Personal Experiences of the Rowers Themselves.* London: Macmillan & Co., 1873.

115. Mosso, A. *Life of Man on the High Alps.* London: T. Fisher Unwin, 1898.

116. Moyse, Y. A brief outline of some activities of the Ling physical education association. *J. Phys. Educ. [Lond]* 41:31–43, 1949.

117. Müller, N. *Von Paris bis Baden-Baden: Die Olympischen Kongresse, 1894–1981.* Niedernhausen: Schors-Verlag, 1981.

118. Myhre, L. G. David Bruce Dill: pioneer and leader in the study of physiological responses to environmental and work stresses. M. K. Yousef (ed.). *Milestones in Environmental Physiology.* The Hague: SPR Academic Publishers, 1989, pp. xviii–xii.

119. Nichols, E. H., and F. R. Richardson. Football injuries of the Harvard squad for three years under the revised rules. *Bost. Med. Surg. J.* 160:33–37, 1909.

120. Nye, R. A. *Crime, Madness and Politics in Modern France: The Medical Concept of National Decline.* Princeton, NJ: Princeton University Press, 1981.

121. Park, R. J. Concern for health and exercise as expressed in the writings of 18th century physicians and informed laymen (England, France, Switzerland). *Res. Q. Exerc. Sport* 47:756–767, 1976.

122. Park, R. J. The Research Quarterly and its antecedents. *Res. Q. Exerc. Sport* 51:1–22, 1980.

123. Park, R. J. Biological thought, athletics and the formation of a "man of character": 1830–1900. J. A. Mangan and J. Walvin (eds.). *Manliness and Morality: Middle-Class Masculinity in Britain and America, 1800–1940.* Manchester, England: Manchester University Press, 1987, pp. 7–34.

124. Park, R. J. Edward M. Hartwell and physical training at the Johns Hopkins University, 1879–1890. *J. Sport Hist.* 14:108–119, 1987.

125. Park, R. J. Athletes and their training in Britain and America, 1800–1914. J. W. Berryman and R. J. Park (eds). *Sport and Exercise Science: Essays in the History of Sports Medicine.* Urbana, IL: University of Illinois Press, 1992, pp. 57–107.

126. Park, R. J. Physiologists, physicians, and physical educators: 19th century biology and exercise, *hygienic* and *educative.* J. W. Berryman and R. J. Park (eds.). *Sport and Exercise Science: Essays in the History of Sports Medicine.* Urbana, IL: University of Illinois Press, 1992, pp. 137–181.

127. Park, R. J. The rise and demise of Harvard's B. S. program in anatomy, physiology, and physical training: a case of conflicts of interest and scarce resources. *Res. Q. Exerc. Sport* 63:1–15, 1992.

128. Parry, N. A. Pioneers of physical education in the 19th century: Mr. Alexander Alexander. *Phys. Educ. Rev. [Lond]* 2:11–24, 1979.

129. Pavy, F. W. *A Treatise on Food and Dietetics, Physiologically and Therapeutically Considered.* Philadelphia: Henry C. Lea, 1874.

130. Peterson, M. J. *The Medical Profession in Mid-Victorian London.* Berkeley, CA: University of California Press, 1978.

131. Physical Education Association of Great Britain and Northern Ireland. *The Physical Education Year Book, 1966–67.* London: Ling House, 1966.

132. Porter, W. T. The growth of St. Louis children. *Transact. Acad. Sci. St. Louis.* 6:263–380, 1894.

133. Quanz, D. R. The impact of North American sport on the Olympic movement in Germany and Austria-Hungary. R. Naul (ed.). *Turnen and Sport: The Cross-Cultural Exchange.* Munster, Germany: Waxmann Verlag, 1991, pp. 147–163.

134. Rabinbach, A. *The Human Motor: Energy, Fatigue and the Origins of Modernity.* Berkeley, CA: University of California Press, 1990.

135. Report of the 1st *national* convention of the A.A.A.P.E., April 4, 5, and 6, 1899. *Am. Phys. Educ. Rev.* 4:139–244, 1899.

136. Richardson, B. W. *Diseases of Modern Life.* New York: D. Appleton & Co., 1876.

137. Rous, S. Foreword. S. S. Knight. *Fitness and Injury in Sport: Care, Diagnosis and Treatment by Physical Means.* New York: Van Nostrand Co., 1953, p. ix.

138. Ryan, A. J. History of the development of sport science and medicine. L. A. Larson (ed.). *Encyclopedia of Sports Sciences and Medicine.* New York: Macmillan & Co., 1971, pp. xxxiii–xlvii.

139. Sargent, D. A. The physical characteristics of the athlete. *Scribner's* 2:541–561, 1887.

140. Savage, W. L. Physiological and pathological effects of severe exercise (the marathon race). *Am. Phys. Educ. Rev.* 15:651–661, 1910.

141. Schmidt, F. A. *Unser Körper: Handbuch der Anatomie, Physiologie und Hygiene der Leibesübungen.* Leipzig, Germany: Voigtländer Verlag, 1909.

142. Schmidt, F. A., and E. H. Miles. *The Training of the Body for Games, Athletics, Gymnastics, and Other Forms of Exercise and for Health, Growth, and Development.* London: Swan Sonneschein & Co., 1901.

143. Schneider, E. C. *Physiology of Muscular Activity.* Philadelphia: W. B. Saunders, 1933.

144. School athletics and boys' races. *Br. Med. J.* 2:890–891, 1909.

145. Simon, J. L'éducation. *Réforme Sociale* 12:676–688, 1887.

146. Sinclair, J. *The Code of Health and Longevity; or, a Concise View of the Principles Calculated for the Preservation of Health and the Attainment of Long Life.* Edinburgh: Arch. Constable & Co., 1807.

147. Skey, F. C. Athletics. *[London] Times,* 10 October, 1867.

148. Smith, W. D. *Stretching Their Bodies: The History of Physical Education.* Newton Abbot, England: David & Charles, 1974.

149. Sperryn, P. At last? (editorial). *Br. J. Sport Med.* 29:3, 1995.

150. Steinhaus, A. H. Chronic effects of exercise. *Physiol. Rev.* 13:103–147, 1933.

151. Storey, T. A. Department organization for the regulation of physical instruction in schools and colleges from the standpoint of hygiene. *Science* 29:527–532, 1909.

152. Sullivan, J. E. Physical culture. D. R. Francis (ed.). *The Universal Exposition of 1904.* St. Louis: Louisiana Purchase Exposition Co., 1913, pp. 57–58.

153. Thibault, J. *Sports et Éducation Physique, 1870–1970.* Paris: Librairie Philosophique J. Vrin, 1972.

154. Thörner, W. Über die Zellelemente des Blutes im Trainingszustand. Untersuchung an Olympiakämpfern in Amsterdam. *Arbeitsphysiologie* 2:116–128, 1929.

155. Tissié, P. A. *La Fatigue et L'Entraînment Physique,* 2nd ed. Paris: F. Alcan, 1903.

156. Tissé, P. A. L'évolution de l'éducation physique en France et en Belgique (1900–1910). *Revue Jeux Scolaires d'Hygiene Sociale* 20:162–166, 1910.

157. Tittel, K. Der deutsche beitrag zur internationalen sportmedizin. K.Tittel, K. H. Arndt and W. Hollmann (eds.). *Sportmedizin: Gestern-Heute-Morgen. Bericht von Jubiläum-symposium des Deutschen Sportärztebundes, Oberhof, 25. bis 27. September 1992.* Leipzig/Berlin/Heidelberg, 1993, pp. 31–42.

158. Tolleneer, J. Gymnastics and religion in Belgium, 1892–1914. *Inter. J. Hist. Sport.* 7:335–347, 1990.

159. Ueberhorst, H. *Sport in Deutschland: Von Turnvater Jahn bis zur Gegenwart.* Dresdner Bank AG, 1991.

160. Ulmann, J. *De la Gymnastique aux Sports Modernes: Histoire des Doctrines de l'Éducation Physique.* Paris: Librairie Philosophique J. Vrin, 1971.

161. Ward, M. P., J. S. Milledge and J. B. West. (eds.). *High Altitude Medicine and Physiology,* 2nd ed. London: Chapman & Hall Medical, 1995.

162. Weber, E. Pierre de Coubertin and the introduction of organized sport in France. *J. Contemp. Hist.* 5:3–26, 1970.

163. Weber, E. *France, Fin de Siècle.* Cambridge, MA: Harvard University Press, 1986, p. 217.

164. Weissbein, S. *Hygiene des Sports: Bibliothek für Sport und Spiel.* Leipzig, Germany: Grethlein & Co., 1911, 2 vols.

165. Weissbein, S., and E. R. Halle. *Bibliographie des Gesamten Sports: Herausgeben von der Internationalen Hygiene-Ausstellung Dresden 1911.* Leipzig, Germany: Verlag von Veit, 1911.

166. Wey, H. D. *Physical and Industrial Training of Criminals.* New York: Industrial Education Association, 1888.
167. White, W. J. A physician's view of exercise and athletics. *Lippencott's Mag.* 39:1008–1033, 1887.
168. Whorton, J. C. Athlete's heart: the medical debate over athleticism, 1870–1920. *J. Sport Hist.* 9:30–52, 1982.
169. Williams, H., and H. D. Arnold. The effects of violent and prolonged muscular exercise upon the heart. *Phila. Med. J.* June 3:1233–1239, 1899.
170. Wolffe, J. B. Future basic research: relating physical education to sports medicine. *59th Annual Proceedings of the College Physical Education Association,* Dayton Beach, FL, 1956, pp. 115–125.
171. Woodgate, W. B. *"Oars and Sculls," and How to Use Them.* London: George Bell & Sons, 1875, p. 148.
172. Zoro, J. *Images de 150 Ans d'E.P.S.: L'Éducation Physique et Sportive a l'École, en France.* Paris: Verdier, 1986.

7
Bone, Exercise, and Stress Fractures

DAVID B. BURR, Ph.D.

EPIDEMIOLOGY OF STRESS FRACTURES

Stress fractures are nontraumatic bone fractures caused by repeated application of loads below the fracture threshold, i.e., they are fatigue fractures. They occur in a variety of skeletal locations (femur, tibia, metarsals, and calcaneus, among others) commonly in physically active individuals (e.g., joggers, soldiers, and ballet dancers). Stress fractures are ranked between the second and eighth most common running injuries [4], with an incidence ranging between 4 [49] and 14.4% [80]. Seventy percent of all stress fractures are reported in runners [76]. Estimates of injury among runners may be too high, because they are based only on those runners who appear in the clinic. Also, estimates rarely include controls for workout intensity or duration, or even for the nature of the physical activity.

The incidence of stress fractures in some of the elite units of the Israeli military are reported as being between 20 and 46% [41, 73, 85, 87, 90]. In a population of 2000 Israeli paratroopers, Milgrom (personal communication) recently found an incidence of 20%.

Rates of occurrence in the U.S. military (1–4%; see ref. 58) are much lower than those reported for Israeli soldiers, although stress fractures still account for more lost duty days among women in the U.S. Army than any other overuse injury [145]. The discrepancy in occurrence in the two military populations may have more to do with the manner in which stress fractures are detected and diagnosed than with inherent differences in the rigor of the training programs [60]. The Israelis diagnose stress fractures based primarily on scintigraphy, whereas the U.S. military relies more heavily on radiographic criteria [124, 154]. The differences in technique could account for a 5-fold higher incidence in the Israeli military, as compared to that in U.S. soldiers [50, 90]. The remaining differences in incidence (about double in the Israeli military) can be accounted for by differences in basic training programs.

Stress fractures most commonly affect the metatarsals, calcaneus, and tibia. The location of the majority of stress fractures has gradually shifted in the past 50 yr from the metatarsals as the predominant site, to the tibia [41, 60]. The incidence of tibial stress fractures in the military now constitutes between 20 [79, 144] and 72% [40, 154] of all stress fractures, whereas calcaneal stress fractures account for about 25% [53]. Tibial stress fractures account for about 50% of stress fractures in runners [55, 76, 101, 137]. They most commonly occur in the medial tibial plateau or in the distal tibial diaphysis [41, 94], the latter at the junction between the middle and distal thirds of the tibia [31, 124]. The tibia is also the most common site for multiple stress fractures, showing an incidence of 1.5 fractures per affected soldier [41].

The location of fracture may vary, depending on the precise activity. For example, metatarsal stress fractures are more common in ballet dancers [36], whereas tibial stress fractures are common among runners [3, 6, 26, 54, 76, 81, 102, 103, 137, 140] and soldiers [40, 41, 46, 50, 73, 87, 90, 91], although some reports from U.S. forces show that stress fractures of the metatarsals and calcaneus may be at least as common [8, 110]. Metatarsal stress fractures account for fewer of the total number of fractures in women than in men [110, 122].

Stress fractures occur early after the onset of training [41, 46, 90]. Rates of occurrence are generally elevated by the second [43, 122, 146] or third [38, 64, 134] wk of training, although there are reports of peak incidence from 5 to 8 wk [40, 112] after the onset of training. Time of onset may differ slightly between men and women. Pester and Smith [110] reported peaks in men during the 2nd and 4th wk after the beginning of training, whereas stress fractures reported in women are elevated in each of the first 3 wk of training.

RISK FACTORS

Many factors have been reported to be associated with the risk of stress fracture. These can be grouped into several general categories of factors, including: demographic (age, gender, race); biomechanical (hip rotation, knee valgus, pelvic width, bone geometry), physical condition (poor strength and flexibility, previous physical activity, aerobic fitness), and factors related to bone density (weight, family history of osteoporosis, low calcium intake, smoking, age at menarche, amenorrhea). It is not the intention here to review all risk factors for stress fractures, but several important risk factors can be identified.

Physical Activity

There are numerous reports that poor physical conditioning is a risk factor for stress fracture [26, 43, 46, 53, 56, 65], but it is problematic as to whether previous physical activity and improved physical fitness actually can reduce the risk for stress fracture. Reports conflict, and most are poorly controlled or rely on self-reporting for prior physical activity [139], rather than on a

TABLE 7.1.
Physical Activity and Stress Fracture Risk

| | Stress Fracture Risk (%) | | |
| | Gardner et al.[b] | Jones et al.[c] | |
Level of Previous Activity[a]	Male	Male	Female
Very active	0.6	3.4	30.7
Active	0.9	15.7	33.3
Average	1.6	35.1	29.7
Below average/inactive	14.2	42.9	30.0

[a]Based on self-reports.
[b]Data are from ref. 39.
[c]Data are from ref. 60, which includes all exercise-related injuries.

standardized physical fitness test before the exercise has started. Barrow and Saha [5] reported only one-half of the prevalence of stress fractures in runners that run regularly (29%), as compared to those that are very irregular runners (49%).

The incidence of stress fractures in U.S. soldiers is higher among those without previous jogging experience [38, 43, 46, 53], although the intensity of the previous physical activity in soldiers who failed to develop a stress fracture is not reported. Garcia et al. [38] report that 72% of the soldiers diagnosed with a stress fracture had no previous running experience, but they do not report how many soldiers who failed to present with a fracture also had no running experience.

In a study of 310 male and female army trainees in which fitness was measured by a battery of tests, including a mile run, push-ups, and sit-ups, Jones et al. [59] found an association between slower mile run times and increased risk for an exercise-related injury in both men and women. The risk of an overuse injury increased as self-assessed activity decreased in men, but there was no relationship between activity levels and injury risk in women. This study reported all overuse injuries, so the specific risk for developing a stress fracture is not reported. However, Gardner et al. [39] found a similar association of physical activity before basic training and stress fracture risk (Table 7.1). Recruits reporting themselves as inactive or below average were nearly nine times more likely to present with a stress fracture, compared to those with average or above-average activity levels.

In the largest study in which physical activity was assessed, 295 infantry recruits between 18 and 20 years old were observed over a 14-wk elite basic training course. No association was found between aerobic physical fitness or pretraining physical activities and risk of later developing a stress fracture [138]. In a separate study of 279 recruits, 31% of the soldiers presented with stress fractures, regardless of whether they had participated in sports before basic training [41]. In a subpopulation that included only runners, no association was found between the distance run each week and stress fracture incidence. Prior physical activity does not seem to explain the occurrence of stress fractures, which is consistent with the observation that stress fractures occur often in those who have been training for years [16].

Age

Age is probably a risk factor for stress fractures in both men and women, but whether stress fractures increase or decrease in older subjects is controversial. Again, the difficulty is quantifying the amount and intensity of activity in different-aged populations.

In a very small sample of women (six runners reporting a history of stress fracture in the tibia and femur and eight runners with no history of fracture), women reporting stress fractures were significantly ($P < 0.05$) younger than those without a history of stress fracture (26.9 vs. 32.8 yr), even though bone mineral density (BMD) in the stress fracture group was greater than that in the nonstress fracture group [48]. Even though the sample was small, the data support the hypothesis that age is a factor contributing to stress fracture incidence, even in the presence of greater overall bone mass.

Based on self-reports from more than 2000 active duty Army women, Friedl et al. [35] found stress fracture prevalence of 19.6% in women 22–23 yr old but 1.4% for women over the age of 40. Stress fracture incidence between the ages of 18 and 34 was consistently between 15 and 20% but fell rapidly to about 5% by age 38. Although the covariate effects of menstrual history, smoking, ethnic origin, and family history were controlled in this study, it did not account for the change in physical activity among women of these different age groups. Therefore, the effect could have been partly the result of reduced physical activity in the older groups.

In a large prospective study of 783 Israeli military recruits between the ages of 17 and 26, Milgrom et al. [89] reported that recruits more than 20 yr old had only a 2.9% incidence of stress fracture, whereas those recruits younger than 20 had an incidence of 26%. Moreover, each year of increased age above 17 yr reduced the risk of a stress fracture by 28%. This is interesting in light of the observation that bone density increases to a maximum between 20 and 30 yr of age [45, 78, 119], and strength would be expected to increase commensurately [24, 29, 27, 131].

This is in direct contrast to data reported from American Marines [39] in whom stress fracture incidence in recruits older than 21 was nearly double that in recruits younger than 20. It is also at odds with data generated from athletes (runners) or from other American military recruits, which show an increase from about 1% between the ages of 17 and 22, to more than 5% between the ages of 29 and 34 [8]. Increased incidence with age occurred in both men and women. Jones et al. [59] showed a higher incidence of overuse injuries of all kinds in men over the age of 23 but did not present data on stress fractures alone. Hulkko and Orava [54] showed a greater stress fracture incidence in athletes between the ages of 20 and 29 than in those of age 19 yr or less. However, they also showed that 40% of all stress fractures in athletes occurred between the ages of 16 and 19, with 78% occurring before the age of 30. Similar data were presented by Orava et al. [102]. However, in neither study was the incidence or prevalence of stress fractures within each age range given, so the age-adjusted risk for stress fracture cannot be determined from these studies.

Gender

Gender is a clear risk factor for the occurrence of stress fractures [8, 39, 53, 58, 60, 70, 86, 96, 107, 112, 113, 122, 140], although the role of gender may not be entirely independent of density. Kowal [64] reported that femoral and tibial stress fractures comprised one third of all musculoskeletal injuries in a group of women undergoing an 8-wk basic training endurance exercise program. Women's smaller body size, lower peak bone density, and tendency to develop menstrual irregularities or even amenorrhea with strenuous and prolonged exercise may be predisposing factors for the occurrence of fracture.

Some studies that suggest that women are more prone to injury than men have not normalized the incidence of injury by using the numbers of male and female runners in the population [56, 104]. Comparisons of men and women undergoing training in the armed forces indicate that rates are much higher in women than in men, although this may be because of a lack of prior physical conditioning and generally lower fitness [4].

In the U.S. Armed Forces, the risk of developing a stress fracture in women is 5–10 times that in men [8, 112, 122], and they may occur earlier [8, 110]. Although the incidence of stress fractures in male soldiers in the U.S. military is reported between 0.9% [8, 51, 110] and 4.8% [134] (mean, 1.8%), that in women in the U.S. military varies between 1.1% [110] and 21% [64] (mean, 9.6%), even with equivalent training regimens [60]. However, these numbers combine racial groups; the relatively low value of 3.4% reported by Brudvig et al. [8] for stress fracture incidence in women, for instance, is increased to 11.83% when only white women are considered. Zernicke et al. [152] report a slightly higher incidence of stress fracture (20–25%) in female collegiate distance runners.

Density

Physical activity can build or maintain bone mass [34]. Greater bone density is positively and exponentially correlated to greater bone strength [27,

28] and stiffness [24, 131]. It is reasonable to conclude from this that greater bone density would reduce the risk for stress fracture.

Some data do, in fact, support this conclusion. Using 50 athletes, one-half of whom had stress fractures and one-half of whom did not and who were matched for sex, age, weight, height, and exercise history, Myburgh et al. [95] found that those with stress fractures had significantly lower bone density in the spine, femoral neck, Ward's triangle, and greater trochanter. However, women in the stress fracture group ($n = 19$ of 25) had a lower calcium intake and lower oral contraceptive use than women in the control group. Moreover, the menstrual status of the women in the stress fracture group was not reported. It is well known that women who are amenorrheic have a higher incidence of stress fractures than that of eumenorrheic women [5, 17, 26, 69]. Pouilles et al. [111] also showed lower BMD in the femoral neck, Ward's triangle, and greater trochanter in 41 military recruits with stress fractures, compared to that of 48 recruits matched for age, height, and weight who did not have fractures.

Grimston et al. [48] found no differences in tibial BMD between runners reporting stress fractures and those without symptoms, even though 7 of the 10 stress fractures reported were localized to the tibia. Although this was an extremely small sample, it is notable that the stress fracture group of women was significantly ($P < 0.05$) younger than that without a history of stress fracture (26.9 vs. 32.8 yr). When age is used as a covariate, BMD in the stress fracture group was greater than that in the nonstress fracture group. These data do not support the hypothesis of a close relationship between low bone density and stress fracture but do support the concept that age is a factor contributing to stress fracture incidence.

In a group of female athletes matched for age, as well as height and weight, Carbon et al. [17] found no significant difference in BMD between women with a stress fracture and those without a stress fracture. Although the authors conclude that bone density does not contribute to the risk for stress fracture, the sample was small, and BMD measurements were not taken at locations where stress fractures occurred. Giladi et al. [41] reported no significant association between tibial bone density and stress fractures at any site ($P > 0.1$) in a study of 295 Israeli military recruits.

Although low bone density can increase the risk for a stress fracture, as demonstrated by irregularly cycling women with low bone mass, stress fracture incidence cannot be explained on this basis in a population in which bone density is within normal limits.

Race

The risk of developing a stress fracture in the U.S. Army is 8.5 times greater for a white woman (11.83%) than for a black woman (1.39%) and about 2.5–4.5 times greater for a white man (1.07–1.56%) than for a black man (0.23–0.60%) [8, 39]. Based on self-reports from more than 2000 active

Army women, 18.5% of white and Asian women reported a history of stress fracture, whereas only 11.3% of black women reported similarly (*P* < 0.001) [35].

Although the data conclusively demonstrate that blacks are less likely to develop stress fractures, this effect is probably not independent of bone mass. It is well known that blacks have higher bone mass and slower turnover than whites [62, 67]. None of the studies demonstrating an effect of ethnicity used bone mass as a covariate in the analysis.

Geometry

Tibial geometry constitutes a risk factor for tibial stress fractures [42, 91]. Tibial width is significantly correlated to stress fracture incidence [42], but the cross-sectional moment of inertia about the anteroposterior axis of bending (IAP), an estimate of bending rigidity, is an even better indicator of risk [91]. Thirty-one percent of recruits with a "low" IAP presented with tibial stress fractures, whereas only 14% of recruits with a "high" IAP presented. No correlation was found between bone mineral content or cortical width of the site and stress fracture [42, 73], although some have proposed that reduced bone mineral content does constitute a risk factor [111, 128]. Shear stresses caused by bending are likely to be a significant causative factor for stress fractures [91, 128], but there are no reported studies in humans comparing the in vivo magnitude or distribution of shear strains to variables that determine stress fracture risk.

ETIOLOGY OF STRESS FRACTURES

Role of Repetitive Loading

It is generally conceded that stress fractures are overuse injuries [7, 74, 77, 136, 139] that result when the skeleton fails to respond quickly enough to stresses and strains imposed upon it [46, 128]. They may be more common when bones are repetitively loaded above a certain stress or strain threshold [97–99], but the kind and magnitude of stress required are not known. The risk of developing a stress fracture increases with greater weekly running mileage [56, 63], suggesting that repetitive loads play some role in the pathogenesis.

Stress fractures can be induced in the tibial diaphysis of an animal model by the repeated application of nontraumatic loads [12]. In this model, the right hindlimb of rabbits is placed in a splint that prevents the contraction of the gastrocnemius and impairs its ability to attenuate tensile loads caused by bending. Skeletally mature rabbits are loaded impulsively at 1 Hz for 40 min/day, 5 days/wk for up to 9 wk. Loads are adjusted to 1.5 times body weight, although because of soft tissue attenuation, loads on the distal tibia are only about 1 times body weight. This loading protocol applies about

FIGURE 7.1.

99mTc scintigram showing the location of the distal stress fracture site in the rabbit model (arrows). This site corresponds to the site of high shear and compressive stresses in the finite element model shown in Figure 7.4.

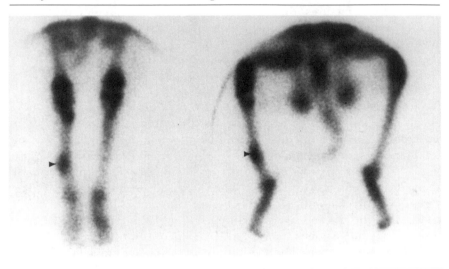

12,000 load cycles/wk at a load equivalent to loads placed on the lower limbs during walking. Within 6 wk, 90% of the animals show scintigraphic or radiographic evidence of a stress fracture in the distal tibia (Fig. 7.1).

Mechanical testing of devitalized bone shows that bone can fail with very few loading cycles when tensile strains are large. Bone may fail within 10^3–10^5 loading cycles at strain ranges of 5,000–10,000 microstrain [20, 21]. Loading in unaxial tension at 3000 microstrain causes bone to fail within 10^6 cycles [18–21]. Strains on the craniomedial cortex of the tibia of rabbits loaded impulsively average about −733 (±233) microstrain, whereas those on the craniolateral cortex average 822 (±428) microstrain (Table 7.2). These strains are much too low to be the sole cause for stress fractures.

Measurements of strain in the human tibia in vivo at a site known to be at risk for stress fracture [13] show that principal compressive strain, even during strenuous physical activities, ranges from −414 microstrain (downhill walk) to −1226 microstrain (zigzag run uphill); principal tensile strain ranges from 381 microstrain (walking on a level surface with a 17-kg pack) to 743 microstrain (zigzag run uphill). Maximum shear strains were greatest for the uphill and downhill zigzag run, reaching nearly 2000 microstrain in each case (Fig. 7.2). Shear strains during sprinting on a level surface were nearly double those during walking with or without a pack (1583 vs. 770 and 871 microstrain). These data show that strains can double or

TABLE 7.2.
Experimentally Measured Strains[a] and Strain Rates

Gauge Location	Principle Strain (microstrain)	Shear Strain (microstrain)	Strain Rate (Shear) (microstrain/s)
Stress fracture site			
Craniomedial	−733 (233)[b]	−426 (358)	6083 (1941)[c]
Craniolateral	822 (428)[b]	−459 (383)	5076 (2592)
Posterior	677 (345)[d]	−478 (285)[b]	5862 (3625)[b]
Tibial midshaft			
Medial	−521 (293)	−345 (374)	3933 (1904)
Lateral	490 (280)	−258 (188)	3338 (2356)
Posterior	270 (66)	−253 (118)	3039 (845)

[a]Strains at stress fracture site larger than strains at tibial midshaft (one-tailed *t* test: [b]$P < 0.05$; [c]$P < 0.01$; [d]$P < 0.005$.

triple during vigorous exercise, compared to those generated in the tibia during walking.

Strains measured on the human tibia during walking show that strains generated at this site are well below the fracture threshold, even during running. Based on cyclic load to failure studies [20, 21] and linearly extrapolating to the range of strains measured in the human tibia, stress fractures should not occur at this stress fracture site for about 10^6 cycles, if failure is caused solely by the repetitive application of load. In real terms, this means that a person would have to perform vigorous activities, such as running for about 1000 miles before bone failure is likely to occur [71]. However, the relationship between the number of loading cycles and failure in bone at a given strain is not linear [106]. Tensile fatigue tests on primary and Haversian bone at 1500 microstrain, similar to the magnitude of strain measured in the human tibia, and strain rates similar to those developed during running [127] show that healthy bone does not fail in tension by fatigue, defined as a 30% loss of stiffness, even after 37 million loading cycles [133] (Fig. 7.3). (Note that subsequent tests showed that bone would not fail for at least 45 million cycles) Yet, stress fractures occur with repeated high-strain loading, suggesting that momentary high strains or strain rates may occur during more vigorous activities, or that factors in addition to repetitive loading, contribute to pathogenesis (e.g., locally high stresses, muscular fatigue or loss of coordination, high-impact loads, or interactions with the remodeling system).

Role of Shear Strain

Milgrom et al. [91] hypothesized that stress fractures occur in regions in which high bending loads are found. This makes bending stress causal and suggests that noninvasive measures of bending rigidity may be one way to

FIGURE 7.2.

Peak engineering shear stains generated on the human tibial midshaft during various activities. Five gait cycles were averaged. In all cases, strains were less than 2,000 microstrain. Error bars represent standard deviations. Reproduced from ref. 15, with permission from Pergamon Press.

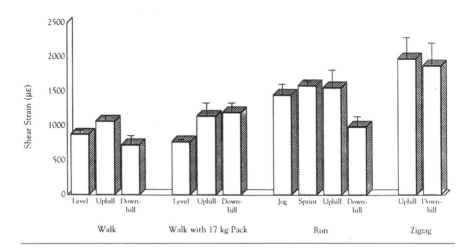

assess risk for fracture. Large bending stresses can create high-shear strains in bone, suggesting the possiblity that it is shear that leads to bone failure.

A finite element analysis (FEA) of experimentally produced tibial stress fractures in a rabbit model of stress fractures [12] predicts locally high-shear and compressive stresses on the anterior cortex of the distal one-third of the rabbit tibia, in the identical location that stress fractures occur (Fig. 7.4; Table 7.2). The correspondence between the location of stress fractures in the experimental model and the prediction by FEA of locally high-shear stresses at this location suggest, in combination, that focal pockets of high-shear stress applied at high rates may contribute to fracture risk.

Experiments in which strain was measured in the human tibia in vivo [13] show compressive and shear strains, and strain rates can double or triple during vigorous activity, compared to walking at a comfortable speed. Strain gauges were applied at the location in which Israeli military recruits develop symptoms of a stress fracture [41]. The result implies an association between elevation of strain magnitude or rate and subsequent development of a stress fracture.

These data are consistent with the hypothesis that stress fractures occur

FIGURE 7.3.

Fatigue-induced modulus decreases vs. number of loading cycles. When bone is loaded in uniaxial tension at physiological strains (1200–1500 microstrain) and strain rates (0.03/s), there is a rapid stiffness loss to about 3 million cycles, after which no further stiffness loss is observed, at least up to 37 million cycles. Data points represent means for the percentage of original specimen modulus; error bars represent standard deviations. Adapted from ref. 133, with permission from Pergamon Press.

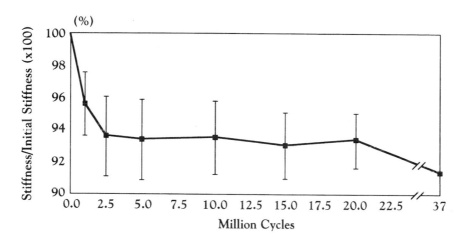

in regions where high bending stresses are found [91]. Shear produced by bending forces is a significant component of the strain induced by normal loading events [129]. Because of varying loading conditions and the complex geometry of the tibia, shear stresses may not be uniform but may be concentrated in specific regions, as the rabbit model suggests. The absolute magnitude of shear strains measured both in the animal model and in humans is low when compared to the fracture strain, however, and may be too low to account for the occurrence of fracture with so few loading cycles.

Bone is generally weak in shear (Table 7.3) [33, 120, 121, 150]. Its transverse breaking strength in shear is similar to that in tension (about 69 mega Pascals (MPa)), which is about one-half of its compressive strength [120, 121]. However, cortical bone shear strength in the longitudinal direction is only about 25% of its strength in tension or transverse shear (17 MPa). Therefore, even relatively small shear stresses may place some bone cortices dangerously close to failure and raises the possibility that shear stresses caused by bending may be partly responsible for some stress fractures.

FIGURE 7.4.

Contour plots of Tresca stress on the anterior cortex of the rabbit tibia. Four of the rabbits for which models were built are shown. The scale is given in MPa. The high shear stress concentrations (> 25 MPa) on the anterior aspect of the distal tibia range from 5 to 30% of tibial length from the distal end, coincident with the region where rabbits presented with stress fractures (see Fig. 7.1).

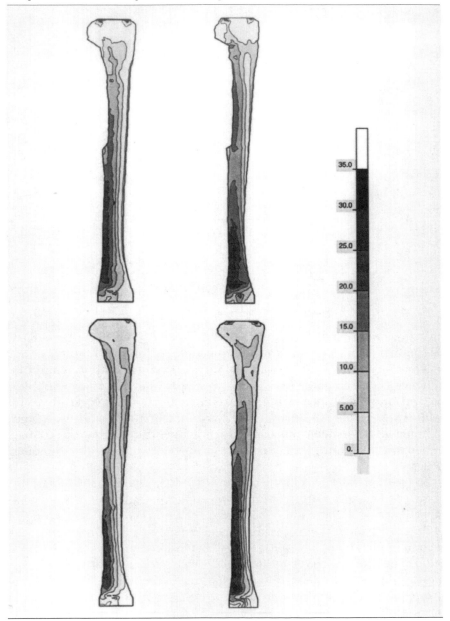

TABLE 7.3.
Bone Strength in Compression, Tension, and Shear

	Transverse Breaking Strength[a]	Longitudinal Breaking Strength[a]
Compression	133 MPa	193 MPa
Tension	51 MPa	133 MPa
Torsion	58 MPa	
Pure shear[b]	62 MPa (Iosepescu)	18 MPa (Arcan)

[a]Data on breaking strength in compression, tension, and torsion from refs. 120 and 121.
[b]Pure shear tests are from quasistatic tests of human femoral midshaft; $n = 12$ in each direction. Pure shear tests in the transverse direction used Iosepescu specimens; those in the longitudinal direction used Arcan specimens. This was necessary because of geometric constraints.

Rules of Musculoskeletal Patterning and Fatigue

During mechanical loading, bones are subject to bending strain [127]. Increased bending of bone causes increased tension and shear, because bending is a combination of compression and tension. Bone is weak in tension and shear [120, 121] and is in the greatest danger of fracturing from high-tensile and shear strains. When muscles on the tensile side of a bone contract, the compression they generate reduces tensile strains [116]. This also reduces shear stress.

Muscles also may dissipate dynamic forces generated in the skeleton by eccentric contraction [52, 83, 108, 109, 115]. They reduce strain rate by absorbing impact energy during movement. Force transients of 5–10 g are produced at heelstrike [68, 108, 135]. These transients send shock waves through the entire skeleton [142, 143, 147, 148]. The leg muscles decelerate the limb before heelstrike [55] and attenuate potentially large ground reaction forces [99, 115, 117, 118]. The time for this reflexive energy-dissipating action of muscles is quick, between 75 and 100 ms [84, 114]. Altered neuromuscular function, such as occurs with muscular fatigue, may slow muscle reaction or otherwise prevent this normal damping mechanism. The transfer of mechanical energy between the eccentric and concentric phases of muscle contraction is reduced during muscular fatigue [44], making the muscle less capable of dissipating impact energy. The absence of appropriate muscle contraction increases the magnitude and rate of application of ground reaction forces at heelstrike [115, 117, 118], and has been linked to the increased risk of fracture in elderly subjects [1, 2, 47, 130].

Clinical observations indicate that stress fractures [32, 63] and other overuse injuries [125, 126] occur most often after muscular fatigue, or with an abrupt change in the normal training routine [26, 56, 81, 82], when the capacity of muscles to protect bone from excessive overloads is compromised. Subjects who have suffered a previous stress fracture produce significantly greater vertical ground reaction and propulsive forces on impact than subjects who have not [48], although whether the greater ground reaction forces were the cause or are the result of the stress fracture is unknown.

It is possible that muscle fatigue, or a change in muscle recruitment patterns associated with fatigue, can increase strain magnitude or rate on a bone significantly. Using a canine model, Yoshikawa et al. [154] showed that muscle fatigue (measured by a shift to lower median electromyogram (EMG) frequencies) was associated with increased peak principal and shear strains on the tibia. Bone strain increased when muscles became fatigued but did not increase when muscles failed to become fatigued. Shear strains increased at a greater rate after muscle fatigue than did either principal tensile or compressive strains. Just as importantly, the *distribution* of strain within the tibia changed.

The magnitude of these changes after fatigue is consistent with those found in human studies. Muscular fatigue leads to a 50% increase in tibial acceleration [141]. This is probably related to an inability of the fatigued muscles to control knee extension and flexion in a way that attenuates impact at heelstrike. Knee extensor/flexor muscle activity is delayed after muscular fatigue. Knee flexion tends to occur earlier [100], reducing stride rate [25] and increasing the amplitude of the heelstrike impact [141]. This increases peak vertical ground reaction forces by about 25% (from 2.35 body weight (BW) to 2.97 BW) [100].

In vivo strain measurements made on seven male subjects between the ages of 23 and 50 yr at a site known to commonly undergo stress fracture indicate that the nature of the change in bone strain after fatigue may vary with age [37]. The subjects walked at 5 km/hr on a treadmill while prefatigue strains were collected for 20 s. Subjects then participated in a 2-hr session of strenuous outdoor exercise that included rapid walking, running up and down hills, and stair climbing. After the outdoor exercise, subjects ran on the treadmill at 11 km/hr until exhausted while muscle activity was monitored using EMG. Strains were measured immediately postfatigue while the subject walked on the treadmill at 5 km/hr.

After fatiguing exercise, tibial strain rates *increased* in younger subjects but *decreased* in older subjects, whereas strain magnitude was *unchanged* in younger subjects but *increased* in older subjects. These data are consistent with previous studies that have examined the effects of age [89] and strain rate [10, 88]. They suggest that (a) the age dependence of stress fracture may result from the age dependency of changes in strain and strain rate after fatiguing exercise and (b) strain rate rather than strain magnitude is implicated in the etiology of stress fracture in subjects younger than 35 yr of age.

Role of Strain Rate and Impact

These data show that alterations in musculoskeletal patterning, coordination, or muscle force production can have a significant effect on the mechanical stimulus to bone. Carter [20, 21] showed that bone fails quickly at strains and strain rates above those normally generated during activities of daily living. Because of the nonlinear relationship among strain magnitude, microdamage accumulation, and bone failure [14, 20, 21, 23], any increase in strain magnitude or rate caused by a reduction of muscular protective reflexes can reduce bone's fatigue life exponentially.

Indeed, high-impact activities generally will be associated with stress fractures. Increased time spent running on concrete or other hard surfaces is correlated with a higher incidence of stress fractures [56]. Because bone is a viscoelastic material, higher loading rates may increase its elastic modulus and material stress [149]. This is correlated with decreased fatigue resistance of compact bone [61, 72, 132]. Relatively few studies have specifically examined the effects of high strain rates on the development of stress fractures. However, measurements at the stress fracture site in the rabbit model show that average shear strain rates on all tibial cortices were >50% higher at the stress fracture site than at midshaft (Table 7.2) [12].

Strain rates can double or triple in the human tibia during strenuous physical activity, reaching 50,000/s. Because these measurements were made at a site at risk for stress fracture, this implies an association between the elevation of strain rate and subsequent development of a stress fracture. Although these strain rates are higher than those previously recorded in humans [66], they are still within the range of strain rates reported for running horses [30] and dogs [127], which can range up to 80,000/s.

However, *if* strain rate is implicated, it may be possible to reduce the risk of a stress fracture through a modification of the training regimen or through the proper use of orthotics. Military training programs that have attempted to eliminate continuous high-impact activities have resulted in a 13% decrease in stress fracture incidence (7% in women and 16% in men) [46]. A randomized prospective study of different types of orthotics on stress fracture incidence in elite infantry recruits ($n = 410$) showed that orthotics could reduce stress fracture incidence to less than one-half of that without orthotics (C. Milgrom and A. Finestone, personal communication). In this case, the use of custom polypropylene modules with neutral rearfoot posts, or with neutral hindfoot posts molded of Pelite reduces stress fracture incidence from 33 to 15%.

This study indicates that a custom-molded orthotically fabricated from a neutral subtalar position, either fabricated from a semirigid or soft material, can significantly lower the incidence of stress fracture. Whether protection afforded by orthotics is the result of a reduction in strain magnitude or rate is not known. However, among athletes at high risk for stress fracture, a polypropylene or Pelite orthotic with neutral hindfoot posts fabricated from neutral subtalar position casts may be warranted.

BIOLOGICAL BASIS FOR STRESS FRACTURES—PATHOGENESIS

The data imply that muscular fatigue may lead to a situation in which locally high shear stresses or impact strains are elevated to the point at which stress fractures can occur but also suggest an interaction with biological processes. Two hypotheses about the pathophysiology of stress fractures are prevalent.

One hypothesis proposes that stress fractures are solely a mechanical result of repeated large-magnitude loads on the bone, i.e., many loading cycles will lead to fatigue failure of the structure. This seems unlikely in view of recent in vivo strain data on the human tibia, which show that strains at a stress fracture site rarely or never exceed 2000 microstrain. Even given the worst case scenario in which there is a linear relationship between strain magnitude and cycles to failure, bone should not fail for at least 10^6 cycles at this strain magnitude [20]. Assuming that 1000 loading cycles are placed on a bone per mile of running [71], 10^6 load cycles would be equivalent to 1000 miles of running (and more of walking). Documentation of training activities in recruits during basic training estimate that they march 70 miles and run 130 miles over 12 wk [60]. The number of loading cycles placed on the lower limb during the entire basic training period is less than 20% of that required to cause fracture solely from bone fatigue. Because we know that there is not a linear relationship between strain magnitude and cycles to failure [133] and that at strains of 2500 microstrain exponentially more cycles are required to cause failure than at 2000 microstrain [106], the discrepancy between the actual training intensity or duration and the fracture threshold is likely to be much greater than this. The majority of fractures occur between 3 and 7 wk in the training regime, when even fewer cycles have been placed on the skeleton, making it even less plausible that loading alone is the cause for stress fractures.

A second hypothesis views the stress fracture as positive feedback between the bone's attempt to adapt to increased strain by remodeling and the continued loading applied to the bone. In this view there is a transient reduction in bone mass caused by the acceleration of remodeling, and fracture is the result of continued repetitive loading superimposed on a significant decrease in bone mass caused by more and larger resorption spaces [57, 128]. Accelerated bone remodeling and increased skeletal fragility may be the consequence of the gradual accumulation and growth of microcracks within the bone [20–22, 24, 27, 153] and their repair [9, 11, 93]. Alternatively, accelerated remodeling may be induced by high strain levels without the introduction of obvious microdamage [15].

Positive Feedback between Loading and Bone Remodeling

It is possible that the "adaptive" response of the bone to repeated loading may accelerate the presentation of a stress fracture. Bone remodeling is strain mediated. Remodeling begins with resorption, and each time a new remodeling unit is begun, it temporarily creates a new resorption space, which increases porosity and reduces bone mass. This decreases bone stiffness and strength exponentially [24, 123, 131]. Because there is less bone to sustain loading, strains on the remaining bone increase, a new remodeling cycle can begin, and more bone is lost. Over time, this leads to a gradual loss of bone and, with repeated overuse, could eventually lead to fracture.

Martin [75] simulated the effects of positive feedback between increased porosity resulting from remodeling, damage accumulation in bone, and repetitive loading. The model showed that, as strain magnitude or the number of load cycles per day increases, a critical threshold is reached at which porosity, damage, and strain begin to grow at a rapidly accelerating rate and without limit. Although periosteal woven bone, in some instances the only radiographic evidence that a stress fracture has occurred, strengthen the bone, this new bone periosteally does not remove the instability. The model shows that porosity introduced by remodeling can contribute via a positive feedback mechanism to an unstable situation in which a stress fracture will occur.

This hypothesis has not been fully tested but is consistent with both the epidemiological and experimental data that exist. In those cases in which it is possible to know, most stress fractures begin within 3 to 7 wk after the initiation of vigorous training [38, 64, 134]. This is coincident with the period when the first phase of bone remodeling (resorption) occurs after the introduction of a higher-than-usual strain stimulus but before new bone formation would be very well established. Generally, after a change in a training regimen, the activation of new remodeling requiring the proliferation and recruitment of new cells will take 5–7 days. The resorption period follows for about 3 wk, whereas the formation phase occurs over the following 3 mo [105]. Thus, fractures occurring between 3 and 7 wk would be well into the resorption phase of bone remodeling and before formation and mineralization caused by the accelerated activity is complete.

Experimental studies with the rabbit model also suggest that positive feedback between loading and remodeling may be a feature of the pathogenesis of stress fractures in this model. Rabbits loaded for 32,400 cycles over the course of 1 day showed no biological evidence of skeletal damage (M. B. Schaffler, personal communication). Rabbits loaded for 36,000 cycles over 3 wk presented with bone microdamage and increased porosity. Eighty percent of these rabbits also have evidence of a stress fracture, and 48% of them showed severe lesions [12]. These data implicate either a damage response or a biological remodeling response, or both, via positive feedback with continued loading, in the pathogenesis of stress fractures.

CONCLUSION

Stress fractures preferentially may occur in regions of high local stress concentration created by repetitive impact loads uncontrolled by synergistic muscle action. Loading alone, at least at magnitudes consistent with normal human activity, is insufficient to cause the development of a stress fracture. It is likely that positive feedback with the normal adaptive remodeling system is a component of the pathogenesis of stress fractures. Any change in training routine, which can lead to uncontrolled remodeling in a region of stress concentration or the loss of muscle coordination, which prevents the normal attenuation of impact loads, will increase the risk for a stress fracture.

REFERENCES

1. Aniansson, A., M. Hedberg, G. Grimby, and M. Krotkiewski. Muscle morphology enzyme activity and muscle strength in elderly men and women. *Clin. Physiol.* 1:73–86 , 1981.
2. Aniansson, A., C. Setterberg, M. Hedberg, and K. G. Henriksson. Impaired muscle function with aging. A background factor in the incidence of fractures of the proximal end of the femur. *Clin. Orthop. Rel. Res.* 191:193–201, 1984.
3. Armstrong, J. R., and W. E. Tucker. *Injury in Sport: The Physiology, Prevention and Treatment of Injuries Associated with Sport.* London: Staples Press, 1964.
4. Atwater, A. E. Gender differences in distance running. P. R. Cavanagh (ed.). *Biomechanics of Distance Running.* Champaign, IL: Human Kinetics, 1990, pp. 321–362.
5. Barrow G. W., and S. Saha. Menstrual irregularity and stress fractures in collegiate female distance runners. *Am. J. Sports Med.* 16:209–216, 1988.
6. Belkin S. C. Stress fractures in athletes. *Orthop. Clin. North Am.* 11:735–741, 1980.
7. Bovens A. M. P., G. M. E. Janssen, H. G. W. Vermeer, J. H. Hoeberigs, M. P. E. Janssen, and F. T. J. Verstappen. Occurrence of running injuries in adults following a supervised training program. *Int. J. Sports Med.* 10:S186–S190, 1989.
8. Brudvig T. J. S., T. D. Gudger, and L. Obermeyer. Stress fractures in 295 trainees: a one-year study of incidence as related to age, sex, and race. *Mil. Med.* 148:666–667, 1983.
9. Burr, D. B. Remodeling and repair of fatigue damage. *Calcif. Tissue Int.* 53(suppl 1):S75–S81, 1993.
10. Burr D. B., M. R. Forwood, M. B. Schaffler, and R. D. Boyd. High strain rates are associated with stress fractures. *Trans. Orthop. Res. Soc.* 20:526, 1995.
11. Burr, D. B., R. B. Martin, M. B. Schaffler, and E. L. Radin. Bone remodeling in response to in vivo fatigue microdamage. *J. Biomech.* 18:189–200, 1985.
12. Burr, D. B., C. Milgrom, R. D. Boyd, W. L. Higgins, G. Robin, and E. L. Radin. Experimental stress fractures of the tibia. Biological and mechanical aetiology in rabbits. *J. Bone Joint Surg. Br.* 72B:370–375, 1990.
13. Burr, D. B., C. Milgrom, D. Fyhrie, et al. In vivo measurement of human tibial strains during vigorous activity. *Bone* 18:405–410, 1996.
14. Burr, D. B., C. H. Turner, P. Naick, M. R. Forwood, and R. Pidaparti. Does microdamage accumulation affect the mechanical properties of bone? *Trans. Orthop. Res. Soc.* 20:127, 1995.
15. Burr, D. B., T. Yoshikawa, and C. B. Ruff. Moderate exercise increases intracortical activation frequency in old dogs. *Trans. Orthop. Res. Soc.* 20:204, 1995.
16. Cameron, K. R., J. D. Wark, and R. D. Telford. Stress fractures and bone loss—the skeletal cost of intense athleticism? *Excel* 8:39–55, 1992.
17. Carbon R., P. N. Sambrook, V. Deakin, et al. Bone density of elite female athletes with stress fractures. *Med. J. Aust.* 153:373–376, 1990.
18. Carter, D. R., and W. E. Caler. Cycle-dependent and time-dependent bone fracture with repeated loading. *Trans. Am. Soc. Mech. Eng.* 105:166–170, 1983.
19. Carter, D. R., and W. E. Caler. A cumulative damage model for bone fracture. *J. Orthop. Res.* 3:84–90, 1985.

20. Carter, D. R., W. E. Caler, D. M. Spengler, and V. H. Frankel. Fatigue behavior of adult cortical bone: the influence of mean strain and strain range. *Acta Orthop. Scand.* 52:481–490, 1981.

21. Carter, D. R., W. E. Caler, D. M. Spengler, and V. H. Frankel. Uniaxial fatigue of human cortical bone. The influence of tissue physical characteristics. *J. Biomech.* 14:461–470, 1981.

22. Carter, D. R., and W. C. Hayes. Compact bone fatigue damage: a microscopic examination. *Clin. Orthop. Rel. Res.* 127:265–274, 1977.

23. Carter, D. R., and W. C. Hayes. Compact bone fatigue damage—I. Residual strength and stiffness. *J. Biomech.* 10:325–337, 1977.

24. Carter, D. R., and Hayes, W. C.: The compressive behavior of bone as a two-phase porous structure. *J Bone Joint Surg Br.* 59A:954–962, 1977.

25. Clarke, T. E., B. L. Cooper, C. L. Hamill, and D. E. Clark. The effect of varied stride rate upon shank deceleration in running. *J. Sports Sci.* 3:41–49, 1985.

26. Clement, D. B., J. Taunton, G. W. Smart, and K. L. McNicol. A survey of overuse running injuries. *Phys. Sports Med.* 9:47–58, 1981.

27. Currey, J. D. Effects of differences in mineralization on the mechanical properties of bone. *Philos. Trans. R. Soc. Lond. Biol.* B304:509–518, 1984.

28. Currey, J. D. The effect of porosity and mineral content on the Young's modulus of elasticity of compact bone. *J. Biomech.* 21:131–139, 1988.

29. Currey, J. D. The mechanical consequences of variation in the mineral content of bone. *J. Biomech.* 2:1–11, 1969.

30. Davies H. M. S., R. N. McCarthy, and L. B. Jeffcott. Surface strain on the dorsal metacarpus of thoroughbreds at different speeds and gaits. *Acta Anat.* 146:148–153, 1993.

31. Devas, M. B. *Stress Fractures.* London: Churchill-Livingstone, 1975.

32. Dressendorfer, R. H., C. E. Wade, J. Claybaugh, S. A. Cucinell, and G. C.Timmis. Effects of 7 successive days of unaccustomed prolonged exercise on aerobid performance and tissue damage in fitness joggers. *Int. J. Sports Med.* 12:55–61, 1991.

33. Evans, F. G. *Mechanical Properties of Bone.* Springfield, IL: Charles C Thomas, 1973.

34. Forwood, M. R., and D. B. Burr. Physical activity and bone mass: exercises in futility? *Bone Miner.* 89–112, 1993.

35. Friedl, K. E., and J. A. Nuovo. Factors associated with stress fracture in young army women: indications for further research. *Mil. Med.* 157:334–338, 1992.

36. Frusztajer, N. T., S. Dhuper, M. P. Warren, J. Brooks-Gunn, and R. P. Fox. Nutrition and the incidence of stress fractures in ballet dancers. *Am. J. Clin. Nutr.* 51:779–783, 1990.

37. Fyhrie, D. P., C. Milgrom, S. J. Hoshaw, et al. Fractional strain changes measured in vivo in humans after fatiguing exercise are age-related. *Trans. Orthop. Res. Soc.* 21:55, 1996.

38. Garcia, J. E., L. L. Grablhorn, and K. J. Franklin. Factors associated with stress fractures in military recruits. *Mil. Med.* 152:45–48, 1987.

39. Gardner, L., J. E. Dsiados, B. H. Jones, et al. Prevention of lower extremity stress fractures: a controlled trial of a shock absorbent insole. *Am. J. Public Health* 78:1563–1567, 1988.

40. Giladi M., Z. Aharonson, M. Stein, Y. L. Danon, and C. Milgrom. Unusual distribution and onset of stress fractures in soldiers. *Clin. Orthop.* 192:142–146, 1985.

41. Giladi, M., C. Milgrom, and Y. L. Danon. Stress fractures in military recruits. *Med. Corps Int.* 3:21–28, 1988.

42. Giladi, M., C. Milgrom, A. Simkin, et al. Stress fractures and tibial bone width. A risk factor. *J. Bone Joint Surg. Br.* 69B:326–329, 1987.

43. Gilbert, R. S., and H. A. Johnson. Stress fractures in military recruits—a review of twelve years' experience. *Mil. Med.* 131:716–721, 1966.

44. Gollhofer, A., P. V. Moki, M. Miyashita, and O. Aura. Fatigue during stretch-shortening cycle exercise: changes in mechanical performance of human skeletal muscle. *Int. J. Sports Med.* 8:71–78, 1987.

45. Gotfredson, A., A. Hadberg, L. Nilas, and C. Christiansen. Total bone mineral in healthy adults. *J. Lab. Clin. Med.* 10:362–368, 1987.

46. Greaney, R. B., F. H. Gerber, R. L. Laughlin, et al. Distribution and natural history of stress fractures in the U.S. Marine recruits. *Radiology* 146:339–346, 1983.
47. Grimby, G., and J. Hannerz. Firing rate and recruitment order of the extensor motor units in different modes of voluntary contraction. *J. Physiol.* 264:865–879, 1977.
48. Grimston, S. K., J. R. Engsberg Jr, R. Kloiber, and D. A. Hanley. Bone mass, external loads, and stress fracture in female runners. *Int. J. Sports Biomech.* 7:293–302, 1991.
49. Gudas, C. J. Patterns of lower-extremity injury in 224 runners. *Compr. Ther.* 6:50–59, 1980.
50. Hallel, T., S. Amit, and D. Segal. Fatigue fractures of tibial and femoral shaft in soldiers. *Clin. Orthop. Rel. Res.* 118:35–43, 1976.
51. *Health in the Army.* Fort Sam Houston, TX: Health Services Command, 1979, pp. 52–53.
52. Hill, D. B. Production and absorption of work by muscle. *Science* 131:897–903, 1962.
53. Hopson, C. N., and D. R. Perry. Stress fractures of the calcaneus in women Marine recruits. *Clin. Orthop. Rel. Res.* 128:159–162, 1977.
54. Hulkko, A., and S. Orava. Stress fractures in athletes. *Int. J. Sports Med.* 8:221–226, 1987.
55. Inman, V. T., H. J. Ralston, and F. Todd. *Human Walking.* New York: Williams & Wilkins, 1981.
56. James, S. L., B. T. Bates, and L. R. Osternig. Injuries to runners. *Am. J. Sports Med.* 6:40–50, 1978.
57. Johnson, L. C., H. T. Stradford, R. W. Geis, J. R. Dineen, and E. Kerley. Histiogenesis of stress fractures. *J. Bone Joint Surg.* 45A:1542, 1963.
58. Jones, B. H., M. W. Bovee, J. McA. Harris, and D. N. Cowan. Intrinsic risk factors for exercise-related injuries among male and female army trainees. *Am. J. Sports Med.* 21:705–710, 1993.
59. Jones, B. H., C. N. Cowan, J. P. Tomlinson, J. R. Robinson, D. W. Polly, and P. N. Frykman. Epidemiology of injuries associated with physical training among young men in the army. *Med. Sci. Sports Exerc.* 25:197–203, 1993.
60. Jones, B. H., J. McA. Harris, T. N. Vinh, and C. Rubin. Exercise-induced stress fractures and stress reactions of bone: epidemiology, etiology, and classification. *Exerc. Sport Sci. Rev.* 17:379–422, 1989.
61. Keller, T. S., J. D. Lovin, D. M. Spengler, and D. R. Carter. Fatigue of immature baboon cortical bone. *J. Biomech.* 18:297–304, 1985.
62. Kleerekoper, M., D. A. Nelson, E. L. Peterson, et al. Reference data for bone mass, calciotropic hormones, and biochemical markers of bone remodeling in older (55–75) postmenopausal white and black women. *J. Bone Joint Surg.* 9:1267–1276.
63. Koplan J. P., K. E. Powell, R. W. Shiriey, and C. C. Campbell. An epidemiologic study of the benefits and risks of running. *J. Am. Med. Assoc.* 248:3118–3121, 1979.
64. Kowal, D. M. Nature and causes of injuries in women resulting from an endurance training program. *Am. J. Sports Med.* 8:265–269, 1980.
65. Kujala, U. M., M. Kvist, K. Osterman, O. Friberg. and T. Aalto. Factors predisposing army conscripts to knee injuries incurred in a physical training program. *Clin. Orthop. Rel. Res.* 210:203–212, 1986.
66. Lanyon, L. E., W. H. J. Hampson, E. Goodship, and J. S. Shah. Bone deformation recorded in vivo from strain gauges attached to the human tibial shaft. *Acta Orthop. Scand.* 46:256–268, 1975.
67. Liel, Y., J. Edwards, J. Shary, K. M. Spicer, L. Gordon, and N. H. Bell. The effects of race and body habitus on bone mineral density of the radius, hip and spine in premenopausal women. *J. Clin. Endocrinol. Metab.* 56:30–35, 1988.
68. Light, L. H., MacClellan, G. E., and L. Klenerman. Skeletal transients on heel strike in normal walking with different footwear. *J. Biomech.* 13:477–480, 1980.
69. Lloyd, T., S. J. Triantafyllou, E. R. Baker, et al. Women athletes with menstrual irregularity have increased musculoskeletal injuries. *Med. Sci. Sports Exerc.* 18:374–379, 1986.
70. Lombardo, S. J., and D. W. Benson. Stress fractures of the femur in runners. *Am. J. Sports Med.* 10:219–227, 1982.

71. Mann, R. A. Biomechanics of running. P. P. Mack (ed.). *Symposium on the Foot and Leg in Running Sports.* St. Louis: C. V. Mosby, 1982, pp. 1–29.
72. Margel-Robertson, D., and D. C. Smith. Compressive strength of mandibular bone as a function of microstructure and strain rate. *J. Biomech.* 11:455–471, 1978.
73. Margulies, J. Y., A. Simkin, I. Leichter, et al. Effect of intense physical activity on the bone-mineral content in the lower limbs of young adults. *J. Bone Joint Surg.* 68A:1090–1093, 1986.
74. Markey, K. L. Stress fractures. *Clin. Sports Med.* 6:405–425, 1987.
75. Martin, R. B. Mathematical model for repair of fatigue damage and stress fracture in osteonal bone. *J. Orthop. Res.* 13:309–316, 1995.
76. Matheson, G. O., D. B. Clement, and D. C. McKenzie. Stress fractures in athletes: a study of 320 cases. *Am. J. Sports Med.* 15:46–58, 1987.
77. Matheson, G. O., J. G. MacIntyre, J. E. Taunton, D. B. Clement, and R. Lloyd-Smith. Musculoskeletal injuries associated with physical activity in older adults. *Med. Sci. Sports Exerc.* 21:379–385, 1989.
78. Matkovich, V. Calcium and peak bone mass. *J. Int. Med.* 231:151–160, 1992.
79. McBryde, A. M., Jr. Stress fractures in athletes. *J. Sports Med.* 3:212–217, 1975.
80. McBryde, A. M. Stress fractures in runners. R. D'Ambrosia and D. Drez (eds.). *Prevention and Treatment of Running Injuries.* Thorofare, NJ: Charles B. Slack, 1982.
81. McBryde, A. M., Jr. Stress fractures in runners. *Clin. Sports Med.* 4:737–752, 1985.
82. McKenzie, D. C., D. B. Clement, and J. E. Taunton. Running shoes, orthotics, and injuries. *Sports Med.* 2:334–347, 1985.
83. McMahon, T. *Muscles, Reflexes and Locomotion.* Princeton, NJ: University Press, 1984.
84. McMahon, T. A., and P. R. Greene. The influence of track compliance on running. *J. Biomech.* 12:893–904, 1979.
85. Meurman, K. O., and S. Elfving. Stress fractures in soldiers: a multifocal bone disorder: a comparative radiological and scintigraphic study. *Radiology* 134:483–487, 1980.
86. Micheli, L. Female runners. R. D'Ambrosia and D. Drez (eds.). *Prevention and Treatment of Running Injuries.* Thorofare, NJ: Charles B. Slack, 1982, pp. 125–134.
87. Milgrom C., R. Chisin, M. Giladi, et al. Multiple stress fractures: a longitudinal study of a soldier with 13 lesions. *Clin. Orthop. Rel. Res.* 192:174–179, 1985.
88. Milgrom C., A. Finestone, N. Shlamkovitch, et al. Prevention of overuse injuries of the foot by improved shoe shock attenuation. *Clin. Orthop. Rel. Res.* 281:189–192, 1992.
89. Milgrom C., A. Finestone, N. Shlamkovitch, et al. Youth is a risk factor for stress fracture. *J. Bone Joint Surg.* 76B:20–22, 1994.
90. Milgrom C., M. Giladi, M. Stein, et al. Stress fractures in military recruits: a prospective study showing an unusually high incidence. *J. Bone Joint Surg.* 67B:732–735, 1985.
91. Milgrom C., M. Giladi, A. Simkin, et al. The area moment of inertia of the tibia: a risk factor for stress fractures. *J. Biomech.* 22:1243–1248, 1989.
92. Mizrahi, J., and Z. Susak. Analysis of parameters affecting impact force attenuation during landing in human vertical free fall. *Eng. Med.* 11:141–147, 1982.
93. Mori S., and D. B. Burr. Increased intracortical remodeling following fatigue damage. *Bone* 14:103–109, 1993.
94. Morris, J. M., and C. D. Blickenstaff. *Fatigue Fractures: A Clinical Study.* Springfield, IL: Charles C Thomas, 1967.
95. Myburgh, K. H., J. Hutchins, A. B. B. Fataar, S. F. Hough, and T. D. Noakes. Low bone density is an etiologic factor for stress fractures in athletes. *Ann. Intern. Med.* 113:754–759, 1990.
96. Noakes, T. D., J. A. Smith, G. Lindenberg, and C. E. Wills. Pelvic stress fractures in long distance runners. *Am. J. Sports Med.* 13:120–123, 1985.
97. Nunamaker, D. M., D. M. Butterweck. Fatigue fractures in thoroughbred racehorses: relationship with age and strain. *Trans. Orthop. Res. Soc.* 12:72, 1987.
98. Nunamaker, D. M. Stress fractures and bone fatigue in racehorses. Presented at the Sun Valley International Workshop on Bone Biology, August 1987.

99. Nunamaker, D. M., D. M. Butterweck, and M. T. Provost. Fatigue fractures in thorough-bred racehorses: relationships with age, peak bone strain, and training. *J. Orthop. Res.* 8:604–611, 1990.

100. Nyland, J. A., R. Shapiro, R. L. Stine, T. S. Horn, and M. L. Ireland. Relationship of fatigued run and rapid stop to ground reaction forces, lower extremity kinematics, and muscle activation. *J. Sports Phys. Ther.* 20:132–137, 1994.

101. Orava, S. Stress fractures. *Br. J. Sports Med.* 14:40–44, 1980.

102. Orava, S., J. Puranen, and L. Ala-Ketola. Stress fractures caused by physical exercise. *Acta Orthop. Scand.* 49:19–27, 1978.

103. Orava, S., and A. Hulkko. Stress fractures of the mid-tibial shaft. *Acta Orthop. Scand.* 55:35–37, 1984.

104. Pagliano, J., and D. Jackson. The ultimate study of running injuries. *Runner's World* 15:42–50, 1980.

105. Parfitt, A. M. The cellular basis of bone remodeling: the quantum concept reexamined in light of recent advances in the cell biology of bone. *Calcif. Tissue Int.* 36(suppl 1):S37–S45, 1984.

106. Pattin, C. A., W. E. Caler, and D. R. Carter. Cyclic mechanical property degradation during fatigue loading of cortical bone. *J. Biomech.* 29:69–79, 1996.

107. Paty, J. G., and D. Swafford. Adolescent running injuries. *J. Adolesc. Health Care* 5:87–90, 1984.

108. Paul, I. L., M. Munro, P. J. Abernethy, S. R. Simon, E. L. Radin, and R. M. Rose. Musculoskeletal shock absorption: relative contribution of bone and soft tissues at various frequencies. *J. Biomech.* 11:237–239, 1978.

109. Pauwels, F. *Contributions on the Functional Anatomy of the Locomotor Apparatus. Biomechanics of the Locomotor Apparatus.* Berlin: Springer-Verlag, 1980.

110. Pester, S., and P. C. Smith. Stress fractures in the lower extremities of soldiers in basic training. *Orthop. Rev.* 21:297–303, 1992.

111. Pouilles, J. M., J. Bernard, F. Tremollieres, J. P. Louvet, and C. Ribot. Femoral bone density in young male adults with stress fractures. *Bone* 10:105–108, 1989.

112. Protzman, R. R., and C. G. Griffis. Comparative stress fracture incidence in males and females in an equal training environment. *Athletic Training* 12:126–130, 1977.

113. Protzman, R. R., and C. G. Griffis. Stress fractures in men and women undergoing military training. *J. Bone Joint Surg.* 59A: 525, 1977.

114. Radin, E. L. Nature of mechanical factors causing degeneration of joints in the hip. *Proceedings of the 2nd Open Scientific Meeting of the Hip Society, 1974.* St. Louis: C.V. Mosby, 1974, pp. 786–781.

115. Radin, E. L. Role of muscles in protecting athletes from injury. *Acta Med. Scand. Suppl.* 711:143–147, 1986.

116. Radin, E. L., S. R. Simon, R. M. Rose, and I. L. Paul. *Practical Biomechanics for the Orthopedic Surgeon.* New York: John Wiley & Sons, 1979, pp. 43–44.

117. Radin, E. L., M. W. Whittle, K. H. Yang, et al. The heelstrike transient, its relationship with the angular velocity of the shank and the effects of quadriceps paralysis. S. A. Lantz and A. I. King (eds.). *1986 Advances in Bioengineering.* New York: The American Society of Mechanical Engineers, BED, 1986, vol. 2, pp. 121–123.

118. Radin, E. L., K. Yang, C. Riegger, V. L. Kish, and J. J. O'Connor. Relationship of repetitive impulsive loading of the leg to knee pain. Paper presented at the 101st Annual Meeting of the American Orthopaedic Association, June, 1988.

119. Recker, R. R ., M. Davies, S. M. Hinders, R. P. Heaney, M. R. Stegman, and D. B. Kimmel. Bone gain in young adult women. *J. Am. Med. Assoc.* 268:2403–2408, 1992.

120. Reilly, D. T., and A. H. Burstein. The mechanical properties of cortical bone. *J. Bone Joint Surg.* 56A:1001–1021, 1974.

121. Reilly, D. T., and A. H. Burstein. The elastic and ultimate properties of compact bone tissue. *J. Biomech.* 8:393–405, 1975.

122. Reinker, K. A., and S. Ozburne. A comparison of male and female orthopaedic pathology in basic training. *Mil. Med.* 144:532–536, 1979.
123. Rice, J. C., S. C. Cowin, and J. A. Bowman. On the dependence of the elasticity and strength of cancellous bone on apparent density. *J. Biomech.* 21:155–168, 1988.
124. Roub, L. W., L. W. Gumerman, and E. N. Hanley, Jr. Bone stress: a radionuclide imaging perspective. *Radiology* 132:431–438, 1979.
125. Roy, S. H., C. J. DeLuca, and D. A. Casavant. Lumbar muscle fatigue and chronic lower back pain. *Spine* 14:992–1001, 1989.
126. Roy, S. H., C. J. DeLuca, L. Snyder-Mackler, M. S. Emley, R. L. Crenshaw, and J. P. Lyons. Fatigue, recovery and low back pain in varsity rowers. *Med. Sci. Sports Exerc.* 22:463–469, 1990.
127. Rubin, C. T., and L. E. Lanyon. Limb mechanics as a function of speed and gait: a study of functional strains in the radius and tibia of horse and dog. *J. Exp. Biol.* 101:187–211, 1982.
128. Rubin, C. T., McA. Harris, B. H. Jones, H. B. Ernst, and L. E. Lanyon. Stress fractures: the remodeling response to excessive repetitive loading. *Trans. Orthop. Res. Soc.* 9:303, 1984.
129. Rubin, C. T., R. Vasu, J. Tashman, H. Seeherman, and K. McLeod. The non-uniform distribution of shear strains in functionally loaded bone: implications for a complex mechanical milieu. *Trans. Orthop. Res. Soc.* 14:313, 1989.
130. Scelci, R., C. Marchetti, and P. Poggi. Histochemical and ultrastructural aspects of m. vastus lateralis in sedentary old people (age 65–89 years). *Acta Neuropathol.* 51:99–105, 1980.
131. Schaffler, M. B., and D. B. Burr. Stiffness of compact bone: effects of porosity and density. *J. Biomech.* 21:13–16, 1988.
132. Schaffler, M. B., E. L. Radin, and D. B. Burr. Mechanical and morphological effects of strain rate on fatigue of compact bone. *Bone* 10:207–214, 1989.
133. Schaffler, M. B., E. L. Radin, and D. B. Burr. Long-term fatigue behavior of compact bone at low strain magnitude. *Bone* 11:321–326, 1990.
134. Scully, T. J., and G. Besterman. Stress fracture—a preventable training injury. *Mil. Med.* 147:285–287, 1982.
135. Simon, S. R., I. L. Paul, J. Mansour, J. Munro, P. J. Abernethy, and E. L. Radin. Peak dynamic force in human gait. *J. Biomech.* 14:817–822, 1981.
136. Stanish, W. D. Overuse injuries in athletes: a perspective. *Med. Sci. Sports Exerc.* 16:1–7, 1984.
137. Sullivan, D., R. F. Warren, H. Pavlov, and G. Kelman. Stress fractures in 51 runners. *Clin. Orthop. Rel. Res.* 187:188–192, 1984.
138. Swissa, A., C. Milgrom, M. Giladi, et al. The effect of pretraining sports activity on the incidence of stress fractures among military recruits. *Clin. Orthop. Rel. Res.* 245:256–260, 1989.
139. Taimela, S., U. M. Kujala, and K. Osterman. Stress injury proneness: a prospective study during a physical training program. *Int. J. Sports Med.* 11:162–165, 1990.
140. Taunton, J. E., D. B. Clement, and D. Webber. Lower extremity stress fractures in athletes. *Phys. Sports Med.* 9:77–86, 1981.
141. Verbitsky, O., J. Mizrahi, A. Voloshin, J. Treiger, and E. Isakov. Shock absorption and fatigue in humans. *J. Biomech.*, submitted for publication, 1996.
142. Voloshin, A., J. Wosk, and M. Brull. Force wave transmission through the human locomotor system. *J. Biomech. Eng.* 103:48–50, 1981.
143. Voloshin, A., and J. Wosk. An *in vivo* study of low back pain and shock absorption in the human locomotor system. *J. Biomech.* 15:21–27, 1982.
144. Walter, N. E., and M. D. Wolf. Stress fractures in young athletes. *Am. J. Sports Med.* 5:165–170, 1977.
145. Westphal, K. A., K. E. Friedl, M. A. Sharp, et al. *Health, Performance, and Nutritional Status of U.S. Army Women during Basic Combat Training.* U.S. Army Research Institute of Environmental Medicine, Tech. Report No. T96–2. Natick, MA: U.S. Army Medical Research and Materiel Command, 1995.

146. Wilson, E. S., and F. N. Katz. Stress fractures. *Radiology* 92:481–486, 1969.
147. Wosk, J., and A. S. Voloshin. Wave attenuation in skeletons of young healthy persons. *J. Biomech.* 14:261–268, 1981.
148. Wosk, J., and A. S. Voloshin. Low back pain: conservative treatment with artificial shock absorbers. *Arch. Phys. Med. Rehabil.* 66:145–148, 1985.
149. Wright, T. M., and W. C. Hayes. The fracture mechanics of fatigue crack propagation in compact bone. *J. Biomed. Mater. Res. Symp.* 7:637–648, 1976.
150. Yamada, H. *Strength of Biological Materials.* Baltimore: Williams & Wilkins, 1970.
151. Yoshikawa, T., S. Mori, A. J. Santiesteban, et al. The effects of muscle fatigue on bone strain. *J. Exp. Biol.* 188:217–233, 1994.
152. Zernicke, R. F., G. Finerman, and O. C. McNitt-Grey. Stress Fracture Risk Assessment among Elite Collegiate Women Runners. Final report to the NCAA, 1993.
153. Zioupos, P., and J. D. Currey. The extent of microcracking and the morphology of microcracks in damaged bone. *J. Mater. Sci.* 29:978–986, 1994.
154. Zwas, S. T., R. Elkanovitch, and G. Frank. Interpretation and classification of bone scintigraphic finds in stress fractures. *J. Nucl. Med.* 28:452–457, 1987.

8
Physical Activity among Persons with Disabilities—A Public Health Perspective

GREGORY W. HEATH, D.H.Sc., M.P.H.
PETER H. FENTEM, M.B.Ch.B.

Participation in regular physical activity, sport, and active recreation is known to reduce mortality from all causes and to prevent coronary heart disease (CHD), noninsulin-dependent diabetes mellitus (NIDDM), and selected cancers [180]. Current estimates indicate that a substantial proportion of the population in Western countries, such as the United States, United Kingdom, and Canada, are either physically inactive or, at best, are active during leisure time on an irregular basis [206]. Epidemiological studies have identified several subgroups of the population that are more likely to have low levels of physical activity. These groups include women, persons of lower socioeconomic status, and selected racial/ethnic minorities [39]. Persons with disabilities belong to another such subgroup for which levels of participation in regular physical activity are low. This is a somewhat heterogeneous group for which regular physical activity is of great importance but has received relatively little attention.

In general, people with disabilities are less active and have a lower work capacity than persons without disabilities. An inactive life-style compounds the effects of the disability itself and makes this a major public health issue. Poor stamina, reduced muscle strength, and limited flexibility restrict functional ability and, therefore, personal independence. This loss of autonomy through inactivity further amplifies its importance, but above everything else it deserves attention because there may be an element of this loss of autonomy that may not be inevitable and may well be, in part, reversible.

The long-term effects of inactivity among persons with disabilities should be a legitimate concern for the public health community. Improvements in medical care, assistive technology, and the removal of social and environmental barriers for persons with disabilities have brought the prospect of a longer and more productive life for those with chronic disabling conditions. Because an inactive life-style increases the risk of CHD, high blood pressure, thromboses, osteoporosis, obesity, and NIDDM among the general population, the importance of regular physical activity among persons with disabilities may be even more critical to their health and well-being than to that of persons without disabilities. Persuading people with a disability to adopt a more active life-style poses a major challenge, including the need to raise the expectations of the people themselves, their caregivers, and the professional groups that support them.

TABLE 8.1.
Major National Surveys on Disability

Name of Survey	Country of Origin	Year of Survey	Age Range (yr)	Definition of Disability	% with Disability
HALS	Canada	1987	15+	Functional limitation	13.3
NHIS	U.S.	1991–1992	18+	Limitation in major life activity	15.0
OPCS on Disability	U.K.	1988	16+	Functional limitation	13.0

Data are from refs. 90, 127, and 143.
Functional limitation—difficulty in walking, using stairs, bending and reaching, reading ordinary newsprint; limitation in major life activities—adults 18–69 yr old, unable or limited in working a job or in a business; in keeping house; or in attending school. Adults 70 yr and older, limited in carrying out ADL and IADL.

This review seeks to understand the scope of disabilities as they occur in the United States, United Kingdom, and Canada and the extent to which people with these disabilities engage in health-promoting levels of regular physical activity. Because there appears to be a profound effect of inactivity on the disabling process per se, the disabling effects of inactivity will also be discussed. Finally, the benefits of regular physical activity with regard to specific disabling conditions will be outlined with particular reference to improvements in the quality of life and maintenance of functional independence of persons with these particular conditions.

DISABILITY

Definitions

Disability traditionally has connoted limitations in ability to perform life activities because of an impairment, including activities of daily living (ADL) and instrumental activities of daily living (IADL) [128]. For example, disability has been characterized by deleterious anatomical or structural changes or the loss of mental or physiological function as a result of active disease, residual losses from formerly active disease, or congenital losses or injury not associated with active disease [128]. The Americans with Disabilities Act (ADA) of 1991 defines disability as either a person with a physical or mental impairment that substantially limits one or more of the major life activities, a person with a medical record of such an impairment, or a person regarded as having such an impairment [Public Law 101-336].

Definitions used for surveillance and assessment of disability are more clearly understood by linking them to a conceptual framework of the consequences of disease and injury. The International Classification of Im-

FIGURE 8.1.

Prevalence of major conditions causing activity limitations—United States, 1992. Reproduced from ref. 127.

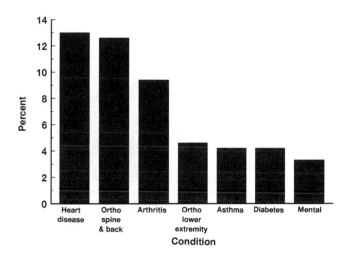

pairments, Disabilities, and Handicaps (ICIDH) is such a conceptual framework [230]. In the ICIDH, three concepts define the consequences of disease and injury: (a) impairment (i.e., the loss of psychological, physiological, or anatomical structure or function), (b) disability (i.e., the limitation in functional performance resulting from an impairment), and (c) handicap (i.e., the disadvantage experienced by a person as a result of impairments and/or disabilities, which limits interaction of the person with their physical and social environment) [32].

Patterns and Current Prevalence

The surveys referred to in this review all use the concept of disability of the ICIDH when describing disabilities. The sources of data are from the 1992 National Health Interview Survey (NHIS) from the United States [127], the 1986–1987 Health and Activity Limitation Surveys (HALS) from Canada [91], and Report 1 on the Prevalence of Disability among Adults of the Office of Population Censuses and Surveys (OPCS), Her Majesty's Statistical Office (HMSO) of the United Kingdom Table 8.1 [143].

According to results from the 1992 NHIS, 15%, or 37.7 million of the noninstitutionalized U.S. adult (18 yr and older) population, report having a disability. The 37.7 million people with a disability report 1.6 conditions per person, on average, for a total of 61 million disabling conditions. Heart disease ranks first in causing disability among 7.9 million Americans (Fig. 8.1). Heart disease is followed by back disorders (7.7 million), arthritis (5.7

FIGURE 8.2.
Percentage of persons with activity limitations, by age group—United States, 1992. Reproduced from ref. 127.

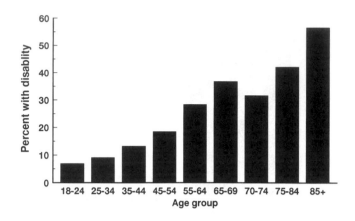

million), orthopedic impairments of the lower extremity (2.8 million), and asthma (2.6 million) [127]. Women are more likely to have a disability, as compared to men (15.4% vs. 14.6%, respectively). American Indians have the highest levels of disability (17.6%), followed by non-Hispanic blacks (15.9%), non-Hispanic whites (15.8%), white Hispanics (10.4%), and Asian and Pacific Islanders (7.2%). The proportion of the population with a disability increases with age (Fig. 8.2) and the mean number of disabling conditions also increases with increasing age (Fig. 8.3).

The HALS in Canada reported an estimated 3.3 million (13%) persons with some level of disability [91]. The survey also showed a significant increase in disability with age, with 5% of children 14 yr old and younger, 11% of adults aged 15–64, and 46% of those aged 65 yr and older reporting a disability [91]. More than 60% of the disabled population 15 yr and older had more than one disability. The HAPS classified disabilities by function. Disabilities associated with mobility impairments were the most prevalent (65%), with 30% reporting a hearing impairment, 18% a visual impairment and 8% an impairment of speech or communication.

The first report of the OPCS on disability in Great Britain was published in 1988 [143]. The results of this survey show that in Great Britain approximately 5 million adults (10%), i.e., those 15 yr and older, have a disability that seriously limits their ability to carry out normal activities. Scales were determined to measure, among other things the individual's capacity to walk, reach, and stretch, as well as to perform fine motor activities. The amount of discomfort suffered in performing these activities was also in-

FIGURE 8.3.

Mean number of conditions per person causing an activity limitation—United States, 1992. Reproduced from ref. 127.

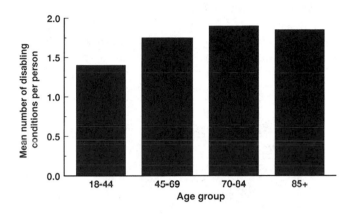

cluded in the score. The prevalence of disability varied according to type and category of disability. The most prevalent type of disabilty was associated with locomotion (mobility), with more than 4 million adults reporting this type of disability. Other more prevalent types of disability included hearing (2.6 million), personal care (2.5 million), visual (1.7 million), and dexterity 1.4 million). Survey results permitted the scoring of the severity of disability, using a 10-point scale. The least severe category was the most common but represents a significant limitation in the individual's ability to perform ADL. Two-thirds of people classified as having a disability were over the age of 60 yr [143] (Fig. 8.4).

Primary Disabling Conditions

A consistent finding across these national surveys is that the most prevalent chronic conditions and impairments causing disability include orthopedic impairments, arthritis, heart disease, hypertension, visual impairments, diabetes, mental disorders, asthma, intervertebral disc disorders, and nervous disorders. In addition, the proportion of persons reporting a disability resulting from chronic health conditions and impairments appears to have increased since the early 1980s [91, 127, 143]. Finally, a disproportionate number of persons above the age of 65 report having a disability.

Thus, trying to understand and describe the patterns of regular physical activity, sports, and active recreation among these subgroups of the population who report having a disability assumes growing importance. There is little information available to shed light on the question of to what extent

FIGURE 8.4.

Estimated numbers of disabled adults according to severity—United Kingdom, 1988. Severity is scored according to a 10-point scale for the following categories: Locomotion, People who "cannot walk 400 yd without stopping for severe discomfort" score 0.5 points. People who can only walk up and down one flight of stairs if they go sideways or one step at a time score 1.5 points. Reaching and stretching, People who cannot put one arm behind their backs to put on their jackets or tuck their shirts in (but can with other arm)/have difficulty putting one arm behind their backs to put on jacket or tuck shirt in, or putting one arm out in front or up to head (but no difficulty with other arm) score 1.0 point. Reproduced from ref. 143.

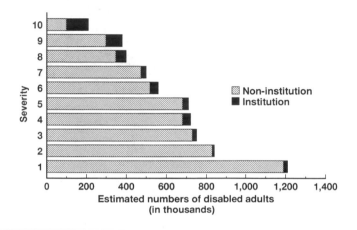

reported disability is a consequence of a chronic condition per se or results from self-imposed physical inactivity, or a combination of both. Examining the patterns of regular physical activity among persons with disabilities not only provides some insight into this question but also helps define the role of physical activity in maintaining function and preventing the progression of the primary disabling condition itself, preventing complications of disabilities associated with physical inactivity, and preventing the compounding of disability.

PHYSICAL ACTIVITY

Definitions

Caspersen [37] has defined physical activity as "any bodily movement produced by skeletal muscles that results in caloric expenditure." The assessment of physical activity is a difficult task because of the complexity of this behavior [37]. Oftentimes, the terms exercise and physical activity are used interchangeably; however, Caspersen [37] has distinguished their differences by defining exercise as a subcategory of physical activity that is "planned, structured, and repetitive, and results in the improvement or maintenance of one or more facets of physical fitness." Physical fitness has been defined as "something that people possess or achieve such as aerobic power, muscular endurance, muscular strength, body composition, and flexibility" [37]. Thus, physical activity, and exercise are behaviors that can potentially influence selected aspects of physical fitness [38]. In describing the physical activity patterns of persons with and without disabilities, this review concentrates on relevant behavior, participation in physical activity, and exercise, rather than on physical fitness. However, in discussing the role of physical activity and exercise in promoting health among persons with selected disabling conditions, alterations in physical fitness will be taken as markers for changes in habitual levels of physical activity and exercise.

Measurement of Physical Activity

Most often, survey questions about physical activity are used to determine the relationship between physical activity and health in a population [38]. Surveys are a convenient method of collecting such information, because they are relatively inexpensive, cause minimal disruption to the respondents' behavior, are modifiable for a particular population, and provide an acceptable level of validity and reliability [37]. Physical activity surveys often use various methods of data collection. These include activity diaries, self-administered questionnaires, or interviewer-administered questionnaires. The mode of collection can also vary from mail-back and telephone-based to face-to-face surveys [37]. Physical activity has been assessed using a single question, recall of 1 wk, 1 mo, or 1 yr or lifetime physical activity [37]. Caspersen [37] has identified surveys with a short timeframe as easy to validate and less likely to suffer from recall bias compared to surveys attempting to examine information over a longer period of time. However, Caspersen et al. [38] have also recognized that assessment over a short period may not reflect usual behavior, because activity may vary by season or as a result of an acute illness. This limitation may be a particular problem when surveying persons with disabilities, because these people are more likely compared to those without disabilities to develop complications of their primary disabling condition that may interfere with their regular patterns of physical activity.

Most questionnaires to explore participation in physical activity inquire primarily about leisure time physical activities requiring energy expenditure at or above the energy cost of tasks of daily living. These leisure time activities often include leisure walking, gardening, household maintenance activities, sports, recreation, and conditioning exercises. Physical activity questionnaires infrequently include questions about ADL and IADL. Some larger survey instruments that include physical activity questions also contain questions about ADL and IADL in other sections of the survey [157]. The omission of questions about ADL and IADL limits the usefulness of surveys of the physical activity patterns of persons with disabilities, because many of these tasks, ADLs and IADLs, may represent a maximum effort for many of them. In addition, such tasks may require a greater energy expenditure than the same task performed by a person without their disability. Thus, the full spectrum of physical activity that may have an impact on the health and well-being of people may not, with some surveys, be assessed adequately, and relevant levels of physical activity will be understated.

Physical Activity Patterns

Recent surveys in Canada [150], England [12], and the United States [39, 51, 157] indicate that only about 10–20% of the adult population in each of these countries reports physical activity and exercise at a level high enough to convey some cardiorespiratory benefit. Generally, this level of activity involves engaging in rather intense dynamic large muscle group (aerobic) activities for 20 min or more per occasion on three or more occasions per wk. Stephens and Caspersen [206] have recently reported on the demography of physical activity from an international perspective. Examining levels of activity that are less than vigorous, the United States, United Kingdom, and Canada report approximately 30–35% of their adult population engaging in these levels of physical activity. Depending on the survey, the definition of "regularly active" is dependent on a variety of methods of factoring duration, frequency, and mode of physical activity. Despite these differences, the distinction between active and inactive persons in each of the surveys can be assessed readily. Persons reporting no physical activity in these surveys ranges from about 25–30% of adults. Most of these surveys assess leisure time physical activity only, with the exception of the U.K. surveys, which assess leisure time physical activity, occupational activity, and ADL. Stephens and Caspersen [206] suggest that the occupational component of these surveys is rather inconsequential to the comparability with the U.S. and Canadian surveys, because occupational activity typically does not add much to total energy expenditure.

Generally, men are more likely than women to engage in both vigorous and moderate levels of physical activity across each of the national surveys. Conversely, women, in all three surveys, are more likely to report no physical activity or irregular levels of physical activity, compared to that of their male counterparts.

Each of the national surveys consistently report that the prevalence of vigorous and/or moderate physical activity declines with age among adults. Compared to younger adults, older adults engage in physical activity less often and tend to choose activities which are lower in energy cost [206]. The Canadian data do demonstrate a tendency for the oldest age group to increase their physical activity levels relative to the next youngest age group;

however, this difference is partially explained by the age-adjusted energy costs of selected physical activities.

Physical Activity Measures among Persons with Disabilities

Many people, because of their impairment, expend more energy in the normal ADLs. The extra metabolic cost of performing physical tasks may arise because of the reduced mass of the muscles, because of inefficient locomotion and abnormal posture attributable to paralysis, or because of high ventilatory effort from respiratory impairment. For example, a person with an amputation above the knee uses about 50% more energy than a person without such an impairment to walk at an average pace [54]. Although there have been substantial attempts, summarized in current reviews [54, 152, 185, 196] to document fitness levels among persons with disabilities, very little information exists regarding the physical activity levels and patterns of persons with disabilities. Dearwater and colleagues [57] recognized the absence of such information and attempted to document the activity levels of persons at what they considered the lowest level of the physical activity spectrum, postspinal cord injured (SCI). Recognizing the difficulty of using conventional physical activity questionnaires, these investigators used physical activity movement counters in order to document the physical activity patterns of persons with paraplegia and quadriplegia. Comparing college students, blue-collar men, and older women to persons with SCI, researchers found that the mean counts per hr were 126.7, 33.2, 32.3, 24.2 (wrist), and 4.0 (ankle), respectively. No subsequent studies among persons with disabilities have been conducted using this method of assessment. In addition, the values obtained from these movement measures may not accurately reflect actual energy expenditure. Godin et al. [83] used a questionnaire to assess the physical activity levels of 62 adults with a lower-limb disability and found the cause of disability to be a stong predictor of physical activity. Other studies have attempted to document the physical activity or exercise behavior of persons with SCI [163]; multiple sclerosis [185]; mental retardation [72]; and arthritis [152], with each of these studies documenting a lower participation rate in physical activity, compared with that of persons free from these disabilities. Unfortunately, few studies among persons with disabilities have used standardized, valid, and reliable measures to assess physical activity, thus leaving little room for comparison with persons without disabilities.

Physical Activity Prevalence among Persons with Disabilities

Canada and the United States have collected at the national level self-reported information about the physical activity and recreational patterns of persons with disabilities. The earliest data from Canada were collected in 1981 as part of the Canada Fitness Survey [11]. The prevalence of persons with disabilities in this survey was 13.7%. Each of the respondents was asked about

TABLE 8.2.
Participation in Leisure-Time Physical Activity among Persons with Disabilities

Data Source	Physical Activity Status	%
NHIS—1991 Health Promotion Disease Prevention Supplement (HPDP)	Low-level LTPA (no reported LTPA + irregular LTPA)	72.8
	Regular moderate/intense LTPA	27.2
HALS—1987	Low LTPA (no reported + irregular LTPA)	65.0

Data are from refs. 90 and 97.
Regular/moderate/intense leisure time physical activity (LTPA)—physical activity ≤6 metabolic equivalents (METS), 5 or more days/wk and accumulation of 30 min or more per day and/or physical activity >6 mets, 3 or more days/wk, ≥20 min/session.

selected leisure time physical activities. Based on their having participated at least once in the past year, 58% reported walking; 29% gardening; 24% bicycling; 22% home exercises; 22% swimming; 9% dancing; 9% jogging; 8% skating; 9% individual sports; and 8% team sports. The nature and extent of the disability was not explored in any detail. In a subsequent survey, the Canadian HALS, 65% of respondents with a disability did not report any physical activities such as walking, swimming, bicycling, or jogging [59, 91] on a regular basis, that is, at least once per wk. (Table 8.2).

Thirty-five percent of people with disabilities reported that they would have liked to have participated more in walking, swimming, bicycling, or jogging but were prevented by their condition. In the United States it is estimated from the results of the NHIS that more than 30% of persons with disabilities report not doing any leisure time physical activity [95, 157]. Heath [95] reported that 27% of persons with a disability, compared to 37% of persons without a disability, engaged in regular moderate physical activity, whereas 9.6 and 14% of persons with and without a disability, respectively, engaged in regular intense or vigorous physical activity. These differences in activity patterns comparing persons with and without disabilities are often confounded by age, socioeconomic status, and health status, suggesting several potentially effective physical activity intervention points for persons with disabilities. As in the Canadian studies, the U.S. surveys have, to date, not determined the physical activity patterns among persons with disabilities according to condition or impairment status, that is, by type of disability, e.g., mobility impairment, sensory impairment, etc.

THE DISABLING CONSEQUENCES OF INACTIVITY

Conditions Attributable to Inactivity

Prolonged physical inactivity is associated with long-term risks of disease in persons with or without a disability. To date, no studies have been conducted to determine whether the long-term benefits of physical activity seen among persons without disabilities, such as lower risks of CHD [186], osteoporosis [44], and obesity [26], also apply to persons with disabilities. It is reasonable to argue that the greater life expectancy of those with even the most severe disabilities now places them at risk from these diseases in later life. Thus, it makes sense for people who have a disability to seek to protect themselves from inactivity-determined conditions that may either exacerbate existing disabilities or contribute to a premature death.

Physical activity is important in preventing weight gain and in managing weight reduction for those who become overweight. Because persons with disabilities are often less active, their risk of gaining weight is greater. Excess body weight may itself have a disabling effect, further restricting mobility, particularly when leg muscles may be weak already. Severe obesity, that is, being more than 30% above desirable weight for height, exacerbates the effects of other conditions and increases the risk of death before age 65 [26]. Regular physical activity can reduce weight. This has been established among persons with [193] and without a disability [74, 133].

It has been argued that, for the general population, physical inactivity is as great a risk factor for CHD as hypertension, hypercholesterolemia, or smoking [186]. With greater longevity, CHD has become a significant cause of death in people who are paraplegic or bilateral lower limb amputees because of trauma [142]. Physical activity appears to lower risk by its favorable effect on blood lipid levels [229], arterial blood pressure [23], blood clotting factors [227], and glucose tolerance and insulin sensitivity among persons without disabilities.

There is strong evidence that high concentrations of high-density lipoprotein (HDL) in the blood are inversely related to the incidence of CHD [40]. There is also strong evidence of a positive relationship between levels of physical activity and plasma levels of HDL [229]. Levels of HDL are generally lower among people who use manual or electric wheelchairs than among persons who do not use wheelchairs [27]. This has been shown to be associated with their inactivity [27]. These authors estimate that among those with SCI, men are at a 60% and women at a 90% greater than average risk of suffering a myocardial infarction [27]. Increased levels of physical activity appear to lead to higher HDL levels among people with SCI [27]. This same finding has been demonstrated among other persons with disabilities, incuding those with rheumatoid arthritis [152] and those with visual impairments [198]. Brenes et al. [27] have shown that athletes who train and compete using manual wheelchairs have higher levels of HDL and lower levels of total cholesterol than control subjects who do not participate in regular wheelchair physical activity. The levels of HDL of the wheelchair athletes were similar to those found among active persons without disabilities [27].

Hypertension is the most common manifestation of cardiovascular disease among persons with SCI [49]. Physical activity has been shown to reduce arterial blood pressure in persons without disabilities who have mild or moderate hypertension [34, 89]. Although no reports were found regarding the effects of regular physical activity on arterial blood pressure among persons with disabilities, it seems plausible to suppose that the effect is similar.

While it seems likely that chronic physical inactivity of persons with disabilities contributes to an increased risk of CHD and that increased levels of physical activity can reduce this risk, the role of multiple risk factors for CHD should be acknowledged. As with the population of persons without disabilities, physical activity of moderate-to-vigorous intensity is no absolute guarantee against developing CHD.

Because prolonged physical inactivity is associated with the development of lower-limb, deep-vein thrombosis, this is an important potential complication of prolonged immobility [104]. Regular physical activity has been shown to reduce this risk and, consequently, that of pulmonary embolus, the more serious related complication.

There is strong evidence that bone density and bone mass are partially determined by habitual levels of physical activity among persons with disabilities [49] as in persons without disabilities [44]. Bone is lost rapidly during bed rest or immobility. The rate of loss can be as high an average loss of 5% of mass per month [192]. Studies have shown that moderate physical activity can reverse this loss. Two factors in maintaining bone emerge from studies among persons without disabilities: (a) the effect appears to be quite specific to the bones which are load bearing during the particular physical activity [156]; (b) gravity and the impact of weight bearing appear to be important factors [115, 192]. No reports were found describing the effects of physical activity on bone density with weight-bearing physical activity among persons with disabilities, but it is a reasonable hypothesis that the effect will be the same as that observed in older adults [200]. Walking appears to be an ideal form of physical activity for the purpose of maintaining bone mass. Walking provides a gravity-dependent stimulus to the bones of the back and lower limbs. These bones are most at risk from osteoporotic fracture. According to what is known of the mechanisms [231], the impact of walking with crutches, braces, or orthoses, even for brief periods, should trigger the osteogenic activity of the bone building cells and maintain density. Maintaining bone density presents a particular problem for people who cannot stand. Paralyzed limbs are most at risk from osteoporotic fracture. Bone can become so fragile that fractures occur with little or no trauma [49]. These problems are not, however, insurmountable. An ingenious method of using a tiltboard for persons with tetraplegia (quadriplegia) to gain the effects of weight bearing and gravity during strengthening exercises showed a significant reduction in calcium loss [117]. The same strengthening exercises performed without the tiltboard showed no such reduction [117]. The reduction of calcium loss may also reduce the incidence of kidney stones common among people with SCI [49].

The Role of Physical Activity in the Prevention of Disability and Secondary Complications

Regular physical activity and exercise training will never restore the capacity lost through damage or disease completely, but some improvement is possible and within the reach of many persons with a disability [160] and older adults [194]. The high levels of "fitness" of participants in the Paralympics and other similar competitions [140, 196], demonstrates what can be achieved by some persons with disabilities. However, even small increases in stamina, strength, and flexibility can lead to large improvements in the quality of life of persons with disabilities [142]. Increases in stamina have been achieved with a modest increase in physical activity by previously inactive older adults who have taken up walking [78]. This is equivalent to jogging in younger people in terms of the production of worthwhile improvement in maximal work capacity [58, 213]. Given a suitable and interesting physical activity program, such improvements will occur among people who have a variety of disabilities, including those where walking or standing is impossible [103, 160, 199].

Low physical work capacity is reversible. The physiological and biochemical improvements that occur in the muscles, the heart, and vascular function with regular physical activity do not depend on enormous physical effort. They depend on a physical effort that is greater than that to which an individual is accustomed. Although athletes may require work at a high intensity to improve their fitness and performance, sedentary or relatively inactive individuals require little exertion for improvement. Training occurs when the effort of an activity is somewhat greater than that to which the individual is accustomed. The degree of improvement depends on the intensity, duration, and frequency of the activity [100]. In people with low exercise tolerance, improvements have resulted from rhythmic physical activity of very short duration (i.e., less than 2 min.) performed frequently enough [93]. Greater reserve capacity will compensate for the increased energy expenditure caused by an impairment. Training can also improve the skill with which a maneuver can be performed and reduce the inefficiency of the movements. This will also reduce the effort. Thus, physical activity training-induced improvements in reserve capacity are especially important.

When muscle strength is decreased and the mass of functional muscle is reduced by paralysis or disease, it is of benefit when the strength of the remaining muscle is increased. Indeed, it is vital that residual capacities are both strengthened and maintained. Evidence from studies with both older adults and persons with disabilities demonstrates that brief contractions of the muscles repeated at frequent intervals [63] lead to an increase in the size of the muscle cells [79, 121] and the strength of the muscles being used [80, 160]. Improvements in muscle strength protect against damage to joints, ligaments and the muscles themselves by stabilizing the joints and by minimizing the damaging effects of sudden movements and unexpected strain.

It appears that long-term regular use of a joint has a beneficial effect. Rather than wearing out joint surfaces, regular movement increases joint nutrition and lubrication, protecting the surfaces and so preventing degenerative joint disease [4, 30]. Gentle motion, accomplished by lubricating the joint, will make movement less painful, which is particularly beneficial to those with joint disease [162, 219]. Suppleness or range of joint movement becomes reduced with inactivity resulting from joint diseases, paralysis, or aging per se. Muscles and tendons shorten if the full range of joint movement is not regularly used. Simple daily stretching exercises help to avoid this. Habitual sitting leads to flexion contractures, which make the individual rigid. This rigidity leads to problems in changing position and makes personal hygiene and transfer from bed to chair and similar movements difficult [2]. Walking exercises or stretching exercises, performed when walking is impossible, appear helpful in avoiding joint contractures (2, 92). Children with paralysis from spina bifida who were able to walk and did so had virtually no joint contractures, while for those consistently using a wheelchair, contractures were a severe problem [2]. Improvements in stamina, strength, and flexibility widen the range of activities an individual can undertake. The importance of being able to walk a little farther, transfer into and out of a chair, or brush one's own hair cannot be overestimated.

Success in overcoming physical impairments and psychological and social barriers helps people adjust to a disability. There are also benefits to self-image. In a society that can devalue individuals for having a disability, the individual could devalue himself or herself. Physical achievement can provide an important opportunity for people with disabilities to gain more control over their bodies and lives. In doing so, their own perception of their disabilities and abilities may change. This can provide a tremendous psychologicial boost [149, 196].

For persons with disabilities who are not interested in sport or exercise, a physical activity plan may be based on customary activities [81]. For example, getting out of a chair with minimal use of one's arms can maximize quadriceps strength training. Many such activities have been designed for older adults and can be adapted for use among persons with disabilities [71].

In addition to the risk of decline in physical capacities resulting from a gradual decline in activities, there is risk of deterioration, even with relatively brief periods of bed rest [50, 198]. Periods of bed rest must be as short as the impairment or intercurrent illness will allow, and subsequent rehabilitation must be energetic.

Inactivity and Aging

As people grow older they generally become less active. This reduced activity contributes to a lowering of capacity over and above that which is age related (Fig. 8.5). A negative spiral of deterioration is established, leading to loss of autonomy and reduction in the quality of life. Cross-sectional

FIGURE 8.5.

Changes in cardiorespiratory fitness (VO$_2$max) and physical inactivity with age. Reproduced from ref. 96.

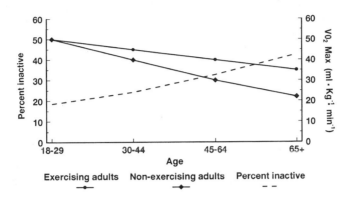

[129] and longitudinal studies [88, 118, 184] of individuals who have maintained high activity levels over many years provide strong evidence that many of the expected declines in physical capacity with increasing age are not inevitable.

Several long-term studies of people who remained very active have not shown the expected deterioration in stamina with age [97, 184]. Athletes 50–70 yr of age had a maximum work capacity which was 60% higher than that of untrained middle-aged men. There are physiological changes in cardiovascular function with age which limit exercise capacity. Older people do have lower maximal heart rates than younger people [97, 189], but maximal cardiac output and maximal work rate can, in general, still be preserved through increases in stroke volume, provided health is good and activity is maintained [88, 184, 189]. Athletes who have trained to peak capacity may, over years, experience a decline [97] but, for the majority of active people work capacity can be maintained certainly at levels well above the average. With good stamina, a wide range of activities, including the occasional demands of extra exertion, may be continued safely and comfortably. Some deterioration is inevitable. The number of muscle cells decreases with increasing age [86], an effect that is thought to result from loss of motor neurons, causing muscles to become weaker and contract more slowly [53]. Regular physical activity, however, appears to moderate this loss. In a 5-yr study of 70 yr olds, those engaged in moderate physical activity had greater muscle strength and, therefore, greater reserves of strength than their sedentary peers [10]. A reserve muscle strength is vital to independent life. To rise from the lavatory or a chair, the average healthy 80-yr-old woman uses maximum quadriceps strength [232]. If the reserve capacity is already close to such a critical threshold, an illness or other periods of inactivity may place an individual below the threshold at which independent function may be resumed.

Impairment of the range of movement of joints and pain on movement are the most frequent health problems among older adults. Thirty-one percent of all people classified as having a disability have some form of arthritis or joint disorder [143]. Joints tend to degenerate with age [18] and that there is an average reduction in joint flexibility of 25–30% [1]. This results in a decline in the ability to perform many of the normal ADLs. Inability to accomplish such tasks as dressing or climbing onto the step of a bus or entering a vehicle seriously restrict independent living.

Long-term physical activity may reduce the risk of degenerative noninflammatory joint disease, with resulting severe restrictions on independent living occurring in later years [30]. A sedentary occupation or low activity in leisure were both associated with greater joint disability in later life [21].

Improvements in stamina, as measured by maximum work capacity [194], have been documented in older people when they engage in regular physical activity. Greater functional strength, attributable to either better neural recruitment or to intrinsic changes in the exercised muscle cells, is common [3, 78]. Improvements in flexibility resulted from physical activity programs in both older women [188] and men [43]. These improvements have been documented to some extent among the frail elderly as well, leading to the conclusion that frailty itself can possibly be prevented by instituting early remedial programs of physical activity among older adults [73].

Most intervention studies involving physical activity exclude older people who have physical impairments arising from chronic and degenerative diseases. A recent study was conducted exclusively involving people representing this subgroup of persons. Although the results of the study did not demonstrate any significant changes in maximal capacity after 16 wk of intervention, there were favorable changes in many of the measured parameters, including workload, strength, blood pressure, and plasma lipids [217]. Another study of older men, which did not exclude those with disabilities, a 4-mo long physical activity program, led to significant favorable changes. Although there was a high dropout rate, 76% of those who completed the program had one or more chronic diseases. Those who completed the program showed increases in treadmill time, abdominal strength, and hip flexibility; decreases in both resting and submaximal heart rate; and a reduction in body fat [154]. There were no adverse reactions to the program in either study, and participants reported subjective improvements and were enthusiastic about continuing to be physically active [217].

Walking for most older people is equivalent to jogging in younger people in terms of relative effort. Improvements in stamina are possible with a modest walking program or some physical activity equivalent for those who cannot use their legs to get about. Walking or its equivalent will also be beneficial for maintaining or improving bone density. A prospective study concluded that walking at least 1 mile three times/wk reduced risk by one-third of suffering a fracture among older women [202]. A program can be devised based on sitting and standing exercises that can load the bones adequately when walking is impossible [200]. Swimming is also beneficial as it maintains both range and strength of a large number of joints and muscles [213] without loading damaged joint surfaces. However, as swimming is ineffective for maintaining bone density [115], some other exercise should also be performed regularly.

HEALTH BENEFITS OF PHYSICAL ACTIVITY AMONG PERSONS WITH SPECIFIC DISABLING CONDITIONS

Persons with Paralysis or Amputation

Paralysis leaves the individual with less functioning muscle mass. Amputation of one or both of the lower limbs poses similar difficulties. For many of the affected persons their paralysis is a result of poliomyelitis, stroke, injury, or of conditions present from birth, such as cerebral palsy or neural-tube defects. With the possible exception of long-standing poliomyelitis or postpolio syndrome [226], these conditions are not progressive and, with current improvements in medical care and technology, the prospect for a longer life is quite promising.

The psychological and physical effects of inactivity and the curtailed mobility resulting from an impairment are major concerns in promoting the health of persons with disabilities. In addition to the nonspecific effects of inactivity, people with paralysis face the consequences of substantial reductions in functioning muscle tissue. Active muscle acts as a pump and contributes to vascular function by facilitating venous return [31]. The impaired vascular function leads to poor peripheral circulation in the nonfunctioning limbs and places an individual at greater risk of pressure sores and thrombosis in the lower-extremity veins [182]. Physical activity provides some protection against these conditions. Active people with SCI have been reported to have fewer of these health problems than those who are inactive [142].

Persons with SCI

With a serious SCI (complete transection of the spinal column), movement and mobility become very restricted. In the absence of adequate social support and personal motivation, a relatively sedentary life-style is oftentimes inevitable. The degree of physical effort attempted in the course of normal daily life by persons with paraplegia living at home is generally modest. There is evidence for this. In one study the increase in heart rate evoked by effort was never more than a 15–24% increase above that which was physiologically possible for persons who were already deconditioned [102]. It appears that these low levels of exertion will lead to a decline in physical capacity over and above that imposed by the injury. The maximum work capacity, as tested by arm ergometry, of a group of men in their early 30s without a mobility impairment was 100 watts. None of the men with paraplegia of the same age could work at that rate, and only 2 of 12 subjects could work at 80 watts [107]. With low energy expenditure, weight gain occurs as fat stores increase and muscle tissue decreases [49, 114, 182]. Stamina among persons with SCI can be improved with regular physical activity and exercise training. The maximal work capacities were 22% higher among athletically active persons with quadriplegia, compared to those of their nonathletic counterparts [64]. The maximal capacities of persons with paraplegia engaging in athletics were 38% higher than those of physically inactive persons of the same age with similar impairments [64]. Significant improvements in work capacity [54, 66, 120, 160, 216], submaximal heart rate [15, 54], and power output [54] have been recorded after as little as 5 wk of exercise training. People who participated in a 3-yr program of daily swimming in addition to conventional rehabilitation exercise showed a 4-fold increase in cardiorespiratory capacity. During this time no change occurred in the group that undertook only conventional rehabilitation [173]. An analysis of 13 intervention studies involving exercise training showed average improvements in physical work capacity of 20 and 40% for people with paraplegia or quadriplegia, respectively, after 4–20 wk [103]. Improvements in dynamic muscle strength of an average of about 20% have also been recorded after people with SCI trained for 7 wk [160]. Flexibility also increased after a program of regular physical activity [177]. The benefits of regular physical activity appear to potentially be long-term for most persons with SCI. In the case of one exercise training program, after 16 yr, 70% of those persons with complete lesions from T-6 downwards were still able to climb and descend stairs with crutches, and 59% were still used [145]. Improvements in strength and stamina can potentially improve the quality of life of many persons with SCI by extending the range of daily activities that can be undertaken safely and comfortably. The degree of improvement will vary with the age of the individual and the time since and extent of the injury. Some wheelchair users have trained to such a level that they have completed marathons in less than 3 hr [140]. The effects of such improvements may extend beyond improvements in physical capacities. A study of self-concept among people with a long-standing SCI established that those who, in their own view, were as physically independent as they were capable of being, scored higher on physical self, personal self, social self, and total self subscales than those whose perceived independence was lower [84]. The determining factor appeared to be not the absolute degree of injury or independence but the degree of independence attained relative to that which was possible. Thus, exercise and sport, as well as providing opportunities for achievement, are important factors in maximizing personal autonomy and self-concept. Active wheelchair users appear to be healthier than their less physically active peers. Regular participants in wheelchair sports had an absentee rate 2% lower (and a monthly wage 22% higher), compared to those of their less active colleagues [156]. In another study, athletes with an SCI had an annual rate of hospital admissions one-third that of nonathletic wheelchair users. Nearly four times as many of the nonathletic group had pressure sores, and nearly five times as many had kidney complications, when compared to the athletic group. These complications tended to be more severe among the less active group [209]. Walking, even for brief periods on crutches or with prostheses [178], also appears to lower the incidence of pressure sores [145].

Persons Postpoliomyelitis and Persons with Cerebral Palsy

With some small exceptions, information about the importance of physical activity for persons with SCI is relevant to people paralyzed by other conditions such as poliomyelitis and cerebral palsy. Persons with quadriplegia caused by polio appear to have a somewhat higher level of physical activity capacity and may be able to tolerate longer bouts of physical activity than those whose paralysis was the result of cervical traumatic spinal injury [225]. There may also be some partial impairment of the functioning muscle of persons paralyzed by cerebral palsy, and in severe cases progress during exercise training may be slower than that of persons paralyzed by traumatic injury [66].

With both poliomyelitis and cerebral palsy, however, the level of impairment is not necessarily as severe as total paralysis. Although there are not the limitations imposed by total paralysis, physical activity may be affected by muscle weakness, spasticity, or rigidity.

Even a small disability can limit involvement in physical activity. Finding it difficult to be active for social or physical reasons, people often settle for an inactive life-style. Children with disabilities spend more time each day in quiet activities [29] and less time with a heart rate greater than 150 beats/min than children without disabilities and, consequently, children with disabilities have a lower physical working capacity [15]. As these children grow into adolescence a decline in physical work capacity has been noted to occur at an earlier age [138].

Practical improvements in the ADLs result from improvements in the health-related components of physical fitness. A 2-yr exercise program for young adults with polio and cerebral palsy improved regular walking speeds by 30% [203]. The affected limbs were also used more in the ADL after a swimming program [179]. Favorable changes in attention levels at school were recorded in motor-impaired children after their exercise levels improved [15]. Many sports have been adapted for persons with motor disabilities. Horseback riding [153] and swimming have proved to be popular and effective [94].

Recently, a new phenomenon has been observed among survivors of polio causing great concern, there is evidence for progression of the paralysis many years after the acute illness. Twenty or 30 yr after the onset of the disease, many individuals experience a progressive weakness and atrophy in muscles that had been rehabilitated [226]. These late complications result in a sudden reduction in functional capacity. The exact cause of this condition is not well understood. It may be the result in part of long-term abnormal strain on muscles and joints because of residual paralysis or deformity. Inactivity resulting from increasing age or other complications also leads to further losses in strength and stamina [56]. Programs of nonfatiguing muscle strength training have been devised to combat these late sequelae of poliomyelitis [63, 172]. A walking program also demonstrated improvements in persons with postpolio symptoms. The authors suggest that in comparison with specific muscle training, walking will strengthen a variety of muscles and bring about practical improvements in functional capacity. After 8 wk of a very modest walking program, patients showed reductions in heart rate, oxygen consumption, and blood pressure. Fatigue and pain were also substantially reduced [63]. There remains a question as to whether the short-term improvement in muscle strength can be maintained or whether the deterioration in muscle strength is inevitably progressive [63].

Persons with Stroke

The annual death rate for stroke in the United Kingdom is about 100 per 100,000, with the incidence of first strokes about 200 per 100,000 people in Britain [141]. The age-adjusted death rate in the United States is 52.6 per 100,000, whereas the incidence rate of first stroke is 220 per 100,000 [32]. Whereas the incidence increases drastically with age, studies have reported 0.08 and 1.73 cases of first stroke per 1000 in people under 45 yr of age and between the ages of 46 and 64, respectively [141]. As fatalities in the first 6 mo are much higher among older people [141], more younger people are left among the survivors. Of the survivors, 10% will have such a severe disability, no improvement is likely, whatever the treatment [205]. Many of the remaining 80% of survivors will show improvement spontaneously within 6 mo [221] but will be left with some disability. These people can benefit from increases in physical activity. Many people who are left with some disability after a stroke will find that the ADL require more effort and are consequently more fatiguing than they were previously [168]. Many will resign themselves to doing less, and a cycle of inactivity often begins. These persons are often left with a very low work capacity [105] and weak muscles long after the initial stroke. Loss of stamina compounds the effects of the stroke. This occurs even in younger adults [101].

The goals of an exercise program soon after a stroke are to restore lost functional capacity as much as possible and to maximize independence. As spasticity, or resistance to movement, often occur with paralysis, flexibility exercises are important. Muscle function returns differentially. In the upper limbs, flexor muscles predominate initially; therefore, exercises should concentrate on strengthening the weaker functioning extensor muscles. In the lower limbs the situation is reversed, and exercise should focus on the flexor muscles [205]. Most people appear to reach a peak in performance within a few months of therapy [205]. There is often a decline in function when the structured program terminates. As individuals return to their peak with recommencement of therapy, one researcher argues for a "booster" dose of therapy every few months [16]. "Booster" therapy would, however, be unnecessary if individuals became interested and motivated enough to participate in some form of physical activity regularly after discharge. In doing so, the longer-term goals of maintaining optimal functional capacity and personal autonomy would be achieved. In addition, participation in physical activity or sport would provide much-needed social contacts. A 4-yr study reported that the greatest deterioration in quality of life after a stroke occurred in the sphere of leisure activities [159]. The effects of long-term physical activity programs for persons who have sustained a stroke have not been studied. In order to provide the most benefit, an activity program must assess each person's abilities. Hemiplegia may cause difficulties in the performance of the rhythmic movements necessary in doing some conventional exercises. Even if muscle function returns, neural damage may have impaired memory, spatial awareness, or the ability to coordinate movement or regulate fine motor activities. Within these constraints, a suitable and enjoyable program can be constructed. Because, in general, work capacity is low and health is often poor, exercise should be of low intensity initially. A recent study found that 89% of a group of stroke patients was too frail or ill to participate in daily therapy [159]. Physical activity that involves sustained isometric contractions and precipitates a rise in blood pressure should be avoided in the presence of a history of cerebrovascular disease or mild or moderate hypertension.

Persons with Neuromuscular Disease

Muscle atrophy, manifesting itself as muscle weakness, is common to many neuromuscular diseases. Fatigue occurs even at very low levels of exertion. Poor fitness and low aerobic capacity are all too readily attributed to the existing medical condition, but exercise training has been shown to improve strength, flexibility, and physical work capacity. The maintenance of maximum possible muscle strength and work capacity enables those persons with neuromuscular disease to enjoy greater independence. Improvements in work capacity help individuals gain increased confidence in their ability to undertake a wider range of activities. They also notice improvement in their symptoms. Many diseases and conditions manifest as muscle weakness. Most are relatively rare. Many studies have, therefore, been conducted on small numbers of subjects having different disorders and differing degrees of disability. Not surprisingly, the results are variable, with some subjects improving greatly and others showing no benefit. Thus it has been difficult to amass sufficient evidence and to collect results for every specific condition. It is likely that relevant information about the effects of particular forms of physical activity on individuals with specific diseases and at various stages in their natural history will only accumulate slowly.

In muscular dystrophies, of which Duchenne muscular dystrophy is the most common, there is a direct loss of muscle fiber, leading to progressive muscle weakness. Some of the congenital myopathies are the result of disorders of muscle energy metabolism; the muscle may function normally at rest and during low-intensity stimulation, but with increased demand for muscle work, abnormalities show up in the metabolic pathways, and energy metabolism fails or the muscle develops a structural weakness. People with nonprogressive dystrophies and those who are in the early stages of slowly progressing conditions, in general, gain the most from muscle strengthening exercise programs. Those in the later stages or whose disease is progressing rapidly are less likely to show improvements. Whenever individuals find that activities such as walking or stair climbing cause fatigue, they change their life-styles and avoid such exertion. Reduced physical activity leads to weaker muscles; fatigue occurs more readily; and activity is reduced further—the vicious cycle to which reference was made earlier. This results in lower capacity. The maximal work capacity of boys with muscular dystrophy was about one-third that of controls without this condition matched for age and weight [201]. Anaerobic performance is also greatly impaired [14].

An exercise program designed for people who either had nonprogressive congenital weaknesses or slow progressive diseases produced a 25% improvement in both maximal and submaximal work capacities after 12 wk of exercise [76]. A 1-yr muscle strengthening program was most successful with limb girdle and facioscapulohumeral dystrophy. Those with Duchenne muscular dystrophy showed the least improvement, but even they compared favorably with the control group. During the experimental year, the control group had lost 8% of muscle strength, whereas the exercise group experienced 1% improvement, despite having suffered losses similar to those of the control group during the previous year [220]. Three years of weight training for two people with muscular dystrophy doubled both their arm strength and their work capacity [151]. It has been suggested that, in some cases, exercise may slow down the course of muscular dystrophy by depressing the degradation of muscle protein [151]. When boys who had already lost, or were about to lose, the ability to walk were fitted with lightweight orthoses, 80% were able to continue walking. Thirty-five percent were still walking 4 yr later [98]. By continuing to walk, people prevented the onset of scoliosis, joint contractures, and other deformities and, most importantly, independence was prolonged. Weight training has been used successfully for people with muscle weaknesses, including muscular dystrophy [151]. In a variety of disorders of muscle metabolism, dynamic or isometric muscle strength training is most effective [90]. Improvements in respiratory muscle strength and endurance have been documented with training and may be of benefit in reducing the incidence of respiratory infections by aiding the draining of secretions [67].

Persons with Neurological Diseases

One of the most common progressive neurological diseases is multiple sclerosis (MS). MS involves patterns of episodic neurological deterioration affecting movement, with remissions. Physical capacity often declines; the muscles become weak or "rigid," leading to abnormal gait, general clumsiness and, eventually, general paralysis. There is no cure for MS, but patients may survive for many decades after the diagnosis. Thus, even with a low incidence, the prevalence rate of the disease in the population will be high. Estimates of prevalence of MS range from 50,000–100,000 cases in the United Kingdom [143] and 150,000–200,000 cases in the United States [127]. Because of extended survival, prolongation of functional capacity and maintenance of personal independence for the longest possible time are of primary importance. Exercise has proved a beneficial adjunct. Exercise started soon after diagnosis has the greatest likelihood of being effective [185].

As with myopathies, the muscle weaknesses and lack of coordination resulting from neurological diseases cause strain and fatigue during physical activity. Unlike with the myopathies there is a rigidity of muscles that, when leg and trunk muscles are affected, leads to a very high energy cost for walking. Walking, even at slow speeds, causes fatigue and breathlessness [167]. When the individual walks less, there is a progressive loss of work capacity, resulting from inactivity over and above the losses resulting from the disease itself [166]. Individuals with MS who took part in a 10-wk moderate exercise program in water showed increases in work performance of upper and lower limbs of, on average, 82 and 330%, respectively. Although not all individuals showed improvements, none of the subjects were adversely affected by the program [80]. Improvements in walking performance, in both distance and speed, resulted from 3–4 wk of training in persons with MS [166]. As fatigue is a major debilitating factor in MS, the ability to be more active in daily life without distress is of real benefit.

There is no evidence that exercise can affect the progress of this disease. The main goal of an exercise program should be to maintain quality of life by maximizing functional independence. This can be accomplished through a program that focuses on improving muscle strength and flexibility. Because many activities have a high energy cost among persons with MS, training should encompass energy-saving maneuvers.

Persons with Joint Disease

Osteoarthritis is commonly considered a "wear-and-tear" disease for which there is little effective therapy. Estimates are that approximately 5.0 million people in the United States are significantly limited in their life activities by osteoarthritis [127]. A disproportionate number of these persons are above 65 yr of age [127].

A person may have a genetic predisposition to osteoarthritis, and the disease may be initiated and/or perpetuated by biomechanical factors such as excess body weight and abnormal joint shape. Risk factors and disease outcomes vary widely with respect to different joints and even at separate locations within a given joint.

Osteoarthritis is an age-related condition. Disease onset most commonly occurs between the ages of 50 and 60 yr. The disease tends to affect the knees, hips, thumb base joints, distal interphalangeal joints of the fingers, first metatarsophalangeal joints, and intervertebral apophyseal joints (often with degenerative intervertebral disc changes). Symptoms may include joint pain, disability, stiffness (particularly after activity), movement restriction, or instability. Symptoms may spontaneously remit and relapse. It is not uncommon for osteoarthritis to remain asymptomatic until injury or unusual exertion stresses the joint.

Many persons with osteoarthritis and some caregivers are concerned that physical activity will damage joints further. However, evidence exists that physical activity, particularly moderate levels of exercise, may indeed reduce the symptoms associated with osteoarthritis. In a trial involving 102 patients with osteoaarthritis of the knee, walking exercises improved function and reduced arthritic pain better than did routine care [119]. Peterson et al. [181] demonstrated, in a group of similar patients, that regular moderate walking could improve gait pattern. Quadriceps-strengthening exercises can reduce pain and disability caused by osteoarthritis of the knee [42, 187].

Weight loss may prevent onset of symptomatic osteoarthritis of the knee, although no data currently exist providing evidence that this will slow ongoing joint damage [68].

Rheumatoid arthritis and ankylosing spondylitis are diseases of the joints that often affect younger people. We have previously described the benefits of regular physical activity for persons with osteoarthritis. Joint pain and deformity result in restriction of movement and consequent muscle wastage. Improvement in joint flexibility and strength achieved by physical activity result in reduction of symptoms and greater participation in the independent ADLs. Building up stamina and strength also creates a margin such that the inevitable loss during acute inflammatory phases, when rest is advised, is less likcly to reduce capacities below the threshold at which functional independence is impaired. Most people with rheumatoid arthritis have low muscle strength and poor general fitness [17]. Work capacity and muscle strength are lost rapidly during acute inflammatory phases, when rest is recommended.

During nonacute phases, pain and stiffness limit movement, resulting in further inactivity and further loss of capacity. The rate of loss of muscle strength may be as great as 30% per wk when pain severely inhibits activity [13]. People with rheumatoid arthritis, particularly those with a mild-to-moderate disability (functional Classes II and III) have shown improvements in several well-controlled training studies [152]. These have included increases in aerobic capacity [52, 93, 161] and reductions in blood lipids. A 38% improvement in isometric quadriceps muscle strength resulted from 2 mo of warm-water swimming [52]. Strengthening muscles around joints can minimize the stress on these joints during daily activities [81]. There is some evidence that regular physical activity increases the thickness of articular cartilage and strengthens ligaments and tendons [162]. This is supported by animal studies that have found that movement facilitates regeneration of articular cartilage [190]. Improvements in the clinical symptoms among persons with RA following participation in an exercise program support this evidence. These have included increases in range of movement at affected joints [162, 219] and decreases in the rate of joint deterioration as determined radiologically [162] in the number of painful or swollen joints [93] and a decrease in the degree of pain and swelling of these joints [93].

Ankylosing spondylitis (AS) involves inflammation of the spine, sacroiliac, and large peripheral joints.

The amount of regular physical activity undertaken was correlated with independent ADLs over a 5-yr period for persons with RA [162]. By the end of the study the exercisers were three times more active in daily life, compared to the control group [162]. In addition, the exercise group took less sick leave, took less medication, and were hospitalized half as much as the control group [162]. Other studies have documented improvements in activities that relate to independent living, such as walking times, and stair climbing [65, 161] and perceived exertion [65]. Subjects have frequently reported being able to move more freely and being more self-sufficient after a regular physical activity program [52].

Participants have been enthusiastic about gains in fitness and decreases in symptoms. A follow-up of 23 patients 6 mo after the termination of their formal exercise program found that 22 had a very positive attitude toward the training program [65]. Many noted that they were able to go out with confidence as they could now negotiate obstacles such as steps on buses [65]. Some participants with AS were able to return to work after previously giving up their job [64].

Persons with CHD

Referring to the national data from the United States, the United Kingdom, and Canada on the prevalence of disability, CHD and the associated complications of angina and congestive heart failure are the most prevalent conditions cited as primary causes of disability [91, 127, 143]. Most people with CHD tend to be in their middle or later years of life, and physical activity may not have been a regular part of their lives previous to the diagnosis of CHD [175]. As there have been many exercise rehabilitation studies for people with CHD, and the results have been widely documented, these provide a model for the type of improvements that may be possible with other impairments.

The functional limitation arising from CHD is exacerbated by inactivity. A 10-yr study of survivors of myocardial infarction (MI) found that 44% reduced their participation in physical activity substantially, particularly vigorous exercise, after their event and maintained this low level over the long term. Only 9% took more exercise after their event. The control people who had not had an MI maintained a fairly stable level of exercise over the same time period [224]. A vicious cycle of inactivity and progressive deterioration is initiated. Oftentimes, the patients with the greatest risk of further complications, are those who are least likely to participate in regular physical activity. In a number of studies, even those randomized at the beginning, the intervention group becomes a self-selected sample of motivated people. The 43% of patients who did not continue to attend a cardiac rehabilitation program were more likely to have multiple risk factors, including chronic inactivity, and they had experienced two or more previous episodes of MI, compared with those who complied with the program [165]. Training has had variable effects on the maximum working capacity of cardiac patients. Studies are difficult to control: the degree of impairment and exercise tolerance differs among subjects, and progress may be so slow as to be not significant during the period of observation. Some studies have reported improvements in maximal working capacity [61, 62], even with low-intensity exercise (less than 45% of maximal capacity) [25]. However, others, although showing increases in submaximal work tolerance, found no change in maximum capacity [60].

The improvements in submaximal exercise tolerance and capacity enable persons with CHD to cope better with everyday activities, dealing safely with the occasional demands for brief vigorous efforts that occur in daily life [99]. Significant improvements in effort tolerance of the normal ADLs have been reported [60, 99]. The person with CHD gains confidence in his/her ability to engage in physical activity safely, and this has been shown to reduce the depression which is associated often with CHD [207].

Regular physical activity can reduce many of the risk factors associated with CHD among cardiac patients. Increases in HDL cholesterol levels [25, 211] and reduction in platelet aggregation have been observed with training [116]. Whether this results in a reduction in mortality has not yet been established conclusively. A recent meta-analysis of six controlled studies among persons with documented CHD showed a reduction in the risk of death from CHD of 19% with exercise-based rehabilitation [144]. In one study of 782 patients with CHD, those persons who were exercising and burning less than 2000 kcal per wk were approximately 1.5 times more likely to have a fatal MI than those active at or above this level [174].

Persons with Respiratory Disease

When respiratory function is impaired, exercise is limited by ventilatory capacity. With any increase in physical effort, muscles use more energy, and ventilation is increased. In contrast with persons without respiratory disease, in whom the cardiovascular response is often the limiting factor in maximal exercise [169], persons with respiratory impairment have difficulty in meeting this ventilatory demand. Exertion causes breathlessness, which is both uncomfortable and frightening. To avoid a recurrence, individuals exert themselves less. The capacity for physical activity diminishes, and breathlessness occurs at a lower level of exertion. Again, the downward spiral of physical inactivity is entered.

When the respiratory impairment is not severe or can be controlled through medication, large measurable improvements in cardiorespiratory fitness and pulmonary function can be achieved. The training of large muscles is of benefit to those with respiratory impairments, as it puts less strain on respiratory muscles during ADLs. Indoor swimming appears to be the most effective physical activity for persons with respiratory disease, as it is effective for cardiorespiratory training and benefits the respiratory muscles.

Cystic fibrosis is an hereditary disease of abnormal secretions of the exocrine glands, including thick mucous secretions, pancreatic insufficiency, and increased salt concentrations in sweat. Repeated lung infections in which lung tissue is destroyed lead to poor pulmonary function and are the most serious consequence of the disease. Those with cystic fibrosis suffer from excessive dead space ventilation [82], limiting alveolar ventilation and, in turn, limiting exercise capacity [41]. Compensation during exertion is by hyperventilation [41, 82]. Insufficient pancreatic symptoms of fatigue, leading to reductions in activity levels, often occurs. As progress has been made with the medical management of these conditions, many people with cystic fibrosis are surviving well into adulthood. Therefore, a lifetime emphasis on regular physical activity should be promoted among these persons by integrating young people into physical and sports activities at school and in the community. Despite the respiratory impairment among persons with cystic fibrosis, the cardiovascular response to exercise is similar to that of persons without the disorder, even when symptoms are severe [41]. Improvements in physical capacity are possible with exercise training [170]. Weight training has also been adapted for persons with this condition, with marked improvements in muscle strength [210]. Respiratory muscle endurance improves with training [170], often resulting in increases in exercise tolerance [9, 170]. With regular physical activity, improvements in pulmonary function among persons with cystic fibrosis have been documented in response swimming [233] and running [170]. Improvements in pulmonary function in response to regular physical activity have been reported in follow-up studies of 5 years and longer [9].

Asthma is a condition that is a primary cause of disability among children and adolescents. The accompanying exercise-induced bronchospasm results in reduced levels of exercise tolerance among these young people [171, 195], with young people who have the most severe conditions registering over 2 SDs below the mean values for maximal work capacity [137]. Regular physical activity has been shown to benefit persons with asthma with as much as 21% improvement being reported in children after 3–4 mo of training [215]. Similar results have been shown among adults with asthma [87, 158, 171]. Athletes with asthma have won major competitions at national and international levels [87]. Regular physical activity and sports participation have resulted in fewer episodes of wheezing and other symptoms among persons with asthma [55, 87, 215].

Chronic obstructive pulmonary disease (COPD) is the end stage of a number of different conditions, including chronic bronchitis and emphysema. COPD is a prevalent chronic disabling condition in the United Kingdom, Canada, and the United States [91, 127, 143], with estimates between 6 and 10% of persons with a disability identifying COPD as a primary cause of disability. COPD is characterized by restricted expiratory airflow and chronic breathlessness [208]. The results of exercise training among persons with COPD is equivocal. Because of initial low work tolerance, studies have been unable to detect significant cardiorespiratory improvements after regular physical activity among persons with COPD [7, 19, 36, 110], whereas others provide evidence of moderate improvement [20, 31, 35]. The most profound improvements among persons with COPD in response to regular physical activity have been in gains in completing ADL such as stair climbing [147] and level walking [199]. Much of the benefit to persons with COPD has come from improvement in symptoms and greater efficiency in carrying out many of the ADLs [35, 46, 147, 148, 199].

Persons with Mental Disabilities

"Mental disabilities" encompasses a wide range of conditions, but most research has been conducted among persons with intellectual impairments, of which Down's syndrome comprises the most common condition. Many individuals with a mental impairment experience slower physical development [214], and they are less spontaneously active than those without such an impairment. Children with mental impairment have physical impairments, including poor muscle tone, balance, and motor coordination, which makes it difficult for these persons to integrate into routine play and games [125]. Clearly, among those children who are not encouraged and stimulated to play and be active, their levels of fitness have been shown to be low [45]. Studies have repeatedly demonstrated lower levels of strength, power, agility, and cardiorespiratory endurance among young people with Down's syndrome, compared to those without the condition [72]. In response to regular physical activity individuals with Down's syndrome have demonstrated improvements in strength, balance, and posture [6, 72]. Improvements in maximal and submaximal working capacity have been documented among children and adults with Down's syndrome [72, 218]. Significant weight loss and a reduction in obesity were noted in response to exercise training among persons with mental impairment [72, 193].

Persons with Visual Impairments

To a large extent, sport and exercise rely on sight for both learning and orientation. Thus, people with a visual impairment may find it difficult to participate in physical activity. The resulting inactivity leads to poor physical capacity. A number of studies have demonstrated poor working capacity [106, 197, 219] and muscle strength [197] among persons with a visual impairment. Children with blindness had, on average, one-half of the work capacity and muscle strength of age-matched controls without visual impairments [197]. The work capacity of children who had partial sight appears better than those with complete blindness but significantly below that of children with a visual impairment [104]. A couple of studies have shown improvement in cardiorespiratory fitness among persons with visual impairments [197, 198]. There are many paired or team activities that are particularly suitable for individuals with visual impairments. These include rowing and cycling in tandem [155], as well as modified ball games, including rugby and baseball/softball [155].

Persons with Hearing Impairment

Hearing impairments do not appear to affect physical activity levels adversely. Some hearing impaired persons do have difficulty with balance because of associated damage to the vestibular apparatus [134]. Improvements in balance were documented among persons with hearing impairment, where the mode of physical activity consisted of the gymnastics training of floor work and work on a balance beam [134]. Motor skills have also been shown to have improved among persons with hearing impairment exposed to a regular physical activity program of walking, strengthening, and balance activities [123].

SUMMARY

Regular physical activity, sports participation, and active recreation are essential behaviors for the prevention of disease, promotion of health, and maintenance of functional independence. This health behavior is essential for persons with and without disabilities. Population-based surveys have consistently demonstrated that persons with disabilities are less likely to be physically active, compared to persons without such limitations. However, these observations are based on relatively few surveys and are dependent on physical activity assessment methods that may not be sensitive and specific enough for persons with disabilities.

Studies clearly demonstrate that many persons, representing a variety of selected disabilities, can adapt to increased levels of physical activity, as evidenced by alterations in various components of physical fitness. More importantly, other studies consistently provide evidence that participation in regular physical activity among persons with selected impairments and disabilities results in improved functional status and quality of life.

Further efforts are critically needed in the area of the development of physical activity assessment methodology for persons with disabilities. Methods need to be developed that will provide survey researchers and those in public health the capacity to measure and monitor activity patterns of persons with disabilities. This information is important not only for public health officials but also health policy analysts, service providers, and disability advocacy groups. Further understanding of the role of physical activity in the maintenance of function and independence among persons with disabilities is needed. The understanding of environmental and social barriers to physical activity among persons with disabilities needs further exploration. Finally, physical activity determinants research among persons with disabilities, including the role of assistive technology as well as maximizing the intrinsic capacity of functional anatomy and physiology, needs to be addressed.

ACKNOWLEDGMENTS

We are grateful to Mrs. N. B. Turnbull for her contributions in the preparation of portions of this manuscript, as well as for her efforts in organizing a number of the citations used in this review.

REFERENCES

1. Adrian, M. J. Flexibility in the aging adult. E. L. Smith and R. C. Serfass (eds.). *Exercise and Aging: The Scientific Basis.* Hillside, NJ: Enslow Publishers, 1981, pp. 45–57.
2. Agre, J. C., T. W. Findley, M. C. McNally, R. Habeck, A. S. Leon, L. Stradel, R. Birkebak, and R. Schmalz. Physical activity capacity in children with myelomeningocele, *Arch. Phys. Med. Rehabil.* 68:372–377, 1987.
3. Agre, J. C., L. E. Pierce, D. M. Raab, M. McAdams, and E. L. Smith. Light resistance and stretching exercise in elderly women: effect upon strength, *Arch. Phys. Med. Rehabil.* 69:273–276, 1988.
4. Ahlqvist, J. On the structural and physiological basis of the influence of exercise, movement and immobilization in inflammatory joint diseases., *Ann. Chir. Gynaecol. Suppl.* 198:10–18, 1985.
5. Ainsworth, B. E., W. L. Haskell, A. S. Leon, D. R. Jacobs, Jr., H. J. Montoye, J. F. Sallis, and

R. S. Paffenbarger, Jr. Compendium of physical activities: classification of energy costs of human physical activities. *Med. Sci. Sports Exerc.* 25:71–80, 1993.

6. Alexander, J., G. E. Molnar, and L. Rotkin. Exercise program for mildly retarded children. *Arch. Phys. Med. Rehabil.* 59:536, 1978.

7. Alpert, J. S., H. Bass, M. M. Szucs, J. S. Banas, J. E. Dalen, and L. Dexter. Effects of physical training on hemodynamics and pulmonary function at rest and during exercise in patients with chronic obstructive pulmonary disease, *Chest* 66:647–651, 1974.

8. Andersen, P., and J. Henriksson. Capillary supply of the quadriceps femoris muscle of man: adaptive response to exercise. *J Physiol.* 270:677–690, 1977.

9. Andréasson, B., B. Jonson, R. Kornfält, E. Nordmark, and S. Sandström. Long-term effects of physical exercise on working capacity and pulmonary function in cystic fibrosis. *Acta Paediatr Scand.* 76:70–75, 1987.

10. Aniansson, A., L. Sperling, K. Rundgren, and E. Lehnberg. Muscle function in 75-year-old men and women. A longitudinal study. *Scand J Rehabil Med Suppl* 9:92–102, 1983.

11. Anonymous. *Canada Fitness Survey: Physical Activity among Activity-Limited and Disabled Adults in Canada.* Ottawa: Canadian Fitness and Lifestyle Research Institute, 1986.

12. Anonymous. Allied Dunbar National Fitness Survey. The Department of Health, The Sports Council, Health Education Authority, UK, Allied Dunbar plc., 1992.

13. Bardwick, P. A., and R. L. Swezey. Physical therapies in arthritis. *Postgrad. Med.* 72:223–234, 1982.

14. Bar-Or, O. Pathophysiological factors which limit the exercise capacity of the sick child. *Med. Sci. Sports Exerc.* 18:276–282, 1986.

15. Bar-Or, O., O. Inbar, and R. Spira. Physiological effects of a sports rehabilitation program on cerebral palsied and post-poliomyelitic adolescents. *Med. Sci. Sports Exerc.* 8:157–161, 1976.

16. Basmajian, J. V., C. A. Gowland, A. J. Finalyson, A. L. Hall, et al. Stroke treatment: comparison of integrated behavioral-physical therapy vs traditional physical therapy programs. *Arch. Phys. Med. Rehabil.* 68:267–272, 1987.

17. Beals, C. A., R. M. Lampman, B. F. Banwell, E. M. Braunstein, et al. Measurement of exercise tolerance in patients with rheumatoid arthritis and osteoarthritis. *J. Rheumatol.* 12:458–461, 1985.

18. Bell, R. D., and T. B. Hoshizaki. Relationships of age and sex with range of motion of seventeen joint actions in humans. *Can. J. Appl. Sport Sci.* 6:202–206, 1981.

19. Belman, M. J., and B. A. Kendregan. Exercise training fails to increase skeletal muscle enzymes in patients with chronic obstructive pulmonary disease. *Am. Rev. Respir. Dis.* 123:256–261, 1981.

20. Belman, M. J., and B. A. Kendregan. Physical training fails to improve ventilatory muscle endurance in patients with chronic obstructive pulmonary disease. *Chest* 81:440–443, 1982.

21. Bergstrom, G., A. Aniansson, A. Bjelle, G. Grimby, et al. Functional consequences of joint impairment at age 79. *Scand. J. Rehabil. Med.* 17:183–190, 1985.

22. Bertoti, D. B. Effects of therapeutic horseback riding on posture in children with cerebral palsy. *Phys. Ther.* 68:1505–1512, 1988.

23. Blair, S. N., N. N. Goodyear, L. W. Gibbons, and K. H. Cooper. Physical fitness and incidence of hypertension in healthy normotensive men and women. *J. Am. Med. Assoc.* 252:487–490, 1984.

24. Blomquist, M., U. Freyschuss, L-G. Wiman, and B. Strandvik. Physical activity and self treatment in cystic fibrosis. *Arch. Dis. Child.* 61:362–367, 1986.

25. Blumenthal, J. A., W. J. Rejeski, M. Walsh-Riddle, et al. Comparison of high- and low-intensity exercise training early after acute myocardial infarction. *Am. J. Cardiol.* 61:26–30, 1988.

26. Bouchard C., J. P. Depres, and A. Trembley. Exercise and obesity. *Obes. Res.* 1:133–147, 1993.

27. Brenes, G., S. Dearwater, R. Shapera, R. E. LaPorte, and E. Collins. High density lipopro-

tein cholesterol concentrations in physically active and sedentary spinal cord injured patients. *Arch. Phys. Med. Rehabil.* 67:445–450, 1986.

28. Breslow, L., and N. Breslow. Health practices and disability: some evidence from Alameda County. *Prev. Med.* 22:86–95, 1993.
29. Brown, M., and W. A. Gordon. Impact of impairment on activity patterns of children. *Arch. Phys. Med. Rehabil.* 68:828–832, 1987.
30. Burry, H. C. Sport, exercise and arthritis. *Br. J. Rheumatol.* 26:386–388, 1987.
31. Busch, A. J., and J. D. McClements. Effects of a supervised home exercise program on patients with severe chronic obstructive pulmonary disease. *Phys. Ther.* 68:469–474, 1988.
32. CDC. Prevalence of disabilities and associated health conditions—United States, 1991–1992. *MMWR Morb. Mortal. Wkly. Rep.* 43:730–739, 1994.
33. CDC. Prevalence of mobility and self-care disability—United States, 1990. *MMWR Morb. Mortal. Wkly. Rep.* 42:760–768, 1993.
34. Cade, R., D. Mars, H. Wagemaker, et al. Effect of aerobic exercise training on patients with systemic arterial hypertension. *Am. J. Med.* 77:785–790, 1984.
35. Carter, R., B. Nicotra, L. Clark, et al. Exercise conditioning in the rehabilitation of patients with chronic obstructive pulmonary disease. *Arch. Phys. Med. Rehabil.* 69:118–122, 1988.
36. Casaburi, R., and K. Wasserman. Exercise training in pulmonary rehabilitation (Editorial). *N. Engl. J. Med.* 314:1509–1511, 1986.
37. Caspersen, C. J. Physical activity epidemiology: concepts, methods, and applications to exercise science. K. Pandolf (ed.). *Exercise and Sport Sciences Reviews*. Baltimore: Williams & Wilkins, 1989, vol. 17, pp. 423–473.
38. Caspersen, C. J., A. M. Kriska, and S. R. Dearwater. Physical activity epidemiology applied to elderly populations. *Baillieres Clin. Rheumatol.* 8:7–27, 1994.
39. Caspersen, C. J., and R. K. Merritt. Physical activity trends among 26 states, 1986–1990. *Med. Sci. Sports Exerc.* 27:713–720, 1995.
40. Castelli, W. P., R. J. Garrison, and P.W.F. Wilson. Incidence of coronary heart disease and lipoprotein cholesterol levels The Framingham Study. *J. Am. Med. Assoc.* 256:2835–2838, 1986.
41. Cerny, F. J., T. P. Pullano, and G.J.A. Cropp. Cardiorespiratory adaptations to exercise in cystic fibrosis. *Am. Rev. Respir. Dis.* 126:217–220, 1982.
42. Chamberlain, M. A., G. Care, and B. Harfield. Physiotherapy in osteoarthritis of the knees: a controlled trial of hospital versus home exercises. *Int. Rehabil. Med.* 4:101–106, 1982.
43. Chapman, E. A., H. A. deVries, and R. Swezey. Joint stiffness: effects of exercise on young and old men. *J Gerontol.* 27:218–221, 1972.
44. Chow, R. K., J. E. Harrison, C. F. Brown, and V. Hajek. Physical fitness effect on bone mass in postmenopausal women. *Arch. Phys. Med. Rehabil.* 67:231–234, 1986.
45. Churton, M. W. Selected measures of physical fitness for a group of learning disabled children. *Percept. Mot. Skills.* 61:678, 1985.
46. Cockcroft, A. E., M. J. Saunders, and G. Berry. Randomised controlled trial of rehabilitation—chronic respiratory disability. *Thorax* 36:200–203, 1981.
47. Compton, D. M., P. A. Eisenman, and H. L. Henderson. Exercise and fitness for persons with disabilities. *Sports Med.* 7:150–162, 1989.
48. Coutts, K. D., and J. L. Strogryn. Aerobic and anaerobic power of Canadian wheelchair track athletes. *Med. Sci. Sports Exerc.* 19:62–65, 1987.
49. Cowell, L. L., W. G. Squires, and P. B. Raven. Benefits of aerobic exercise for the paraplegic: a brief review. *Med. Sci. Sports Exerc.* 18:501–508, 1986.
50. Coyle, E. F., W. H. Martin, S. A. Bloomfield, O. H. Lowry, and J. O. Holloszy. Effects of detraining on responses to submaximal exercise. *J. Appl. Physiol.* 59:853–859, 1985.
51. Crespo, C. J., S. J. Keteyian, G. W. Heath, and C. T. Sempos. Leisure-time physical activity among U.S. adults: results from the Third National Health and Nutrition Examination Survey. *Arch. Intern. Med.* 156:93–98, 1996.
52. Danneskiold-Samsøe, B., K. Lyngberg, T. Risum, and M. Telling. The effect of water ex-

ercise therapy given to patients with rheumatoid arthritis. *Scand. J. Rehabil. Med.* 19:31–35, 1987.

53. Davies, C.T.M., D. O. Thomas, and M. J. White. Mechanical properties of young and elderly human muscle. *Acta Med. Scand.* 220(suppl 711):219–226, 1986.

54. Davis, G. M. Exercise capacity of individuals with paraplegia. *Med. Sci. Sports Exerc.* 25:423–432, 1993.

55. Dean, M., E. Bell, C. R. Kershaw, B. M. Guyer, and D. W. Hide. A short exercise and living course for asthmatics. *Br. J. Dis. Chest* 82:155–161, 1988.

56. Dean, E., and J. Ross. Modified aerobic walking program: effect on patients with postpolio syndrome symptoms. *Arch. Phys. Med. Rehabil.* 69:1033–1038, 1988.

57. Dearwater, S. R., R. E. LaPorte, R. J. Robertson, G. Brenes, L. L. Adams, and D. Becker. Activity in the spinal cord-injured patient: an epidemiologic analysis of metabolic parameters. *Med. Sci. Sports.* 18:541–544, 1986.

58. deVries, H. A. Physiological effects of an exercise training regimen upon men aged 52–88. *J. Gerontol.* 4:325–336, 1979.

59. Dowler, J. M., and D. A. Jordan-Simpson. Participation of people with disabilities in selected activities. *Health Rep.* 2:269–277, 1990.

60. Dressendorfer, R. H., J. L. Smith, E. A. Amsterdam, and D. T. Mason. Reduction of submaximal exercise myocardial oxygen demand post-walk training program in coronary patients due to improved physical work efficiency. *Am. Heart J.* 103:358–362, 1982.

61. Ehsani, A. A., G. W. Heath, W. H. Martin, 3rd, J. M. Hagberg, and J. O. Holloszy. Effects of intense exercise training on plasma catecholamines in coronary patients. *J. Appl. Physiol.* 57:154–159, 1984.

62. Ehsani, A. A., W. H. Martin, 3rd, G. W. Heath, and E. F. Coyle. Cardiac effects of prolonged and intense exercise training in patients with coronary artery disease. *Am. J. Cardiol.* 50:246–254, 1982.

63. Einarsson, G. Muscle adaptation and disability in late poliomyelitis. *Scand. J. Rehabil. Med.* 25(suppl):1–76, 1991.

64. Eriksson, P., L. Löfström, and B. Ekblom. Aerobic power during maximal exercise in untrained and well-trained persons with quadriplegia and paraplegia. *Scand. J. Rehabil. Med.* 20:141–147, 1988.

65. Ekblom, B., O. Lövgren, M. Alderin, M. Fridström, and G. Sätterström. Effect of short-term physical training on patients with rheumatoid arthritis: a six month follow-up. *Scand. J. Rheumatol.* 4:87–91, 1975.

66. Ekblom, B., and A. Lundberg. Effect of physical training on adolescents with severe motor handicaps. *Acta Paediatr. Scand.* 57:17–23, 1968.

67. Estrup, C., S. Lyager, N. Nœraa, and C. Olsen. Effect of respiratory muscle training in patients with neuromuscular diseases and in normals. *Respiration* 50:36–43, 1986.

68. Felson, D. T., Y. Zhang, J. M. Anthony, A. Nalmark, and J. J. Anderson. Weight loss reduces risk for symptomatic knee osteoarthritis in women: the Framingham Study. *Ann. Intern. Med.* 116:535–539, 1992.

69. Fentem, P. H. Exercise in the prevention of disease. *Br. Med. Bull.* 48:630–650, 1992.

70. Fentem, P. H. Benefits of exercise in health and disease. *Br. Med. J.* 308.1291–1295, 1994.

71. Fentem, P. H., and E. J. Bassey. 50+ All to Play For: A Guide for Those in Charge of Activity Groups. London: British Sports Council, 1985.

72. Fernhall, B., K. H. Pitetti, J. H. Rimmer, J. A. McCubbin, P. Rintala, and A. L. Millar. Cardiorespiratory capacity of individuals with mental retardation including Down's syndrome. *Med. Sci. Sports Exerc.* 28:366–371, 1996.

73. Fiaterone, M. A., E. F. O'Neill, N. D. Ryan, et al. Exercise training and nutritional supplementation for physical frailty in very elderly people. *N. Engl. J. Med.* 330:1769–1775, 1994.

74. Findlay, I. N., R. S. Taylor, H. J. Dargie, et al. Cardiovascular effects of training for a marathon run in unfit middle aged men. *Br. Med. J.* 295:521–524, 1987.

75. Fletcher, B. J., S. B. Dunbar, J. M. Felner, B. E. Jensen, L. Almon, G. Cotsonis, and G. F.

Fletcher. Exercise testing and training in physically disabled men with clinical evidence of coronary artery disease. *Am. J. Cardiol.* 73:170–174, 1994.

76. Florence, J. M., and J. M. Hagberg. Effect of training on the exercise responses of neuromuscular disease patients. *Med. Sci. Sports Exerc.* 16:460–465, 1984.

77. Fries, J. F., G. Singh, D. Morfeld, H. B. Hubert, N. E. Lane, and B. W. Brown, Jr. Running and the development of disability with age. *Ann. Intern. Med.* 121:502–509, 1994.

78. Frontera, W. R., C. N. Meredith, K. P. O'Reilly, H. G. Knuttgen, and W. J. Evans. Strength conditioning in older men: skeletal muscle hypertrophy and improved function. *J. Appl. Physiol.* 64:1038–1044, 1988.

79. Gaffney, F. A., G. Grimby, B. Danneskiold-Samsøe, and O. Halskov. Adaptation to peripheral muscle training. *Scand. J. Rehabil. Med.* 13:11–16, 1981.

80. Gehlsen, G. M., S. A. Grigsby, and D. M. Winant. Effects of an aquatic fitness program on the muscular strength and endurance of patients with multiple sclerosis. *Phys. Ther.* 64:653–657, 1984.

81. Gloag, D. Rehabilitation in rheumatic diseases. *Br. Med. J.* 290:132–136, 1985.

82. Godfrey, S., and M. Mearns. Pulmonary function and response to exercise in cystic fibrosis. *Arch. Dis. Child.* 46:144–151, 1971.

83. Godin, G., A. Colantonio, G. M. Davis, R. J. Shephard, and C. Simard. Prediction of leisure time exercise behavior among a group of lower-limb disabled adults. *J. Clin. Psychol.* 42:272–279, 1986.

84. Green, B. C., C. C. Pratt, and T. E. Grigsby. Self concept among persons with long-term spinal cord injury. *Arch. Phys. Med. Rehabil.* 65:751–754, 1984.

85. Grimby, G., G. Einarsson, M. Hedberg, and A. Aniansson. Muscle adaptive changes in post-polio subjects. *Scand. J. Rehabil. Med.* 21:19–26, 1989.

86. Grimby, G., and B. Saltin. The ageing muscle: mini-review. *Clin. Physiol.* 3:209–218, 1983.

87. Haas, F., S. Pasierski, N. Levine, et al. Effect of aerobic training on forced expiratory airflow in exercising asthmatic humans. *J. Appl. Physiol.* 63:1230–1235, 1987.

88. Hagberg, J. M. Effect of training on the decline of VO2 max with aging. *Fed. Proc.* 46:1830–1833, 1987.

89. Hagberg, J. M., D. Goldring, A. A. Ehsani, et al. Effect of exercise training on the blood pressure and hemodynamic features of hypertensive adolescents. *Am. J. Cardiol.* 52:763–768, 1983.

90. Haller, R. G., and S. F. Lewis. Pathophysiology of exercise performance in muscle disease. *Med. Sci. Sports Exerc.* 16:456–459, 1984.

91. Hamilton, M. K. The health and activity limitation survey. *Health Rep.* 1:175–187, 1989.

92. Hardy, L., and D. Jones. Dynamic flexibility and proprioceptive neuromuscular facilitation. *Res. Q. Exerc. Sport* 57:150–153, 1986.

93. Harkcom, T. M., Lampman, R. M., Banwell, B. F., and Castor, C. W. Therapeutic value of graded aerobic exercise training in rheumatoid arthritis. *Arthritis Rheum.* 28:32–39, 1985.

94. Harris, S. R. Children with motor handicaps. M. J. Guralnick and F. C. Bennett (eds.). *The Effectiveness of Early Intervention for At-Risk and Handicapped Children.* London: Academic Press, 1987, pp. 175–212.

95. Heath, G.W. Physical activity promotion in persons with disabilities: clinical applications, public health implications (abstract). *Med. Sci. Sports Exerc.* 26(suppl 5):51, 1993.

96. Heath, G.W. Physical fitness and aging: effects of deconditioning. *Science Sports* 9:197–200, 1994.

97. Heath, G. W., J. M. Hagberg, A. A. Ehsani, and J. O. Holloszy. A physiological comparison of young and older endurance athletes. *J. Appl. Physiol.* 51:634–640, 1981.

98. Heckmatt, J. Z., V. Dubowitz, S. A. Hyde, J. Florence, A. C. Gabain, and N. Thompson. Prolongation of walking in Duchenne muscular dystrophy with lightweight orthoses: review of 57 cases. *Dev. Med. Child Neurol.* 27:149–154, 1985.

99. Hertanu, J. S., L. Davis, and M. Focseneanu. Cardiac rehabilitation exercise program: outcome assessment. *Arch. Phys. Med. Rehabil.* 67:431–435, 1986.

100. Hickson, R. C., C. Kanakis, Jr., J. R. Davis, A. M. Moore, and S. Rich. Reduced training duration effects on aerobic power, endurance, and cardiac growth. *J. Appl. Physiol.* 53:225–229, 1982.

101. Hjeltnes, N. Capacity for physical work and training after spinal injuries and strokes. *Scand J Soc Med* suppl. 29:245–51, 1982.

102. Hjeltnes, N., and Z. Vokac. Circulatory strain in everyday life of paraplegics. *Scand. J. Rehabil. Med.* 11:67–73, 1979.

103. Hoffman, M. D. Cardiorespiratory fitness and training in quadriplegics and paraplegics. *Sports Med.* 3:312–330, 1986.

104. Hopkins, W. G., H. Gaeta, A. C. Thomas, and P. McN. Hill. Physical fitness of blind and sighted children. *Eur. J. Appl. Physiol.* 56:69–73, 1987.

105. Hoskins, T. A. Physiologic responses to known exercise loads in hemiplegic patients. *Arch. Phys. Med. Rehabil.* 56:544, 1975.

106. Housley, E. Treating claudication in five words. *Br. Med. J.* 296:1483, 1988.

107. Huang, C. T., A. B. McEachran, K. V. Kuhlemeier, M. J. DeVivo, and P. R. Fine. Prescriptive arm ergometry to optimize muscular endurance in acutely injured paraplegic patients. *Arch. Phys. Med. Rehabil.* 64:578–582, 1983.

108. Hubert, H. B., D. A. Bloch, and J. F. Fries. Risk factors for physical disability in an aging cohort: the NHANES I epidemiologic follow-up study. *J. Rheumatol.* 20:480–488, 1993.

109. Huddleston, A. L., D. Rockwell, D. N. Kulund, and B. Harrison. Bone mass in lifetime tennis athletes. *J. Am. Med. Assoc.* 244:1107–1109, 1980.

110. Hughes, R. L., and R. Davison. Limitations of exercise reconditioning in COLD. *Chest* 83:241–249, 1983.

111. Ike, R. W., R. M. Lampman, and C. W. Castor. Arthritis and aerobic exercise: a review. *Phys. Sports Med.* 17:128–138, 1989.

112. Inglis, J., M. W. Donald, T. N. Monga, M. Sproule, and M. J. Young. Electromyographic biofeedback and physical therapy of the hemiplegic upper limb. *Arch. Phys. Med. Rehabil.* 65:755–759, 1984.

113. Ivy, J. L. The insulin-like effect of muscle contraction. *Exerc. Sports Sci. Rev.* 15:29–51, 1987.

114. Jackson, R. W., and G. M. Davis. The value of sports and recreation for the physically disabled. *Orthop. Clin. North Am.* 14:301–315, 1983.

115. Jacobson, P. C., W. Beaver, S. A. Grubb, T. N. Taft, and R. V. Talmage. Bone density in women: college athletes and older athletic women. *J. Orthop. Res.* 2:328–332, 1984.

116. Joye, J., A. N. DeMaria, J. Giddens, R. Kaku, E. A. Amsterdam, D. T. Mason, and G. Lee. Exercise induced decreases in platelet aggregation: comparison of normals and coronary patients showing similar physical activity related effects. *Am. J. Cardiol.* 41:432, 1978.

117. Kaplan, P. E., W. Roden, E. Gilbert, L. Richards, and J. W. Goldschmidt. Reduction of hypercalciuria in tetraplegia after weight-bearing and strengthening exercises. *Paraplegia* 19:289–293, 1981.

118. Kasch, F. W., and J. P. Wallace. Physiological variables during 10 years of endurance exercise. *Med. Sci. Sports* 8:5 8, 1976.

119. Kovar, P. A., I. P. Allegrante, C. R. MacKenzie, M.G.E. Peterson, B. Gutin, and M. E. Charlson. Supervised walking in patients with osteoarthritis of the knee: a randomized controlled trial. *Ann. Intern. Med.* 116:529–534, 1992.

120. Knutsson, E., E. Leuenhaupt Olsson, and M. Thorsen. Physical work capacity and physical conditioning in paraplegic patients. *Paraplegia* 11:205–216, 1976.

121. Kristensen J. H., T. I. Hansen, and B. Saltin. Cross-sectional and fiber size changes in the quadriceps muscle of man with immobilization and physical training. *Muscle Nerve* 3:275–276, 1980.

122. LaCroix, A. Z., J. M. Guralnik, L. F. Berkman, R. B. Wallace, and S. Satterfield. Maintaining mobility in late life. II. Smoking, alcohol consumption, physical activity, and body mass index. *Am. J. Epidemiol.* 137:858–869, 1993.

123. Lagerstrøm, D. Sports for the deaf. The First International Medical Congress on Sports

for Disabled, Ustaoset. H. Natvig (ed.). Royal Ministry of Church Education State Office for Youth and Sports, Oslo, 1980, pp. 100–105.

124. Lagomarcino, A., D. H. Reid, M. T. Ivancic, and G. D. Faw. Leisure-dance instruction for severely and profoundly retarded persons:teaching an intermediate community-living skill. *J. Appl. Behav. Anal.* 17:71–84, 1984.

125. Lakatta, E. G. Cardiovascular reserve capacity in healthy older humans. *Aging* 6:213–223, 1994.

126. Lapidus, L., and C. Bengtssen. Socioeconomic factors and physical activity in relation to cardiovascular disease and death. *Br. Heart J.* 55:295–301, 1986.

127. LaPlante, M., and D. Carlson. Disability in the United States: prevalence and causes, 1992. *Disability Statistics Report,* No. 7, Washington, D.C.: U.S. Department of Education, National Institute of Disability and Rehabilitation Reseach, 1996.

128. LaPlante, M. P. Medical conditions associated with disability. S. Thompson-Hoffman and I. Fitzgerald Storck (eds.). *Disability in the United States: A Portrait from National Data.* New York: Springer Publishing Company, 1991, pp. 34–72.

129. Larsson, B., P. Renstrom, K. Svardsudd, L. Welin, G. Grimby, H. Eriksson, L.-O. Ohlson, L. Wilhelmson, and P. Bjorntorp. Health and ageing characteristics of highly physically active 65-year-old men. *Eur. Heart J. (suppl E)* 5:31–35, 1984.

130. Laukkanen, P., E. Heikkinen, and M. Kauppinen. Muscle strength and mobility as predictors of survival in 75–84-year-old people. *Age Ageing* 24:468–473, 1995.

131. Launer, L. J., T. Harris, C. Rumpel, and J. Madans. Body mass index, weight change, and risk of mobility disability in middle-aged and older women: the epidemiologic follow-up study of NANES I. *J. Am. Med. Assoc.* 271:1093–1098, 1994.

132. Lee, P., A. Helewa, H. A. Smythe, C. Bombardier, and C. H. Goldsmith. Epidemiology of musculoskeletal disorders (complaints) and related disability in Canada. *J. Rheumatol.* 12:1169–1173, 1985.

133. Leon, A. S., J. Conrad, D. B. Hunninghake, and R. Serfass. Effect of a vigorous walking program on body composition, and carbohydrate and lipid metabolism of obese young men, *Am. J. Clin. Nutr.* 33:1776–1787, 1979.

134. Lewis, S., L. Higham, and D. B. Cherry. Development of an exercise program to improve the static and dynamic balance of profoundly hearing-impaired children. *Am. Ann. Deaf* 130:278–284, 1985.

135. Logigian, M. K., M. A. Samuels, and J. Falconer. Clinical exercise trial for stroke patients. *Arch. Phys. Med. Rehabil.* 64:364–367, 1983.

136. Lorig, K. R., P. D. Mazonsoll, and H. R. Holmall. Evidence suggesting that health education for self-management in patients with chronic arthritis has sustained health benefits while reducing health care costs. *Arthritis Rheum.* 36:439–446, 1993.

137. Ludwick, S. K., J. W. Jones, T. K. Jones, J. Fukuhara, and R. C. Strunk. Normalization of cardiopulmonary endurance in severely asthmatic children after bicycle ergometry therapy. *J. Pediatr.* 109:446–451, 1986.

138. Lundberg, Å. Changes in the working pulse during the school year in adolescents with cerebral palsy. *Scand. J. Rehabil. Med.* 5:12–17, 1973.

139. Lundberg, Å., C. O. Ovenfors, and B. Saltin. Effect of physical training on school-children with cerebral palsy. *Acta Paediatr. Scand.* 56:182–188, 1967.

140. Madorsky, J. G., and A. Madorsky. Wheelchair racing: an important modality in acute rehabilitation after paraplegia. *Arch. Phys. Med. Rehabil.* 64:186–187, 1983.

141. Malmgren, R., J. Bamford, C. Warlow, P. Sandercock, and J. Slattery. Projecting the number of patients with first ever strokes and patients newly handicapped by stroke in England and Wales. *Br. Med. J.* 298:656–660, 1989.

142. Marge, M. M. Health promotion for persons with disabilities: moving beyond rehabilitation. *Am. J. Health Promotion* 2:29–35, 1988.

143. Martin, J., H. Meltzer, and D. Elliot. The Prevalence of Disability among Adults. Office of Population Censuses and Surveys, HMSO, Report 1, 1988.

144. May, G. S., K. A. Eberlein, C. D. Furberg, E. R. Passamani, and D. L. DeMets. Secondary prevention after myocardial infarction: a review of long-term trials. *Prog. Cardiovasc. Dis.* 24:331–352, 1982.

145. McAdam, R., and H. Natvig. Stair climbing and ability to work for paraplegics with complete lesions—a sixteen year follow-up. *Paraplegia* 18:197–203, 1980.

146. McCartney, N., D. Moroz, S. H. Garner, and A. J. McComas. The effects of strength training in patients with selected neuromuscular disorders. *Med. Sci. Sport Exerc.* 20:362–368, 1988.

147. McGavin, C. R., S. P. Gupta, E. L. Lloyd, and G.J.R. McHardy. Physical rehabilitation for the chronic bronchitis; results of a controlled trial of exercises in the home. *Thorax* 32:307–311, 1977.

148. Mertens, D. J., R. J. Shephard, and T. Kavanagh. Long-term exercise therapy for chronic obstructive lung disease. *Respiration* 35:96–107, 1978.

149. Meyer, C.M.H. Sport and recreation for the severely disabled. *S. Afr. Med. J.* 60:868–871, 1981.

150. Millar, W. J. Report on the 1991 General Social Survey. Ottawa: Statistics Canada, March 1992.

151. Milner-Brown, H. S., and R. G. Miller. Muscle strengthening through high-resistance weight training in patients with neuromuscular disorders. *Arch. Phys. Med. Rehabil.* 69:14 19, 1988.

152. Minor, M. A., and J.F. Hewett. Physical fitness and work capacity in women with rhematoid arthritis. *Arthritis Care Res.* 8:146–154, 1995.

153. Molnar, G. Rehabilitative benefits of sports for the handicapped. *Conn. Med.* 45:574–577, 1981.

154. Morey, M. C., P. A. Cowper, J. R. Feussner, R. C. DiPasquale, G. M. Crowley, D. W. Kitzman, and R. J. Sullivan. Evaluation of a supervised exercise program in a geriatric population. *J. Am Geriatr. Soc.* 37:348–354, 1989.

155. Morisbak, I. Sports for the Blind and Partially Sighted. The First International Medical Congress on Sports for Disabled, Ustaoset. H. Natvig (ed.). Royal Ministry of Church Education State Office for Youth and Sports, Oslo, 1980, pp. 93–99.

156. Nakamura, Y. Working ability of the paraplegics. *Paraplegia* 11:182–193, 1973.

157. National Center for Health Statistics. Healthy People 2000 Review, 1993. Hyattsville, MD: Public Health Service, 1994, pp. 7–13.

158. Nickerson, B. G., D. B. Bautista, M. A. Namey, W. Richards, and T. G. Keens. Distance running improves fitness in asthmatic children without pulmonary complications or changes in exercise-induced bronchospasm. *Pediatrics* 71:147–151, 1983.

159. Niemi, M. L., R. Laaksonen, M. Kotila, and O. Waltimo. Quality of life 4 years after stroke. *Stroke* 19:1101–1107, 1988.

160. Nilsson, S., P. H. Staff, and E.D.R. Pruett. Physical work capacity and the effect of training on subjects with long-standing paraplegia. *Scand. J. Rehabil. Med.* 7:51–56, 1975

161. Nordemar, R., U. Berg, B. Ekblom., and L. Edstrom. Changes in muscle fibre size and physical performance in patients with rheumatoid arthritis after 7 months' physical training. *Scand. J. Rheumatol.* 5:233–238, 1976.

162. Nordemar, R., B. Ekblom, L. Zachrisson, and K. Lundqvist. Physical training in rheumatoid arthritis: a controlled long-term study. *Scand. J. Rheumatol.* 10:17–23, 1981.

163. Noreau, L., R. J. Shephard, C. Simard, G. Pare, and P. Pomerleau. Relationship of impairment and functional ability to habitual activity and fitness following spinal cord injury. *Int. J. Rehabil. Res.* 16:265–275, 1993.

164. O'Brien, B. Multiple Sclerosis, Office of Health Care Economics, 1987.

165. Oldridge, N. B., J. R. Wicks, C. Hanley, J. R. Sutton, and N. L. Jones. Noncompliance in an exercise rehabilitation program for men who have suffered a myocardial infarction. *Can. Med. Assoc. J.* 118:361–364, 1978.

166. Olgiati, R., and P. E. di Prampero. Effect of physical exercise on adaptation to energy expenditure in multiple sclerosis. *Schweiz. Med. Wochenschr.* 116:374–377, 1986.

167. Oligiati, R., J.-M. Burgunder, and M. Mumenthaler. Increased energy cost of walking in multiple sclerosis: effect of spasticity, ataxia, and weakness. *Arch. Phys. Med. Rehabil.* 69:846–849, 1988.

168. Olney, S. J., T. N. Monga, and P. A. Costigan. Mechanical energy of walking of stroke patients. *Arch. Phys. Med. Rehabil.* 67:92–98, 1986.

169. Orenstein, D. M. Exercise tolerance and exercise conditioning in children with chronic lung disease. *J. Pediatr.* 112:1043–1047, 1988.

170. Orenstein, D. M., B. A. Franklin, C. F. Doershuk, H. K. Hellerstein, K. J. Germann, J. G. Horowitz, and R. C. Stern. Exercise conditioning and cardiopulmonary fitness in cystic fibrosis: the effects of a three-month supervised running program. *Chest* 80:392–398, 1981.

171. Orenstein, D. M., M. E. Reed, F. T. Grogan, and L. V. Crawford. Exercise conditioning in children with asthma. *J. Pediatr.* 106:556–560, 1985.

172. Owen, R. R., and D. Jones. Polio residuals clinic: conditioning exercise program. *Orthopedics* 8:882–883, 1985.

173. Pachalski, A., and T. Mekarski. Effect of swimming on increasing of cardio-respiratory capacity in paraplegics. *Paraplegia* 18:190–196, 1980.

174. Paffenbarger, R. S., and R. T. Hyde. Exercise in the prevention of coronary heart disease. *Prev. Med.* 13:3–22, 1984.

175. Paffenbarger, R. S., Jr., A. L. Wing, and R. T. Hyde. Physical activity as an index of heart attack risk in college alumni. *Am. J. Epidemiol.* 108:161–175, 1978.

176. Painter, P., and G. Blackburn. Exercise for patients with chronic disease. *Postgrad. Med.* 83:185–196, 1988.

177. Pandavela, J., S. Gordon, G. Gordon, and C. Jones. Martial arts for the quadriplegic. *Am. J. Phys. Med.* 65:17–29, 1986.

178. Patrick, J. H., and M. R. McClelland. Low energy cost reciprocal walking for the adult paraplegic. *Paraplegia* 23:113–117, 1985.

179. Peganhoff, S. A. The use of aquatics with cerebral palsied adolescents. *Am. J. Occup. Ther.* 38:469–473, 1984.

180. Pate, R. R., M. Pratt, S. N. Blair, W. L. Haskell, C. A. Macera, C. Bouchard, D. Buchner, W. Ettinger, G. W. Heath, et al. Physical activity and public health: a recommendation from the Centers for Disease Control and Prevention and the American College of Sports Medicine. *J. Am. Med. Assoc.* 273:402–407, 1995.

181. Peterson, M.G.E., P. A. Kovar-Toledano, J. C. Otis, et al. Effect of a walking program on gait characteristics in patients with osteoarthritis. *Arthritis Care Res.* 6:11–16, 1993.

182. Petrofsky, J.S., H. Heaton, 3rd., and C. A. Phillips. Outdoor bicycle for exercise in paraplegics and quadriplegics. *J. Biomed. Eng.* 5:292–296, 1983.

183. Phillips, W. T., and W. L. Haskell. Muscular Fitness —easing the burden of disability for elderly adults. *J. Aging Phys. Activity* 3:261–289, 1995.

184. Pollock, M. L., C. Foster, D. Knapp, J. L. Rod, and D. H. Schmidt. Effect of age and training on aerobic capacity and body composition of master athletes. *J. Appl. Physiol.* 62:725–731, 1987.

185. Ponichtera-Mulcare, J. A. Exercise and multiple sclerosis. *Med. Sci. Sports Exerc.* 25:451–465, 1993.

186. Powell, K. E., P. D. Thompson, C. J. Casperson, and J. S. Kendrick. Physical activity and the incidence of coronary heart disease. *Ann. Rev. Public Health* 8:253–287, 1987.

187. Puett, D. W., and M. R. Griffin. Published trials of nonmedical and noninvasive therapies for hip and knee osteoarthritis. *Ann. Intern. Med.* 121:133–140, 1994.

188. Raab, D. M., J. C. Agre, M. McAdams, and E. L. Smith. Light resistance and stretching exercise in elderly women: effect upon flexibility. *Arch. Phys. Med. Rehabil.* 69:268–272, 1988.

189. Rodeheffer, R. J., G. Gerstenblith, L. C. Becker, J. L. Fleg, M. L. Weisfeldt, and E. G. Lakatta. Exercise cardiac output is maintained with advancing age in healthy human subjects: cardiac dilatation and increased stroke volume compensate for a diminished heart rate. *Circulation* 69:203–213, 1984.

190. Salter, R. B. Prevention of arthritis through preservation of cartilage. *J. Can. Assoc. Radiol.* 32:5–7, 1981.

191. Santiago, M. C., C. P. Coyle, and W. B. Kinney. Aerobic exercise effect on individuals with physical disabilities. *Arch. Phys. Med. Rehabil.* 74:1192–1198, 1993.

192. Schneider, V. S., and J. McDonald. Skeletal calcium homeostasis and countermeasures to prevent disuse osteoporosis. *Calcif. Tissue Int.* 36(suppl):S151–S154, 1984.

193. Schurrer, R., A. Weltman, and H. Brammell. Effects of physical training on cardiovascular fitness and behavior patterns of mentally retarded adults. *Am. J. Ment. Defic.* 90:167–170, 1985.

194. Seals, D. R., J. M. Hagberg, B. F. Hurley, A. A. Ehsani, and J. O. Holloszy. Endurance training in older men and women I. Cardiovascular responses to exercise. *J. Appl. Physiol.* 57:1024–1029, 1984.

195. Shephard, R. J. Training and the respiratory system—therapy for asthma and other obstructive diseases? *Ann. Clin. Res.* 14(suppl 34):86–96, 1982.

196. Shephard, R. J. Benefits of sport and physical activity for the disabled: implications for the individual and for society. *Scand. J. Rehabil. Med.* 23:51–59, 1991.

197. Shindo, M., S. Komagai, and H. Tanaka. Physical work capacity and effect of endurance training in visually handicapped boys and young male adults. *Eur. J. Appl. Physiol.* 56:501–507.

198. Siegel, W., C. Blomqvist, and J. H. Mitchell. Effects of a quantitated physical training program on middle-aged sedentary men. *Circulation* 41:19–29, 1970.

199. Sinclair, D. J. M., and C. G. Ingram. Controlled trial of supervised exercise training in chronic bronchitis. *Br. Med. J.* 1:519–521, 1980.

200. Smith, E. L., Jr., W. Reddan, and P. E. Smith. Physical activity and calcium modalities for bone mineral increase in aged women. *Med. Sci. Sports Exerc.* 13:60–64, 1981.

201. Sockolov, R., B. Irwin, R. H. Dressendorfer, and E. M. Bernauer. Exercise performance in 6-to-11 year old boys with Duchenne muscular dystrophy. *Arch. Phys. Med. Rehabil.* 58:195–201, 1977.

202. Sorock, G. S., T. L. Bush, A. L. Golden, L. P. Fried, B. Breuer, and W. E. Hale. Physical activity and fracture risk in a free-living elderly cohort. *J. Gerontol.* 43: M134–139, 1988.

203. Spira, R. Sport activities in severe motor paralysis in adolescents: their therapeutic and preventive value The First International Medical Congress on Sports for Disabled, Ustaoset. H. Natvig (ed.). Royal Ministry of Church Education State Office for Youth and Sports, Oslo, 1980, pp. 200–205.

204. Stanghelle, J. K., H. Michalsen, and D. Skyberg. Five-year follow-up of pulmonary function and peak oxygen uptake in 16-year-old boys with cystic fibrosis, with special regard to the influence of regular physical exercise. *Int. J. Sports Med.* 9:19–24, 1988.

205. Steinberg, F. U. Rehabilitating the older stroke patient: what's possible? *Geriatrics* 41:85–97, 1986.

206. Stephens, T., and C. J. Caspersen. The demography of physical activity. C. Bouchard, R. Shephard, and T. Stephens (eds.). *Physical Activity, Fitness, and Health.* Champaign, IL: Human Kinetics, 1994, pp. 204–213.

207. Stern, M. J., P. A. Gorman, and L. Kaslow. The group counselling v exercise therapy study. A controlled intervention with subjects following myocardial infarction. *Arch. Intern. Med.* 143:1719–1725, 1983.

208. Stewart, R. I. Exercise in patients with chronic obstructive pulmonary disease. *S. Afr. Med. J.* 67:87–89, 1985.

209. Stotts, K. M. Health maintenance: paraplegic athletes and nonathletes. *Arch. Phys. Med. Rehabil.* 67:109–114, 1986.

210. Strauss, G. D., A. Osher, C.-I. Wang, E. Goodrich, F. Gold, W. Colman, M. Stabile, A. Dobrenchuk, and T. G. Kenns. Variable weight training in cystic fibrosis. *Chest* 92:273–276, 1987.

211. Streja, D., and D. Mymin. Moderate exercise and high-density lipoprotein-cholesterol: observations during a cardiac rehabilitation program. *J. Am. Med. Assoc.* 242:2190–2192, 1979.

212. Sundberg, S. Maximal oxygen uptake in relation to age in blind and normal boys and girls. *Acta Paediatr. Scand.* 71:603–608, 1982.

213. Suominen, H., E. Heikkinen, and T. Parkatti. Effect of eight weeks' physical training on muscle and connective tissue of the m. vastus lateralis in 69-year-old men and women. *J. Gerontol.* 32:33–37, 1977.

214. Svendsen, D. Physical activity in the treatment of mentally retarded persons. *Scand. J. Soc. Med.* 29(suppl 711):253–257, 1982.

215. Svenonius, E., R. Kautto, and M. Arborelius, Jr. Improvement after training of children with exercise-induced asthma. *Acta Paediatr. Scand.* 72:23–30, 1983.

216. Taylor, A. W., E. McDonell, and L. Brassard. The effects of an arm ergometer training programme on wheelchair subjects. *Paraplegia* 24:105–114, 1986.

217. Thompson, R. F., D. M. Crist, M. Marsh, and M. Rosenthal. Effects of physical exercise for elderly patients with physical impairments. *J. Am. Gerontol. Soc.* 36:130–135, 1988.

218. Tomporowski, P. D., and N. R. Ellis. The effects of exercise on the health, intelligence, and adaptive behavior of institutionalized severely and profoundly mentally retarded adults: a systematic replication. *Appl. Res. Ment. Retard.* 6:465–473, 1985.

219. Van Deusen, J. The efficacy of ROM dance program for adults with rheumatoid arthritis. *Am. J. Occup. Ther.* 41:90–95, 1987.

220. Vignos, P. J., and M. P. Watkins. Effect of exercise in muscular dystrophy. *J. Am. Med. Assoc.* 197:121–126, 1966.

221. Wade, D. T., C. E. Skilbeck, R. L. Hewer, and V. A. Wood. Therapy after stroke: amounts, determinants and effects. *Int. Rehabil. Med.* 6:105–110, 1984.

222. Wagner E. H., and A. Z. LaCroix. Effects of physical activity on health status in older adults. I. Observational studies. *Ann. Rev. Public Health* 13:451–468, 1992.

223. Weinberger, M., W. M. Tierney, P. Booher, and B. P. Katz. Can provision of information to patients with osteoarthritis improve functional status?: a randomized, controlled trial. *Arthritis Rheum.* 32:1577–1583, 1989.

224. West, R. R., and D. A. Evans. Lifestyle changes in long term survivors of acute myocardial infarction, *J. Epidemiol. Commun. Health* 40:103–109, 1986.

225. Wicks, J. R., B. J. Cameron, N. B. Oldreidge, B. J. Cameron, and N. L. Jones. Arm cranking and wheelchair ergometry in elite spinal cord injured athletes. *Med. Sci. Sports Exerc.* 15:224–231, 1983.

226. Wiechers, D. O. Acute and latent effects of poliomyelitis on the motor unit as revealed by electromyography. *Orthopedics* 8:870–872, 1985.

227. Williams, R. S., E. E. Logue, J. L. Lewis, T. Barton, N. W. Stead, A. G. Wallace, and S. V. Pizzo. Physical conditioning augments the fibrinolytic response to venous occlusion in healthy adults. *N. Engl. J. Med.* 302:987–991, 1980.

228. Wolf, S. L., and S. A. Binder-Macleod. Electromyographic biofeedback applications to hemiplegic patient: changes in upper extremity neuromuscular and functional status. *Phys. Ther.* 63:1393–1403, 1983.

229. Wood, P. D., W. L. Haskell, S. N. Blair, P. T. Williams, R. N. Krauss, F. T. Lindgren, J. J. Albers, P. H. Ho, and J. W. Farquhar. Increased exercise level and plasma lipoprotein concentrations: a one-year, randomized, controlled study in sedentary, middle-aged men. *Metabolism* 32:31–39, 1983.

230. World Health Organization. *International Classification of Impairments, Disabilities, and Handicaps.* Geneva: WHO, 1980.

231. Yeh, C-K, and G. A. Rodan. Tensile forces enhance prostaglandin E synthesis in osteoblastic cells grown on collagen ribbons. *Calcif. Tissue Int.* 36(suppl):S67–S71, 1984.

232. Young, A. Exercise physiology in geriatric practice. *Acta Med. Scand.* 711(suppl):S227–S232, 1986.

233. Zach, M. S., B. Purrer, and B. Oberwaldner. Effect of swimming on forced expiration and sputum clearance in cystic fibrosis. *Lancet* ii:1201–1203, 1981.

9
Exercise Testing and Training in Patients with Malignant Arrhythmias

FREDRIC J. PASHKOW, M.D.
ROBERT A. SCHWEIKERT, M.D.
BRUCE L. WILKOFF, M.D.

For years, the presence of premature ventricular contractions (PVCs) during exercise has been disquieting to both exercise and medical professionals. The assumption, until relatively recently, was that such ectopy is a hallmark of pathology. Although there was some effort made to distinguish between ectopic rhythm conditions that are "benign" (meaning no negative immediate hemodynamic effect or prognosis) or "malignant" (meaning an association with immediate or future hemodynamic instability or sudden death), the mere presence of any ventricular ectopy warranted concern and often resulted in attempts at suppression. This notion was applied especially to patients who had experienced myocardial infarction (MI). It was a predominant influence in the development of procedural codes in the 1970s for cardiac rehabilitation that specified the need for continuous electrocardiogram (ECG) monitoring and a physician's presence while coronary disease patients participated in diagnostic or therapeutic exercise.

However, observant clinicians began to report that there were particular conditions predisposing patients to untoward arrhythmia-induced events. The presence or absence of ventricular ectopic activity during monitoring is actually a poorer predictor of future outcomes than documentation of predisposing conditions or clinical concomitants. The circumstances include the presence of active ischemia, especially when adjacent to a region of prior myocardial injury; compromised left ventricular (LV) function; or the occurrence of sudden death, except in the recent aftermath of an acute MI. When these circumstances are present, the current approach is to assess the patient carefully with noninvasive and/or invasive studies to determine both the need for and the appropriate type of therapy. The therapy of malignant or potentially malignant arrhythmia has changed radically in recent years.

Until relatively recently, antiarrhythmic drugs were the approach of choice when suppression was deemed appropriate. However, the Cardiac Arrhythmia Suppression Trial (CAST) study taught us that the proarrhythmic effects of antiarrhythmic drugs may produce greater harm than the desired outcome of ectopy suppression [110]. In addition, there was a growing body of evidence supporting clinical suspicion that compromised LV function predisposes to bad outcome. Several studies demonstrated that patients with poor LV function are particularly at risk for proarrhythmia [111, 116]. Although initially appearing to be a more radical approach, implanted antiarrhythmic devices may have better efficacy and overall cost-effectiveness than what is observed with antiarrhythmic drugs. This controversial subject is being evaluated in several large multicenter trial, including Antiarrhythmics Versus Implantable Defibrillators (AVID) [9], Canadian Implantable Defibrillation Study (CIDS) [24], Cardiac Arrest Study Hamburg (CASH) [106], and Multicenter Automatic Defibrillator Implantation Trial (MADIT) [8].

In this review, we will examine the relevant physiology of exercise and arrhythmia in the context of exercise testing and training of patients in whom malignant arrhythmia is suspected or already identified as a problem. We will discuss the indications for exercise testing and, for those who undertake testing of people at risk, some appropriate measures and guidelines. We will then apply these findings to the patient's management and the formulation of activity guidelines and the exercise prescription. We will also provide an introduction to implantable cardioverter-defibrillators (ICDs), including a description of the features of the devices and directions for programming and management.

This is a dynamic field of medicine; it has literally evolved into an entire superspecialty (electrophysiology) within the last decade. The details of the application and the technology of the antiarrhythmic devices change almost weekly. However, the fundamental principles and virtues of exercise remain the same for both the evaluation and treatment of those burdened with malignant arrhythmias.

PHYSIOLOGY OF ARRHYTHMIA AND EXERCISE

In order to understand the important role of exercise testing in the evaluation of patients with malignant arrhythmias, one must understand the proposed mechanisms responsible for the initiation of arrhythmia and the complex interaction among the myocardial substrate and the sympathetic and parasympathetic nervous system, circulating catecholamines, and other metabolic and mechanical factors that are influenced by exercise. In general, arrhythmias occur as a result of abnormalities of impulse formation and/or impulse conduction [128]. Three principal mechanisms have been proposed to explain the cause of arrhythmia [28]: (a) reentry; (b) enhanced automaticity; and (c) triggered automaticity. Reentrant arrhythmia is a disorder of impulse conduction resulting from continuous movement of electrical activity around a physiological circuit. This requires a myocardial substrate with differing properties of conduction velocity and refractoriness. Enhanced automaticity of ectopic foci results from the increased rate of spontaneous (Phase 4) depolarization of myocardial tissue, as may occur within regions damaged by cardiac disease. Triggered automaticity results from delayed afterpotentials [122].

Cardiac disease can, therefore, provide conditions whereby arrhythmias are more likely to occur, and these conditions may be fixed or relatively transient. Coronary artery disease can result in myocardial scar secondary to infarction, or produce transient effects secondary to ischemia. Cardiomyopathies, such as those secondary to an idiopathic process, hypertrophy, multiple infarcts, infections, or infiltrative diseases like sarcoidosis, also provide substrate that can promote arrhythmias via these mechanisms. Disruption of myocardial tissue, such as postsurgical states (e.g., that after aneurysmectomy or repair of congenital malformations), may also play a role in the genesis of arrhythmias.

Any of these mechanisms may be potentiated by transient changes in factors such as the autonomic nervous system, circulating catecholamines [51], serum electrolytes, oxygen saturation, and pH. The sympathetic nervous system and catecholamines, in particular, have a significant effect on many physiological factors that play a role in arrhythmogenesis, including mechanical, metabolic, and electrophysiological factors [91, 92]. Catecholamines increase myocardial conduction velocity and decrease membrane refractory periods [51]. In fact, for this reason isoproterenol is useful in the facilitation of ventricular arrhythmia induction during electrophysiology studies [43]. Activation of the sympathetic nervous system results in an increase in the spontaneous automaticity (Phase 4 spontaneous depolarization) of myocardial tissue. There is also an increase in the amplitude of delayed afterpotentials as the result of an increase in the influx of calcium ions, which can potentiate triggered automaticity [123]. Patients with abnormal ventricular function may be particularly susceptible to provocation of arrhythmias resulting from activation of the sympathetic nervous system [92].

In addition, changes in various metabolic factors may lead to electrolyte imbalance, acidosis, or ischemia that can favor arrhythmogenesis. Mechanical alterations, such as increased inotropy, heart rate, blood pressure, and afterload, can lead to an increase in myocardial oxygen demand. In the presence of significant coronary artery disease, these changes could result in myocardial ischemia, which can lead to arrhythmias [93].

Exercise produces complex physiological changes that can potentiate or suppress arrhythmias. The increased heart rate may suppress ventricular ectopic activity, thereby eliminating a potential trigger for arrhythmia. However, exercise results in the withdrawal of vagal tone, and activation of the sympathetic nervous system with a concomitant increase in circulating serum catecholamines. Figure 9.1 illustrates the interaction of the parasympathetic and sympathetic nervous systems during exercise, which can lead to initiation of arrhythmia [91]. This withdrawal of vagal tone and activation of the sympathetic nervous system serves to potentiate arrhythmia, particularly in patients with the proper substrate from cardiac disease [27]. Is-

FIGURE 9.1.
Physiological effects of exercise. Modified from ref. 91.

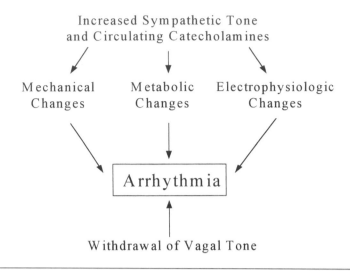

chemia is thought to be a precipitating factor in many ventricular arrhythmias associated with exercise as well [6, 38].

With our interest focused on electrical phenomena, we often forget about the interrelationship between the ECG and the mechanical ejection of blood from the heart. There may be no effective ejection of blood after a PVC and, thus, no pressure pulse generated from the premature beat. The beat after the PVC may produce a larger stroke volume related to the prolonged filling time, but the net effect of increasing PVCs during exercise could be the compromise of cardiac output during exercise stress. A patient who develops ventricular bigeminy at a high level of exercise could theoretically experience a 50% reduction in cardiac output. There has been very little published in the clinical literature regarding the hemodynamic implications of frequent ventricular ectopy during exercise, but preliminary observations from our laboratory suggest that an increasing frequency of PVCs during exercise is associated with a decrease in achieved workload, even after multivariables are controlled (R. A. Schweikert, unpublished observations).

SIGNIFICANCE OF EXERCISE-INDUCED VENTRICULAR ECTOPIC ACTIVITY

The clinical significance of exercise-induced ventricular ectopic activity, however, is unclear. Table 9.1 [89] summarizes the findings of selected

TABLE 9.1.
Prevalence of Ventricular Arrhythmia during Exercise

| | % with Arrhythmia | | | |
| | Simple VPBs[a] | | Repetitive VPBs | |
Study	Normal	Heart Disease	Normal	Heart Disease
Beard and Owen [13]	8.0		0.3	
Master [72]	18.0		0.3	
Whinnery [121]	5.0	50.0	0	15.0
McHenry et al. [74]	34.0	50.0	6.0	22.0
Poblete et al. [89]	7.0	62.0	0	31.0
Cordini et al. [26]			0.1	0.7
Ryan et al. [96]		55.0		20.0
Gooch and McConnell [46]		45.0		
Califf et al. [20]	14.0	23.0	2.4	8.2
Weiner et al. [118]		19.0		
Detry et al. [32]				0.58[b]
Jelinek and Lown [56]	19.0	36.0	1.8	3.6

From ref. 91.
[a]VPB, ventricular premature beats.
[b]Ventricular tachycardia or ventricular fibrillation.

studies that examined the incidence of ventricular ectopic activity during exercise [13, 20, 26, 32, 46, 56, 72, 74, 89, 96, 118, 121]. Both simple and more complex repetitive ventricular ectopy occurred more frequently in patients with heart disease than in those without heart disease.

The observation that exercise-induced ventricular arrhythmias occur more frequently in patients with heart disease raised questions as to their impact on subsequent mortality. The prognostic importance of exercise-induced ventricular ectopic activity has been studied in various patient populations. Table 9.2, expanded from the original table published by Podrid, summarizes the findings of several studies [17, 20, 22, 41, 44, 47, 52, 65, 77, 80, 85, 99, 112, 117–119, 126]. Patients with coronary artery disease and exercise-induced ventricular arrhythmias, particularly those with a recent myocardial infarction or evidence of ischemia on exercise testing, were shown by some studies to have a higher subsequent mortality rate than those patients without coronary artery disease. However, other studies do not corroborate this. Sami et al. retrospectively reviewed 1486 patients with stable coronary artery disease included in the multicenter registry for the Coronary Artery Surgery Study who underwent exercise stress testing and were followed for an average of 4.3 yr. The event-free survival was not significantly different for those patients with exercise-induced ventricular arrhythmia and those without, regardless of the presence or absence of significant coronary artery disease [99]. Weiner et al. reported similar findings

TABLE 9.2.
Prognostic Significance of Exercise-induced Ventricular Premature Beats

Study	Population	No. of Patients	Follow-up (yr)	Mortality %			Signifi-cant
				No VPBs[a]	Simple VPBs	Complex VPBs	
Califf et al. [20]	No sig. CAD	673	3.0	<2	<2	<2	No
Califf et al. [20]	CAD	620	3.0	10	17	25	Yes
Weiner et al. [118]	Significant CAD	335	4.3	NR	13	NR	No
Weiner et al. [118]	Minimal CAD	111	5.0	NR	9	NR	No
Udall and Ellestad [112]	CAD (−ST)	758	5.0	1.4	8		Yes
Udall and Ellestad [112]	CAD (+ST)	569	5.0	NR	22		Yes
Weld et al. [119]	Early post-MI	236	1	1	12	?	Yes
Krone et al. [66]	Early post-MI	667	1	NR	7	13	Yes
Henry et al. [52]	Early post-MI	163	2	8	25	NR	Yes
Graboys et al. [47]	SCD survivors	123	2.6		2.3	43.6	Yes
Weaver et al. [117]	SCD survivors	90	2.0	41	15	44	No
Sami et al. [99]	Minimal CAD	245	4.3	12	24		No
Sami et al. [99]	Significant CAD	1241	4.3	24	29		No
Yang et al. [126]	Suspected CAD	3351	2.2	5.1	3.6		No
Peduzzi et al. [85]	CAD	245	11	25	48		Yes
Fioretti et al. [41]	Early post-MI	408	1		7	17	No
O'Hara et al. [80]	VT/VF post-MI	150	2.8		14	35	Yes
Casella et al. [22]	Late post-MI	777	2	3.4	1.8	3.2	No
Busby et al. [17]	Asymptomatic	1160	5.6		±10	±10	No
Morris et al. [77]	Known or suspected CAD	588	5	NR	26	5	No
Froelicher [44]	Early post-MI	258	7.9	NR	NR	NR	No

Adapted from ref. 91.
[a]VPB, ventricular premature beats; CAD, coronary artery disease; SCD, sudden cardiac death; +ST, ST-segment depression; −ST, no ST-segment. changes; NR, not reported.

in a study of 446 patients who underwent exercise stress testing and cardiac catheterization. Exercise-induced ventricular arrhythmias were associated with three-vessel or left main coronary artery disease, ischemic ST-segment depression, lower ventricular ejection fraction, and more severe regional wall motion abnormalities. However, exercise-induced ventricular arrhythmias were not associated with a higher cardiac mortality at a mean follow-up of 5.3 yr [118].

We prospectively examined 2743 consecutive adults without heart failure, valve disease, prior invasive procedures, known severe resting ventricular ectopic activity, or use of β-blockers or digitalis who underwent maximal exercise thallium studies and were followed for 2 yr. Frequent ventricular ectopy or nonsustained ventricular tachycardia occurred in 128 patients (4.7%) during exercise and was associated with male gender, older age, and lower exercise capacity. There was no association with angina, diuretic use, or other standard risk factors. Exercise-induced ventricular ectopic activity was predictive of thallium defects but did not predict cardiac or all cause mortality. Interestingly, for those patients who subsequently underwent cardiac catheterization, exercise-induced ventricular arrhythmias were not associated with the presence or anatomical extent of coronary artery disease (R. A. Schweikert, unpublished data).

HEART RATE VARIABILITY AND ITS POTENTIAL RELATIONSHIP TO ARRHYTHMIA AND EXERCISE

Heart rate variability (HRV) has been shown to be a predictor of mortality after MI [61]. Kleiger et al. followed 808 patients after MI and found a 34.4% mortality rate in those patients with a HRV less than 50 ms, whereas patients with a HRV greater than 100 ms had only a 9% mortality rate. HRV was defined by Kleiger as the standard deviation of all normal RR intervals in a 24-hr continuous ECG done 11 ± 3 days after MI. Using a Cox Proportional Hazard Model, Kleiger noticed a stronger association between HRV and mortality than other Holter variables, including PVC frequency, runs of PVCs, or couplets. The relative risk for these Holter variables were 3.4, 2.6, 2.7, and 2.5, respectively. Cripps et al. [29] corroborated Kleiger's findings by demonstrating a relative risk of 7.0 for the occurrence of sudden death or ventricular arrhythmia in those patients with a HRV index less than 25.

Kleiger and associates have demonstrated that patients with a shorter cycle length variability (CLV) of <50 ms have a relative mortality risk five times as high as those with a CLV >100 ms [62]. Kleiger suggests that the increased sympathetic tone, the decreased parasympathetic tone, or both cause the low CLV values that are independently associated with the increased mortality. Bigger and associates found that a variety of other indices of heart period variability are reduced in patients with a low CLV [15], suggesting that patients with low heart period variability after MI have reduced parasympathetic (vagal) activity. Multiple measures of vagal activity appear to increase with atenolol administration but not with diltiazem, possibly explaining the improved mortality observed in those treated with β-blockers and not with calcium-channel blockers after MI [25].

Exercise training increases vagal activity [115]. Exercise training of dogs after MI increased the baroreceptor reflex slope (which had decreased after MI) and decreased susceptibility to ventricular fibrillation [103]. Lombardi and colleagues found that in the early weeks after infarction, patients had smaller high-frequency (HF) peaks (representing vagal activity) and larger low-frequency (LF) peaks (representing sympathetic activity), when compared to the controls [69]. Late studies suggest that autonomic balance returned by 6 mo.

Seals has shown that physical training may influence HRV [104]. Subjects were studied before and after a period of regular endurance exercise and showed that, in general, HRV was greater after training, but there was no significant alteration in baroreflex control of heart rate.

Mazzuero et al. have examined the effects of physical training on the multiple indices of HRV in patients with previous anterior MI [73]. At 4–6 wk after MI, patients were randomly assigned to a training group ($n = 22$) or to a control group ($n = 16$) and studied again 6 mo later. HRV was almost in normal range or slightly decreased in a few subjects initially and increased on average at 6 mo without significant differences between that of training and control groups. However, analysis of 24-hr dynamics of HRV in single patients showed different patterns and adaptations 6 mo after anterior MI [73]. Thus, the question of whether the reduction in cardiac sudden death observed in rehabilitation patients undergoing exercise training is a result of improvements in HRV remains an open one. However, the findings suggest that the alteration of vagal activity associated with physical training may have positive theoretical benefit in patients with ectopic arrhythmia.

SAFETY OF EXERCISE TESTING AND TRAINING IN NORMAL PATIENTS AND THE REHABILITATION POPULATION

The safety of exercise stress testing and training has been evaluated in populations thought to be at low risk for cardiovascular complications. Exercise stress testing has been demonstrated to be safe, and more recent studies indicate increased safety over the years. This trend reflects the improvements in cardiac care. The evolving medical and surgical therapy of ischemia has achieved significant success. Ischemia, a known precipitant of arrhythmia, is now better controlled by the time patients arrive in the cardiac rehabilitation setting than it was during the previous decade. This is a reflection of improved medical therapies for coronary artery disease, as well as increased use of coronary revascularization.

The improvement in the safety of exercise may also be related to advances in appropriate patient selection, as well as to better monitoring techniques during and after the study. Furthermore, there is more judicious use of antiarrhythmic drugs in light of the lessons learned from trials such as CAST. This trend should continue as more trials demonstrate the potential for antiarrhythmic drugs to worsen patient outcome. A more recent example is the premature termination of the Survival with Oral *d*-Sotalol (SWORD) trial because of excess mortality. This was a study of the use of *d*-sotalol, a Class III antiarrhythmic drug, for the treatment of ventricular arrhythmias in patients with LV dysfunction after MI [116]. In addition, drug therapy for congestive heart failure has improved, as medications with proven efficacy and safety in large clinical trials become more widely used.

There have been many reports documenting the safety of exercise stress testing in low-risk patient populations. Table 9.3 summarizes the findings of several of these studies [11, 18, 33, 45, 55, 109, 126, 127]. These studies demonstrate the low morbidity and mortality rates of exercise testing in these patient groups. Irving and Bruce reported the experience with 10,700 maximal treadmill exercise tests performed in 15 centers as part of the Seattle Heart Watch Study. There were six cases (0.06%) of ventricular fibrillation, each of which were successfully resuscitated [55]. Gibbons et al. reported on 71,914 maximal exercise tests conducted at a single medical center from 1971 through 1987, in a population with a low prevalence of known coronary artery disease. There were six major cardiac complications, including one death, all occurring before 1979. The complication rate was reported to be 0.008%, with no complications reported in the final 10 yr involving 45,000 tests [45]. It is interesting, as Gibbons and coworkers point out, that no complications occurred at their facility after 1978 when there was initiation of a 3-min gradual cool-down after normal exercise tests and a 5-min gradual cool down after abnormal tests.

We have examined the incidence of serious arrhythmic complications during approximately 50,000 consecutive stress tests performed at the Cleveland Clinic Foundation from 1988 through June 1996. Serious arrhythmic complications were defined as the occurrence of ventricular fibrillation or ventricular tachycardia, resulting in hemodynamic instability or arrest necessitating the termination of the study. There were 24 (0.05%) episodes of sustained ventricular tachycardia and 7 (0.01%) episodes of ventricular fibrillation (F. J. Pashkow et al., unpublished data). This data is comparable to that reported from other published reports (Table 9.3).

The history of cardiac arrest with exercise in rehabilitation also shows a dramatically improved trend. From 1960 to 1977, one cardiac arrest per 33,000 patient hr of exercise was reported [50]. From 1980 to 1984, the

TABLE 9.3.
Complications of Exercise Stress Testing in Low-Risk Populations

Study	No. of Exercise Tests	Sustained VT[a] per 10,000 Tests (%)	VF per 10,000 Tests (%)	Morbidity per 10,000 Tests (%)	Mortality per 10,000 Tests (%)
Atterhog, et al. [11]	50,000	5.8 (0.06)	0.2 (0.002)	5.2 (0.05)	0.4 (0.004)
Cahalin et al. [18]	10,577	2.8 (0.03)	0	3.8 (0.04)	0.9 (0.009)
Irving and Bruce [55]	10,700	Not reported	5.6 (0.05)		0
Detry et al. [33]	7,500	17.3 (0.17)	8 (0.08)		0
Gibbons et al. [45]	71,914	0	0.28 (0.003)	0.8 (0.008)	0.1 (0.001)
Stuart and Ellestad [109]	518,448	4.78 (0.05)		8.36 (0.08)	0.5 (0.01)
Yang et al. [126]	3,351 pts	14.9 (0.15)	3 (0.03)	11.9 (0.12)	0
Young et al. [127]	8,221	0	4.9 (0.05)		0

[a]VT, ventricular tachycardia; VF, ventricular fibrillation.

odds improved to the occurrence of one arrest during 112,000 patient hr [113]. Again, this is likely a reflection of the improvements in the medical and surgical treatment of heart disease, as well as technological advancements in the monitoring of patients during and after the study.

It is possible that better understanding of the complex physiological changes that occur during exercise has also led to increased safety. For example, the literature suggests that it is the early recovery period when patients are most susceptible to serious complications, including arrhythmia. Measurements of plasma catecholamines during and after exercise have demonstrated a significant surge in catecholamines, particularly norepinephrine, in the early recovery period [34]. Minimizing this surge in catecholamines with a "cool-down" period, that is, a gradual cessation of exercise, would be prudent, particularly in patients who are at high risk for developing sustained tachyarrhythmias.

In light of the physiological effects of exercise, stress testing is useful as an adjunctive technique to the other methods used to evaluate arrhythmia, as a diagnostic tool for the exposure of arrhythmia in patients thought to be at high risk, and also as a method of evaluating the response to therapy. Exercise may counteract or enhance the effects of antiarrhythmic drugs used in the treatment of arrhythmias. Membrane-active antiarrhythmic drugs result in decreased velocity of membrane conduction (Phase 0), prolongation of myocardial refractory period (Phase 3), decreased excitability, and decreased automaticity (Phase 4). These effects are in opposition to, and therefore possibly counteracted by, the physiological effects of catecholamines. This is supported by studies whereby administration of isoproterenol or epinephrine has been shown to reverse the effects of certain antiarrhythmic agents [1, 76].

However, the complex physiological changes that occur during and after exercise may also result in enhancement of antiarrhythmic drug action. The Class I antiarrhythmic drugs, or the sodium-channel blocking drugs, have a property called use dependence. This refers to the enhancement of drug action at higher heart rates. Myocardial depolarization results in sodium-channel activation (opening), then inactivation, which facilitates drug binding. Myocardial repolarization results in the sodium-channel returning to its resting state, which facilitates drug dissociation. An increase in heart rate results in more time spent in the activated/inactivated states, which may lead to enhancement of antiarrhythmic drug action. In addition, each antiarrhythmic drug has a particular time constant or time interval during which the drug binds and unbinds to the sodium channel. Drugs with a longer time constant, such as the Class IC agents, may have a more enhanced effect with exercise than those agents with shorter time constants and, therefore, may be more prone to proarrhythmia during exercise [53, 54, 95].

This is an important concept to recognize in the management of a patient with malignant arrhythmias. The efficacy and safety of an antiarrhythmic drug may not be the same during exercise as they are during rest, particularly with Type IC drugs such as flecainide. In fact, some authorities have recommended routine exercise testing to assess the proarrhythmic potential of patients treated with flecainide [7].

EXERCISE STRESS TESTING IN THE DIAGNOSIS AND MANAGEMENT OF ARRHYTHMIAS

Indications for Exercise Stress Testing

Exercise stress testing plays an important role in the evaluation of patients with heart disease, particularly in those patients with malignant ventricular arrhythmias. Table 9.4 summarizes the indications for exercise stress testing for patients with symptoms or signs suggestive of coronary artery disease or with known coronary artery disease, as recommended by The American Heart Association/American College of Cardiology Task Force on Assessment of Cardiovascular Procedures [100]. Note that the evaluation of patients with suspected exercise-induced cardiac arrhythmias is a Class I indication for exercise stress testing.

Contraindications to Exercise Stress Testing

Table 9.5 summarizes the absolute and relative contraindications to exercise testing according to the American Heart Association report on exercise standards [42]. Patients with uncontrolled cardiac arrhythmias, particularly those patients with severely symptomatic or hemodynamically unstable arrhythmias, should not undergo exercise stress testing or training.

TABLE 9.4.
Indications for Exercise Testing in Patients with Symptoms or Signs Suggestive of Coronary Artery Disease or with Known Coronary Artery Disease

Class I: Exercise Testing Justified
1. To assist in the diagnosis of coronary artery disease in male patients with symptoms that are atypical for myocardial ischemia
2. To assess functional capacity and to aid in assessing the prognosis of patients with known coronary artery disease
3. To evaluate patients with symptoms consistent with recurrent, exercise-induced cardiac arrhythmias

Class II: Exercise Testing Controversial
1. To assist in the diagnosis of coronary artery disease in women with a history of typical or atypical angina pectoris
2. To assist in the diagnosis of coronary artery disease in patients taking digitalis
3. To assist in the diagnosis of coronary artery disease in patients with complete right bundle branch block
4. To evaluate the functional capacity and response to therapy with cardiovascular drugs in patients with coronary artery disease or heart failure
5. To evaluate patients with variant angina
6. To follow serially (at 1-yr or longer intervals) patients with known coronary artery disease

Class III: Exercise Testing Not Justified
1. To evaluate patients with simple premature ventricular depolarizations on resting ECG but no other evidence of coronary artery disease
2. To evaluate functional capacity serially in the course of an exercise cardiac rehabilitation program
3. To assist in the diagnosis of coronary artery disease in patients who demonstrate preexcitation (Wolff-Parkinson-White) syndrome or complete left bundle branch block on the resting ECG

Adapted from ref. 100.

Tachyarrhythmias and bradyarrhythmias constitute a relative contraindication to exercise testing; however, there are several situations in which exercise testing can provide valuable information. Exercise testing is useful in the assessment of the risk of arrhythmia recurrence, antiarrhythmic drug efficacy and safety/proarrhythmic potential, and the chronotropic response to exercise. The chronotropic response to exercise, in particular, is valuable information for the management of a patient with an ICD. Although the reproducibility of exercise-induced arrhythmias has been questioned [30, 37, 39, 105, 108], studies have demonstrated the reproducibility of exercise-induced arrhythmias in patients with a history of malignant arrhythmia [47, 90, 97]. Exercise stress testing has been especially useful in the assessment of exercise-induced ventricular tachycardia [81, 124, 125].

THE SAFETY OF EXERCISE STRESS TESTING IN PATIENTS WITH MALIGNANT ARRHYTHMIA

Data have also been published regarding the safety of exercise stress testing in patient populations thought to be at high risk for cardiovascular

TABLE 9.5.
Absolute and Relative Contraindications to Exercise Testing

Absolute
    Acute myocardial infarction (within 3–5 days)
    Unstable angina
    Uncontrolled cardiac arrhythmias causing symptoms or hemodynamic compromise
    Active endocarditis
    Symptomatic severe aortic stenosis
    Uncontrolled symptomatic heart failure
    Acute pulmonary embolus or pulmonary infarction
    Acute noncardiac disorder that may affect exercise performance or be aggravated by
        exercise (e.g., infection, renal failure, thyrotoxicosis)
    Acute myocarditis or pericarditis
    Physical disability that would preclude safe and adequate test performance
    Thrombosis of lower extremity
Relative[a]
    Left main coronary stenosis or its equivalent
    Moderate stenotic valvular heart disease
    Electrolyte abnormalities
    Significant arterial or pulmonary hypertension
    Tachyarrhythmias or bradyarrhythmias
    Hypertrophic cardiomyopathy
    Mental impairment leading to inability to cooperate
    High-degree atrioventricular block

From ref. 42.
[a]Relative contraindications can be superseded when benefits outweigh risks of exercise.

complications, such as those patients with unstable angina, recent myocardial infarction, congestive heart failure, or a history of malignant arrhythmias. Table 9.6 summarizes some of the published data regarding the complications of exercise stress testing in patients with a history of malignant ventricular arrhythmias or aborted sudden cardiac death [2, 40, 47, 117, 127].

Young and colleagues reported on their experience with 1377 maximal exercise stress tests in 263 patients with a history of malignant ventricular arrhythmias, 71% of whom had ventricular fibrillation or hemodynamically unstable ventricular tachycardia. Complications, defined as the occurrence of arrhythmia during exercise testing that required medical attention, including ventricular fibrillation, ventricular tachycardia, and bradycardia, occurred in 24 (9.1%) patients during 32 (2.3%) tests. Of the 32 tests, 22 were complicated by ventricular tachycardia, 9 by ventricular fibrillation, and 1 by bradycardia. There were no deaths or myocardial infarctions in this group of patients. The occurrence of a complication was found to be associated with male gender, coronary artery disease, and a history of exertional arrhythmia. Interestingly, complications were not associated with the use of antiarrhythmic drugs at the time of exercise stress testing. In contrast, a reference population of 3444 pa-

TABLE 9.6.
Complications of Exercise Stress Testing in Populations with a History of Malignant Arrhythmia

Study	No. of Exercise Tests	Nonsustained VT[a] per 10,000 Tests (%)	Sustained VT per 10,000 Tests (%)	VF per 10,000 Tests (%)	Mortality per 10,000 Tests (%)
Allen et al. [2]	64	3437.5 (34)	781.3 (7.8)	0	0
Fintel et al. [40]	103	2200.0 (22)	0	0	0
Graboys et al. [47]	60	6500.0 (65)	0	0	0
Weaver et al. [117]	86	814.0 (81)	0	0	0
Young et al. [127]	1,377	?15.6%	159.7 (1.6)	65.4 (0.65)	0

Adapted from ref. 58.
[a]VT, ventricular tachycardia; VF, ventricular fibrillation.

tients without a history of malignant arrhythmias who took part in 8221 exercise tests was also studied. Four (0.12%) of these patients developed ventricular fibrillation during 0.05% of the tests, all of whom were successfully resuscitated [127].

Allen and coworkers reported the results of exercise stress testing in 64 consecutive patients with a history of malignant ventricular arrhythmias, all of whom were off of antiarrhythmic drugs. Of the 64 patients, 22 patients (34%) had nonsustained ventricular tachycardia, and 5 patients (8%) had sustained ventricular tachycardia requiring medical intervention. No patient required electrical cardioversion, and no patient experienced ventricular fibrillation or significant major complications during exercise testing. The results of electrophysiology studies did not correlate with the results of exercise testing, and the presence of ventricular tachycardia on ambulatory monitoring did not predict the occurrence of ventricular tachycardia during exercise. However, the absence of ventricular tachycardia on ambulatory monitoring was predictive of a patient not developing ventricular tachycardia during exercise.

Exercise training for patient populations with malignant arrhythmias has also been shown to be safe and valuable for physical conditioning and relieving psychological stress [58]. Kelly and colleagues reported their experience with more than 1200 hr of inpatient exercise training in a population of 135 patients with malignant arrhythmias [59]. Ventricular arrhythmias during exercise occurred in almost 80% of these patients. Thirty-one patients developed ventricular tachycardia; four episodes were sustained. More than 80% of these arrhythmias were asymptomatic, likely because only 20% of the tachyarrhythmias exceeded a rate of 175 bpm. There were 7 episodes of urgent complications (1 per 173 patient-hr of exercise), including three episodes of symptomatic, sustained ventricular tachycardia. There was one emergent complication (1 per 1214 patient-hr of exercise) involving an episode of cardiac arrest from sustained ventricular tachycardia. This patient was successfully resuscitated. The three patients who experienced symptomatic sustained ventricular tachycardia and the patient who had a cardiac arrest were all being treated with antiarrhythmic drugs at the time of these episodes [59].

Kelly and associates also reported their 9-yr experience with outpatient exercise training in 42 patients previously hospitalized for evaluation of malignant ventricular arrhythmias (1246 patient exercise sessions) [60]. More than 90% of these patients had ventricular arrhythmias during exercise, approximately 30% of whom had ventricular tachycardia. Interestingly, there was a higher rate of urgent complications (1 per 138 patient-hr), including three episodes of symptomatic ventricular tachycardia. There were no emergent complications or deaths in this group [60]. After examining various factors such as age, LV systolic function, presenting arrhythmia, and exercise variables, only the presence of exercise-induced ventricular tachycardia was associated with subsequent urgent complication during exercise training [58].

COMPLEMENTARITY OF EXERCISE TESTING TO OTHER TECHNIQUES

Exercise stress testing can be complementary to other techniques used for the diagnosis and management of arrhythmias, including electrophysiology studies, ambulatory Holter monitoring/event recorders, and signal-averaged electrocardiography. These tests have important limitations when compared with those of exercise testing. Ambulatory monitoring may not detect an arrhythmia in a patient who has infrequent episodes. Lown and colleagues reported that up to 10% of patients with a history of sustained ventricular tachycardia had nonsustained or sustained ventricular tachycardia documented by exercise testing and not by ambulatory monitoring [70]. The electrophysiology laboratory may not reproduce the precise physiological conditions that may be required for the exposure of an arrhythmia. Arrhythmias in some patients may require certain triggers in order to be uncovered. Exercise has the advantage of producing electrophysiological and neurohormonal changes that may facilitate the unmasking of a malignant arrhythmia [91]. In a retrospective review of patients with worsening of arrhythmia while taking either quinidine, mexiletine, or encainide, Slater et al. reported 17 of 51 patients (33%) with arrhythmia exposed only by exercise stress testing, although ambulatory monitoring had shown a reduction in arrhythmia [107]. This underscores the complementary nature of these tests in the evaluation of a patient with malignant arrhythmias.

RELEVANT GUIDELINES AND STANDARDS FOR STRESS TESTING

Equipment, Staff, and Procedures

The safe administration of exercise stress testing and subsequent exercise training for a patient with a history of potentially malignant ventricular arrhythmias requires special attention to the emergency and resuscitative equipment that should be available in every exercise laboratory. Comprehensive guidelines for the initiation and maintenance of a clinical laboratory for administering graded exercise tests to adults have been outlined by the American Heart Association Committee on Exercise and Cardiac Rehabilitation [86]. Especially important is the updating of the proper medications and maintenance of emergency equipment, including a cardioverter-defibrillator with R-wave synchronizing capability. This equipment and medications should be immediately accessible in the event of an arrest before, during, and after exercise. An emergency protocol should be posted and reviewed with the exercise laboratory personnel at least quarterly. There should be a clear, preconceived plan for the transfer of unstable patients to an appropriate hospital for emergency evaluation and treatment [86]. Basic and advanced cardiac life support should be administered as outlined in the American Heart Association published guidelines [35].

Standards and Guidelines for Supervision and Monitoring

A detailed revised report from the American Heart Association providing standards and guidelines for exercise testing and training has been published recently [42]. ECG monitoring of patients with malignant arrhythmias must be more comprehensive than the methods commonly used for patients at low risk for cardiac complications. A complete 12-lead ECG should be available on demand, as well as during each stage of exercise in patients with arrhythmias. Continuous ECG monitoring of at least three leads is recommended [42]. Antman and colleagues demonstrated a 6-fold higher yield of detecting repetitive ventricular arrhythmias (couplets or nonsustained ventricular tachycardia) during exercise stress testing with continuous rather than intermittent ECG monitoring [10].

Early outpatient (Phase II) cardiac rehabilitation programs must also consider which patients warrant continuous ECG monitoring. Table 9.7 summarizes the guidelines provided by the American College of Cardiology to identify patients at high risk for cardiovascular complications during exercise training, and who, therefore, should have continuous ECG monitoring during the session [4]. More detailed guidelines for cardiac rehabilitation of low-, intermediate-, and high-risk patients are available in a recent publication from the American Association of Cardiovascular and Pulmonary Rehabilitation [3].

The American College of Sports Medicine has established guidelines for the proficiency and appropriate training for personnel involved with exer-

TABLE 9.7.
American College of Cardiology Criteria Identifying Patients in Whom ECG Monitoring Should Be Included during Exercise

Criteria for ECG Monitoring
(a) Severely depressed LV function (ejection fraction under 30)
(b) Resting complex ventricular arrhythmia (Lown Type 4 or 5)
(c) Ventricular arrhythmias appearing or increasing with exercise
(d) Decrease in systolic blood pressure with exercise
(e) Survivors of sudden cardiac death
(f) Patients after myocardial infarction complicated by congestive heart failure, cardiogenic shock, and/or serious ventricular arrhythmias
(g) Patients with severe coronary artery disease and marked exercise-induced ischemia
(h) Inability to self-monitor heart rate as a result of physical or intellectual impairment

From ref. 4.

cise testing [5]. These personnel may include exercise physiologists, exercise technicians, nurses, physical therapists, ECG technicians, or physician assistants. Exercise testing should be performed under the supervision of a physician whose qualifications and training meet the requirements outlined in the American College of Physicians/American College of Cardiology/American Heart Association statement on clinical competence [101]. The level of supervision, however, may vary with the type of patient being tested. Patients at higher risk for complications during exercise testing, such as patients with untreated unstable angina, decompensated congestive heart failure, and malignant arrhythmias, should be supervised directly by the physician when exercise testing is considered necessary. For patients not at high risk for exercise induced complications, the physician need only be readily available [86]. Additional personnel may be required to be present or readily available when performing exercise stress testing for a patient with an ICD, including a nurse, physician, or technician with expertise with ICD programming.

CONSIDERATIONS FOR EXERCISE TRAINING AND ACTIVITY RECOMMENDATIONS IN PATIENTS WITH POTENTIALLY MALIGNANT ARRHYTHMIA

Patients with Heart Failure: An Important Subset

The principles of exercise training that apply to any patient apply as well to those with malignant arrhythmia. Exercise prescriptions must deal with the defining parameters of frequency, duration, and intensity. Because a significant number of patients with malignant arrhythmias have LV dysfunction, we will mention first some of the principles relevant to this particular subset of patients.

The patient with poor LV function may show a varying and inconsistent response to exercise [83]. However, despite the inconsistent responses to exercise, there are theoretical as well as demonstrated benefits of exercise in these patients. Patients with severe LV dysfunction can condition safely by gradually raising their heart rates above resting level. With time, they are able to extract more oxygen from the blood during exercise, thus widening the arteriovenous oxygen difference. The effects of exercise training on mortality for these patients is unknown, although the consequence theoretically should be favorable because of the parasympathetic enhancement discussed above in some detail. Exercise tolerance is improved, as illustrated by lower heart rates during submaximal exercise and increased maximal workloads [68]. Endurance and fatigue levels should be considered, in addition to aerobic capacity. Heart failure patients may be able to achieve high aerobic workloads but then experience prolonged fatigue for hours or days after an exercise session. All of these considerations require careful program design and precautions.

Exercise training helps these patients accomplish significant gains in functional capacity below anaerobic threshold. The ability to sustain activity at low metabolic equivalent (MET) levels may mean the difference between living independently vs. requiring custodial care. Cardiac rehabilitation can substantially enhance the quality of these patients' everyday lives.

These patients need continuous supervision by staff trained to recognize the special problems associated with this population. Specific recommendations for supervision are summarized in Table 9.8. Patients with severe LV dysfunction should be on continuous telemetry (ECG monitoring) throughout warm-up, exercise, and cool-down, regardless of the absence of a history of malignant arrhythmia. The absolute contraindications for exercise include critical obstruction to LV outflow, severe concomitant right heart failure, active myocardial inflammation, decompensated clinical congestive heart failure, and hemodynamically unstable arrhythmia. Relative contraindications to exercise training in LV dysfunction include severe chronotropic incompetence, the inability to increase systolic blood pressure during exercise, the inability to maintain stroke volume during exercise (as evidenced by a poor oxygen pulse), changing pattern angina, dyspnea and fatigue, or an unequivocal arrest in progress after 3 wk of exercise training.

These guidelines for exercise training and supervision are eminently appropriate in all patients with potentially malignant arrhythmia. Further consideration for the arrhythmic patient includes the issue of heart rate as a parameter for monitoring intensity. A significant number of patients with a history of malignant arrhythmia are currently treated with antiarrhythmic agents that have significant negative chronotropic effects. Sotalol (Betapace), a Class III antiarrhythmic agent released for clinical use in the United States within the last 2 yr, also has significant β-adrenergic blocking

TABLE 9.8.
Guidelines for Exercising Patients with Left Ventricular Failure

---

- The pretraining evaluation is critical. In addition to the usual medical examination and graded exercise study, these patients may need gas analysis with measurement of VO_2max and AT; assessment of LVEF by MUGA or LV and/or RV function with PA pressures by echocardiography during exercise.
- Patients should be checked for their condition at each session (without rest angina, decompensated heart failure, or arrhythmias that compromise hemodynamic stability) before exercise.
- Patients need to be trained for the use of subjective functional scales of relative perceived exertion (RPE) and know how to apply them during exercise sessions and their normal ADL.
- Patients with LV dysfunction will tolerate increases in duration of exercise better than large increments in workload. Warm-up and cool-down should be extended beyond the usual duration. Use dynamic muscle strengthening in lieu of isometrics. Interval training may be appropriate.
- Follow-up parameters, such as body weight, blood pressure, and pulse, which are collected on a routine basis, are especially significant for tracking the clinical status of these patients.
- Patients' target heart rate range should be adjusted to at least 10 bpm below any significant end points of exercise observed in the pretraining evaluation, e.g., exertional hypotension, significant dyspnea, the onset of sustained arrhythmia.

LVEF, left ventricular ejection fraction; MUGA, multigated acquisition.

effects with a potency similar to that of propranolol. The use of sotalol for the treatment of ventricular arrhythmias has become more popular, particularly after the results of the recently published electrophysiologic study vs. electrocardiographic monitoring (ESVEM) trial. This study compared Holter monitoring to electrophysiology study-guided antiarrhythmic therapy for the treatment of ventricular arrhythmias, and sotalol was found to be more efficacious than Class I antiarrhythmic agents [71]. There has also been increasing use of amiodarone (Cordarone), a unique antiarrhythmic drug with Class III effects, as well as significant negative chronotropic actions. Whereas there has been concern regarding increased mortality with the use of Class I antiarrhythmic agents in certain patient populations, there are indications from some studies that amiodarone may improve mortality in patients treated for ventricular arrhythmias [16, 19, 78]. As a result, it is very likely that an increasing number of patients with malignant arrhythmias will present to the exercise laboratory on one of these medications.

Because these drugs can have such a profound impact on the maximum heart rate achieved during exercise, we strongly suggest these patients undergo formal exercise testing on the drug before starting an exercise training program. In this age of tightening healthcare budgets, clinicians are loathe to repeat tests, but stress studies in these patients performed for the determination of active ischemia generally are done with the patient off the drug, because the reduced maximum heart rate achieved significantly reduces test sensitivity. They should be retested on drug so that the appropriate rate and rating of perceived exertion (RPE) for therapeutic exercise can be determined.

The issue of activity recommendations is common to all patients with a history of malignant arrhythmia. Critical to any recommendation regarding this sensitive and significant issue to patients are the individual characteristics of the patient's arrhythmia problem. When the patient is subject to sudden loss of consciousness or cognitive control related to the onset or offset of their arrhythmia (even when "controlled" by drug therapy), then they should be advised to restrict themselves from exercise activities, where they may be a potential risk to themselves or others.

EXERCISE TESTING AND CARDIAC REHABILITATION: RECOMMENDATIONS SPECIFIC FOR PATIENTS WITH ICDS

Exercise Testing of Patients with ICDs: General Considerations

Patients with ICDs pose a special problem during exercise stress testing. Since the introduction of ICDs in 1980 for clinical use in patients with multiple cardiac arrests [75], it is estimated that more than 100,000 devices have been implanted worldwide. The early devices were relatively simple "shock box" units capable only of detecting ventricular fibrillation and delivering a high-energy defibrillation shock. These ICD systems required implantation of the generator into a subcutaneous abdominal pocket and epicardial patch electrodes placed via thoracotomy. ICDs have now evolved into complex multiprogrammable, tiered therapy systems capable of a wide range of low- and high-energy shocks, antitachycardia pacing, and backup ventricular pacing for bradyarrhythmias [63, 98]. Current ICDs can be programmed to provide progressive therapy dictated by the rate of the tachyarrhythmia and the failure of the previous therapy ("tiered" therapy). Thus, these devices may be programmed to deliver antitachycardia pacing, followed by low-energy shock if unsuccessful, then high-energy shocks if necessary. After charging in preparation for therapy delivery, ICDs reconfirm the continued presence of a tachyarrhythmia before delivering the therapy. This is referred to as noncommitted shocks, and it is designed to help avoid delivery of therapy for nonsustained arrhythmias [36].

Table 9.9 outlines the defibrillator code system for the description of the various capabilities of the ICD, as adopted by the North American Society of Pacing and Electrophysiology, together with the British Pacing and Electrophysiology Group (NASPE/BPEG) [14]. Future developments for the ICD will involve incorporation of sensor-driven, dual-chamber pacing technology, as many patients who receive an ICD also require a pacemaker. This development would virtually eliminate the problem of adverse interaction

TABLE 9.9.
North American Society of Pacing and Electrophysiology/British Pacing and
Electrophysiology Group (NASPE/BPEG) Defibrillator Code (NBD Code)

I: Shock Chamber	II: Antitachycardia Pacing Chamber	III: Tachycardia Detection	IV: Antibradycardia Pacing Chamber
O = none	O = none	E = electrogram	O = none
A = atrium	A = atrium	H = hemodynamic	A = atrium
V = ventricle	V = ventricle		V = ventricle
D = dual (A + V)	D = dual (A + V)		D = dual (A + V)

From ref. 14.

between an ICD and pacemaker. For more details regarding ICDs, Pinski and Trohman have published a comprehensive review of ICDs targeted for the nonelectrophysiologist [88].

Implantation techniques have also evolved, especially with the development of smaller generators. A nonthoracotomy transvenous lead system has been developed, which involves subcutaneous tunneling of the lead system from the pulse generator to the subclavian vein. This newer approach appears to reduce perioperative morbidity, postoperative hospital care requirement, and cost [64, 67, 114]. The transvenous lead system has been recommended by some authorities as the implant technique of first choice [84, 120]. The more compact size of the newer pulse generators permits the use of a prepectoral implantation site, which is considered superior to the abdominal site [21, 49].

Considerations in the Testing and Training of Patients with ICDs

Exercise stress testing and training for patients with ICDs has more associated risk than for the average patient. As discussed above, there is a higher risk of complications because of the history of arrhythmias or cardiac arrest that led to implantation of the device. However, there are also potential problems with ICDs during stress testing that can be circumvented or avoided with proper precautions and training. Important considerations before stress testing include knowing the type and frequency of the patient's arrhythmias, including any history of precipitation by exercise or catecholamines. Knowledge of the characteristics of the previous arrhythmia, such as rate, hemodynamic stability, response to cough or vagal maneuvers and to various therapies such as antiarrhythmic drugs and cardiac medications, antitachycardia pacing, and cardioversion, is very important.

Perhaps most importantly, the supervising physician and exercise lab personnel need to know the type, or model, of ICD and the programmed parameters. Especially important is knowing the detection interval, that is, the interval in milliseconds or heart rate in beats per minute (bpm) at which the device recognizes a tachyarrhythmia. It is important to realize that, in general, ICDs recognize rate, not specific arrhythmia patterns. Any rhythm that becomes sufficiently rapid to reach and/or exceed the detection interval of the ICD, including sinus tachycardia, may be recognized as a tachyarrhythmia and treated according to the programmed therapies for that device. Furthermore, ICDs must not only recognize a particular rate, but also, a certain number of beats at or above that rate must occur before the device detects the presence of arrhythmia and begins to charge. The number of beats that must occur before detection is also programmable in most models. There are now a wide variety of programmable features that attempt to distinguish between regular and irregular tachycardias, as well as the initiation, i.e., gradual vs. rapid onset of the rhythm disturbance.

DEALING WITH THE TECHNOLOGY OF THE DEVICES. Exercise stress testing and training in patients with ICDs, therefore, poses a unique set of potential problems that may require prompt, if not emergent, action on behalf of the exercise laboratory team. There is obviously the risk of ventricular arrhythmia as described above. However, the presence of the ICD adds a level of complexity to the management of these patients before, during, and after exercise. There has been very little published data regarding the safety of exercise stress testing for patients with ICDs. Deborde et al., from The Johns Hopkins University, reported their experience with ICD charges during 12 exercise stress tests in nine patients. In all, 9 charges were secondary to sinus tachycardia, 2 to atrial fibrillation, and 1 to sustained ventricular tachycardia. Shocks were diverted in 10 of 12 patients with application of a magnet. They concluded that the presence of an ICD did not preclude that population from maximal exercise testing and that unnecessary therapy (i.e., a shock) from the ICD could be diverted during the test [31].

Before exercise stress testing, it is imperative to determine the programmed detection interval of the device in order to avoid rate crossover during exercise and subsequent inappropriate therapies (particularly shocks) from the ICD for sinus tachycardia. Inappropriate therapies from an ICD are not only uncomfortable for the patient but also may result in the induction of a malignant arrhythmia [23, 48, 79, 87, 102]. However, exercise testing can be quite useful for determination of the patient's chronotropic response to exercise, particularly for those patients with slower tachyarrhythmias in which sinus rate crossover during routine daily activities is more likely to occur.

There are multiple methods of managing the potential for rate crossover and inappropriate ICD therapies during exercise testing and training. The appropriate method will vary from one patient to another, and consultation with the patient's physician is recommended. It may be prudent in some complex patients to also consult with the patient's cardiologist or electrophysiologist before exercise testing. When the patient has a history of rapid ventricular tachycardia or ventricular fibrillation, the detection interval will most likely be programmed to such a level that sinus tachycardia during exercise will not be detected. In this situation, one need only carefully monitor the heart rate during exercise and terminate the test when the heart rate approaches the detection interval of the device. If the test is being performed for the assessment of chronotropic response to exercise, particularly to determine the risk of sinus rate crossover, then this approach is suitable for any patient, regardless of the programmed detection interval. However, when a maximal stress test is required, such as an evaluation for exercise-induced ischemia, then this approach may not be suitable for those patients with slower tachycardias and, therefore, slower programmed detection rates.

One approach to managing these patients involves deactivation of the ICD just before the test. This requires the appropriate programmer for the device and someone trained in its use to be present in the exercise laboratory during the study. This method may result in the patient being unprotected from malignant arrhythmias and sudden cardiac death during the period of time the test is conducted; therefore, one must be prepared to rapidly reactivate the ICD or use external cardioversion/defibrillation in the event of an emergency. An alternative would be to reprogram the detection interval to a level beyond that expected for sinus tachycardia during exercise. This method may be safer for some patients than inactivating the device, as they would remain protected from faster ventricular tachycardias and ventricular fibrillation, a situation in which rapid defibrillation is crucial. However, these patients would not be protected from slower ventricular tachycardias which, in some patients, may result in injury secondary to syncope.

Perhaps more appropriate is the method of temporarily inactivating or "blinding" the device with a magnet during exercise. All ICDs have a reed switch that closes when a magnetic field of sufficient strength is applied. The response to this maneuver is somewhat variable between ICD models and manufacturers, as summarized in Table 9.10 [88]. However, they all have in common the capability to be disabled from delivering therapies or shocks with application of the magnet. The magnet used must be of sufficient strength. The most common is a standard ring or donut-shaped magnet. In some cases, especially in those patients with excess tissue between the skin surface and pulse generator, a second donut magnet stacked on top of the other will be necessary. One should be aware that most of the ICD manufacturers recommend magnet placement over one end of the device, rather than directly over the center, to ensure reed switch closure.

Devices manufactured by Cardiac Pacemakers, Inc. (St. Paul, MN) are unique in that the application of a magnetic field can be used to permanently inactivate the ICD (turning it "off") without the use of a programmer. Upon application of a magnet over the site of the pulse generator, beeping tones are emitted that indicate the current programmed mode of the device. When R-wave synchronous tones are emitted, the device is programmed to an active mode, which indicates that tachyarrhythmia therapy

TABLE 9.10.

Features and Magnet Response of Implantable Cardioverter-Defibrillators

Manufacturer	ICD Model	Available Therapies	Therapy Commitment	Magnet Response
CPI	Ventak 1500, 1510, 1520, 1550, 1555	Defib	Committed	Inhibiton of detection and therapy (<30 s). Deactivation (≥30 s).
CPI	Ventak P 1600	CV, Defib	Committed	Inhibition of detection and therapy (<30 s). Deactivation (≥30 s).
CPI	Ventak P2 1625	CV, Defib, VVI	Programmable	Inhibition of detection and therapy (<30 s). Deactivation (≥30 s). Programmable.
CPI	Ventak PRx 1700, 1705	ATP, CV, Defib, VVI	Programmable	Inhibition of detection and therapy (<30 s). Deactivation (≥30 sec). Programmable.
CPI	Ventak PRx II 1710, 1715	ATP, CV, Defib, VVI	Programmable	Inhibition of detection and therapy (<30 s). Deactivation (≥30 s). Programmable.
CPI	Ventak PRx III 1720, 1721[b]	ATP, CV, Defib, VVI	Programmable	Inhibition of detection and therapy (<30 s). Deactivation (≥30 s). Programmable.
CPI	Ventak MINI 1740/1745, 1741/1746	ATP, CV, Defib, VVI	Programmable	Inhibition of detection and therapy (<30 s). Deactivation (≥30 s). Programmable.
Intermedics	Res-Q 101–01	ATP,[a] CV, Defib, VVI	Committed	Inhibition of detection and therapy VVI pacing at 100 bpm
Intermedics	Res-Q II 101-07	ATP, CV, Defib, VVI	Programmable for VT Committed for VF	Inhibition of detection and therapy VVI pacing at 100 bpm (programmable)

TABLE 9.10. *(continued)*
Features and Magnet Response of Implantable Cardioverter-Defibrillators

Manufacturer	ICD Model	Available Therapies	Therapy Commitment	Magnet Response
Medtronic	PCD 7217	ATP, CV, Defib, VVI	Noncommitted for VT Committed for VF	Inhibition of detection and therapy
Medtronic	PCD Jewel 7218, 7219	ATP, CV, Defib, VVI	Noncommitted for VT Programmable for VF (first shock), then committed	Inhibition of detection and therapy
Telectronics	Guardian 4211, 4215	ATP, CV, Defib, VVI	Programmable	Inhibition of detection and therapy
Ventritex	Cadence V-100, V-110	ATP, CV, Defib, VVI	Noncommitted	Inhibition of detection and therapy (programmable)
Ventritex	Cadet V-115	ATP, CV, Defib, VVI	Noncommitted	Inhibition of detection and therapy (programmable)
Angeion	Sentinel 2000	ATP, CV, Defib, VVI	Programmable	Inhibition of detection and therapy (programmable)

Adapted from ref. 88.
^aATP, antitachycardia pacing; CV, cardioversion; Defib, defibrillation shock; VVI, ventricular antibradycardia pacing; VT, ventricular tachycardia; VF, ventricular fibrillation.

can be delivered, if detection criteria is met, after removal of the magnet. When a continuous tone is emitted, the device is programmed to an inactive mode, which indicates that tachyarrhythmia therapy will not be available after the magnet is removed. The mode can be changed between these two positions simply by holding the magnet over the pulse generator for at least 30 s, at which time a change in the beeping tones will indicate the new mode. Removal of the magnet for at least 2 s and reapplication of the magnet for at least 30 s will result in a change in the beeping tones, indicating a return to the previous mode.

The newer models from CPI (Models 1625 and higher) have a programmable option that controls whether or not the mode can be changed (active vs. inactive) by a magnet. If this feature has been programmed off, then application of the magnet will not change the beeping tones after 30 s, indicating that the mode cannot be changed. This feature is designed to protect patients with ICDs who may be exposed to strong magnetic fields, such as those in the workplace. However, tachyarrhythmia therapy is inhibited any time the magnet is properly positioned over the pulse generator. Tachyarrhythmia detection continues during this time. When the magnet is applied for more than 1–2 s while the ICD is charging to deliver shock therapy, the charge is diverted into the device's internal test load, and therapy is thereby aborted. When the magnet is applied for more than 1–2 s while the ICD is delivering antitachycardia pacing therapy, the delivery is terminated. Bradycardia pacing is not affected by application of the magnet. Thus, application of a magnet for more than 30 s may disable the ICD before exercise stress testing, providing that the feature has been allowed by previous programming. Otherwise, the magnet will need to be applied and held in place when necessary to circumvent inappropriate therapies, or it can be taped in position over the pulse generator before beginning the test and removed when therapy for a malignant tachyarrhythmia is necessary.

The ICDs manufactured by Medtronic Inc. (Minneapolis, MN), including the models PCD and Jewel and Telectronics Pacing Systems (Englewood, CO), including the model Guardian, are temporarily disabled from tachyarrhythmia detection and therapy upon application of a magnetic field over the pulse generator. Bradycardia pacing is not affected. Upon removal of the magnet, the device is restored to normal operating function. Application of a magnet to ICDs manufactured by Intermedics, Inc. (Angleton, TX), including the Res-Q and Res-Q II, results in inhibition of tachyarrhythmia detection and therapy, however the bradycardia pacing mode is changed to VVI at 100 bpm. ICDs manufactured by Ventritex (Sunnyvale, CA), including the model Cadence, and Angeion (Minneapolis, MN), including the model Sentinel, are also temporarily disabled from tachyarrhythmia detection and therapy when a magnetic field is applied over the pulse generator. Bradycardia pacing is not affected. However, the device can be programmed to ignore the position of the reed switch, and it would not be affected by the application of a magnet. This underscores the necessity of knowing the manufacturer of the ICD and how it is programmed. A patient with a Ventritex Cadence or Angeion Sentinel ICD would need to have the reed switch control function activated in order to allow inhibition of inappropriate therapies with a magnet during exercise, or another method of avoiding sinus rate crossover would have to be used as described above.

EVALUATION AFTER IMPLANTATION. Most of the algorithms currently integrated into the design of commercially released ICDs involve rate dependency. Thus, we again advocate that patients be formally exercise tested to be sure that the patient's intrinsic rate will not exceed the threshold rate of the device and fire inadvertently during physical activity. Many patients

TABLE 9.11.
Typical Distribution of Rate Criterion for Programming of Implantable Cardioverter-Defibrillators

Rate Criterion (bpm)	% Patients Programmed
110–115	0.5
120–125	2.5
130–135	3.8
140–145	8.7
150–155	25.1
160–165	13.5
170–175	25.1
180–185	11.1
190–195	5.4
≥200	3.4

From ref. 82.

are concomitantly being treated with drugs, so although premature activation of the device is generally unlikely, such testing should be done.

In many defibrillator clinics, the patient is ambulated on an informal basis on the assumption that the patient's most strenuous physical activity is walking and that the device only needs to accommodate the heart rate achieved with this activity. Although informal ambulation will often suffice for follow-up purposes, initial programming should be done in conjunction with formal testing. This is especially useful when the patient's threshold is close to the heart rate achieved at MET levels that approximate realistic activity for the patient. Precise measures of the rate required for an adequate margin of safety can have a significant impact on the patient functionally and psychologically.

Patients are aware that they may be shocked by the device during the exercise test, and some are very apprehensive. The device can be programmed to be "off" for the duration of the study, and the patient can be reassured that an inappropriate defibrillation will not occur. Once the device is reprogrammed, they can be shown a printout of the heart rates achieved during exercise study, and the concept of threshold discrimination can be emphasized.

Table 9.11 summarizes the rate criterion observed in more than 100 patients with ICDs [82]. Because the average patient receiving an ICD is 60 yr of age, a training heart rate of 120 bpm will likely exceed the rate criterion in only less than 3% of patients implanted with these devices. However, a patient 35 yr of age may have a training rate of 140 bpm, a value exceeding the rate criterion of about 15% of the patients programmed, so the likelihood that rate ambiguity may be a problem is somewhat greater in younger patients.

Once evaluated by exercise testing, the exercise prescription can then be written to accommodate the heart rate limits of the device. No other major adaptations to the presence of the internal defibrillator are really necessary. Future devices will hopefully incorporate some of the same sensor technologies currently being used in rate-adaptive pacemakers to incorporate hemodynamic parameters such as cardiac output into the therapy delivery algorithms.

ROLE OF CARDIAC REHABILITATION

ICD patients are excellent candidates for rehabilitation programs that have supervision by medical professionals and telemetry monitoring capability, at least until the likelihood of inadvertent defibrillation has been ruled out with sufficient experience [12].

They also benefit from group support and socialization [94]. The implantation of such a potent device into an individual can have significant psychological ramifications [12]. The opportunity to share experiences and to be regarded by others as "normal" is, for many, a significant relief. Formal group psychotherapy can be offered to those who are identified as having significant adjustment problems. Most patients employed before ICD implantation are able to return to work after the procedure [57].

The issue of activity recommendations is analogous to that of patients with a history of malignant arrhythmia. At issue in the ICD patient is the clinical significance of the latent period; the time between the onset of arrhythmia and its detection by a device, the charging of the capacitors, and the delivery of therapy. This typically will require several seconds to occur, and when patients are without a pulse during this time they again must be protected from injury to themselves or others. This may rule out running in close proximity to vehicular traffic, swimming, or cycling, for example, in favor of activities such as a rowing machine or low-impact aerobics on a padded surface. The technical operation of these devices is generally unaffected by the types of exercise activities engaged in by patients for conditioning purposes. These types of concerns are much more frequent regarding vocational and recreational exposure to appliances and machines that may produce radiofrequency interference.

The staff should be aware that the ICD will not harm someone in physical contact with a patient while it is discharging. An understanding of how the device can be temporarily turned off (usually by magnet) is also necessary (see above). An annotated table below summarizes the technical features of the currently available ICDs. Again, availability of this detailed knowledge, as well as an understanding of the underlying disease process, and thorough preparation for the management of emergencies lead to the projection of an air of confidence by the staff that is very reassuring to these often anxious patients.

SUMMARY

Patients with malignant arrhythmias are a challenge when they present to the laboratory for exercise testing and training. The complex metabolic and electrophysiological changes that occur during and after exercise may suppress or potentiate arrhythmias and alter the efficacy and safety of antiarrhythmic agents. The presence of an ICD adds a level of complexity to the study; however, a general understanding of how ICDs function and a review of the programmed parameters before the study will result in a lesser likelihood of complication and more efficient and appropriate action, should a complication occur.

Exercise testing and training are valuable methods for the evaluation and treatment of patients with malignant ventricular arrhythmias. Exercise testing is a useful adjunctive technique in the exposure of arrhythmia and the evaluation of the efficacy and proarrhythmic potential of antiarrhythmic agents. These patients are excellent candidates for rehabilitation and exercise training programs, which may result in increased functional capacity and improved quality of life.

With this knowledge and adherence to the appropriate guidelines for patient selection and testing, exercise testing and training of patients with malignant arrhythmias can be prescribed and conducted in a safe, controlled manner in an atmosphere of confidence and professionalism.

REFERENCES

1. Akhtar, M., I. Niazi, G. V. Naccarelli, et al. Role of adrenergic stimulation by isoproterenol in reversal of effects of encainide in supraventricular tachycardia. *Am. J. Cardiol.* 62:45L–49L, 1988.
2. Allen, B. J., T. P. Casey, M. A. Brodsky, C. R. Luckett, and W. L. Henry. Exercise testing in patients with life-threatening ventricular tachyarrhythmias: results and correlation with clinical and arrhythmia factors. *Am. Heart. J.* 116:997–1002, 1988.
3. American Association of Cardiovascular and Pulmonary Rehabilitation. Guidelines for Cardiac Rehabilitation Programs. Champaign, IL: Human Kinetics Books, 1995, p. 27.
4. American College of Cardiology. Position report on cardiac rehabilitation. *J. Am. Coll. Cardiol.* 7:451–453, 1986.
5. American College of Sports Medicine: Guidelines for Exercise Testing and Prescription. Philadelphia: Lea & Febiger, 1991.
6. Amsterdam, E. A. Relation of silent myocardial ischemia to ventricular arrhythmias and sudden death. *Am. J. Cardiol.* 62:24I–27I, 1988.
7. Anastasiou-Nana, M. I., J. L. Anderson, J. R. Stewart, et al. Occurrence of exercise-induced and spontaneous wide complex tachycardia during therapy with flecainide for complex ventricular arrhythmias: a probable proarrhythmic effect. *Am. Heart J.* 113:1071–1077, 1987.
8. Anonymous: Multicenter automatic defibrillator implantation trial (MADIT): design and clinical protocol. MADIT Executive Committee. *PACE Pacing Clin. Electrophysiol.* 14:920–927, 1991.
9. Anonymous: Antiarrhythmics Versus Implantable Defibrillators (AVID)—rationale, design, and methods. *Am. J. Cardiol.* 75:470–475, 1995.

10. Antman, E., T. B. Graboys, and B. Lown. Continuous monitoring for ventricular arrhythmias during exercise tests. *J. Am. Med. Assoc.* 241:2802–2805, 1979.

11. Atterhog, J. H., B. Jonsson, and R. Samuelsson. Exercise testing: a prospective study of complication rates. *Am. Heart. J.* 98:572–579, 1979.

12. Badger, J. M., and P. L. Morris. Observations of a support group for automatic implantable cardioverter-defibrillator recipients and their spouses. *Heart Lung* 18:238–243, 1989.

13. Beard, E. F., and C. A. Owen. Cardiac arrhythmias during exercise testing in healthy men. *Aerospace Med* 44:286–289, 1973.

14. Bernstein, A. D., and V. Parsonnet. Pacemaker and defibrillator codes. K. A. Ellenbogen, G. N. Kay and B. L. Wilkoff (eds.). *Clinical Cardiac Pacing.* Philadelphia: W. B. Saunders, 1995, pp. 279–283.

15. Bigger, J. J., R. E. Kleiger, J. L. Fleiss, L. M. Rolnitzky, R. C. Steinman, and J. P. Miller. Components of heart rate variability measured during healing of acute myocardial infarction. *Am. J. Cardiol.* 61:208–215, 1988.

16. Burkart, F., M. Pfisterer, W. Kiowski, F. Follath, and D. Burckhardt. Effect of antiarrhythmic therapy on mortality in survivors of myocardial infarction with asymptomatic complex ventricular arrhythmia: Basel Antiarrhythmic Study of Infarct Survival (BASIS). *J. Am. Coll. Cardiol.* 16:1711–1718, 1990.

17. Busby, M. J., E. A. Shefrin, and J. L. Fleg. Prevalence and long-term significance of exercise-induced frequent or repetitive ventricular ectopic beats in apparently healthy volunteers. *J. Am. Coll. Cardiol.* 14:1659–1665, 1989.

18. Cahalin, L., R. L. Blessey, D. Kummer, and M. Simard. The safety of exercise testing performed independently by physical therapists. *J. Cardiopulmonary Rehabil.* 7:269–276, 1987.

19. Cairns, J. A., S. J. Connolly, M. Gent, and R. Roberts. Post-myocardial infarction mortality in patients with ventricular premature depolarization: Canadian Amiodarone Myocardial Infarction Arrhythmia Trial (CAMIAT) pilot study. *Circulation* 84:550–557, 1991.

20. Califf, R. M., R. A. McKinnis, J. F. McNeer, et al. Prognostic value of ventricular arrhythmias associated with treadmill exercise testing in patients studied with cardiac catheterization for suspected ischemic heart disease. *J. Am. Coll. Cardiol.* 2:1060–1067, 1983.

21. Callans, D. J., and M. E. Josephson. Future developments in implantable cardioverter defibrillators: the optimal device. *Prog. Cardiovasc. Dis.* 36:227–244, 1993.

22. Casella, G., P. C. Pavesi, P. Sangiorgio, A. Rubboli, and D. Bracchetti. Exercise-induced ventricular arrhythmias in patients with healed myocardial infarction. *Int. J. Cardiol.* 40:229–235, 1993.

23. Cohen, T. J., W. W. Chien, K. G. Lurie, et al. Implantable cardioverter defibrillator proarrhythmia: case report and review of the literature. *PACE Pacing Clin. Electrophysiol.* 14:1326–1329, 1991.

24. Connolly, S. J., M. Gent, R. S. Roberts, et al. Canadian Implantable Defibrillator Study (CIDS): study design and organization. CIDS Co-Investigators. *Am. J. Cardiol.* 72:103F–108F, 1993.

25. Cook, J. R., J. J. Bigger, R. E. Kleiger, J. L. Fleiss, R. C. Steinman, and L. M. Rolnitzky. Effect of atenolol and diltiazem on heart period variability in normal persons. *J. Am. Coll. Cardiol.* 17:480–484, 1991.

26. Cordini, M. A., L. Sommerfeldt, and L. E. Egbil. Clinical significance and characteristics of exercise-induced ventricular tachycardia. *Cathet. Cardiovasc. Diagn.* 7:227, 1981.

27. Coumel, P., M. Zimmermann, and C. Funck-Brentano. Exercise test: arrhythmogenic or antiarrhythmic? Rate-dependency vs. adrenergic-dependency of tachyarrhythmias. *Eur. Heart J.* 8:7–15, 1987.

28. Cranefield, P. F., A. L. Wit, and B. F. Hoffman. Genesis of cardiac arrhythmias. *Circulation* 47:190–204, 1973.

29. Cripps, T. R., M. Malik, T. G. Farrell, and A. J. Camm. Prognostic value of reduced heart rate variability after myocardial infarction: clinical evaluation of a new analysis method. *Br. Heart J.* 65:14–19, 1991.

30. De Backer, G., D. Jacobs, R. Prineas, R. Crow, J. Vilandre, and H. Blackburn. Ventricular premature beats. Reliability in various measurement methods at rest and during exercise. *Cardiology* 63:53–63, 1978.

31. DeBorde, R., J. H. Levine, L.S.C. Griffith, et al. Exercise testing in patients with automatic implantable cardioverter defibrillators (abstract). *J. Am. Coll. Cardiol.* 9:169A, 1987.

32. Detry, J. M., S. Abouantoun, and W. Wyns. Incidence and prognostic implications of severe ventricular arrhythmias during maximal exercise testing. *Cardiology* 68:35–43, 1981.

33. Detry, J. M., and D. De Jonghe. Exercise testing in the evaluation of ventricular arrhythmias in coronary artery disease. *Eur. Heart J.* 8:55–59, 1987.

34. Dimsdale, J. E., L. H. Hartley, T. Guiney, J. N. Ruskin, and D. Greenblatt. Postexercise peril: plasma catecholamines and exercise. *J. Am. Med. Assoc.* 251:630–663, 1984.

35. Emergency Cardiac Care Committee and Subcommittees, A.H.A. Guidelines for cardiopulmonary resuscitation and emergency cardiac care. *J. Am. Med. Assoc.* 268:2171–2302, 1992.

36. Estes, N. A. M., III. Overview of the implantable cardioverter-defibrillator. N. A. M. Estes, III, A. S. Manolis and P. J. Wang (eds.). *Implantable Cardioverter-Defibrillators: A Comprehensive Textbook.* New York: Marcel Dekker, 1994, pp. 635–653.

37. Fabian, J., I. Stolz, M. Janota, and J. Rohac. Reproducibility of exercise tests in patients with symptomatic ischaemic heart disease. *Br. Heart J.* 37:785–789, 1975.

38. Falcone, C., S. de Servi, E. Poma, et al. Clinical significance of exercise-induced silent myocardial ischemia in patients with coronary artery disease. *J. Am. Coll. Cardiol.* 9:295–299, 1987.

39. Faris, J. V., P. C. McHenry, J. W. Jordan, and S. N. Morris. Prevalence and reproducibility of exercise-induced ventricular arrhythmias during maximal exercise testing in normal men. *Am. J. Cardiol.* 37:617–622, 1976.

40. Fintel, D., L. Griffith, E. Platia, C. Kallman, and P. Reid. Exercise-induced ventricular tachycardia does not predict outcome in patients with recurrent ventricular tachycardia or fibrillation. *PACE Pacing Clin. Electrophysiol.* 7:459, 1984.

41. Fioretti, P., J. Deckers, T. Baardman, et al. Incidence and prognostic implications of repetitive ventricular complexes during pre-discharge bicycle ergometry after myocardial infarction. *Eur. Heart. J.* 8:51–54, 1987.

42. Fletcher, G. F., G. Balady, V. F. Froelicher, L. H. Hartley, W. L. Haskell, and M. L. Pollock. Exercise standards: a statement for healthcare professionals from the American Heart Association. *Circulation* 91:580–615, 1995.

43. Freedman, R. A., C. D. Swerdlow, D. S. Echt, R. A. Winkle, V. Soderholm-Difatte, and J. W. Mason. Facilitation of ventricular tachyarrhythmia induction by isoproterenol. *Am. J. Cardiol.* 54:765–770, 1984.

44. Froelicher, E. S. Usefulness of exercise testing shortly after acute myocardial infarction for predicting 10-year mortality. *Am. J. Cardiol.* 74:318–323, 1994.

45. Gibbons, L., S. N. Blair, H. W. Kohl, and K. Cooper. The safety of maximal exercise testing. *Circulation* 80:846–852, 1989.

46. Gooch, A. S., and D. McConnell. Analysis of transient arrhythmias and conduction disturbances occurring during submaximal treadmill exercise testing. *Prog. Cardiovasc. Dis.* 13:293–307, 1970.

47. Graboys, T. B., B. Lown, P. J. Podrid, and R. DeSilva. Long-term survival of patients with malignant ventricular arrhythmia treated with antiarrhythmic drugs. *Am. J. Cardiol.* 50:437–443, 1982.

48. Grimm, W., B. T. Flores, and F. E. Marchlinski. Shock occurrence and survival in 241 patients with implantable cardioverter-defibrillator therapy. *Circulation* 87:1880–1888, 1993.

49. Hammel, D., M. Block, A. Geiger, et al. Single-incision implantation of cardioverter defibrillators using nonthoracotomy lead systems [see comments]. *Ann. Thorac. Surg.* 58:1614–1616, 1994.

50. Haskell, W. Cardiovascular complications during exercise training of cardiac patients. *Circulation* 57:920–924, 1978.

51. Hauswirth, D., D. Noble, and R. W. Tsien. Adrenaline mechanism of action of the pacemaker potential in cardiac Purkinje fibers. *Science* 162:916, 1968.

52. Henry, R. L., G. T. Kennedy, and M. H. Crawford. Prognostic value of exercise-induced ventricular ectopic activity for mortality after acute myocardial infarction. *Am. J. Cardiol.* 59:1251–1255, 1987.

53. Hondeghem, L. M., and B. G. Katzung. Time- and voltage-dependent interactions of antiarrhythmic drugs with cardiac sodium channels. *Biochim. Biophys. Acta* 472:373–398, 1977.

54. Hondeghem, L. M., and B. G. Katzung. Antiarrhythmic agents: the modulated receptor mechanism of action of sodium and calcium channel-blocking drugs. *Annu. Rev. Pharmacol. Toxicol.* 24:387–423, 1984.

55. Irving, J. B., and R. A. Bruce. Exertional hypotension and postexertional ventricular fibrillation in stress testing. *Am. J. Cardiol.* 39:849–851, 1977.

56. Jelinek, M. V., and B. Lown. Exercise stress testing for exposure of cardiac arrhythmia. *Prog. Cardiovasc. Dis.* 16:497–522, 1974.

57. Kalbfleisch, K. R., M. H. Lehmann, R. T. Steinman, and et al. Reemployment following implantation of the automatic cardioverter-defibrillator. *Am. J. Cardiol.* 64:199–202, 1989.

58. Kelly, T.M. Exercise testing and training of patients with malignant ventricular arrhythmias. *Med. Sci. Sports Exerc.* 28:53–61, 1995.

59. Kelly, T. M., K. Menard-Rothe, C. Callahan, and A. Klapperich. Exercise training in high risk cardiac patients. *J. Cardiopulm. Rehabil.* 8:404, 1988.

60. Kelly, T. M., K. Menard-Rothe, C. Callahan, A. Klapperich, and R. White. Outpatient exercise training in cardiac patients with malignant arrhythmias. *J. Cardiopulm. Rehabil.* 9:395, 1989.

61. Kleiger, R. E., J. P. Miller, J. J. Bigger, and A. J. Moss. Decreased heart rate variability and its association with increased mortality after acute myocardial infarction. *Am. J. Cardiol.* 59:256–262, 1987.

62. Kleiger, R. E., J. P. Miller, R. J. Krone, and J. J. Bigger. The independence of cycle length variability and exercise testing on predicting mortality of patients surviving acute myocardial infarction. The Multicenter Postinfarction Research Group. *Am. J. Cardiol.* 65:408–411, 1990.

63. Klein, L. S., W. M. Miles, and D. P. Zipes. Antitachycardia devices: realities and promises. *J. Am. Coll. Cardiol.* 18:1349–1362, 1991.

64. Kleman, J. M., L. W. Castle, G. A. Kidwell, et al. Nonthoracotomy- versus thoracotomy-implantable defibrillators. Intention-to-treat comparison of clinical outcomes. *Circulation* 90:2833–2842, 1994.

65. Krone, R. J., E. M. Dwyer, Jr., H. Greenberg, J. P. Miller, and J. A. Gillespie. Risk stratification in patients with first non-Q wave infarction: limited value of the early low level exercise test after uncomplicated infarcts. The Multicenter Post-Infarction Research Group. *J. Am. Coll. Cardiol.* 14:31–37; discussion 38–39, 1989.

66. Krone, R. J., J. A. Gillespie, F. M. Weld, J. P. Miller, and A. J. Moss. Low-level exercise testing after myocardial infarction: usefulness in enhancing clinical risk stratification. *Circulation* 71:80–89, 1985.

67. Lawton, J. S., K. A. Ellenbogen, M. A. Wood, et al. Clinical experience with nonthoracotomy cardioverter defibrillators. *Ann. Thor. Surg.* 59:1092–1098; discussion 1098–1099, 1995.

68. Lee, A., and et al. Long-term effects of physical training in coronary patients with impaired ventricular function. *Circulation* 60:1519, 1979.

69. Lombardi, F., G. Sandrone, S. Pernpruner, and et al. Heart rate variability as an index of sympathovagal interaction after acute myocardial infarction. *Am. J. Cardiol.* 60:1239–1245, 1987.

70. Lown, B., P. J. Podrid, R. A. DeSilva, et al. Sudden cardiac death: management of the patient at risk. *Curr. Probl. Cardiol.* 4:1, 1980.

71. Mason, J. W. A comparison of seven antiarrhythmic drugs in patients with ventricular tachyarrhythmias. Electrophysiologic study versus electrocardiographic monitoring investigators (comments). *N. Engl. J. Med.* 329:452–458, 1993.

72. Master, A.M. Cardiac arrhythmias elicited by the two-step exercise test. *Am. J. Cardiol.* 32:766–771, 1973.

73. Mazzuero, G., P. Lanfranchi, R. Colombo, P. Giannuzzi, and A. Giordano. Long-term adaptation of 24 hour heart rate variability after myocardial infarction. The EAMI Study Group. Exercise training in anterior myocardial infarction. *Chest* 101:304S–308S, 1992.

74. McHenry, P. L., C. Fisch, and J. W. Jordan. Cardiac arrhythmia observed during maximal exercise testing in clinically normal men. *Am. J. Cardiol.* 39:311, 1978.

75. Mirowski, M., P. R. Reid, M. M. Mower, et al. Termination of malignant ventricular arrhythmias with an implanted automatic defibrillator in human beings. *N. Engl. J. Med.* 303:322–324, 1980.

76. Morady, F., W. H. Kou, A. H. Kadish, et al. Antagonism of quinidine's electrophysiologic effects by epinephrine in patients with ventricular tachycardia. *J. Am. Coll. Cardiol.* 12:388–394, 1988.

77. Morris, C. K., K. Morrow, V. Froelicher, et al. Prediction of cardiovascular death by means of clinical and exercise test variables in patients selected for cardiac catheterization. *Am. Heart J.* 125:1717–1726, 1993.

78. Nademanee, K., B. N. Singh, W. G. Stevenson, and J. N. Weiss. Amiodarone and post-myocardial infarction patients. *Circulation* 88:764–774, 1993.

79. Nunain, S. O., M. Roelke, T. Trouton, et al. Limitations and late complications of third-generation automatic cardioverter-defibrillators. *Circulation* 91:2204–2213, 1995.

80. O'Hara, G., P. Brugada, L. M. Rodriguez, et al. Incidence, pathophysiology and prognosis of exercise-induced sustained ventricular tachycardia associated with healed myocardial infarction. *Am. J. Cardiol.* 70:875–878, 1992.

81. Palileo, E. V., W. W. Ashley, S. Swiryn, et al. Exercise provocable right ventricular outflow tract tachycardia. *Am. Heart J.* 104:185–193, 1982.

82. Pashkow, F. J. Populations with special needs for exercise rehabilitation: patients with implanted pacemakers or implanted cardioverter-defibrillators. N. K. Wenger and H. Hellerstein (eds.). *Rehabilitation of the Coronary Patient.* New York: Churchill Livingstone, 1992, pp. 431–438.

83. Pashkow, F. J. Rehabilitation of the cardiologically complex patient—left ventricular dysfunction, arrhythmia, and valvular heart disease. F. J. Pashkow and W. A. Dafoe (eds.). *Clinical Cardiac Rehabilitation: A Cardiologist's Guide.* Baltimore: Williams & Wilkins, 1993, pp. 143 155.

84. PCD Investigator Group. Clinical outcome of patients with malignant ventricular tachyarrhythmias and a multiprogrammable implantable cardioverter-defibrillator implanted with or without thoracotomy: an international multicenter study. *J. Am. Coll. Cardiol.* 23:1521–1530, 1994.

85. Peduzzi, P., H. Hultgren, J. Thomsen, and W. Angell. Prognostic value of baseline exercise tests. *Prog. Cardiovasc. Dis.* 28:285–292, 1986.

86. Pina, I. L., G. J. Balady, P. Hanson, A. J. Labovitz, D. W. Madonna, and J. Myers. Guidelines for clinical exercise testing laboratories. A statement for healthcare professionals from the Committee on Exercise and Cardiac Rehabilitation, American Heart Association. *Circulation* 91:912–921, 1995.

87. Pinski, S. L., and G. J. Fahy. The proarrhythmic potential of implantable cardioverter-defibrillators. *Circulation* 92:1651–1664, 1995.

88. Pinski, S. L., and R. G. Trohman. Implantable cardioverter defibrillators: implications for the nonelectrophysiologist. *Ann. Intern. Med.* 122:770–777, 1995.

89. Poblete, P. F., H. L. Kennedy, and D. G. Caralis. Detection of ventricular ectopy in patients with coronary heart disease and normal subjects by exercise testing and ambulatory electrocardiography. *Chest* 74:402–407, 1978.

90. Podrid, P. J. Treatment of ventricular arrhythmia. Applications and limitations of noninvasive vs invasive approach. *Chest* 88:121–128, 1985.

91. Podrid, P. J., F. Bumio, and R. I. Fogel. Evaluating patients with ventricular arrhythmia. Role of the signal-averaged electrocardiogram, exercise test, ambulatory electrocardiogram, and electrophysiologic studies. *Cardiol. Clin.* 10:371–395, 1992.

92. Podrid, P. J., T. Fuchs, and R. Candinas. Role of the sympathetic nervous system in the genesis of ventricular arrhythmias. *Circulation* 82:1103, 1990.

93. Podrid, P. J., F. J. Venditti, P. A. Levine, and M. D. Klein. The role of exercise testing in evaluation of arrhythmias. *Am. J. Cardiol.* 62:24H–33H, 1988.

94. Pycha, C., and et al. Psychological responses to the implantable defibrillator. *Psychosomatics* 27:841–845, 1986.

95. Ranger, S., M. Talajic, R. Lemery, D. Roy, C. Villemaire, and S. Nattel. Kinetics of use-dependent ventricular conduction slowing by antiarrhythmic drugs in humans. *Circulation* 83:1987–1994, 1991.

96. Ryan, M., B. Lown, and H. Horn. Comparison of ventricular ectopic activity during 24-hour monitoring and exercise testing in patients with coronary heart disease. *N. Engl. J. Med.* 292:224–229, 1975.

97. Saini, V., T. B. Graboys, V. Towne, and B. Lown. Reproducibility of exercise-induced ventricular arrhythmia in patients undergoing evaluation for malignant ventricular arrhythmia. *Am. J. Cardiol.* 63:697–701, 1989.

98. Saksena, S., R. B. Krol, and R. R. Kaushik. Innovations in pulse generators and lead systems: balancing complexity with clinical benefit and long-term results. *Am. Heart J.* 127:1010–1021, 1994.

99. Sami, M., B. Chaitman, L. Fisher, D. Holmes, D. Fray, and E. Alderman. Significance of exercise-induced ventricular arrhythmia in stable coronary artery disease: a coronary artery surgery study project. *Am. J. Cardiol.* 54:1182–1188, 1984.

100. Schlant, R. C., C. G. Blomqvist, R. O. Brandenburg, et al. Guidelines for exercise testing. A report of the Joint American College of Cardiology/American Heart Association Task Force on Assessment of Cardiovascular Procedures (Subcommittee on Exercise Testing). *Circulation* 74:653A–667A, 1986.

101. Schlant, R. C., G. C. I. Friesinger, and J. J. Leonard. Clinical competence in exercise testing: a statement for physicians from the ACP/ACC/AHA Task Force on Clinical Privileges in Cardiology. *J. Am. Coll. Cardiol.* 16:1061–1065, 1990.

102. Schmitt, C., M. Montero, and J. Melichercik. Significance of supraventricular tachyarrhythmias in patients with implanted pacing cardioverter defibrillators. *PACE Pacing Clin. Electrophysiol.* 17:295–302, 1994.

103. Schwartz, P. J. Manipulation of the autonomic nervous system in the prevention of sudden cardiac death. P. W. Brugada and H. J. Wellens (eds.). *Cardiac Arrhythmias: Where Do We Go From Here?* New York: Futura, 1987, pp. 741–765.

104. Seals, D. R., and P. B. Chase. Influence of physical training on heart rate variability and baroreflex circulatory control. *J. Appl. Physiol.* 66:1886–1895, 1989.

105. Sheps, D. S., J. C. Ernst, F. R. Briese, et al. Decreased frequency of exercise-induced ventricular ectopic activity in the second of two consecutive treadmill tests. *Circulation* 55:892–895, 1977.

106. Siebels, J., R. Cappato, R. Ruppel, M. A. Schneider, and K. H. Kuck. Preliminary results of the Cardiac Arrest Study Hamburg (CASH). CASH Investigators. *Am. J. Cardiol.* 72:109F–113F, 1993.

107. Slater, W., S. Lampert, P. J. Podrid, and B. Lown. Clinical predictors of arrhythmia worsening by antiarrhythmic drugs. *Am. J. Cardiol.* 61:349–353, 1988.

108. Starling, M. R., M. H. Crawford, G. T. Kennedy, and O. R. RA. Treadmill exercise tests predischarge and six weeks post-myocardial infarction to detect abnormalities of known prognostic value. *Ann. Intern. Med.* 94:721–727, 1981.

109. Stuart, R. J., Jr., and M. H. Ellestad. National survey of exercise stress testing facilities. *Chest* 77:94–97, 1980.
110. The Cardiac Arrhythmia Suppression Trial (CAST) Investigators. Preliminary report: Effect of flecainide and encainide on mortality in a randomized trial of arrhythmia suppression after myocardial infarction. *N. Engl. J. Med.* 321:406–412, 1989.
111. The Encainide-Ventricular Tachycardia Study Group. Treatment of life-threatening ventricular tachycardia with encainide hydrochloride in patients with left ventricular dysfunction. *Am. J. Cardiol.* 62:571, 1988.
112. Udall, J. A., and M. H. Ellestad. Predictive implications of ventricular premature contractions associated with treadmill stress testing. *Circulation* 56:985–989, 1977.
113. Van Camp, S., and R. A. Peterson. Cardiovascular complications of outpatient cardiac rehabilitation programs. *J. Am. Med. Assoc.* 256:1160–1163, 1986.
114. Venditti, F. J., Jr., O. C. M, D. T. Martin, and D. M. Shahian. Transvenous cardioverter defibrillators: cost implications of a less invasive approach. *PACE Pacing Clin. Electrophysiol.* 18:711–715, 1995.
115. Victor, R. G., D. R. Seals, and A. L. Mark. Differential control of heart rate and sympathetic nerve activity during dynamic exercise. Insight from intraneural recordings in humans. *J. Clin. Invest.* 79:508–516, 1987.
116. Waldo, A. L., A. J. Camm, H. de Ruyter, et al. Survival with oral d-sotalol in patients with left ventricular dysfunction after myocardial infarction: rationale, design, and methods (the SWORD trial). *Am. J. Cardiol.* 75:1023–1027, 1995.
117. Weaver, W. D., L. A. Cobb, and A. P. Hallstrom. Characteristics of survivors of exertion- and nonexertion- related cardiac arrest: value of subsequent exercise testing. *Am. J. Cardiol.* 50:671–676, 1982.
118. Weiner, D. A., S. R. Levine, M. D. Klein, and T. J. Ryan. Ventricular arrhythmias during exercise testing: mechanism, response to coronary bypass surgery and prognostic significance. *Am. J. Cardiol.* 53:1553–1557, 1984.
119. Weld, F. M., K. L. Chu, J. T. Bigger, Jr., and L. M. Rolnitzky. Risk stratification with low-level exercise testing 2 weeks after acute myocardial infarction. *Circulation* 64:306–314, 1981.
120. Wellens, F., P. Brugada, G. Guiraudon, Y. De Grieck, R. De Geest, and H. Vanermen. The implantable cardioverter defibrillator: the end of the thoracotomy approach. *Eur. J. Cardiothorac. Surg.* 8:628–634, 1994.
121. Whinnery, J. E. Dysrhythmia comparison in apparently healthy males during and after treadmill and acceleration stress testing. *Am. Heart J.* 105:732–737, 1983.
122. Wit, A. L., and P. F. Cranefield. Triggered activities in cardiac muscle fibers of the simian mitral valve. *Circ. Res.* 38:85–92, 1976.
123. Wit, A. L., and M. R. Rosen. Afterpotentials and triggered activity. II. A. Fozzard, E. Haber, R. B. Jennings, A. M. Katz, and H. E. Morgan (eds.). *The Heart and Cardiovascular System.* New York: Raven Press, 1986, pp. 1449–1490.
124. Woelfel, A., J. R. Foster, R. J. Simpson, Jr., and L. S. Gettes. Reproducibility and treatment of exercise-induced ventricular tachycardia. *Am. J. Cardiol.* 53:751–756, 1984.
125. Wu, D., H. C. Kou, and J. S. Hung. Exercise-triggered paroxysmal ventricular tachycardia. A repetitive rhythmic activity possibly related to afterdepolarization. *Ann. Intern. Med.* 95:410–414, 1981.
126. Yang, J. C., R. C. Wesley, Jr., and V. F. Froelicher. Ventricular tachycardia during routine treadmill testing. Risk and prognosis. *Arch. Intern. Med.* 151:349–353, 1991.
127. Young, D. Z., S. Lampert, T. B. Graboys, and B. Lown. Safety of maximal exercise testing in patients at high risk for ventricular arrhythmia. *Circulation* 70:184–191, 1984.
128. Zipes, D. Genesis of cardiac arrhythmias: electrophysiological considerations. E. Braunwald (ed.). *Heart Disease: A Textbook of Cardiovascular Medicine.* Philadelphia: W. B. Saunders, 1992, vol. 1, pp. 588–627.

10
Visceral Obesity, Insulin Resistance, and Dyslipidemia: Contribution of Endurance Exercise Training to the Treatment of the Plurimetabolic Syndrome

JEAN-PIERRE DESPRÉS, Ph.D.

Obese patients are frequently characterized by an insulin-resistant dyslipidemic state. However, not every obese patient shows a substantial disturbance in the metabolic profile predictive of cardiovascular disease (CVD) risk, which suggests that obesity is a heterogeneous condition. In this regard, regional adipose tissue (AT) distribution has been recognized as an important factor involved in the etiology of metabolic disturbances found among obese patients. Studies that have used imaging techniques such as magnetic resonance imaging or computed tomography, in order to discriminate precisely subcutaneous from intraabdominal (visceral) AT, have shown that visceral AT accumulation is a significant correlate of an altered metabolic profile that includes hyperinsulinemia, insulin resistance and glucose intolerance, hypertriglyceridemia, reduced high-density lipoprotein (HDL) cholesterol concentrations, and increased apolipoprotein B levels, as well as an elevated proportion of small, dense low-density lipoprotein (LDL) particles. Recent results have suggested that the hyperinsulinemic state that characterizes visceral obesity and insulin resistance not only increases the risk of noninsulin-dependent diabetes mellitus but also is associated with an increased risk of ischemic heart disease. Thus, visceral obesity is now recognized as an additional component of the insulin-resistant dyslipidemic syndrome, which has been described extensively in several previous reviews. It is suggested that this cluster of metabolic abnormalities may represent the most prevalent cause of coronary artery disease in developed countries. However, residual metabolic heterogeneity is noted among obese patients with similar levels of visceral AT. Variation in genes involved in the metabolic phenotypes, such as relevant enzymes and apolipoproteins, could alter the relationship of body fat distribution to the metabolic profile. This phenomenon may explain the marked susceptibility to insulin resistance, dyslipidemia, and premature coronary artery disease in some visceral obese patients and the relative resistance to complications found among other visceral obese subjects. Thus, visceral obesity should be considered a permissive factor that exacerbates an individual sus-

271

ceptibility to insulin resistance and Type II diabetes, as well as to dyslipidemia and coronary artery disease.

It is believed that these notions have considerable public health implications. Indeed, it is known that regular endurance exercise training can potentially improve insulin action, leading to a reduction in plasma insulin concentrations. Furthermore, endurance exercise training can improve plasma lipoprotein levels when the increase in energy expenditure associated with the exercise program is sufficient. Under those circumstances, reductions in plasma triglyceride and in apo B-associated lipoprotein concentrations, as well as an increase in HDL cholesterol levels, especially in the HDL_2 subfraction, are noted. Several beneficial alterations in lipoprotein subphenotypes are observed, contributing to the improved lipoprotein lipid profile found among physically active individuals. Furthermore, it appears that the energy expenditure associated with exercise training may be the most important factor explaining the metabolic improvements noted with endurance exercise training. Indeed, a dissociation between cardiorespiratory fitness and what has been described as metabolic fitness has been reported. Indeed, most metabolic improvements associated with endurance exercise training in obese patients appear to be related to the volume of exercise and to the amount of body weight (fat) loss, rather than to the increase in $\dot{V}O_2$ max, a common indicator of cardiorespiratory fitness. Therefore, from a metabolic and public health perspective, it appears more important to emphasize the need to increase substantially the energy expenditure related to a given exercise training program, rather than to focus on its intensity. Indeed, improvements in cardiorespiratory fitness do not appear to be required in order to reduce the risk of Type II diabetes and coronary heart disease (CHD) among insulin-resistant dyslipidemic patients with an excess of visceral AT. However, no prospective studies are currently available to support this model. Although such studies would require considerable expenses, their public health implications are such that their financial burden appears largely justified.

OBESITY AND CARDIOVASCULAR DISEASE (CVD) RISK: IMPORTANCE OF VISCERAL AT

Obesity is highly prevalent in developed countries and has been generally associated with complications such as hypertension, diabetes, and dyslipidemia, as well as with an increased risk of cerebral and vascular diseases, and obese patients are more prone to alterations in free fatty acid metabolism as well as to atherosclerosis [5, 13, 61, 84]. However, not every obese patient is confronted by these deleterious alterations, suggesting that it is a heterogeneous condition [8]. Indeed, studies conducted over the last 15 yr have emphasized the heterogeneous nature of obesity, not only in terms of its etiology but also regarding its complications [7, 8, 25, 59, 61]. In this regard, epidemiological studies conducted in the mid-1980s [40, 41, 72, 73, 88] have largely contributed to reemphasize a notion introduced in 1947 by Jean Vague [114], who was the first to suggest that body fat topography was much more important to consider than AT mass per se in the clinical assessment of obese patients. Indeed, Vague suggested that a preferential abdominal fat accumulation, a condition that he described as android obesity, was a much more prevalent condition among overweight patients with hypertension, diabetes, or coronary heart disease (CHD), whereas what he referred to as gynoid obesity or female type obesity was rarely associated with major complications [115]. However, it took more than 35 yr before these remarkable clinical observations were confirmed by epidemiological and metabolic studies. Among the researchers of those studies, Kissebah et al. [60] were the first, in 1982, to suggest that a high proportion of abdominal fat, simply assessed by an elevated ratio of waist/hip circumferences, was associated with glucose intolerance and hypertriglyceridemia, a finding that was almost simultaneously confirmed by Krotkiewski and colleagues [66]. Furthermore, in 1984, two papers [72, 73] were published by the obesity research group of Per Björntorp in Göteborg, reporting that a high waist/hip ratio was an independent predictor of mortality from cardiovascular disease in both men and women. Furthermore, the same group also reported 1 yr later [88] that a high waist/hip ratio was associated with an increased risk of developing diabetes over a 13½-yr follow-up period and that a tremendous synergy was found between a high body mass index (BMI) and an elevated waist/hip ratio in modulating the increased probability of developing diabetes mellitus (Fig. 10.1). Indeed, in this study, men in both the third body mass index (BMI) and waist/hip ratio tertiles were more than 30 times at risk of developing diabetes than subjects who were in both the first BMI and waist/hip ratios tertiles. Furthermore, among men in the first waist/hip ratio tertile, an increase in the BMI was not associated with an increased risk of developing diabetes mellitus. Therefore, among all men in the third BMI tertile, considering the waist/hip ratio was critical in evaluating the risk of diabetes mellitus. From these results, one can conclude that assessing the risk of developing diabetes solely on the basis of BMI is not sufficient and completely misleading [33].

Although the assessment of the risk related to obesity can be further refined by taking into account the distribution of body fat with the use of the waist/hip ratio, this variable only provides a crude index of AT distribution. With the development of imaging techniques such as magnetic resonance imaging or computed tomography, it has been possible to measure, with a high level of precision, body fat distribution and, more particularly, to assess the amount of fat located in the abdominal cavity, the so-called intraabdominal or visceral AT [12, 46, 68, 105, 112]. With the use of computed tomography, one can precisely measure visceral AT accumulation

FIGURE 10.1.

Percent probability of developing diabetes mellitus over a 13½-yr follow-up period in men of the Göteborg prospective study classified into tertiles of BMI and waist-to-hip ratio (WHR). Reproduced from ref. 88.

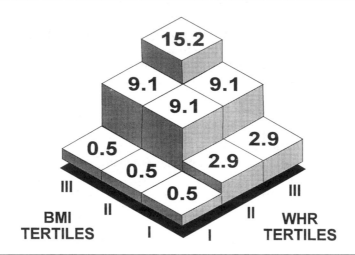

and sort out the independent contributions of visceral fat accumulation vs. those of total body fat as correlates of the common metabolic complications found among overweight patients.

In order to examine this issue, we have previously performed a very simple analysis in which we matched individuals with the same amount of total body fat but with either a low or high accumulation of visceral AT measured by computed tomography [25, 32, 38, 97]. We then compared these two subgroups to a group of lean controls. In both men and women, we found that obesity per se was associated with moderate metabolic alterations, which mainly included moderate increases in fasting insulin and triglyceride concentrations [25, 32, 38, 97]. However, in both men and women, excess visceral AT tissue accumulation was clearly associated with increased plasma triglyceride concentrations, reduced HDL cholesterol levels, increased plasma insulin concentrations measured in the fasting state, as well as after an oral glucose load and with a greater glycemic response to standard 75 g oral glucose load [25, 32, 38, 97] (Figs. 10.2–10.4). These results clearly indicated that excess visceral AT accumulation was a correlate of the common metabolic complications of obesity, which included hyperinsulinemia, glucose intolerance, hypertriglyceridemia, elevated apo B concentrations, and reduced HDL cholesterol levels [25, 30, 32, 34, 35, 37–39, 97]. Further measurements of HDL subfractions revealed that the reduced HDL cholesterol

FIGURE 10.2.

Plasma glucose and insulin levels measured after a 75-g oral glucose load in three groups of premenopausal women. Adapted from ref. 38.

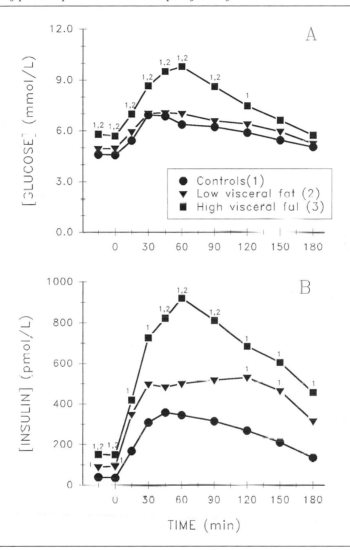

levels found in visceral obesity mainly resulted from a reduction in the cholesterol content of the HDL_2 subfraction [31]. We have also previously reported that this reduction in HDL_2 cholesterol levels in visceral obesity was the consequence of reciprocal changes in the activity of two enzymes involved in HDL metabolism, namely, lipoprotein lipase (LPL), whose activ-

FIGURE 10.3.

Plasma insulin concentrations measured in the fasting state after an oral glucose load (area under the curve) in three groups of men. The two groups of obese patients were matched for percent body fat but were characterized by either low or high levels of visceral AT measured by computed tomography. 1, significantly different from lean controls; 2, significantly different from obese men with low levels of visceral adipose tissue, p < 0.05. Adapted from ref. 97.

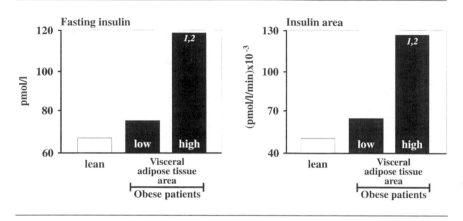

ity is reduced in visceral obesity, and hepatic lipase (HL), whose activity that has been found to be substantially increased in this condition [31]. Accordingly, we found that the greater the accumulation of visceral AT was, the greater the activity of hepatic lipase was and the lower were the plasma HDL_2 cholesterol levels [31]. Thus, the reciprocal changes noted in the activity of LPL and HL is an important factor for the modulation of HDL_2 cholesterol levels in visceral obesity.

GENDER DIFFERENCES IN VISCERAL AT ACCUMULATION

We have also been interested in the well-known gender difference in AT distribution, with men being obviously more prone to abdominal fat accumulation than premenopausal women. In order to quantify this phenomenon precisely, we have examined the relationship between total body fat mass and visceral AT accumulation measured by computed tomography in both men and premenopausal women [77]. For any level of total body fat, we found that men had, on average, twice the amount of visceral AT found in premenopausal women [77] (Fig. 10.5). As excess visceral AT accumulation is a significant correlate of a cluster of metabolic complications [25, 30, 32, 34, 35, 37–39, 50–52, 92, 97, 107], we had previously proposed that the

FIGURE 10.4.
Plasma triglyceride and HDL-C levels in a group of nonobese men and in two groups of obese men matched for percent body fat but with either low or high levels of visceral AT measured by computed tomography. 1, significantly different from lean controls, p < 0.05. Adapted from ref. 29.

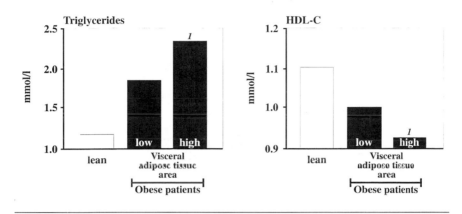

greater accumulation of visceral AT found in men than in premenopausal women could explain the greater susceptibility of men to metabolic complications for a given excess of AT. To examine this possibility further, we matched men and women for the same amount of visceral AT, and this procedure largely eliminated the well-known gender difference in the CVD risk profile [76]. Therefore, we believe that the relative protection of women against visceral AT accumulation before menopause is a factor contributing to explain their more favorable CVD risk profile, compared to that of men. However, at menopause, in the absence of hormonal replacement therapy, an acceleration of abdominal fat accumulation is noted [53], which is likely to be associated with the development of metabolic disturbances. Further work in this area is clearly warranted to verify whether prevention of visceral AT accumulation at menopause by hormonal replacement therapy or by life-style modifications is important for the primary prevention of diabetes and CHD in women.

CHOLESTEROL AND LDL-CHOLESTEROL LEVELS IN VISCERAL OBESITY: POTENTIALLY MISLEADING INFORMATION

Despite the presence of insulin resistance and hyperinsulinemia in visceral obesity, these individuals are most often characterized by nearly normal cholesterol and LDL cholesterol levels [32, 34, 35, 37, 39]. However, one

FIGURE 10.5.

Relationship of total body fat mass assessed by underwater weighing to visceral AT accumulation, measured by computed tomography in men and in premenopausal women. Adapted from ref. 77.

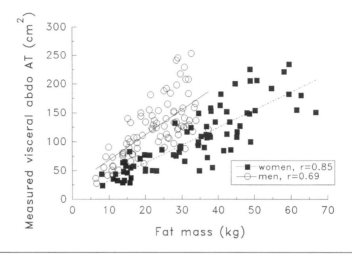

should not be misled by these apparently normal concentrations. Indeed, by using additional techniques such as density gradient ultracentrifugation or polyacrylamide gradient gel electrophoresis, one could reach the conclusion that visceral obesity is associated with a greater proportion of small, dense, cholesterol ester-depleted LDL particles [110] that cannot be appropriately assessed on the basis of plasma LDL cholesterol levels. However, as there is one apo B molecule per LDL particle, irrespective of its cholesteryl ester content, we suggest that measurements of apo B or LDL apo B levels in visceral obesity provide a more adequate estimate of the number of atherogenic particles than LDL-cholesterol levels [29]. Indeed, by using this methodology we have reported a 15–20% increase in apo B and LDL apo B concentrations in visceral obesity despite the fact that these subjects were characterized by apparently normal LDL cholesterol levels [29]. Thus, for any level of plasma LDL cholesterol, visceral obese men and women are generally characterized by an increased LDL particle number. We have further examined this issue by measuring the proportion of small dense LDL particles by 2–16% polyacrylamide gel electrophoresis [110]. We assessed LDL peak particle diameter, as well as derived an LDL particle score that was calculated as a continuous variable, using the migration distance of each LDL peak identified on the gel multiplied by its respective relative area. The LDL peak particle size and the LDL particle score showed a highly significant correlation, with the shared variance between the two measurements just below 60% [110]. However, the LDL particle score, which provides a global index of the proportion of small dense LDL particles [110], was not significantly correlated with plasma LDL cholesterol and LDL apo B levels, whereas it was positively correlated with the LDL apo B:LDL cholesterol ratio, with fasting plasma triglyceride levels, and with the cholesterol: HDL cholesterol ratio. We then performed additional analyses that revealed that the high triglyceride-low HDL cholesterol dyslipidemia found in visceral obese patients was the best correlate of the proportion of small, dense LDL particles found in visceral obese-insulin-resistant patients [110]. Thus, visceral obesity is associated with metabolic disturbances predictive of an increased risk of developing Type II diabetes, as well as with complications also contributing to an increase in the risk of CHD. It is also relevant to point out that the prevalence of visceral obesity in sedentary men has been estimated to reach approximatively 25% of the population [29, 32, 39], a finding that is remarkably similar to the estimated prevalence of the insulin resistance syndrome among nondiabetic men [100], as well as to the proportion of men with the atherogenic phenotype [3, 4], which includes the high triglyceride-low HDL cholesterol dyslipidemia, as well as an increased proportion of small, dense LDL particles.

AN ANTHROPOMETRIC CORRELATE OF VISCERAL AT: THE WAIST CIRCUMFERENCE CONCEPT

We have also been interested in identifying a critical value of visceral AT accumulation associated with an increased likelihood of finding metabolic abnormalities [28]. In order to examine this issue, we have performed a very simple procedure in which our sample of men and women were divided into quintiles of visceral AT accumulation measured at the L4-L5 level [28]. Our findings suggested that subjects with cross-sectional areas of visceral adipose tissue below 100 cm^2 were characterized by a relatively normal metabolic profile, whereas subjects with a visceral AT accumulation above 130 cm^2 were generally characterized by a cluster of metabolic abnormalities predictive of an increased risk of noninsulin-dependent diabetes mellitus (NIDDM) and coronary heart disease. Thus, we believe that a visceral adipose tissue accumulation above approximatively 130 cm^2 is predictive, in both men and women, of an increased probability of finding disturbances in the cardiovascular disease risk profile. However, as imaging techniques are obviously not available to most clinicians and for reasons such as cost and the irradiation related to the procedure, we have been interested in identifying anthropometric correlates of visceral AT accumulation [95]. We first examined the relationship between the commonly used waist-to-hip ratio and visceral AT accumulation and we found that the common variance between the two variables did not reach 50% in both men and women [95].

However, although the relationship was not perfect, visceral AT accumulation showed a correlation with the waist circumference which was of higher magnitude than with the waist/hip ratio [95]. Indeed, by using age and the waist circumference, we were able to predict up to 75% of the variance in visceral AT accumulation [95]. Inclusion of additional anthropometric variables failed to improve our ability to predict visceral AT accumulation. Thus, the waist circumference appears to be the best anthropometric correlate of visceral AT currently available. It is also relevant to point out that the correlation of waist girth to height was not significantly different from zero in both men and women, suggesting that there is no need to adjust the waist circumference for height. Thus, we believe that the measurement of waist girth is justified from a public health standpoint. Furthermore, the health professionals should be much more interested in reducing waist girth than in normalizing body weight through an exercise program. Indeed, any increase in muscle mass in response to an exercise program may potentially mask changes in AT distribution which, however, will be revealed by changes in waist circumference. Therefore, it is possible to envision a situation in which visceral obese subjects could lose 2–3 cm of waist circumference without any change in body weight when a given exercise program produces a significant increase in muscle mass. However, a reduction in waist circumference clearly indicates a mobilization of abdominal (probably visceral) AT.

Finally, we have also found that the relationship of waist circumference to visceral AT accumulation is influenced by age. Indeed, there is with age a selective accumulation of visceral AT that cannot always be adequately assessed by changes in the waistline [79]. Therefore, we have proposed that among subjects below 40 yr of age, a waist circumference of 1 m would be associated with a visceral AT accumulation predictive of an increased risk of finding metabolic complications [95]. However, among men and women between 40 and 60 yr of age, a waist circumference above 90 cm would be associated with an increased likelihood of finding an accumulation of visceral AT of 130 cm^2 and above [79]. Thus, in older adults, we have to be more careful regarding the critical waist circumference value likely to be associated with metabolic complications.

Furthermore, although visceral AT increases with age, no longitudinal data was, until recently, available on the potential metabolic impact of this age-related selective accumulation of visceral fat. We have recently completed a study in which 7-yr follow-up data was available in a sample of 32 initially premenopausal women [78]. Over the 7-yr follow-up period, these women showed a significant increase in visceral AT accumulation that was not accompanied by a significant increase in total body fat mass. However, waist circumference increased by 4 cm and was significantly correlated with the change in visceral AT cross-sectional area as assessed by computed tomography (0.81; $P < 0.0001$). Despite the fact that body fat mass did not change significantly over the follow-up period, the increased visceral AT accumulation was associated with an increase in the glycemic response to a 75-g oral glucose load [78]. We also compared two subgroups of women who were matched for their change in total body fat mass but who showed little change or substantial increase in visceral AT over 7 yr. Women who did not present any significant change in visceral adipose tissue over 7 yr did not show any deterioration in the glycemic response to the oral glucose load. However, despite the fact that the other group of women studied also showed no change in total body fat mass, these women were characterized by an increase of 50 cm^2 of visceral AT, which was associated with a highly significant deterioration in the glycemic response to the oral glucose challenge [78]. Thus, results from this longitudinal study indicate that the increase in visceral AT noted with age is associated with a significant deterioration in the metabolic profile, suggesting that the prevention of visceral fat deposition is also an important issue from a public health standpoint.

THE HYPERINSULINEMIC/DYSLIPIDEMIC STATE OF VISCERAL OBESITY: AN ATHEROGENIC COMBINATION

Visceral obesity is associated with an insulin-resistant hyperinsulinemic state that may lead to glucose intolerance and, eventually, to Type II diabetes in the presence of genetic factors presently poorly understood [7, 59, 75]. Furthermore, this insulin-resistant hyperinsulinemic state is associated with a dyslipidemia that includes hypertriglyceridemia, low HDL cholesterol levels, elevated apo B concentrations, and an increased proportion of small dense LDL particles [25, 27, 29, 32, 34, 36, 37]. Prospective studies have shown that this dyslipidemic profile is also associated with an increased risk of CHD [2, 83]. However, until recently, whether or not hyperinsulinemia was an independent predictor of CHD had remained controversial. Four prospective studies found that fasting hyperinsulinemia was associated with an increased risk of ischemic heart disease in men [43, 99, 118, 125], but these findings had not been confirmed in all studies [120]. Furthermore, whether the association between hyperinsulinemia and ischemic heart disease remained significant after control for the concomitant dyslipidemic state was uncertain. For example, Fontbonne et al. [47–49] found that only hyperinsulinemic men of the Paris Prospective Study who also had hypertriglyceridemia showed an increased rate of mortality from CHD. In this regard, recent observations from our prospective study conducted in Québec City have allowed us to examine this issue [24]. Indeed, in the Québec Cardiovascular Study, a sample of 2103 men initially free from ischemic heart disease were followed for a period of 5 yr, from 1985 to 1990 [24, 69]. Over the 5-yr follow-up period, 114 cases of ischemic heart disease were noted, which included myocardial infarction, effort angina, and mortality from CHD. The first question that we examined in this study was the prevalence of various dyslipidemic states in men who developed ischemic heart disease, compared to that of those who remained healthy [69]. Results indicated that about 50% of the 1989 men who remained free from ischemic heart disease had a normal lipoprotein lipid profile. However, less than one-third of the 114 men who developed ischemic heart disease had normal plasma lipoprotein concentrations. Thus, the various dyslipidemic phenotypes were associated with an increased risk of ischemic heart disease in this cohort. We then performed stepwise regression analyses to predict ischemic heart disease, examining lipoprotein concentrations as continuous variables [71]. Results revealed that diabetes, apolipoprotein B, age, smoking, and systolic blood pressure were significant predictors of the risk of ischemic heart disease in this cohort [71]. However, apolipoprotein B concentration was the best metabolic predictor of the risk of ischemic heart disease in this sample of French-Canadian men [71]. Indeed, after inclusion of apo B concentration in the prediction model, no other lipoprotein lipid variable was able to contribute to further explaining the risk of ischemic heart disease in this cohort.

We also examined the relationship of hyperinsulinemia to ischemic heart disease by measuring fasting insulin concentrations in men who eventually developed ischemic heart disease and then matching them for age, BMI, smoking, and alcohol consumption with a group of subjects who remained healthy over the 5-yr follow-up period [24]. We measured fasting insulin concentrations in these subjects by using an assay that did not cross-react with proinsulin [24]. After exclusion of men with diabetes, an 18% increase in fasting insulin concentrations was found in men who eventually developed ischemic heart disease, compared to that of men who remained healthy [24]. We have also observed that a 1 SD increase in fasting insulin concentration was associated with a 70% increase in the risk of ischemic heart disease, with this relationship being essentially unaltered by adjustment for concomitant variation in triglyceride, HDL cholesterol, or apo B levels [24]. Thus, this prospective study was the first to report that hyperinsulinemia is an independent predictor of the risk of ischemic heart disease in men. Furthermore, as apolipoprotein B concentration was found to be the best predictor of ischemic heart disease in this group [71], we also examined the potential interaction or synergy between hyperinsulinemia and elevated apo B levels in the modulation of ischemic heart disease risk in this cohort [24]. For this purpose, we divided the sample into tertiles of fasting insulin concentrations and used the median of the distribution of apo B concentrations to arbitrarily identify subjects with either low or elevated apo B concentrations (Fig. 10.6). Among subjects with low apo B concentrations, hyperinsulinemia per se was associated with a 3-fold increase in the risk of ischemic heart disease [24]. However, the combination of hyperinsulinemia and elevated apo B concentration was associated with more than a 10-fold increase in the risk of ischemic heart disease [24]. It is important to point out that hyperinsulinemia combined with elevated apo B levels rep-

FIGURE 10.6.

Odds ratios for ischemic heart disease over a 5-yr follow-up in initially healthy men classified on the basis of fasting insulin and apolipoprotein B concentrations. Adapted from ref. 24.

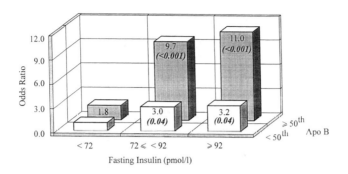

resents a pattern of metabolic abnormalities commonly found in visceral obese patients, even in the absence of elevated plasma cholesterol or LDL-cholesterol levels [25, 27, 29, 32, 34, 36, 37]. Results of the Québec Cardiovascular Study indicate that the hyperinsulinemic/hyperapo B condition of visceral obesity is associated with a marked increase in the risk of ischemic heart disease [24]. Thus, although no prospective study has shown that visceral AT accumulation is an independent predictor of ischemic heart disease, the cluster of metabolic abnormalities found in visceral obesity not only increases the probability of developing Type II diabetes but also the risk of developing ischemic heart disease.

VISCERAL OBESITY AND THE PLURIMETABOLIC SYNDROME: A CAUSAL RELATIONSHIP?

Although it is well established that visceral AT is a strong correlate of metabolic abnormalities increasing the risk of Type II diabetes and ischemic heart disease, such evidence should not be considered as supporting a cause-and-effect relationship. Indeed, the possibility cannot be excluded that visceral obesity is only a marker of this cluster of metabolic abnormalities (Fig. 10.7). For example, Björntorp [9] has suggested that visceral obesity may be a marker of a civilization syndrome associated with a maladaptive response to stress. Indeed, inability to adequately cope with stress would be associated with an activation of the hypothalamic-pituitary-adrenal axis [9]. This activation would contribute to an increase of the control of carbohydrate and lipid metabolism by glucocorticoids [14, 15] and to a re-

FIGURE 10.7.

Simplified working model emphasizing the potential contribution of endocrine abnormalities to the relationship between visceral obesity and dyslipidemia. VLDL, very low-density lipoprotein. TG, triglycerides; apo B, apolipoprotein B; LDL-apo b/CHOL, low-density lipoprotein apo B over LDL-cholesterol ratio.

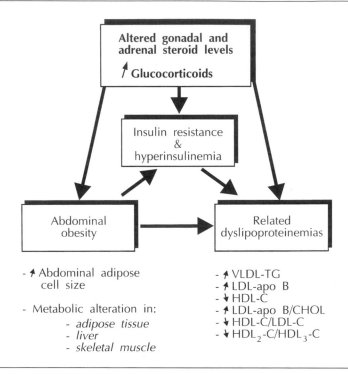

duction of the production of gonadal steroids [9]. In concordance with this model, women with a high proportion of abdominal fat, as estimated by an elevated waist/hip ratio, have been characterized by reduced sex hormone binding globulin (SHBG) levels and increased free testosterone levels [44, 62, 93]. Reduced SHBG levels have also been associated with increased plasma glucose and insulin levels, as well as with hypertriglyceridemia in women [44, 62]. Thus, in women, visceral obesity appears to be associated with reduced SHBG levels and with an increased concentration of free testosterone, with these endocrine abnormalities contributing to further exacerbation of the insulin-resistant dyslipidemic state. In men, reduced plasma testosterone concentrations were found, along with decreased SHBG levels [104, 108]. These reduced testosterone concentrations are accompanied by increased estrogen levels [108]. We have also reported that visceral obesity in men is associated with reduced levels of adrenal steroids such as Δ5-DIOL and DHEA. However, in order to examine whether the concomitant variation in adrenal and gonadal steroid concentrations plays a role in the etiology of the hyperinsulinemic insulin-resistant condition found in visceral obese men, we have compared glycemic and insulinemic responses of two subgroups of men who were matched for DHEA levels but had either high or low levels of visceral fat [109]. Even after matching for DHEA levels, we found that men with a high accumulation of visceral AT were characterized by greater glycemic and insulin responses to an oral glucose load [109]. However, after matching subjects for visceral AT accumulation, men with low vs. high DHEA levels were not characterized by any difference in indices of plasma glucose insulin homeostasis. These results suggest that the relationship of visceral obesity to insulin resistance and hyperinsulinemia in men is probably largely independent of the concomitant variation in adrenal and gonadal steroid levels.

GENETIC SUSCEPTIBILITY TO DYSLIPIDEMIA IN VISCERAL OBESITY

There is, therefore, overwhelming evidence that visceral AT accumulation is a much closer correlate of metabolic abnormalities than is an excess of total body fat per se. Thus, it is critical to assess or at least estimate visceral AT accumulation in the evaluation of the obese patient's risk profile. However, two individuals with similar levels of visceral AT may remain quite heterogeneous in terms of metabolic complications. In this regard, we have been very much interested in the residual metabolic heterogeneity found among visceral obese patients. Indeed, the shared variance between visceral AT deposition and plasma lipoprotein levels varies between 10 and 30%, depending on the variable examined [20]. Thus, we have proposed that genetic susceptibility to diabetes, dyslipidemia, and CHD may modulate the risk of chronic diseases in visceral obese patients [20, 25]. Hence, subjects with a positive family history of premature CHD or diabetes may develop metabolic complications at a much lower excess of visceral AT deposition [20, 25]. Thus, some genes can modulate susceptibility to dyslipidemia and premature CHD in visceral obesity. In this regard, we have been first interested by the contribution of known polymorphisms found in apolipoprotein genes. For example, apo E and apo B are two apoliproteins playing important roles in lipoprotein metabolism. For instance, we have reported that the apo E polymorphism substantially modified the relationship of visceral AT accumulation and hyperinsulinemia to hypertriglyceridemia [19, 96]. Indeed, we found that abdominal obesity in women was positively associated with fasting triglyceride concentrations among apo E2 carriers but that this relationship was absent in apo E4 carriers [96]. Accordingly, hyperinsulinemia was associated with hypertriglyceridemia in apo E2 carriers but not in apo E4 carriers [19]. Thus, abdominal obesity and hyperinsulinemia were only associated with hypertriglyceridemia in the absence of the apo E4 allele. We have also studied a polymorphism in the apo B-100 gene identified by the restriction enzyme EcoRI [98]. Individuals heterozygous for the absence of this restriction site had higher apo B and LDL apo B levels in the presence of visceral obesity [98]. Furthermore, a significant correlation was observed between visceral AT accumulation and LDL apo B concentrations among heterozygous men for the absence of the EcoRI restriction site, whereas this association could not be found among men who were homozygous for the presence of the restriction site. Furthermore, among heterozygous men, hyperinsulinemia was positively correlated with the proportion of small, dense LDL particles, but this association was not found among the homozygotes [117]. Thus, the absence of this EcoRI restriction site in the apo B gene may be an important modulator of the susceptibility to hyperapo B and to the dense LDL phenotype in visceral obesity.

We also examined a LPL gene Hind III polymorphism recently that also appears to be a potent modulator of the susceptibility to develop hypertriglyceridemia in visceral obesity [116]. Indeed, among homozygous men for the presence of the Hind III restriction site, we found the expected positive correlation between visceral obesity and hypertriglyceridemia, whereas this relationship could not be found among heterozygous subjects for the absence of the restriction site [116]. Thus, polymorphisms for these candidate genes (apo E, apo B, LPL) provide simple examples of the potential interaction between genetic and environmental factors in the modulation of susceptibility to develop a dyslipidemic profile in visceral obesity. Thus, the magnitude of the relationship between visceral obesity, metabolic complications, and CHD may be determined, to some extent, by variation in candidate genes involved in lipoprotein metabolism [20, 25]. Some individuals, therefore, may be at a greater risk of developing severe complications and may require more aggressive preventive therapies than other individuals with no family history of chronic disease and who do not show variants in relevant candidate genes.

THE VISCERAL OBESITY CONCEPT: IMPLICATIONS FOR THE PREVENTION OF RELATED METABOLIC COMPLICATIONS

Thus, the hyperinsulinemic dyslipidemic profile of visceral obesity results from a complex network of hormonal and metabolic variables interacting with mostly unknown genetic factors (Fig. 10.8). Visceral obesity may, therefore, be a marker of a cluster of metabolic abnormalities that may include an activated hypothalamic pituitary adrenal axis, leading to an increased control of lipid metabolism by glucocorticoids, altered sex steroid levels, in-

FIGURE 10.8.

Summary of the complex endocrine and metabolic interactions involved in the regulation of the dyslipidemic state found in visceral obesity. VLDL, very low-density lipoprotein; FFA, free fatty acid. LCAT, lecithin cholesterol acyl transferase; TG, triglycerides; CE, cholesteryl ester.

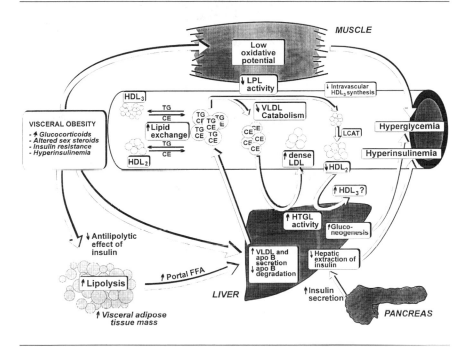

sulin resistance, hyperinsulinemia, and dyslipidemia. This cluster of metabolic abnormalities is so prevalent in our affluent societies, it may represent the most prevalent cause of CHD [39]. It is, therefore, critically important to identify potential sites for intervention in order to treat this condition or to prevent its development. The simplified schematic representation of Figure 10.9 illustrates this concept. First of all, as an increased turnover of free fatty acids has been reported in abdominal obesity [57], a reduced fat intake should theoretically reduce the flux of lipids into a system that is already quite disturbed and insulin resistant [101]. However, the literature is clearly deficient regarding the treatment of the insulin-resistant dyslipidemic syndrome of visceral obesity by an ad libitum low-fat diet, and intervention studies are clearly warranted in this area [28]. Secondly, it is also important to examine approaches that would lead to reduction in visceral AT mass. From a metabolic standpoint, a reduction in visceral AT accumulation

FIGURE 10.9.

Simplified scheme emphasizing the critical sites for interventions aimed at treating the complications of visceral obesity. See text for further details. FFA, free fatty acid.

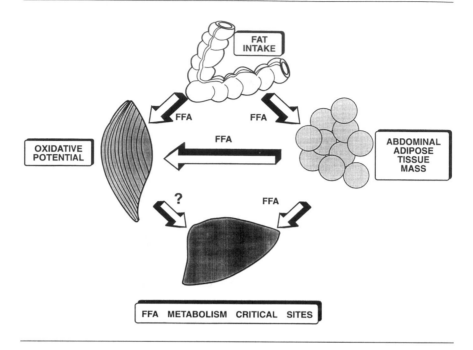

should be associated with improvements in the metabolic profile [29]. Studies conducted so far have indicated that a loss of visceral AT induced either by diet or exercise is indeed associated with improvements in the CVD risk profile [28, 50, 74]. Finally, a role for the skeletal muscle in the etiology of the complications of visceral obesity has been suggested recently [17], as an impaired potential to oxidize lipids in the skeletal muscle could obviously contribute to the etiology of this condition [17]. In this regard, regular endurance exercise training can potentially improve in vivo insulin action in skeletal muscle and increase its oxidative potential [6, 10, 16, 18, 65, 87, 89, 111]. Thus, investigation of the potential contribution of endurance exercise as an approach to treating visceral obesity and the related insulin-resistant state clearly appear warranted. However, what should be the optimal exercise prescription for the treatment of this condition remains unknown. Indeed, epidemiological studies have shown that physically active individuals are at lower risk of coronary heart disease and related mortality, compared to sedentary individuals [80, 85, 86, 90, 91, 102]. The exact mechanisms by which regular physical activity may reduce the risk of ischemic heart disease have not been identified. However, it has been suggested that the high level of cardiorespiratory fitness found in physically active individuals could be an important factor explaining their reduced ischemic heart disease risk [11, 42, 82, 94, 106]. Thus, it has been proposed that a physically active life-style could reduce the risk of ischemic heart disease via an improved cardiorespiratory fitness. However, from the literature on endurance training vs. CVD risk factors such as plasma lipoprotein levels, we concluded that the improvement in cardiorespiratory fitness is not critical in order to reduce the risk of ischemic heart disease by regular exercise [26, 28].

EXERCISE TRAINING AND ITS EFFECT ON INSULIN ACTION AND PLASMA LIPOPROTEIN LEVELS

Exercise training is generally considered to have significant beneficial effects on CVD risk factors, as it improves blood pressure [67, 103], insulin action [10, 111], and the plasma lipoprotein-lipid profile [55, 56, 64, 121–124]. There is, however, some controversy regarding the exercise modalities that should be recommended to improve the CVD risk profile optimally.

The American College of Sports Medicine (ACSM) has defined the minimal amount of exercise required to improve cardiorespiratory fitness [1]; it includes 20 min of continuous exercise performed at a minimum of 50% of $\dot{V}O_2$max (maximal oxygen consumption), 3 days/wk, for several weeks. The ACSM has recognized, however, that a different minimal exercise stimulus may be required to improve health-related fitness, including plasma insulin levels, insulin sensitivity, plasma lipoprotein levels, and glucose tolerance [1], a concept largely emphasized at a Canadian conference on exercise, fitness, and health [45]. Thus, although the improvement of exercise tolerance is a relevant goal for the health professional dealing with dyslipidemic visceral obese patients, the potential effect of regular exercise on the health-related variables should also be considered. The literature currently available suggests that metabolic variables predictive of diabetes and CHD risk may be altered to a greater extent by the volume of exercise, rather than by its intensity (for reviews, see refs. 26 and 28).

Several studies have shown that exercise training programs performed at 70% of subjects' maximal oxygen uptake produce favorable changes in cardiorespiratory fitness and in the metabolic condition when the net increase in energy expenditure is sufficient [26, 55, 56, 64, 121, 122, 124]. Generally, reduction in plasma triglyceride and apo B levels and an increase in plasma high-density lipoprotein cholesterol (HDL-C) concentrations have been reported, although some discrepant results have been published [1, 55, 56, 64, 103, 121, 122]. It is also important to point out that the more deteriorated the initial lipoprotein profile, the greater generally, is, the likelihood of finding significant improvements with regular exercise training [26, 28].

In addition, exercise training programs that did not report any significant change in plasma lipid profiles may not have been adequate in duration and frequency of sessions to yield improvements in plasma lipids levels [26]. In this regard, it is relevant to note that the exercise training studies that induced the largest increases in energy expenditure were those that reported the largest weight losses and the most substantial improvements in plasma lipoprotein levels [26, 55, 56, 64, 121, 122, 124].

We have recently examined, in a review study, whether the critical issue was to improve fitness or to induce a large energy expenditure when dealing with diabetogenic and atherogenic metabolic complications [26]. Overall, the improvement in plasma lipoprotein levels produced by exercise training is poorly related to changes in treadmill performance or changes in $\dot{V}O_2max$ that are commonly used as fitness indexes [26]. In this regard, Williams et al. [119] have shown that improvements in both $\dot{V}O_2max$ and treadmill duration in response to exercise training were poor correlates of changes in plasma HDL-C levels. However, a closer association between the increase in plasma HDL-C concentrations and the training volume (as estimated by the number of miles run per week) was noted [119], a finding in accordance with recent observations [63]. Thus, these results suggest that metabolic changes noted with training are more related to the training volume (and to the related increase in energy expenditure) than to the improvement in cardiorespiratory fitness. Thus, it is relevant to increase energy expenditure substantially, rather than to focus on improving cardiorespiratory fitness when the main therapeutic objective is to improve the CVD risk profile of the visceral obese patient by regular endurance exercise. Thus, exercise intensity does not appear to be critical to generating favorable changes in metabolic variables relevant to CVD risk.

In this regard, studies that used moderate-intensity endurance exercise reported favorable improvement in plasma lipoprotein levels when the exercise volume was sufficient [26]. Exercise training conducted at about 50–70% of maximal aerobic power induced significant reductions in body weight, plasma insulin levels, and LDL concentrations, as well as significant increases in HDL-C levels, particularly in the cardioprotective HDL_2 subfraction [21–23, 70]. It is relevant to note that, in these studies, changes in cardiorespiratory fitness did not show any relationship to improvement in plasma lipid profile [21–23, 70]. Thus, the insulin-resistant, dyslipidemic patient with visceral obesity may particularly benefit from low-to-moderate intensity endurance exercise. Optimal results are likely to be obtained by doing prolonged exercise performed on an almost daily basis [26, 28]. With this approach, the increased energy expenditure will be such that a negative energy balance more likely will be produced, generating losses of total and visceral AT and improvements in the CVD risk profile [26, 28].

Our high-fat intake, combined with our sedentary life-style, are two contributing factors that explain the high prevalence of hyperinsulinemia and insulin resistance in our population [28, 100]. As insulin resistance is a significant correlate of a dyslipidemic profile predictive of an increased risk of CHD [100], it has been proposed that the insulin-resistant, dyslipidemic state frequently observed in subjects with visceral obesity may be the most prevalent cause of CHD in North America [29, 32, 39, 70, 100]. Consequently, maintaining an adequate level of insulin sensitivity through regular exercise may not only reduce the risk of developing Type II diabetes but also it may be associated with a more favorable plasma lipid profile, thereby contributing to reduction of the risk of CHD [26, 28]. Indeed, prolonged endurance exercise, which is associated with an increased oxidation of lipids and mobilization of glycogen stores, has been shown to improve insulin sensitivity acutely, an effect that may last for 48–72 hr [16, 87]. Thus, rapid improvement in the plasma lipoprotein lipid profile of the sedentary visceral obese dyslipidemic patient may be obtained through the daily improvement in insulin action generated by repeated daily bouts of prolonged exercise. Thus, a moderate-intensity endurance exercise program in which subjects exercised for more than 1 hr on an almost daily basis induced significant improvements in insulin sensitivity and in plasma lipoprotein levels (Fig. 10.10). These changes include reductions in plasma triglyceride and apo B levels, increases in HDL-C levels (particularly in the HDL_2 subfraction), and reciprocal changes in the activity of two enzymes that play critical roles in the regulation of plasma triglyceride and HDL-C levels, namely, plasma postheparin LPL (which is low in visceral obesity but generally increases with training) and hepatic triglyceride lipase (HTGL) (which is high in visceral obesity but markedly reduced in exercise-trained individuals) [26]. These reciprocal changes in postheparin LPL and HTGL activities are important correlates of the increased proportion of HDL-C found in physically active people [26]. Furthermore, these metabolic adaptations also appear to be dissociated from the improvement in physical fitness, as they appeared rather to be related to the degree of weight loss [23], an indicator of the increased energy expenditure associated with the exercise program (Fig. 10.11).

In this regard, Oshida et al. [89] showed that a moderate-intensity jogging program inducing no significant increase in maximal aerobic power produced substantial improvements in insulin sensitivity. Furthermore, in a landmark randomized study, Wood et al. [123] reported that diet-induced weight loss led to similar increases in plasma HDL-C levels, when compared to weight loss produced by exercise training. This result emphasized the importance of concomitant weight loss (and, therefore, of producing a negative energy balance by means of exercise) as a determinant of the metabolic improvement produced by endurance exercise, a concept that has been further supported by results from a recent randomized controlled trial of weight loss vs. aerobic exercise training [58].

FIGURE 10.10.

Overview of the metabolic response of visceral obese patients to an endurance exercise training program. Adapted from ref. 26. TG, triglycerides; CHOL, cholesterol; LDL-B/CHOL, low density lipoprotein-apo B over LDL-cholesterol ratio.

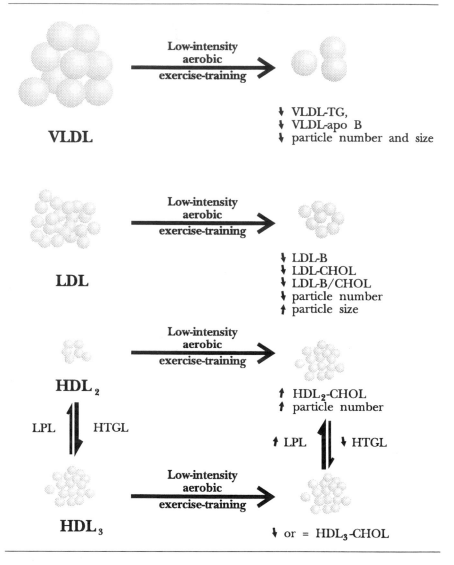

Regarding visceral AT, we reported that moderate-intensity training generating a large increase in energy expenditure can induce a reduction in the level of visceral fat [28]. Further analyses have suggested that the magnitude of visceral AT loss was correlated with improvement in insulin sen-

FIGURE 10.11.

Overview of some of the complex interrelationships found in the metabolic adaptation to endurance exercise training. Adapted from ref. 26.

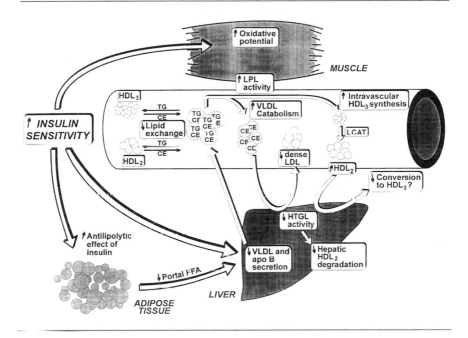

sitivity and in the plasma lipid profile induced by moderate-intensity endurance exercise [28]. Thus, moderate-intensity endurance exercise may be a relevant prescription for the visceral obese patient with insulin resistance and dyslipidemia.

However, it is also important to point out that although we have evidence that the hyperinsulinemic-dyslipidemic state of visceral obesity increases the risk of ischemic heart disease, no prospective study has compared the contribution of improved metabolic fitness vs. that of cardiorespiratory fitness as a correlate of the reduced CHD risk resulting from regular endurance exercise in these high-risk subjects. There is enough evidence available, however, to suggest that improvement in the metabolic condition of dyslipidemic patients may be much more effective than improvement in cardiorespiratory fitness in reducing CHD risk. Therefore, although there is overwhelming evidence that attending the exercise club to perform 25–30 min of endurance exercise, three times/wk, will eventually improve physical fitness, the net increase in energy expenditure associated with such a program is rather trivial and is unlikely to induce substantial weight loss and metabolic improvement [26, 28]. On the other hand, reducing the intensity of exercise and prescribing an almost daily and prolonged exercise regimen (with the simplest form being brisk walking) is more likely to generate a large increase in energy expenditure and, thus, more substantial improvement in insulin sensitivity and in the plasma lipoprotein profile. Therefore, it has been proposed that regular, moderate-intensity daily exercise may be the most efficient and relevant form of exercise that can be followed by the largest number of sedentary dyslipidemic visceral obese patients. In this regard, studies have documented the benefits of regular walking on CHD risk factors [54, 81, 113]. However, it is hoped that a prospective randomized study on endurance exercise in insulin-resistant dyslipidemic patients will be conducted in order to test the hypothesis that exercise can indeed reduce the incidence of NIDDM and CHD.

ACKNOWLEDGMENTS

Results from the author's laboratory presented in this review paper have been obtained with the financial support of the Medical Research Council of Canada, the Canadian Diabetes Association, the Heart and Stroke Foundation of Canada, and the Natural Sciences and Engineering Research Council of Canada.

REFERENCES

1. American College of Sports Medicine. Position stand on the recommended quantity and quality of exercise for developing and maintaining cardiorespiratory and muscular fitness in healthy adults. *Med. Sci. Sports Exerc.* 22:265–274, 1990.
2. Assmann, G., and H. Schulte. Relation of high-density lipoprotein cholesterol and triglycerides to incidence of atherosclerotic coronary artery disease (The PROCAM Experience). *Am. J. Cardiol.* 70:733–737, 1992.
3. Austin, M. A., M. C. King, K. M. Vranizan, and R. M. Krauss. Atherogenic lipoprotein phenotype: a proposed genetic marker for coronary heart disease. *Circulation* 82:495–506, 1990.
4. Austin, M. A. Plasma triglyceride and coronary heart disease. *Arterioscler. Thromb.* 11:1–14, 1991.
5. Barrett-Connor, E. Obesity, atherosclerosis, and coronary artery disease. *Ann. Intern. Med.* 103:1010–1019, 1985.
6. Björntorp, P., K. De Jounge, L. Sjöström, and L. Sullivan. The effect of physical training on insulin production in obesity. *Metabolism* 19:631–638, 1970.
7. Björntorp, P. Abdominal obesity and the development of non-insulin dependent diabetes mellitus. *Diabetes Metab. Rev.* 4:615–622, 1988.
8. Björntorp, P. Hazards in subgroups of human obesity. *Eur. J. Clin. Invest.* 14:239–41, 1984.
9. Björntorp, P. Visceral fat accumulation: the missing link between psychosocial factors and cardiovascular disease? *J. Intern. Med.* 230:195–201, 1991.
10. Björntorp, P: Effects of exercise on plasma insulin. *Int. J. Sports Med.* 2:125–129, 1981.
11. Blair, S. N., H. W. Kohl, III, R. S. Paffenbarger, et al. Physical fitness and all-cause mortality. A prospective study of men and women. *J. Am. Med. Assoc.* 262:2395–2401, 1989.
12. Borkan, G. A., S. G. Gerzof, A. H. Robbins, D. E. Hults, C. K. Silbert, and J. E. Silbert. As-

sessment of abdominal fat content by computed tomography. *Am. J. Clin. Nutr.* 36:172–177, 1982.

13. Bray, G. A. Complications of obesity. *Ann. Intern. Med.* 103:1052–1062,1985.
14. Brindley, D. N., and Y. Rolland. Possible connections between stress, diabetes, obesity, hypertension, and altered metabolism that may result in atherosclerosis. *Clin. Sci.* 77:453–461, 1989.
15. Brindley, D. N. Neuroendocrine regulation and obesity. *Int. J. Obes.* 16:S73–S79, 1992.
16. Burnstein, R., C. Polychronakos, C. J. Toews, et al. Acute reversal of the enhanced insulin action in trained athletes: association with insulin receptor changes. *Diabetes* 34:756–760, 1985.
17. Colberg, S. R., J. A. Simoneau, F. L. Thaete, et al. Skeletal muscle utilization of free fatty acids in women with visceral obesity. *J. Clin. Invest.* 95:1846–1853, 1995.
18. Costill, D. L., W. J. Fink, L. H. Getchell, J. L. Ivy, and F. A. Witzman. Lipid metabolism in skeletal muscles of endurance-trained males and females. *J. Appl. Physiol.* 47:787–791, 1979.
19. Després, J. P., M. F. Verdon, S. Moorjani, et al. Apolipoprotein E polymorphism modifies relation of hyperinsulinemia to hypertriglyceridemia. *Diabetes* 42:1474–1481, 1993.
20. Després, J. P., S. Moorjani, P. J. Lupien, A. Tremblay, A. Nadeau, and C. Bouchard. Genetic aspects of susceptibility to obesity and related dyslipidemias. *Mol. Cell. Biochem.* 113:151–169, 1992.
21. Després, J. P., S. Moorjani, A. Tremblay, et al. Heredity and changes in plasma lipids and lipoproteins afetr short-term exercise training in men. *Arteriosclerosis* 8:402–409, 1988.
22. Després, J. P., A. Tremblay, S. Moorjani, et al. Long-term exercise training with constant energy intake. 3. Effects of plasma lipoprotein levels. *Int. J. Obes.* 14:85–94, 1990.
23. Després, J. P., M. C. Pouliot, S. Moorjani, et al. Loss of abdominal fat and metabolic response to exercise training in obese women. *Am. J. Physiol. (Endocrinol. Metab.)* 261:E159–E167, 1991.
24. Després, J. P., B. Lamarche, P. Mauriège, et al. Hyperinsulinemia as an independent risk factor for ischemic heart disease. *N. Engl. J. Med.* 334:952–957, 1996.
25. Després, J. P., S. Moorjani, P. J. Lupien, A. Tremblay, A. Nadeau, and C. Bouchard. Regional distribution of body fat, plasma lipoproteins, and cardiovascular disease. *Arteriosclerosis* 10:497–511, 1990.
26. Després, J. P., and B. Lamarche. Low-intensity endurance exercise training, plasma lipoproteins and the risk of coranary heart disease. *J. Intern. Med.* 236:7–22, 1994.
27. Després, J. P., and A. Marette. Relation of components of insulin resistance syndrome to coronary disease risk. *Curr. Opin. Lipidol.* 5:274–289, 1994.
28. Després, J. P., and B. Lamarche. Effects of diet and physical activity on adiposity and body fat distribution: implications for the prevention of cardiovascular disease. *Nutr. Res. Rev.* 6:137–159, 1993.
29. Després, J. P., S. Lemieux, B. Lamarche, et al. The insulin resistance-dyslipidemic syndrome: contribution of visceral obesity and therapeutic implications. *Int. J. Obes.* 19:S76–S86, 1995.
30. Després, J. P., A. Nadeau, A. Tremblay, M. Ferland, and P. J. Lupien. Role of deep abdominal fat in the association between regional adipose tissue distribution and glucose tolerance in obese women. *Diabetes* 38:304–309, 1989.
31. Després, J. P., M. Ferland, S. Moorjani, et al. Role of hepatic-triglyceride lipase activity in the association between intra-abdominal fat and plasma HDL-cholesterol in obese women. *Arteriosclerosis* 9:485–492, 1989.
32. Després, J. P. Abdominal obesity as an important component of insulin resistance syndrome. *Nutrition* 9:452–459, 1993.
33. Després, J. P. Assessing obesity: beyond BMI. *NIN Rev.* 7[19]:1–4, 1992.
34. Després, J. P. Dyslipidemia and obesity. *Ballieres Clin. Endocrinol. Metab.* 8:629–660, 1994.
35. Després, J. P., S. Moorjani, M. Ferland, et al. Adipose tissue distribution and plasma

lipoprotein levels in obese women: importance of intra-abdominal fat. *Arteriosclerosis* 9:203–210, 1989.

36. Després, J. P. Lipoprotein metabolism in visceral obesity. *Int. J. Obes.* 15:45–52, 1991.

37. Després, J. P. Obesity and lipid metabolism: relevance of body fat distribution. *Curr. Opin. Lipidol.* 2:5–15, 1991.

38. Després, J. P. Visceral obesity, insulin resistance, and related dyslipoproteinemias. H. Rifkin, J. A. Colwell, and S. I. Taylor (eds.). *Diabetes.* Amsterdam: Elsevier Science Publishers, 1991, pp. 95–99.

39. Després, J. P. Visceral obesity: a component of the insulin resistance-dyslipidemic syndrome. *Can. J. Cardiol.* 10:17B–22B, 1991.

40. Donahue, R. P., R. D. Abbott, E. Bloom, D. M. Reed, and K. Yano. Central obesity and coronary heart disease in men. *Lancet* April:822–824, 1987.

41. Ducimetière, P., J. Richard, and F. Cambien. The pattern of subcutaneous fat distribution in middle-aged men and the risk of coronary heart disease: the Paris Prospective study. *Int. J. Obes.* 10:229–240, 1986.

42. Ekelund, L. G., W. L. Haskell, J. L. Johnson, et al. Physical fitness as a predictor of cardiovascular mortality in asymptomatic North American men: The Lipid Research Clinic Mortality Follow-up Study. *N. Engl. J. Med.* 319:1379–1384, 1988.

43. Eschwège, E., J. L. Richard, N. Thibult, P. Ducimetière, J. M. Warnet, and G. Rosselin. Coronary heart disease mortality in relation with diabetes, blood glucose and plasma insulin levels: the Paris Prospective Study, ten years later. *Horm. Metab. Res.* 15(suppl.):41–46, 1985.

44. Evans, D. J., R. G. Hoffmann, R. K. Kalkhoff, and A. H. Kissebah. Relationship of androgenic activity to body fat topography, fat cell morphology, and metabolic aberrations in premenopausal women. *J. Clin. Endocrinol. Metab.* 57:304–310, 1983.

45. Exercise, fitness, and health. The consensus statement. C. Bouchard, R. J. Shephard, T. Stephens, J. R. Sutton, B. D. McPherson (eds.). *Exercise, Fitness, and Health.* Champaign, IL: Human Kinetics, 1990, pp. 3–28.

46. Ferland, M., J. P. Després, A. Tremblay, et al. Assessment of adipose tissue distribution by computed axial tomography in obese women: association with body density and anthropometric measurements. *Br. J. Nutr.* 61:139–148, 1989.

47. Fontbonne, A., E. Eschwège, F. Cambien, et al. Hypertriglyceridemia as a risk factor of coronary heart disease mortality in subjects with impaired glucose tolerance or diabetes: results from the 11-year follow-up of the Paris Prospective study. *Diabetologia* 32:300–304, 1989.

48. Fontbonne, A. Why can high insulin levels indicate a risk for coronary heart disease? *Diabetologia* 37:953–955, 1994.

49. Fontbonne, E., M. A. Charles, N. Thibult, J. L. Richard, J. M. Claude, J. M. Warnet, G. E. Rosselin, and E. Eschwège. Hyperinsulinemia as a predictor of coronary heart disease mortality in a healthy population: the Paris Prospective Study. 15-year follow-up. *Diabetologia* 34:356–361, 1991.

50. Fujioka, S., Y. Matsuzawa, K. Tokunaga, et al. Improvement of glucose and lipid metabolism associated with selective reduction of intra-abdominal visceral fat in premenopausal women with visceral fat obesity. *Int. J. Obes.* 15:853–859, 1991.

51. Fujioka, S., Y. Matsuzawa, K. Tokunaga, and S. Tarui. Contribution of intra-abdominal fat accumulation to the impairment of glucose and lipid metabolism in human obesity. *Metabolism* 36:54–59, 1987.

52. Fujioka, S., Y. Matsuzawa, K. Tokunaga, Y. Kano, T. Kobatake, and S. Tarui. Treatment of visceral obesity. *Int. J. Obes.* 15:59–65, 1991.

53. Haarbo, J., U. Marslew, A. Gotfredsen, and C. Christiansen. Post-menopausal hormone replacement therapy prevents central distribution of body fat after menopause. *Metabolism* 40:1323–1326, 1991.

54. Hardman, A. E., A. Hudson, P. R. M. Jones, et al. Brisk walking and plasma high-density

lipoprotein cholesterol concentration in previously sedentary women. *Br. Med. J.* 299: 1204–1205, 1989.

55. Haskell, W. L. Exercise-induced changes in plasma lipids and lipoproteins. *Prev. Med.* 13:23–36, 1984.

56. Haskell, W. L. The influence of exercise training on plasma lipids and lipoproteins on health and disease. *Acta Med. Scand.* 711(suppl):25–37, 1986.

57. Jensen, M. D., M. W. Haymond, R. A. Rizza, P. E. Cryer, and P. E. Miles. Influence of body fat distribution on free fatty acids metabolism in obesity. *J. Clin. Invest.* 83:1168–1173, 1989.

58. Katzel, L. I., E. R. Bleecker, E. G. Colman, E. M. Rogues, J. D. Sorkin, and A. P. Goldberg. Effects of weight loss vs aerobic exercise training on risk factors for coronary disease in healthy, obese, middle-aged and older men. A randomized controlled trial. *J. Am. Med. Assoc.* 274:1915–1921, 1995.

59. Kissebah, A. H., and A. N. Peiris. Biology of regional body fat distribution: relationship to non-insulin-dependent diabetes mellitus. *Diabetes Metab. Rev.* 5:83–109, 1989.

60. Kissebah, A. H., N. Vydelingum, R. Murray, D. J. Evans, A. J. Hartz, R. K. Kalkhoff, and P. W. Adams. Relation of body fat distribution to metabolic complications of obesity. *J. Clin. Endocrinol. Metab.* 54:254–260, 1982.

61. Kissebah, A. H., D. S. Freedman, and A. N. Peiris. Health risks of obesity. *Med. Clin. North Am.* 73:111–138, 1989.

62. Kissebah, A. H., D. J. Evans, A. Peiris, and C. R. Wilson. Endocrine characteristics in regional obesities: role of sex steroids. J. Vague, P. Björntorp, B. Guy-Grand, et al. (eds.). *Metabolic Complications of Human Obesities*. Amsterdam: Elsevier Science Publishers, 1985, pp. 115–130.

63. Kokkins, P. F., J. C. Holland, P. Narayan, J. A. Colleran C. O. Dotson, and V. Papademetriou. Miles run per week and high-density lipoprotein cholesterol levels in healthy, middle-aged men. *Arch. Intern. Med.* 155:415–420, 1995.

64. Krauss, R. M. Exercise, lipoproteins and coronary heart disease. *Circulation* 79:1143–1145, 1989.

65. Krotkiewski, M., and P. Björntorp. Muscle tissue in obesity with different distribution of adipose tissue: effects of physical training. *Int. J. Obes.* 10:331–341, 1986.

66. Krotkiewski, M., P. Björntorp, L. Sjöström, and U. Smith. Impact of obesity on metabolism in men and women. Importance of regional adipose tissue distribution. *J. Clin. Invest.* 72:1150–1162, 1983.

67. Krotkiewski, M., K. Mandroukas, L. Sjöström, et al. Effects of long-term physical training on body fat, metabolism and blood pressure in obesity. *Metabolism* 28:650–658, 1979.

68. Kvist, H., B. Chowdhury, U. Grangard, U. Tylén, and L. Sjöström. Total and visceral adipose tissue volumes derived from measurements with computed tomography in adult men and women: predictive equations. *Am. J. Clin. Nutr.* 48:1351–1361, 1988.

69. Lamarche, B., J. P. Després, S. Moorjani, B. Cantin, G. Dagenais, and P. J. Lupien. Prevalence of dyslipidemic phenotypes in ischemic heart disease (prospective results from the Québec Cardiovascular study). *Am. J. Cardiol.* 75:1189–1195, 1995.

70. Lamarche, B., J. P. Després, M.C. Pouliot, et al. Is body fat loss a determinant factor in the improvement of carbohydrate and lipid metabolism following aerobic exercise training in obese women? *Metabolism* 41:1249–1256, 1992.

71. Lamarche, B., S. Moorjani, P. J. Lupien, et al. Apolipoprotein A-I and B levels and the risk of ischemic heart disease during a five-year follow-up of men in the Québec Cardiovascular Study. *Circulation* 94:273–278, 1996.

72. Lapidus, L., C. Bengtsson, B. Larsson, K. Pennert, E. Rybo, and L. Sjöström. Distribution of adipose tissue and risk of cardiovascular disease and death: a 12 year follow-up of participants in the population study of women in Gothenburg, Sweden. *Br. Med. J.* 289: 1261–1263, 1984.

73. Larsson, B., K. Svardsudd, L. Welin, L. Wilhemsen, P. Björntorp, and G. Tibblin. Abdominal adipose tissue distribution, obesity and risk of cardiovascular disease and death: 13

year follow-up of participants in the study of men born in 1913. *Br. Med. J.* 288:1401–1404, 1984.

74. Leenen, R., K. Van der Kooy, P. Deurenberg, et al. Visceral fat accumulation in obese subjects: relation to energy expenditure and response to weight loss. *Am. J. Physiol. (Endocrinol. Metab.)* 263:E913–E919, 1992.

75. Lemieux, S., and J. P. Després. Metabolic complications of visceral obesity: contribution to the actiology of type 2 diabetes and implications for prevention and treatment. *Diabete Metab.* 20:375–393, 1994.

76. Lemieux, S., J. P. Després, S. Moorjani, et al. Are gender differences in cardiovascular disease risk factors explained by the level of visceral adipose tissue? *Diabetologia* 37:757–64, 1994.

77. Lemieux, S., D. Prud'homme, C. Bouchard, A. Tremblay, and J. P. Després. Sex differences in the relation of visceral adipose tissue accumulation to total body fatness. *Am. J. Clin. Nutr.* 58:463–467, 1993.

78. Lemieux, S., D. Prud'homme, A. Nadeau, A. Tremblay, C. Bouchard, and J. P. Després. Seven-year changes in body fat and visceral adipose tissue in women. Associations with indexes of plasma glucose-insulin homeostasis. *Diabetes Care,* 19(9):983–991, 1996.

79. Lemieux, S., D. Prud'homme, C. Bouchard, A. Tremblay, and J. P. Després. A single threshold value of waist girth to identify non-obese and overweight subjects with excess visceral adipose tissue. *Am. J. Clin. Nutr.,* 64:685–693, 1996.

80. Leon, A. S., J. Connet, D. R. Jacobs, Jr., et al. Leisure-time physical activity levels and risk of coronary heart disease and death. The Multiple Risk Factor Intervention Trial. *J. Am. Med. Assoc.* 258:2388–2395, 1987.

81. Leon, A. S., J. Conrad, D. B. Hunninghake, et al. Effects of vigorous walking program on body composition, and carbohydrate and lipid metabolism of obese young men. *Am. J. Clin. Nutr.* 32:1776–1787, 1979.

82. Lie, H., R. Mundal, and J. Ericksson. Coronary risk factors and incidence of coronary death in relation to physical fitness: seven years follow-up study of middle-aged and elderly men. *Eur. Heart J.* 6:147–157, 1985.

83. Manninen, V., L. Tenkanen, P. Koskinen, et al. Joint effects of serum triglyceride and LDL-cholesterol and HDL-cholesterol concentrations on coronary heart disease risk in the Helsinki Heart Study. Implications for treatment. *Circulation* 85:37–45, 1992.

84. Manson, J. E., W. C. Willett, M. J. Stampfer, et al. Body weight and mortality among women. *N. Engl. J. Med.* 333:677–685, 1995.

85. Morris, J. N., M. G. Everitt, R. Pollard, et al. Vigorous exercise in leisure-time: protection against coronary heart disease. *Lancet* 2:1207–1210, 1980.

86. Morris, N., P. W. Chave, C. Adam, et al. Vigorous exercise in leisure-time and the incidence of coronary heart disease. *Lancet* 1:333–339, 1973.

87. National Institute of Health. Consensus development conference on diet and exercise in non insulin-dependent diabetes mellitus. *Diabetes Care* 10:639–644, 1987.

88. Ohlson, L. O., B. Larsson, K. Svärdsudd, L. Welin, H. Eriksson, L. Wilhelmsen, P. Björntorp, and G. Tibblin. The influence of body fat distribution on the incidence of diabetes mellitus—13.5 years of follow-up of the participants in the study of men born in 1913. *Diabetes* 34:1055–1058, 1985.

89. Oshida, Y., K. Yamamouchi, S. Hayamizu, and Y. Sato. Long-term mild jogging increases insulin action despite no influence on body mass index or $\dot{V}O_2$ max. *J. Appl. Physiol.* 66:2206–2210, 1989.

90. Paffenbarger, R. S., A. L. Wing, and R. Hyde. Physical activity as an index for heart attack risk in college alumni. *Am. J. Epidemiol.* 108:161–175, 1978.

91. Paffenbarger, R. S., Jr., and W. E. Hale. Work activity and coronary heart mortality. *N. Engl. J. Med.* 292:545–550, 1976.

92. Peiris, A. N., M. S. Sothmann, M. I. Hennes, et al. Relative contribution of obesity and body fat distribution to alterations in glucose insulin homeostasis: predictive values of selected indices in premenopausal women. *Am. J. Clin. Nutr.* 49:758–764, 1989.

93. Peiris, A. N., R. A. Mueller, M. F. Struve, G. A. Smith, and A. H. Kissebah. Relationship of androgenic activity to splanchnic insulin metabolism and peripheral glucose utilization in premenopausal women. *J. Clin. Endocrinol. Metab.* 64:162–169, 1987.

94. Peters, R. K., L. D. Cady, Jr., D. P. Bischoff, et al. Physical fitness and subsequent myocard infarction in healthy workers. *J. Am. Med. Assoc.* 249:3052–3056, 1983.

95. Pouliot, M. C., J. P. Després, S. Lemieux, et al. Waist circumference and abdominal sagittal diameter: best simple anthropometric indexes of abdominal visceral adipose tissue accumulation and related cardiovascular risk in men and women. *Am. J. Cardiol.* 73:460–468, 1994.

96. Pouliot, M. C., J. P. Després, S. Moorjani, P. J. Lupien, A. Tremblay, and C. Bouchard. Apolipoprotein E polymorphism alters the association between body fatness and plasma lipoprotein in women. *J. Lipid Res.* 31:1023–1029, 1990.

97. Pouliot, M. C., J. P. Després, A. Nadeau, et al. Visceral obesity in men. Associations with glucose tolerance, plasma insulin, and lipoprotein levels. *Diabetes* 41:826–834, 1992.

98. Pouliot, M. C., J. P. Després, F. T. Dionne, et al. Apolipoprotein B-100 gene *Eco*RI polymorphism: relations to the plasma lipoprotein changes associated with abdominal visceral obesity. *Arterioscler. Thromb.* 14:527–533, 1994.

99. Pyörälä, K. Relationship of glucose tolerance and plasma insulin to the incidence of coronary heart disease: results from the two population studies in Finland. *Diabetes Care* 2:131–141, 1979.

100. Reaven, G. M. Role of insulin resistance in human disease. *Diabetes* 37:1595–1607, 1988.

101. Roust, L. R., and M. Jensen. Postprandial free fatty acid kinetics are abnormal in upper body obesity. *Diabetes* 42:1567–1573, 1993.

102. Salonen, J. T., J. S. Slater, J. Tuomilehto, et al. Leisure-time occupational physical activity: risk of death from ischaemic heart disease. *Am. J. Epidemiol.* 127:87–94, 1988.

103. Seals, D. R., and J. M. Hagberg. The effect of exercise training on human hypertension: a review. *Med. Sci. Sports Exerc.* 16:207–215, 1984.

104. Seidell, J. C., P. Björntorp, L. Sjöström, H. Kvist, and R. Sannerstedt. Visceral fat accumulation is positively associated with insulin, glucose and C-peptide levels, but negatively with testosterone levels. *Metabolism* 39:897–901, 1990.

105. Sjöström, L., H. Kvist, A. Cederblad, and U. Tylen. Determination of total adipose tissue and body fat in women by computed tomography, ^{40}K, and tritium. *Am. J. Physiol. (Endocrinol. Metab.)* 250:E736–E745, 1986.

106. Slattery, M. L., and D. R. Jacobs, Jr. Physical fitness and cardiovascular disease mortality: the US railroad Study. *Am. J. Epidemiol.* 127:571–580, 1988.

107. Sparrow, D., G. A. Borkan, S. G. Gerzof, and C. K. Wisniewski. Relationship of body fat distribution to glucose tolerance. Results of computed tomography in male participants of the normative aging study. *Diabetes* 35:411–415, 1986.

108. Tchernof, A., J. P. Després, A. Bélanger, et al. Reduced testosterone and adrenal C$_{19}$ steroid levels in obese men. *Metabolism* 4:513–519, 1994.

109. Tchernof, A., J. P. Després, A. Dupont, et al. Importance of body fatness and adipose tissue distribution in the relation of steroid hormones to glucose tolerance and plasma insulin levels in men. *Diabetes Care* 18:292–299, 1995.

110. Tchernof, A., B. Lamarche, D. Prud'homme, et al. The dense LDL phenotype: association with plasma lipoprotein levels, visceral obesity, and hyperinsulinemia in men. *Diabetes Care* 19[6]:9[6]:629–637, 1996.

111. Technical Review. Exercise and NIDDM. *Diabetes* 14(suppl):52–56, 1991.

112. Tokunaga, K., Y. Matsuzawa, K. Ishikawa, and S. Tarui. A novel technique for the determination of body fat by computed tomography. *Int. J. Obes.* 7:437–445, 1983.

113. Tucker, L. A., and G. M. Freeman. Walking and serum cholesterol in adults. *Am. J. Public Health* 80:1111–1113, 1990.

114. Vague, J. La différenciation sexuelle, facteur déterminant des formes de l'obésité. *Presse Med.* 30:339–340, 1947.

115. Vague, J. The degree of masculine differentiation of obesities: a factor determining predisposition to diabetes, atherosclerosis, gout and uric-calculous disease. *Am. J. Clin. Nutr.* 4:20–34, 1956.

116. Vohl, M. C., B. Lamarche, S. Moorjani, et al. The plasma lipoprotein lipase *Hind*III polymorphism modulates plasma triglyceride levels in visceral obesity. *Arterioscler. Thromb. Vasc. Biol.* 15:714–720, 1995.

117. Vohl, M. C., A. Tchernof, F. T. Dionne, et al. The apoB-100 gene EcoRI polymorphism influences the relationship between features of the insulin resistance syndrome and the hyperapoB and dense LDL phenotype in men. *Diabetes Care* 45:1405–1411, 1996.

118. Welborn, T. A., and K. Wearne. Coronary heart disease incidence and cardiovascular mortality in Busselton with reference to glucose and insulin concentrations. *Diabetes Care* 2:154–160, 1979.

119. Williams, P. T., P. D. Wood, R. M. Krauss, et al. The effect of running mileage and duration on plasma liporotein levels. *J. Am. Med. Assoc.* 247:2674–2679, 1982.

120. Wingard, D. L., E. L. Barrett-Connor, and A. Ferrara. Is insulin really a heart disease risk factor? *Diabetes Care* 18:1299–1304, 1995.

121. Wood, P., and W. Haskell. The effect of exercise on plasma high-density lipoproteins. *Lipids* 14:417–427, 1979.

122. Wood, P. D., P. T. Williams, and W. L. Haskell. Physical activity and high-density lipoproteins. N. E. Miller and G. J. Miller (eds.). *Clinical and Metabolic Aspects of High-Density Lipoproteins.* Amsterdam: Elsevier Science Publishers, 1984, pp. 133–165.

123. Wood, P. D., M. L. Stefanick, D. M. Dreon, et al. Changes in plasma lipids and lipoproteins in overweight men during weight loss through dieting as compared with exercise. *N. Engl. J. Med.* 319:1173–1169, 1988.

124. Wood, P. D., and M. L. Stefanick. Exercise, fitness and atherosclerosis. C. Bouchard, R. J. Shephard, T. Stephens, J. R. Sutton, and B. D. McPherson (eds.). *Exercise, Fitness and Health. A Consensus of Current Knowledge.* Champaign, IL: Human Kinetics, 1988, pp. 409–420.

125. Yarnell, J. W. G., P. M. Sweetnam, V. Marks, J. D. Teale, and C. H. Bolton. Insulin in ischemic heart disease: Are associations explained by triglyceride concentrations? The Caerphilly Prospective Study. *Br. Heart J.* 171:293–296, 1994.

11
The Regulation of Gene Expression in Hypertrophying Skeletal Muscle

JAMES A. CARSON, Ph.D.

Compensatory growth in response to an imposed load is an important, but not well understood, biological adaptation of skeletal muscle. This increase in muscle mass is primarily the result of the enlargement of existing muscle fibers, allowing the muscle greater force-generating capacity (see review, ref. 23). Since humankind's beginning skeletal muscle's ability to undergo overload-induced growth has contributed to our species' proficiency for adapting and thriving in inhospitable environments. However, currently there is not a clear understanding as to how functional overload signals skeletal muscle enlargement.

Humankind's survival and welfare during the next millennium will probably not be dependent on having a large amount of skeletal muscle; however, there are numerous reasons for increasing muscle mass beyond making our clothing fit better. Competitors in all types of athletic events have discovered the benefits individuals involved in occupations having a significant strength component. This is especially true for women in today's society who are pursuing careers in previously male dominated occupations and must possess a basal strength level to be effective (i.e., firefighter, construction, law enforcement, military service). Skeletal muscle mass enlargement also benefits our general population by both preventing and rehabilitating orthopaedic injuries. Physical therapy after an injury often involves muscle strengthening to provide greater integrity to the injured joint [31].

An individual's skeletal muscle mass decreases with advancing age, and this fact directly impacts an older individual's ability to maintain an independent life-style (see reviews, refs. 13 and 52). Thus, aged individuals can also benefit from interventions such as resistance exercise, which function to maintain or improve their muscle mass. The increasing population of elderly individuals in the United States poses many challenges to our healthcare system, including the management of consistently increasing medical costs. Older adults that have maintained or increased their skeletal muscle mass should be able to sustain independent, productive, and fulfilling life-styles. These healthy, active elderly individuals should be less of a financial burden on our society. Resolving the mechanisms involved in signaling overload-induced skeletal muscle hypertrophy will clearly benefit our society as a whole.

FIGURE 11.1.

Potential levels of gene expression control during skeletal muscle hypertrophy.

	Investigated During Overload
Pre-Translational	
Transcriptional Regulation	Yes
RNA Processing	No
RNA Stability	No
Translational	
Translation Initiation	No
Peptide Elongation	No
Post-Translational	
Protein Processing	No
Protein Degradation	Yes

The focus of this literature review is to examine alterations in the molecular biology of functionally overloaded skeletal muscle. Understanding the mechanisms of skeletal muscle hypertrophy at the molecular level will provide insight into the cellular mechanisms inducing enlargement. This research will eventually impact clinically relevant problems, such as the development of more efficient rehabilitative protocols used by individuals recovering from injury and also will provide the basis for resistance training regimes that maximize efficiency and minimize risk of injury in older individuals trying to maintain or gain skeletal muscle mass.

DEFINING MOLECULAR EVENTS DURING HYPERTROPHY

Skeletal muscle proteins have specific half-lives and are constantly subjected to degradation and replacement [19]. A specific protein's quantity in a muscle fiber is attributable to its synthesis and degradation rates (see review, ref. 20). Protein synthesis and degradation are altered in overloaded hypertrophying muscle [17, 19, 34]. The vast majority of molecular biology techniques available today examine factors involved in the capacity of skeletal muscle to synthesize protein; less is understood about protein degradation and the specificity of this process (see reviews, refs. 20 and 30).

The quantity of a specific protein can be altered by pretranslational, translational, and posttranslational regulation (Fig. 11.1). Assembly, folding, packaging, and degradation of a protein can be defined as either translational or posttranslational events and reflect an alteration in the expression of the protein for a given quantity of RNA (RNA activity). Pretranslational events include factors altering the abundance of a specific mRNA. Mechanisms in-

FIGURE 11.2.

Regulation of transcription by DNA-binding proteins.

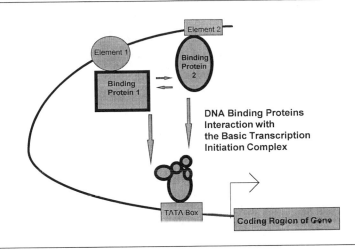

volved in altering mRNA abundance include the synthesis, processing, and stability/degradation of mRNA. mRNA synthesis is controlled by the transcription rate of the gene encoding the mRNA. A gene's transcription rate is affected by *cis*-acting DNA sequences in nontranslated regions of the gene that bind nuclear proteins with a high degree of specificity. This 5' untranslated region containing DNA regulatory sequences is often referred to as the gene's promoter region. DNA binding proteins are often described as transcription factors, and their binding to DNA sequences allows interaction with the basic transcription initiation complex through protein-protein interactions (Fig. 11.2). These interactions serve to either stabilize or destabilize the basic transcription machinery, altering the transcription rate of a gene.

CHANGES IN TOTAL RNA DURING SKELETAL MUSCLE HYPERTROPHY

The passive stretching of skeletal muscle induces hypertrophy of myofibers and myotubes in vitro [50] and in vivo [44]. Total RNA, consisting of rRNA, tRNA, and mRNA, is increased in the hypertrophying chicken anterior latissimus dorsi (ALD) muscle after chronic stretch overload [4, 34, 45] (Fig. 11.3). This increase in RNA content occurs at the onset of hypertrophy and peaks at 10 days of stretch overload [34]. The hypertrophying muscle's increased total RNA in large part represents an increase in 18s and 28s ribo-

FIGURE 11.3.

The chicken anterior latissimus dorsi muscle's time course of molecular adaptation to 1 wk of stretch overload. ↑, *increase;* ———, *no change;* ☆, *not measured.*

	Duration of Stretch Overload		
	1 Day	3 Days	6-7 Days
Protein Synthesis	↑	↑	↑
Protein Degradation	↑	↑	↑
Actin Protein Synthesis	↑	↑	☆
RNA activity	↑	—	—
Total RNA abundance	↑	↑	↑
Total mRNA / total RNA	—	↑	☆
Actin mRNA abundance	☆	—	↑

somal RNAs. The enlarged pool of 18s and 28s rRNAs increases the ribosomal capacity for translation of mRNAs in the hypertrophying muscle.

RNA activity represents the quantity of protein synthesized per day for a given quantity of RNA. RNA activity is increased in the hypertrophying ALD muscle at the onset of overload but returns to control levels as the stretch overload stimulus is continued [34]. These data imply that increases in the translational capacity and/or translational efficiency are responsible for increased protein synthesis at the onset of hypertrophy. Increased RNA abundance does not appear to be a significant factor for increasing protein synthesis until later in the time course of hypertrophy.

There is additional evidence for translational regulation at the onset of hypertrophy in the chronically stretch-overloaded chicken ALD muscle. The mRNA:total RNA ratio in the muscle is not increased at 24 hr of overload, whereas actin protein synthesis is increased [24]. Stretch overloading the muscle for 48 and 72 hr increases the mRNA:total RNA ratio to 2.5 and 3 times greater than control levels [24], and actin protein synthesis remains elevated. The increased mRNA:total RNA ratio demonstrates that after the onset of hypertrophy the mRNA pool is increasing to a greater extent than the ribosomal capacity of the muscle. Actin mRNA levels, corrected for total RNA changes, have been shown not to increase in 3-day overloaded ALD muscle but are increased by day 6 of overload [3]. Although protein synthesis remains elevated during the first week of stretch overload, the molecular events regulating increased protein synthesis are altered during this same period. Increased translational capacity and efficiency are important regulators for increasing protein synthesis at the onset of stretch overload, but an increased mRNA abundance seems to become more important as the overload stimulus is continued.

Chronic stretching also induces hypertrophy in rat and rabbit hindlimb muscle [21, 22]. Protein synthesis rates in the rat EDL muscle are increased after 6 hr of stretch. The initial increase in protein synthesis is most likely the result of translational or posttranslational mechanisms, because RNA activity also increases (23%). Total RNA content in the hypertrophying EDL did increase after 24 hr (15%) and 7 days (22%); however, RNA activity also remained elevated in the stretched muscle at 24 hr (32%) and 7 days (63%) [21]. The increase in RNA activity without the increase in total RNA indicates that increases in translational efficiency, rather than translational capacity, are important for the increased protein synthesis in the hypertrophying muscle.

Stretching of the rabbit EDL muscle causes more dramatic changes than those in the stretched rat EDL muscle. Total protein synthesis (milligrams per day) increased 191% in the rabbit EDL after 3 days of stretch; RNA activity did not significantly increase (27%), even though total RNA increased 128% [22]. The simultaneous application of stretch and chronic low-frequency stimulation to the EDL muscle for 3 days had a more dramatic response than stretch alone [22]. Protein synthesis and total RNA were increased (452 and 300%, respectively); however, RNA activity did not significantly change (45%). These data imply that by the 3rd day of either stretch or stretch/stimulation, increased protein synthesis rates in the rabbit EDL are closely correlated with increased total RNA, which represents an increased translational capacity in the muscle.

Animal models mimicking human resistance exercise have been used to examine molecular changes during overload-induced hypertrophy [56, 57]. These models, unlike passive stretch, involve muscle contraction against a resistance. Isotonic plantar flexion resistance exercise training for 16 wk increased rat gastrocnemius (GAS) and plantaris (PLAN) wet weight (18%) and RNA content (26%) [56]. The increased RNA content in the hypertrophied muscle could be attributed to the increased muscle wet weight, because RNA concentration was unchanged by training. Acute high-frequency, low-resistance exercise training increased myofibril protein synthesis rate in the rat GAS (47%) 17 hr postexercise; however, protein synthesis rates had returned to control levels 41 hr postexercise [57]. The exercised muscle's concentration of total RNA was increased at both 12 and 36 hr postexercise and RNA activity (milligrams of protein synthesized per day per milligrams of RNA) was increased at both 12 and 36 hr postexercise (23 and 45%). Skeletal α-actin mRNA concentration did not change after one resistance training bout, and 10 wk of training only moderately increased (12–14%) α-actin mRNA content. The increased RNA activity, without a change in α-actin mRNA abundance, implies translational or posttranslational mechanisms mediate increased actin protein synthesis in resistance-exercised rat GAS muscle.

MUSCLE PHENOTYPE TRANSITIONS DURING HYPERTROPHY

Hypertrophy induced by synergist ablation causes a fast-to-slow phenotype transition in the rat plantaris (PLAN) muscle and a slow-to-fast phenotype transition in the rat soleus (SOL) muscle (see review, ref. 1). Shifts in the myosin protein profile of the hypertrophying rat SOL and rat PLAN muscles are accompanied by corresponding changes in the abundance of the appropriate mRNA [25]. The overloaded mouse PLAN muscle also increases mRNA levels for slow β-myosin heavy-chain, slow-myosin light-chain 1, and slow-myosin light-chain 2 mRNA levels after 3 wk of compensatory overload [54]. Myosin isoform transitions in overloaded skeletal muscle appear to be regulated, at least partially, by pretranslational mechanisms serving to increase the abundance of specific mRNAs.

Negative gene regulation can also be found in the compensatory overloaded mouse PLAN muscle. Muscle creatine kinase (MCK) mRNA and protein levels are decreased after 2 days (240 and 158%) and remain decreased after 6 wk (150 and 120%) of overload [47]. The rapid decrease in MCK mRNA suggests that pretranslational regulation is involved in this muscle phenotype switch. The changes in MCK gene expression appear complete after 48 hr of overload, even though the fast-to-slow conversion of the PLAN phenotype takes several wk.

These studies demonstrate that pretranslational regulation is important for phenotype shifts in hypertrophying rodent muscle. The increased mRNA abundance during muscle phenotype shifts is likely related to mRNA synthesis and/or stability. Interestingly, myosin type IIa mRNA abundance appears to be regulated via opposite mechanisms during compensatory overload-induced hypertrophy, decreasing in the slow rat soleus while increasing in the fast rat plantaris [24, 26]. The synergist ablation hypertrophy model induces both a growth and a phenotype switch in rodent hindlimb skeletal muscle, which are the result of the combination of the compensatory overload stimulus and the hypertrophying muscle's altered functional role [16]. In this context the underlying stimulus inducing the myosin shifts must be examined carefully, because the altering of a muscle's activity pattern can induce phenotype shifts [25].

Stretch overload-induced hypertrophy of the chicken ALD muscle causes an accelerated developmental shift in the muscle's slow myosin composition, decreasing the proportion of slow myosin-1 (SM1) isoform and increasing the content of slow myosin-2 isoform [25]. Stretch overloading the ALD muscle for 24 hr causes a reduction in the synthesis rate of both SM1 and SM2 isoforms, although the muscle's overall protein synthesis rate and actin synthesis rate are increased in the hypertrophying ALD. Fifty percent of the stretched ALD's SM1 protein is lost by 72 hr of overload; however, muscle mass increased 50% over this same period, suggesting that specific protein degradation occurs at the onset of overload-induced hypertrophy. Unlike regulation of the rat skeletal muscle myosin profile during compensatory overload, the stretch-induced acceleration of myosin isoform shifts in the chicken ALD muscle may be regulated by translational and/or posttranslational mechanisms. However, the specific slow myosin isoform mRNA levels have not been reported.

Stretch overload also induces a reexpression of mRNAs encoding embryonic MHC isoforms in the hypertrophying chicken patagialis (PAT) muscle [15]. Embryonic MHC mRNAs are expressed in the PAT at the highest levels in the embryo and 1 wk posthatching. Two wk of stretch overload-induced expression of one type of embryonic MHC mRNA isoform (p110) to levels found in newly hatched chicks. The abundance of another embryonic MHC (p251) mRNA was not induced. These data demonstrate that during stretch overload-induced hypertrophy there are selective alterations in the expression of developmentally regulated embryonic MHC isoforms. Activated satellite cells are reported to function in overloaded skeletal muscle by contributing to de novo synthesis of muscle fibers, fusion with regenerating muscle fibers, and fusion with growing fibers to maintain the nuclear:cytosolic ratio within the fiber (see review, ref. 43). Activated satellite cells that have fused with existing fibers may progress through a developmental pattern of gene expression before expressing adult isoforms. However, nonsatellite cell-derived myonuclei have been shown to express developmental MHC isoforms during stretch-induced hypertrophy [36]. Further work is needed to understand why some nonsatellite cell-derived myonuclei reexpress embryonic MHC isoforms in hypertrophying fibers.

CHANGES IN SIGNALING PROTEINS DURING HYPERTROPHY

Proto-oncogenes

c-*fos*, c-*myc* and c-*jun* are examples of proto-oncogenes involved in mitosis and cell cycle regulation [28]. These proto-oncogenes are known as immediate early genes and are induced rapidly in a variety of cell types after an assortment of stimuli. Immediate early genes function as the targets of intracellular signaling cascades, and their gene products function as DNA-binding proteins regulating transcription in the cell.

Overload- or β-agonist-induced cardiac muscle hypertrophy induces the mRNA transcripts of some immediate early genes [29, 41]. Overload-induced hypertrophy of rat skeletal muscle increases c-*myc* mRNA levels [53]; however, the time course and the extent of the change in c-*myc* mRNA in hypertrophying muscle is affected by the muscle's fiber type distribution

[53]. An increase in c-*myc* mRNA abundance occurs transiently at the onset of hypertrophy, and by 48 hr of overload the mRNA has returned to control levels. The abundance of c-*fos* mRNA is increased at the onset of cardiac hypertrophy [29, 41]; however, c-*fos* mRNA levels have been shown not to increase during skeletal muscle hypertrophy induced by either tetonomy or clembuterol administration [53]. c-*fos* induction during hypertrophy of the rat skeletal muscle may have been missed, because the muscle was not analyzed until 3 hr postoverload. c-*fos* and c-*jun* mRNA levels are induced in the passively stretched or simultaneously stretched/stimulated rabbit EDL muscle, and this induction of mRNA peaks at 1 hr posttreatment [22]. The rabbit latissimus dorsi muscle also increases c-*fos* and c-*jun* mRNA during passive stretching peaking at 1 hr and, despite the maintenance of the stretch stimulus mRNA, returns to basal levels by 3 hr [11]. The duration, degree, and timing of passive stretch all appear to influence the extent of c-*fos* and c-*jun* mRNA induction in the rabbit latissimus dorsi muscle [11].

There is a possibility that increased proto-oncogene expression at the early onset of overload-induced hypertrophy could signal changes that affect the translational or posttranslational capacity of the muscle. Increased protein synthesis at the onset of hypertrophy appears to be regulated by translational or posttranslational mechanisms [21, 34]. Additionally, during the first 12 hr of chronic low-frequency stimulation, c-*fos* and c-*jun* mRNA abundance is increased in the rabbit EDL without subsequent growth or hypertrophy to the muscle [22]. However, c-*fos* and c-*jun* are mainly expressed in the nuclei of interstitial cells during chronic stimulation, and during stretch these oncoproteins are mainly found in myonuclei [38]. The functional role of proto-oncogene induction during the onset of skeletal muscle hypertrophy has yet to be established.

Insulin-like Growth Factors

Insulin-like growth factors I and II (IGF-I and II) are polypeptide growth factors exerting their biological actions on skeletal muscle through receptor binding on the sarcolemma of the muscle fiber (see reviews, refs. 7 and 9). IGF binding to its receptor activates tyrosine kinase residues in the cytosolic domain of the receptor, initiating signaling cascades within the cytosol of the fiber. These cascades act through protein-protein interactions, altering a target protein's activity via phosphorylation of specific amino acids on the protein. IGF's effect on cells includes the stimulation of cellular growth and differentiation.

IGF's stimulation by growth hormone and its affect on protein synthesis suggest an important function in skeletal muscle growth. Transgenic mice having a high level of human IGF-1 expression in skeletal muscle exhibit myofiber hypertrophy [8]. Cultured chick myotubes in serum-free media undergo hypertrophy in response to exogenous IGF-1 administration [49]. Hypertrophy induced in cultured myotubes by repetitive stretch-relaxation stimulates the autocrine secretion of IGF-1 [39]. Endogenously produced IGFs from skeletal muscle appear to play an important role in regulating subsequent muscle growth.

IGF gene expression is increased in skeletal muscle induced to hypertrophy by mechanical stimuli [10, 12, 22]. Compensatory overloading of either the rat SOL or PLAN muscles for 2 days induces a 3-fold increase in IGF-I mRNA abundance, and this increase remains at 4 and 8 days of overload [12]. The compensatory overloaded SOL and PLAN muscles also increase their abundance of IGF-II mRNA after 2 days, but IGF-II mRNA in the PLAN continued to increase the 2nd and 8th days of overload [12]. Passive stretching the rabbit EDL muscle for 3 days increases IGF-1 mRNA content 12-fold, as determined by quantitative polymerase chain reaction (PCR) assay [22]. The simultaneous imposition of stretch and chronic low-frequency stimulation on the rabbit EDL for 3 days produced hypertrophy to the muscle and a 40-fold induction of IGF-1 mRNA, as determined by quantitative PCR [22]. The stretch-overloaded chicken patagialis muscle does not increase IGF-mRNA abundance per microgram of total RNA after 2 days, but 11 days of stretch-overload produced a 4- to 5-fold increase in IGF-1 mRNA [10]. Removal of the stretch stimulus after 11 days of stretch overload caused a regression in the mass of the hypertrophied patagialis and a subsequent decline in IGF mRNA levels. The correlation between increased IGF-I and II mRNA levels in hypertrophying skeletal muscle suggests the importance of endogenously synthesized IGFs. The endogenously produced IGFs may act in an autocrine fashion and participate in the signaling of mechanical overload-induced muscle growth.

The incidence of increased IGF-I mRNA and, to some extent, IGF-II mRNA in hypertrophying rat muscle do not appear to be dependent on pituitary hormone factors [12]. Overloaded skeletal muscle from hypophysectomized rats still undergoes hypertrophy, and IGF-1 mRNA levels are increased above the control levels [12]. The induction of IGF-II mRNA during hypertrophy of the PLAN muscle is reduced in hypophysectomized rats, compared to that in nonhypophysectomized rats. These data imply that the muscle has an intrinsic capacity to activate IGF gene expression in overloaded skeletal muscle. This intrinsic mechanism could be related to the muscle sensing the imposed mechanical overload which, in turn, activates signaling cascades, serving to alter gene expression in the nucleus.

IGF-I mRNA can be induced in skeletal muscle without the muscle undergoing increased loading. Testosterone administration to nonexercising elderly men increased muscle strength and muscle protein synthesis without changing the peripheral growth hormone IGF-I system [48]. The testosterone administration also increased IGF-1 mRNA abundance in skeletal muscle. Muscle biopsy samples revealed that the men had a 2-fold increase in IGF-I mRNA concentration, and that insulin-like growth factor binding-protein 4 mRNA concentration decreased 50% [48]. Data were not presented about alterations in muscle fiber cross-sectional area. These results demonstrate that IGF gene expression can be activated in skeletal muscle by hormonal administration in the absence of increased external loading. IGF gene expression can be increased in skeletal muscle in the absence of circulating growth hormone. Whether or not testosterone administration and mechanical overload induce IGF gene expression through similar cellular mechanisms remains to be investigated.

GENE REGULATION DURING HYPERTROPHY

Muscle Creatine Kinase

The enzyme muscle creatine kinase (MCK) plays an important role in skeletal muscle energy metabolism. MCK maintains adenosine triphosphate (ATP) levels during intense periods of contraction and is also functionally coupled to glycolysis. MCK enzymatic activity differs in muscles of different fiber types, being 2-fold higher in fast muscle, when compared to slow muscle [58]. Compensatory overload of the rat PLAN muscle induces a fiber-type shift from fast-to-slow properties (see review, ref. 1). There is a corresponding change in MCK mRNA levels during compensatory hypertrophy of the PLAN muscle, which could be the result of decreased MCK gene transcription [47].

Cis-acting DNA regulatory elements responsible for MCK gene regulation during compensatory hypertrophy of mouse plantaris muscle have been investigated [47]. Transgenic mice containing one of three lengths of the MCK 5'-promoter sequence directing the reporter gene chloramphenicol acetyltransferase (CAT) were used to determine the region of the MCK promoter important for regulation during compensatory overload. Six weeks of compensatory overload did not alter CAT activity directed from the −1256 to +7 base pair (bp) MCK promoter, when compared to control activity; however, the −3300 to +7 MCK promoter demonstrated a 400–460% decrease in CAT activity [47]. These data demonstrate that the region of the MCK promoter between −3300 and −1256 bps from the transcription start site appears to contain DNA regulatory sequences critical for repressing the mouse MCK gene during compensatory overload [47].

The length of MCK DNA (−3300 to −1256) responsible for gene repression during compensatory overload does not include a critical enhancer region (−1256 to −1050) that contains many previously described *cis*-acting DNA regulatory elements important for basal MCK expression. It will be interesting to delineate the specific elements or sequences responding to compensatory overload in the −3300 to −1257 region of the MCK promoter.

Once the responding DNA regulatory elements have been identified, the specificity of their response would be interesting to ascertain. This may provide information as to whether the elements are responding to signaling related to the overload stimulus or to the fast-to-slow phenotype transition occurring in the muscle. Fast-to-slow phenotype transitions can occur in rodent muscle without being accompanied by muscle hypertrophy [24]. Studies attempting to identify cis-acting DNA regulatory elements that sense overload signals inducing hypertrophy must be interpreted carefully. Hypertrophy models can produce multiple stimuli, such as signaling pathways activated by alterations in the contractile pattern of the muscle.

β-Myosin Heavy Chain

Gene regulation involved in myosin isoform switching during surgical ablation of synergists has been investigated using transgenic mice [54]. β-MHC is induced in the enlarging fast-type plantaris muscle. After synergist ablation the PLAN undergoes a conversion in its functional, biochemical, and histological properties toward a slow twitch muscle (see review, ref. 1).

Multiple independent lines of transgenic mice were generated for four different lengths of the human β-MHC transgene [54]. Multiple lines of transgenic animals are used in transgenic experiments to control for the influences that different gene integration sites and gene copy numbers have on transgene expression. The four lengths of the human β-MHC promoter used in the study were from +120 to either −141, −450, −988, or −1285 bps from the transcription start site.

Compensatory overload for 7 wk increased CAT expression 3- to 20-fold from the −1285, −988, and −450 lengths of the β-MHC promoter [54]. CAT activity from the −141 β-MHC promoter was not detected in either control or overloaded muscles. These data suggest that activity is increased in the mouse PLAN after 7 wk of compensatory overload. A region of the β-MHC promoter located between −451 and −142 bps appeared necessary for this induction. Further deletions of the β-MHC promoter have demonstrated that the −293 to +120 bps region is sufficient to up regulate the gene during compensatory hypertrophy [55]. More information is needed to determine what DNA regulatory elements between −293 and +120 bps are sufficient for β-MHC induction during compensatory overload. Several highly conserved *cis*-acting DNA regulatory elements are located between −293 and −181 bps of the human β-MHC promoter. Three discrete regions are present from −293 to −142 bps of the human β-MHC promoter, including an MCAT region, a C-rich region, and a βe3 region; however, mutations to these conserved regions did not alter the β-MHC promoter's response to compensatory overload [46]. Regulatory elements found in one or more of these regions could require interaction with other regulatory elements located between −141 and +120 bps of the β-MHC promoter. Combinatorial regulation between regulatory elements in the β-MHC promoter could be mediated by specific protein-protein interactions.

The specific element(s) in the β-MHC promoter from −293 to +120 that are necessary for compensatory overload induction should provide important insights into the signaling of the β-MHC isoform switch during compensatory overload. However, multiple signaling pathways may be activated as the function of the PLAN is altered with surgical ablation of synergists, and distinguishing between signals influencing fast-to-slow isoform transitions and those signaling muscle growth may be difficult.

Skeletal α-Actin

Chicken ALD muscle enlargement occurs rapidly when the muscle is chronically stretch overloaded. Studying gene regulation during hypertrophy induced by the avian stretch overload model has several advantages. An intraanimal control can be employed using the unweighted contralateral wing, and stretch overloading the ALD does not induce a change in the function of the hypertrophying muscle. There are also advantages to studying skeletal α-actin gene regulation. Skeletal muscle hypertrophy does not appear to induce an actin protein isoform shift, as in hypertrophying cardiac muscle; hence, the gene regulatory phenomena is related to growth and not isoform switching. Skeletal α-actin protein is the primary component of the thin filament in skeletal muscle; thus, a muscle undergoing functional enlargement will need to increase the expression of skeletal α-actin protein. These reasons make skeletal α-actin an excellent marker for studying the regulation of skeletal muscle hypertrophy.

Stretch overloading the chicken ALD muscle results in both an increase in the synthesis rate of skeletal α-actin protein [24] and an increase in the quantity of actin mRNA [3, 4]. The regulation of the skeletal α-actin gene during hypertrophy of skeletal muscle has been studied in the living animal by directly injecting plasmid DNA into the ALD muscle [3, 4]. Deletions of the −2090 bp chicken skeletal α-actin promoter were subcloned into plasmids directing luciferase expression, injected into the ALD muscle and the muscle stretch overloaded for six days. Six days of chronic stretch overload increased skeletal α-actin directed luciferase expression in the hypertrophying ALD muscle [4]. Subsequent deletion analysis of the skeletal α-actin promoter established that the first 100 bps of the promoter were sufficient for increasing actin directed luciferase expression, and that −99 to −77 bps were necessary for this response. The −99 to −77 bp region corresponds to the location of serum response element 1 (SRE1). SRE1 is necessary for skeletal α-actin expression in cell culture [6].

Actin promoter constructs containing mutations to the SRE1 element and minimal promoter constructs linked to SRE1 have provided evidence that SRE1 is sufficient and necessary for increased actin-directed luciferase expression during stretch overload-induced hypertrophy [3]. A consensus TEF-1 element linked to a minimal promoter construct also demonstrated that it was sufficient to increase promoter activity (2,000%) during stretch

FIGURE 11.4.
Regulation of the skeletal actin gene during stretch overload-induced hypertrophy.

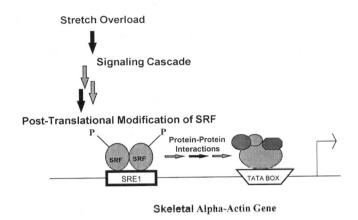

Skeletal Alpha-Actin Gene

overload. The skeletal α-actin promoter contains a TEF-1 site within the first 100 bps of the promoter (−66 to −60 bps). Combinatorial interactions between the TEF-1 site and SRE1 could be involved in conferring stretch overload induction to the skeletal α-actin promoter.

Studies using primary myoblast cultures have demonstrated that SRE1 has strong affinity for 2 *trans*-acting DNA binding proteins: serum response factor (SRF), an activator of actin transcription, and Yin Yang 1 (YY1), a repressor of α-actin transcription [35]. DNA binding proteins interacting with the α-actin promoter from 5-wk old chickens have been analyzed using gel mobility shift assays (GMSAs) on nuclear protein extracts from ALD muscle. GMSAs have demonstrated that SRE1 of the skeletal α-actin promoter binds SRF and YY1 in both control and stretched ALD nuclear protein extracts [3]. However, after nondenaturing gel electrophoresis the SRF-SRE1 complex from hypertrophied ALD muscle demonstrates a slightly faster migration pattern than the SRF-SRE1 complex from control muscle. This faster migrating complex does not appear until the 3rd day of stretch overload and remains present at day 6. Additionally, altered migration of the SRF-SRE1 complex was not apparent in crude protein extracts, consisting mainly of cytosolic protein. SRF protein is found in both the cytosol and nucleus of skeletal muscle. These data imply that stretch overload-induced hypertrophy of the chicken ALD muscle is causing a posttranslational modification in the nuclear population of SRF.

Signaling cascades originating from receptors or channels located on the muscle fibers sarcolemma could be responsible for a posttranslational modification of the nuclear SRF population (Fig. 11.4). There is a possibility that the posttranslational modification of SRF could involve phosphorylation or glycosylation, which would then alter the protein's charge or conformation. Posttranslational modifications, such as a phosphorylation event, could alter SRF's association with other nuclear factors. These enhanced protein-protein interactions with SRF could interact with the transcription initiation complex during hypertrophy. Regulation could also involve a posttranslational modification inducing translocation of cytosolic SRF to the nucleus, where interaction with SRE1 would influence gene transcription. Another possibility is that SRF, which binds SRE1 as a homodimer, could dimerize with different DNA binding proteins to influence gene transcription. The regulation and mechanisms by which DNA binding proteins influence the transcription rate of genes remains a complex event and will take time to be established.

Regulation of nuclear proteins which bind DNA and alter gene transcription could involve several mechanisms, including: phosphorylation, glycosylation, dimerization with other transcription factors, compartmentalization of the protein within the cell, and association with other regulatory proteins. Tremendous insight into the regulation of skeletal muscle hypertrophy can be gained by understanding the regulation of nuclear binding proteins and defining the signaling cascades affecting them; however, this regulation seems to be a very complex event that will not be easily defined.

A MODEL FOR THE REGULATION OF GENE EXPRESSION DURING OVERLOAD INDUCED HYPERTROPHY OF SKELETAL MUSCLE

Overload-induced hypertrophy is a complex event; however, the literature in this area of research supports a model for the regulation of gene expression in overloaded skeletal muscle. This review presents a two-stage model of skeletal muscle adaptation to overload (Fig. 11.5). This model proposes that hypertrophying skeletal muscle is not only sensitive to loading conditions but also is influenced by a muscle fiber's microenviroment. A muscle fiber's microenviroment includes the degree of enlargement that a muscle fiber has undergone. Alterations in cell shape can signal the nucleus to alter gene expression, and integrin receptors may play a prominent role in this pathway (see review, ref. 42).

During the first stage of skeletal muscle hypertrophy, at the onset of overload, RNA activity is increased. The evidence strongly suggests that increased skeletal protein synthesis rates during the onset of hypertrophy are a result mainly of increased RNA activity. Increased protein synthesis at this time point of muscle overload could be attributed to increased translational efficiency and/or increased translational capacity. Increases in the total RNA pool can be regarded as a good indicator of increased translational capacity, because a majority of the RNA pool is ribosomal RNA. Total RNA in-

FIGURE 11.5.

A multistage model for the regulation of gene expression during skeletal muscle hypertrophy.

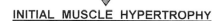

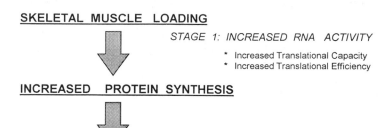

SKELETAL MUSCLE LOADING

STAGE 1: INCREASED RNA ACTIVITY

* Increased Translational Capacity
* Increased Translational Efficiency

INCREASED PROTEIN SYNTHESIS

INITIAL MUSCLE HYPERTROPHY

STAGE 2: INCREASED RNA ABUNDANCE

* Increased Transcriptional Efficiency
  - increased transcription rate per myonuclei
* Increased Transcriptional Capacity
  - satellite cell fusion with muscle fibers
    increasing myonuclei number
* Increased mRNA stability

CONTINUED MUSCLE HYPERTROPHY

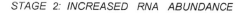

creases at the onset of overload-induced hypertrophy [34], demonstrating that translational capacity is elevated at the onset of hypertrophy.

Currently, the regulation of translation in overloaded skeletal muscle is not well understood. However, the understanding of translational regulation in striated muscle after physiological perturbations is growing rapidly. Increased translational efficiency is thought to be regulated by translational initiation factors whose activity can be modified by their phosphorylation state [18]. Translational initiation factors regulate at the level of peptide chain initiation. The phosphorylation of eIF-4E has been linked to increased protein synthesis in the pressure overloaded canine left ventricle [51]. Decreased skeletal muscle protein synthesis rates during disuse atrophy are related to a decrease in the elongation rate of nascent polypeptide chains [32]. This decreased elongation rate in the atrophying soleus may be related to a decreased association of 70-kd heat-shock cognate/heat shock protein (HSP-70) with the polysome [33]. HSP-70 facilitates translation by stabilizing the translation complex with nascent polypeptide chains. Understanding the molecular signaling involved in increasing translation at the onset of hypertrophy will provide important insights into the overall regulation of skeletal muscle hypertrophy.

The regulation of increased RNA activity during the first stage of hypertrophy seems critical for resistance exercise adaptation in humans. People are more likely to undergo individual bouts of resistance exercise, rather than chronic overload. Wong and Booth [57] have demonstrated that after acute-resistance exercise, the major mediator of increased myofibril protein synthesis in the rat GAS is not RNA abundance but increased RNA activity, implying translational or posttranslational regulation. Increased protein synthesis after a bout of resistance training is driven by translational and posttranslational mechanisms. Protein synthesis then returns to baseline and remains at control levels until stimulated by the next bout of resistance exercise.

mRNA abundance is increased during the second stage of overloaded skeletal muscle adaptation. After an initial lag, mRNA levels for myofibrillar proteins increase in most hypertrophy models. This increase reflects increased transcriptional efficiency, increased transcriptional capacity, and/or increased mRNA stability in the hypertrophying muscle. Increased transciptional efficiency would indicate an increased transcription rate of a given gene per myonuclei. The hypertrophying muscles' transcriptional capacity could be increased by the addition of satellite cell-derived nuclei that fuse with the enlarging fiber. mRNA stability could be affected by specific protein-RNA interactions in the 3′ untranslated region of the RNA. During skeletal muscle hypertrophy several mechanisms could serve, either in concert or in stages, to increase the mRNA template available for translation and protein synthesis.

An increased abundance of myofibril mRNAs per myonuclei becomes critical for maintaining increased protein synthesis rate. There is currently very little information available about the role of RNA processing and stability during hypertrophy of skeletal muscle. A specific mRNA's synthesis rate is controlled by the transcription rate of the given gene. An enlarging fiber would reach a critical size threshold and induce intracellular signaling, which initiates regulation that increases the fiber's transcriptional capacity. Transcriptional capacity would be increased when translational and posttranslational mechanisms can no longer maintain the protein synthesis rates required to sustain fiber enlargement. In addition to translational and posttranslational regulation, hypertrophied muscle would have an increased transcriptional capacity per myonuclei.

The regulation of skeletal muscle hypertrophy also must account for the concept of a myonuclei having a cytosolic domain, or the fiber maintaining a certain nuclei:cytoplasm ratio. A growing muscle fiber adds myonuclei [37] that are thought to be derived from activated satellite cells (see review, ref. 43). Satellite cell nuclei are thought to be recruited into enlarging fibers because a myonuclei's transcriptional machinery can only sustain a finite volume of muscle fiber (see review, ref. 5). Hence, the nuclear domain hypothesis predicts that in order to sustain muscle fiber growth, the enlarging fiber must recruit additional nuclei. Satellite cell activity in the compensatory overloaded mouse EDL muscle is essential for hypertrophy to occur [40]. However, during chronic stretch overload the time course of new fiber formation and increased muscle mass is altered in aged quail, compared to the that in the adult, without any affect of age on satellite cell activation [2]. These data demonstrate the likelihood that the processes of satellite cell replication and satellite cell differentiation/fusion are controlled by different mechanisms, and each is critical to the hypertrophy response.

The signaling that induces satellite cells to become mitotically active and then have the potential to fuse with enlarging fibers is not clearly defined (see review, ref. 43). Increasing myonuclei number in an enlarging fiber expands the transcriptional capacity within the fiber and could possibly reduce the transcription rate per myonuclei. However, increased RNA activity after a bout of resistance exercise continues to be the event that sustains the stimulus that induces muscle fiber growth.

This model for the regulation of gene expression during hypertrophy is drawn from a consensus of literature from muscle adaptation to overload; however, parts of this model still need to be established further. The model does demonstrate that skeletal muscle adaptation to overload is a very complex event. The true understanding of this phenomena will take the combined efforts of researchers studying myofibril assembly, translational regulation, mRNA stability, transcriptional control, satellite cell regulation, and kinase-signaling cascades. A defect in one or several of these areas could possibly contribute to a varied response of the muscle to resistance exercise in different populations, such as elderly individuals. Understanding the molecular events that signal overload-induced skeletal muscle enlargement will impact such clinically relevant problems as maintaining and improving muscle mass in elderly individuals and the rehabilitation of individuals after serious injury.

ACKNOWLEDGMENTS

Dr. Frank W. Booth and David I. Mann are thanked for their critical review of the manuscript. Research funds for this work were provided by the National Institute of Arthritis and Musculoskeletal and Skin Diseases Grants R01-AR-19393 and F32-AR-8328.

REFERENCES

1. Booth, F. W., and K. M. Baldwin. Muscle plasticity: energy demanding and supply processes. L. B. Rowell and J. T. Shepard (eds.). *Handbook of Physiology: Sect. 12; Exercise: Regulation and Integration of Multiple Systems.* New York: Oxford University Press, 1996, pp 1075–1123.

2. Carson, J. A., and S. E. Alway, Stretch overload-induced satellite cell activation in slow tonic muscle from adult and aged Japanese quail. *Am. J. Physiol.* 270:C578–C584, 1996.

3. Carson, J. A., R. J. Schwartz, and F. W. Booth. SRF and TEF-1 control of chicken skeletal α-actin gene during slow-muscle hypertrophy. *Am. J. Physiol.* 270:C1624–C1633, 1996.

4. Carson, J. A., Z. Yan, F. W. Booth, M. E. Coleman, R. J. Schwartz, and C. S. Stump. Regulation of skeletal α-actin promoter in young chickens during hypertrophy caused by stretch overload. *Am J. Physiol.* 268:C918–C924, 1995.

5. Cheek, D. B., A. B. Holt, D. E. Hill, and J. L. Talbert. Skeletal muscle mass and growth: the concept of the deoxyribonucleic acid unit. *Pediatr. Res.* 5:312–328, 1971.

6. Chow, K. L., and R. J. Schwartz. A combination of closely associated positive and negative cis-acting promoter elements regulates transcription of the skeletal α-actin gene. *Mol. Cell Biol.* 10:528–538, 1990.

7. Cohick, W. S., and D. R. Clemmons. The insulin-like growth factors. *Annu. Rev. Physiol.* 55:131–153, 1993.

8. Coleman, M. E., F. DeMayo, K. C. ZYin, H. M. Lee, R. Geske, C. Montgomery, and R. J. Schwartz. Myogenic vector expression of insulin-like growth factor I stimulates muscle cell differentiation and myofiber hypertrophy in transgenic mice. *J. Biol. Chem.* 270(20): 12109–12116, 1995.

9. Czech, M. P. Signal transmission by the insulin-like growth factors. *Cell* 59:235–238, 1989.

10. Czerwinski, S. M., J. M. Martin, and P. J. Bechtel. Modulation of IGF mRNA abundance during stretch-induced skeletal muscle hypertrophy and regression. *J. Appl. Physiol.* 76[5]: 2026–2030, 1994.

11. Dawes, N. J., K. S. Park, V. M. Cox, H. NGA and D. F. Goldspink. The induction of c-fos and c-jun in the stretched rabbit latissimus dorsi muscle: response to duration, degree and re-application of the stretch stimulus. *Exp. Physiol.*, in press, 1996.

12. Devol, D. L., P. Rotwein, J. L. Sadow, J. Novakofski, and P. J. Bechtel. Activation of insulin-like growth factor gene expression during work-induced skeletal muscle growth. *Am. J. Physiol.* 259:E89–E95, 1990.

13. Dipietro, L., and D. R. Seals. Introduction to exercise in older adults. D. R. Lamb, C. V. Gisolfi and E. Nadel (eds.). *Perspectives in Exercise Science and Sports Medicine: Exercise in Older Adults.* Carmel, IN: Cooper Publishing, 1995, vol. 8, pp. 1–10.

14. Essig, D. A., D. L. Devol, P. J. Bechtel, and T. J. Trannel. Expression of embryonic myosin heavy chain mRNA in stretched adult chicken muscle. *Am. J. Physiol.* 260(29):C1325–C1331, 1991.

15. Essig, D. A., S. Kamel-Reid, D. L. DeVol, P. J. Bechtel, R. Zak, and P. K. Umeda. Acceleration of myosin heavy chain isoform transitions during compensatory hypertrophy of developing avian muscles. A. W. Taylor (ed.). *Biochemistry of Exercise VII.* Champaign, IL: Human Kinetics, 1990, vol. 21, pp. 123–131.

16. Fluckey. J. D., T. C. Vary, L. S. Jefferson, and P. A. Farrell. Augmented insulin action on rates of protein synthesis after resistance exercise in rats. *Am. J. Physiol.* 270(33):E313–E319, 1996.

17. Frederickson, R. M., and N. Sonenberg. eIF-4E phosphorylation and the regulation of protein synthesis. J. Ilan (ed.). *Translational Regulation of Gene Expression 2.* New York: Plenum Press, 1993, pp. 143–162.

18. Goldberg, A. L. Protein turnover in skeletal muscle. *J. Biol. Chem.* 244(12):3217–3222, 1969.

19. Goldspink, D. F. Exercise related changes in protein turnover in mammalian striated muscle. *J. Exp. Biol.* 160:127–148, 1991.

20. Goldspink, D. F. The influence of immobilization and stretch on protein turnover of rat skeletal muscle. *J. Physiol.* 264:267–282, 1977.

21. Goldspink, D. F., V. M. Cox, S. K. Smith, L. A. Eaves, N. J. Obaldeston, D. M. Lee, and D. Mantle. Muscle growth in response to mechanical stimuli. *Am. J. Physiol.* 268(31):E288–E297, 1995.

22. Goldspink, G. Cellular and molecular aspects of adaptation in skeletal muscle. P. V. Komi (ed.). *Strength and Power in Sport.* Oxford: England: Blackwell Scientific Publications, 1992, pp. 211–229.

23. Gregory, P, J. Gagnon, D. A. Essig, S. K. Reid, G.Prior, and R. Zak. Differential regulation of actin and myosin isoenzyme synthesis in functionally overloaded skeletal muscle. *Biochem J.* 265:525–532, 1990.

24. Gregory, P, G. Prior, M. Periasamy, J. Gagnon, and R. Zak. Molecular basis of myosin heavy chain isozyme transitions in skeletal muscle hypertrophy. A. W. Taylor (ed.). *Biochemistry of Exercise VII.* Champain, IL: Human Kinetics, 1990, vol. 21, pp. 133–144.

25. Gregory, P., R. B. Low, and W.S. Stirewalt. Fractional synthesis rates in vivo of skeletal-muscle myosin isoenzymes. *Biochem. J.* 245:133–137, 1987.

26. Gregory, P., R. B. Low, and W. S. Stirewalt. Changes in skeletal muscle myosin isoenzymes. *Biochem. J.* 238:55–63, 1986.

27. Hesketh, J. E., and P. A. Whitelaw. The role of cellular oncogenes in myogenesis and muscle cell hypertrophy. *Int. J. Biochem.* 24:193–203, 1992.

28. Izumo, S., B. Nadal-Ginard, and V. Mahdavi. Protooncogene induction and reprogramming of cardiac gene expression produced by pressure overload. *Proc. Natl. Acad. Sci. U. S. A.* 85:339–343, 1988.

29. Jentsch, S., and S. Schlenker. Selective protein degradation: a journey's end within the proteosome. *Cell* 82:881–884, 1995.

30. Kisner, C., and L. A., Colby. *Therapeutic Exercise, Foundations and Techniches,* Philadelphia: F. A. Davis, 1985.

31. Ku, Z., and D. B. Thomason. Soleus muscle nascent polypeptide chain elongation slows protein synthesis rate during non-weight bearing activity. *Am. J. Physiol.* 267:C115–C1126, 1994.

32. Ku, Z., J. Yang, V. Menon, and D. B. Thomason. Decreased polysomal HSP-70 may slow polypeptide elongation during skeletal muscle atrophy. *Am. J. Physiol.* 268:C1369–C1374, 1995.

33. Laurent, G. J., M. P. Sparrow, and D. J. Millward. Turnover of muscle protein in the fowl. Changes in rates of protein synthesis and breakdown during hypertrophy of the anterior and posterior latissimus dori muscle. *Biochem. J.* 176:407–417, 1978.

34. Lee, T. C., K.-L. Chow, P. Fang, and R. J. Schwartz. Activation of skeletal α-actin gene transcription: the cooperative formation of serum response factor-binding complexes over positive cis-acting promoter serum response elements displaces a negative-acting nuclear factor enriched in replicating myoblasts and nonmyogenic cells. *Mol. Cell. Biol.* 11:5090–5100, 1991.

35. McCormick, K. M., and E. Schultz. Role of satellite cells in altering myosin expression during avian skeletal muscle hypertrophy. *Dev. Dyn.* 199:52–63, 1994.

36. Moss, F. P., and C. P. Leblond. Satellite cells as the source of nuclei in muscles of growing rats. *Anat. Rec.* 170:421–436, 1971.

37. Osbaldeston, N. J., D. M. Lee, V. M. Cox, J. E. Hesketh, J. E. Morrison, G. E. Blair, and D F. Goldspink. The temporal and cellular expression of c-fos and c-jun in mechanically stimulated muscle. *Biochem. J.* 308:465–471, 1995.

38. Perrone, C. E., D. Fenwick-Smith, and H. H. Vandenburgh. Collagen and stretch modulate autocrine secretion of insulin-like growth factor-I and insulin-like growth factor binding proteins from differentiated skeletal muscle cells. *J. Biol. Chem.* 270(5):2099–2106, 1995.

39. Rosenblatt, J. D., and D. J. Parry. Gamma irradiation prevents compensatory hypertrophy of overloaded mouse extensor digitorum longus muscle. *J. Appl. Physiol.* 73:2538–2543, 1992.

40. Sadoshima, J., and S. Izumo. Mechanical stretch rapidly activates multiple signal transduction pathways in cardiac myocytes: potential involvement of an autocrine/paricrine mechanism. *EMBO J.* 12(4):1681–1692, 1993.

41. Schwartz, M. A, and D. E. Ingber. Integrating with integrins. *Mol. Biol. Cell* 5(4):389–393, 1994.
42. Shultz, E., and K. M. McCormick. Skeletal muscle satellite cells. *Rev. Physiol. Biochem. Pharmacol.* 123:213–257, 1994.
43. Sola, O. M., D. L. Christensen, and A. W. Martin. Hypertrophy and hyperplasia of adult chicken anterior latissimus dorsi muscles following stretch with and without denervation. *Exp. Neurol.* 41:76–100, 1973.
44. Sparrow, M. P. Regression of skeletal muscle of chicken wing after stretch-induced hypertrophy. *Am. J. Physiol.* 242:C333–C338, 1982.
45. Tsika, G. L., J. L. Wiedenman, L. Gao, J. J. McCarthy, K. Sheriff-Carter, I. D. Rivera-Rivera, and R. W. Tsika. Induction of β-MHC transgene in overloaded skeletal muscle is not eliminated by mutation of conserved elements. *Am. J. Physiol.* 271:C690–C699, 1996.
46. Tsika, R. W., S. D. Hauschka, and L. Gao. M-creatine kinase gene expression in mechanically overloaded skeletal muscle of transgenic mice. *Am. J. Physiol.* 269:C665–C674, 1995.
47. Urban, R. J., Y. H. Bodenburg, C. Gilkison, J. Foxworthy, A. R. Cogan, R. R. Wolfe, and A. Fernando. Testosterone administration to elderly men increases skeletal muscle strength and protein synthesis. *Am. J. Physiol.* 269:E820–E826, 1995.
48. Vandenburgh, H. H., P. Karlisch, J. Shansky, and R. Feldstein. Insulin and IGF-I induce pronounced hypertrophy of skeletal myofibers in tissue culture. *Am. J. Physiol.* 260:C475–C484, 1991.
49. Vandenburgh, H. H., and S. Kaufman. An in vitro model for stretch-induced hypertrophy of skeletal muscle. *Science* 203:265–268, 1979.
50. Wada, H., C. T. Ivester, B. A. Carabello, G. Cooper, and P. J. McDermott. Translational initiation factor eIF-4e, a link between cardiac load and protein synthesis. *J. Biol. Chem.* 271(14):8359–8364, 1996.
51. White, T. P. Skeletal muscle structure and function in older mammals. D. R. Lamb, C. V. Gisolfi, and E. Nadel (eds.). *Perspectives in Exercise Science and Sports Medicine: Exercise in Older Adults.* Carmel, IN: Cooper Publishing, 1995, vol. 8, pp. 115–174.
52. Whitelaw, P. F., and J. E. Hesketh. Expression of c-myc and c-fos in rat skeletal muscle. *Biochem J.* 281:143–147, 1992.
53. Wiedenman, J. L., I. Rivera-Rivera, D. Vyas, G. Tsika, L. Gao, K. Sheriff-Carter, X. Wang, L. Kwan, and R. Tsika. β-MHC and SMLC1 transgene induction in overloaded skeletal muscle of transgenic mice. *Am. J. Physiol.* 270:C1111–C1121, 1996.
54. Wiedenmen, J. L., G. L. Tsika, L. Gao, J. J. McCarthy, I. D. Rivera-Rivera, Vyas, K. Sheriff-Carter, and R. W. Tsika. Muscle-specific and inducible expression of 293-base pair β-myosin heavy chain promoter in transgenic mice. *Am. J. Physiol.* 271:R688–R695, 1996.
55. Wong, T. S., and F. W. Booth. Skeletal muscle enlargement with weight-lifting exercise by rats. *J. Appl. Physiol.* 65(2):950–954, 1988.
56. Wong, T. S., and F. W. Booth. Protein metabolism in rat gastrocnemius muscle after stimulated chronic concentric exercise. *J. Appl. Physiol.* 69(4):1709–1717, 1990.
57. Yamashita, K., and T. Yoshioka. Profiles of creatine kinase isoenzyme compositions in single muscle fibers of different types. *J. Muscle Res. Cell Motil.* 12:37–44, 1991.

12
Force Transmission in Skeletal Muscle: from Actomyosin to External Tendons

TINA J. PATEL, M.S., RICHARD L. LIEBER, Ph.D.

One of the primary functions of skeletal muscle is to generate force and produce movement. Physiological and biomechanical experiments have demonstrated conclusively that actin-myosin interaction is responsible for force generation (Fig. 12.1A), but there is growing evidence that force transmission from this point outward is more complicated than previously thought. For example, force transmission from the myosin filaments to the Z-disk is mediated both by the actin filament and by the titin molecule (Fig. 12.1A). Similarly, although sarcomere force transmission in series is well-accepted, evidence exists for lateral force transmission to adjacent sarcomeres via the intermediate filament system (Fig. 12.1B). These proteins interconnect adjacent myofibrils and then form connections with the cell surface membrane via specialized focal adhesion sites known as "costameres" (Fig. 12.1C) along the fiber length and at the muscle-tendon junction (Fig. 12.1D). Finally, muscle fibers themselves have a complex mode of force transmission to the extracellular matrix via lateral connections to the endomysial connective tissue (Fig. 12.1E) or even via muscle fiber-muscle fiber connections in series. Suffice it to say that the actual path of force transmission from contractile proteins to the "outside world" is not completely understood. An understanding of the force transmission paths is tantamount to developing adequate models of structure-function relationships in skeletal muscle. It also permits more sophisticated interpretation of the functional effects of the injury and repair processes that accompany exercise training.

In this review, we summarize current studies describing the structural arrangement of the proteins within a muscle cell that are involved in such diverse functions as force transmission, force transduction and, perhaps, cellular signaling. Based on this description, we review the significance of this arrangement in muscle contraction. Finally, putative physiological roles for many of these proteins are presented.

INTRACELLULAR FORCE TRANSMISSIONS

While most skeletal muscle micrographs demonstrate the dominant striation pattern that results primarily from actin and myosin, numerous other

FIGURE 12.1.
Schematic representation of potential paths of force generation and transmission in skeletal muscle. In all parts of the figure, arrows with asterisks represent current research areas, whereas solid arrows represent accepted paths of muscle force transmission. (A) Force generation occurs between actin and myosin filaments and is also transmitted to the Z-disk by titin molecules. (B) Force is transmitted serially between sarcomeres but also laterally by the intermediate filament system. (C) Force is transmitted laterally between myofibrils by intermediate filaments and to the surface membrane by costameres and the dystrophin complex. (D) Force is transmitted laterally between myofibrils by intermediate filaments and to the muscle-tendon junction by further specialized adhesion connections. (E) Force is transmitted laterally between fibers to the connective tissue matrix, which is ultimately transmitted to the external muscle tendon.

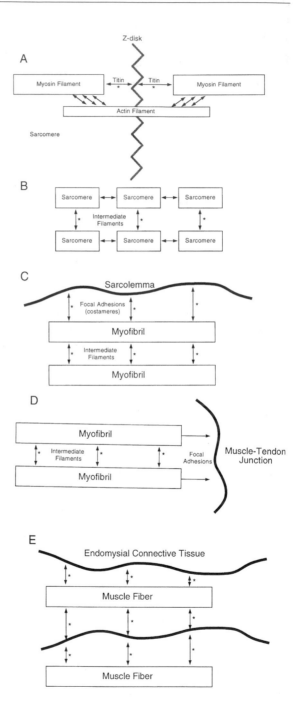

proteins are present within the cell. Specifically, cytoskeletal proteins maintain the structural integrity of the myofibrillar lattice, transmit force generated by actomyosin interaction, and are ubiquitous throughout the muscle cell (Table 12.1). Recent studies demonstrated that the intracellular cytoskeleton is an important cellular component in muscle cells, as has been already demonstrated in many other cell types. We divide the discussion of these structures based on whether they are located within the myofibrillar lattice itself (titin and nebulin) or form a network around the myofibrils and connect to the sarcolemma (intermediate filaments, dystrophin, and focal adhesions).

The Intrasarcomeric Cytoskeleton

The most widely studied of the cytoskeletal proteins are those found in the intrasarcomeric region. Studies of these two proteins, titin (also called connectin) and nebulin, have revolutionized our understanding of muscle passive tension and sarcomere filament assembly. Both proteins appear to have a role in providing a scaffold for assembly of contractile filaments, and recent studies provide insight into their function in passive (titin) and active (nebulin) force generation.

TITIN (CONNECTIN). *Experimental Demonstration of the Role of Titin.* Early evidence for a significant load-bearing structure in skeletal muscle, distinct from the actin and myosin contractile filaments, was provided from measurements of passive tension. Because muscle activation was not required for passive tension, many investigators had assumed that passive tension was a manifestation of noncontractile material, such as the connective tissue matrix or the muscle membrane itself [3, 84]. Recent studies have clearly revealed that this is not the case. In one of the first studies to measure the source of passive tension explicitly, Magid and Law [62] measured the stiffness of intact single muscle fibers, using very slow passive stretches, and compared that to the stiffness measured from chemically skinned single muscle fibers (in which the membrane was permeabilized using a mild detergent). Because they found that the stiffness measured in the two preparations (with and without an intact membrane) was nearly the same [62], this provided evidence that the load bearing capability of the sarcolemma was minimal (Fig. 12.2). Magid and Law then extended this experiment by measuring the stiffness of bundles of muscle fibers, using similar methodology, and compared that to the stiffness of the intact or skinned single fiber. With the bundles intact, and thus with a significant network of endomysial, perimysial and, perhaps, even epimysial connective tissue present, they again demonstrated that stiffness was nearly identical when compared with that of the intact or skinned single fiber. These data provided some of the first mechanical evidence that the structure responsible for bearing muscle passive tension resided within the fiber itself and was not significantly affected by extracellular matrix material or muscle membranes.

TABLE 12.1.
Skeletal Sarcomere Muscle Proteins

Protein		Size Description (MW, L, φ)*	Localization	Putative Function	Selected Refs.
Endosarcomeric Contractile	Actin	40 kd, 7 nm, 7nm	I-Band	Contractile protein; interacts with myosin	[121]
	Myosin	480 kd, 150 nm, 12 nm	A-Band	Contractile protein; generates force by interaction with actin	[121]
	C-protein	140–150 kd, 50 nm	A-Band	Binds to rod region of myosin and actin, may alter myosin cross-bridge movement	[42, 68]
Myosin -associated	Creatine kinase	42 kd × 2	M-Band region	Helps regulate ATP concentration	[107, 108]
	F protein	121 kd	A-Band	Not known	[67]
	H protein	74 kd	near M-line	Not known	[67]
	I protein	50 kd	Edge of A-band	Inhibits ATPase activity	[70]
	M protein	165 kd, 36 nm, 4 nm	M-Band	Links thick filaments to titin	[38, 64]
	Myomesin	185 kd, 36 nm, 4 nm	M-Band	Links thick filaments to titin	[38, 64]
	Titin	3 md, 1μm, 4 nm	A & I-Bands, Z-disc	Supports passive tension and myosin alignment	[54, 112]
Actin -associated	α-Actinin	95 kd × 2, 40 nm	Z-disc	Anchors actin to Z-disk	[4, 7]
	β-actinin	32 + 35 kd	Free end of actin	Caps free end of actin	[28]
	γ-Actinin	35 kd		Inhibits actin polymerization	[51]
	Nebulin	800 kd	Actin filament	Regulates actin length	[15, 50, 53]
	Paratropomyosin	34 kd ×2	A-I Band junction	Inhibits actomyosin interaction	[93]
	Tropomodulin	40.6 kd	Free end of actin	Interacts with tropomyosin to weaken actomyosin connections	[24, 25]
Z-line -associated	eu-actinin	42 kd	Z-Disc	Supports lattice structure	[52]
	Paranemin	280 kd	Z-Disc	Cross-links intermediate filaments	[10, 80]
	Plectin	4 × 446 kd, 190 nm	Z-Disc	Cross-links intermediate filaments	[22, 117, 119]
	Synemin	230 kd	Z-Disc	Cross-links intermediate filaments	[37, 80]
	Z-protein	50 kd	Z-Disc	Forms lattice structure	[69]
	z-nin	400 kd	Z-Disc	Forms lattice structure	[69]
Calcium regulatory	Tropomyosin	64 kd, 40 nm	Actin-associated	Regulates actomyosin binding	[18, 30]
	Troponin	78 kd	Actin associated	Regulates actomyosin binding	[17]

		MW, L, φ*	Location	Function	References
Exosarcomeric Intermediate filaments	Desmin	53 kd × 2, 45 nm, 10 nm	Z-disc	Longitudinal and lateral Z-disk connector	[10, 94]
	Skelemin	200 + 200 kd	M-band	Maintains M-line integrity	[81, 82]
	Vimentin	53 kd, ≤5 nm, 10 nm	Z-disc	Maintains Z-disc periodicity during development	[10]
Cytoskeletal anchor proteins	α-Actinin	95 kd × 2, 40 nm	Z-disc/actin	Anchors actin to Z-disc	[4, 7]
	Ankyrin	202–206 kd	Costamere	Assembles and/or maintains cell surface Proteins in membrane domains	[6]
	Desmin	53 kd × 2, 45 nm, 10 nm	Z-disc	Longitudinal and lateral Z-disc Connector; links to actin filaments	[10, 94]
	Dystrophin	427 kd, 150 nm	Costamere	Binds actin to ECM via DAP complex	[13, 49, 71, 77]
	Integrins		Sarcolemma	Anchors cytoskeletal proteins and ECM	[87]
	Myonexin	30 kd	MT junction	Not known	[96]
	Paxillin	58 kd	Focal adhesion site	Interacts with vinculin to link actin Filaments to sarcolemma	[95, 104]
	Syntrophin	58 kd	Costamere	Links dystrophin to DAP	[1]
	Talin	225–325 kd, 60 nm	Costamere	Anchors thin filaments and vinculin to costamere	[95, 98]
	Vinculin	130 kd, 27 nm	Costamere	Anchors actin and talin to costamere	[31, 32]

*(MW, L, φ), molecular weight, length, diameter; ECM, extracellular matrix; DAP, dystrophin-associated proteins; MT, muscle tendon.

FIGURE 12.2.

(A) Relationship between sarcomere length and passive stress in four different frog muscles at rest. These relationships are nonlinear and are described by the relationship

$$\sigma = \frac{E_o}{\alpha}(e^{\alpha \epsilon_s} - 1),$$ *where σ represents fiber passive stress, α is an empirical constant,*

E_o is initial elastic modulus, and ϵ_s is sarcomere strain. (B) Values for σ and E_o are obtained by plotting natural log of stress vs. strain and interact to produce a value for muscle "stiffness" that varies with sarcomere strain. These values are compared between whole muscles, intact muscle fibers, and skinned single fibers and are shown to be about the same. [Data are taken from ref. 62].

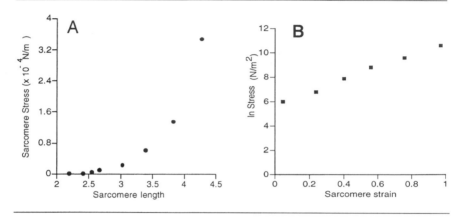

Demonstration of Titin Size. The approximate size of the proteins responsible for passive load bearing was estimated in a study that related the force-generating and force-bearing properties of skinned muscle fiber bundles to their protein composition [43, 44]. These authors used a biophysical method known as target analysis to relate the radiation dose imposed on the muscle to its biological function and protein composition. The method is based on the fact that, the larger the structure, the greater the probability it will be destroyed by radiation. Thus, radiation inactivation was used to impose a specific dose of ionizing radiation onto frozen muscle, and then the resultant structural and functional losses were measured. As an example, force generation induced by bathing the muscle in an exogenous calcium-adenosine triphosphate (ATP) solution was first measured in a small bundle of intact muscle fibers before and after freezing (Fig. 12.3A). Then, passive tension was measured at three different sarcomere lengths. These passive and active data were compared to those of a bundle that was frozen, irradiated at a dose of 0.5 Mrad, thawed, and active and passive force were again measured across a range of sarcomere lengths (Fig. 12.3B). Finally, the quantity of titin and nebulin were estimated from sodium dodecyl sulfate (SDS)-polyacrylamide gels of homogenates from the same mus-

FIGURE 12.3.

Active and passive tension measured from rabbit psoas skeletal muscle fibers stretched across a range of sarcomere lengths. (a) Records from intact muscle. (b) Records from a muscle subjected to freezing, irradiation at 0.5 Mrad, and thawing. Note that both active and passive force generation are compromised after irradiation. Target analysis (see Fig. 12.4) revealed that the structure(s) responsible for the functional loss were in the 3.2- to 3.4-Md range, consistent with titin as the structural basis for the functional loss. Data are taken from ref. 43 and 44.

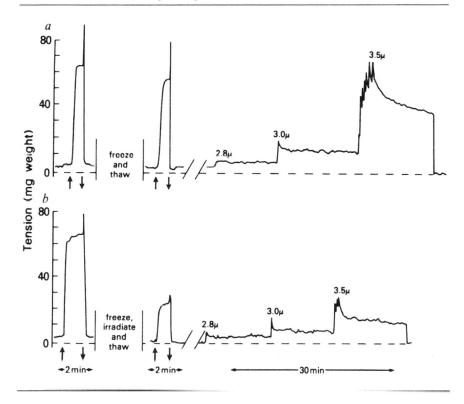

cle fiber bundles. Interestingly, the relationships between active or passive tension and radiation dose was identical (Fig. 12.4). This provided evidence that the size of the structure responsible for the functional loss in both active and passive force generation was similar. The target size of this structure was calculated to be 3.2–3.4 Md (Fig. 12.4). Given this large size, the most likely candidate protein that could fulfill this role was titin. When target size was calculated from the gel electrophoresis pattern of titin, it was shown to be 5–7 Md or two to three times that of the actual estimated molecular weight of titin. This calculation provided indirect evidence that the individual titin peptides might be linked together (for example, by disul-

FIGURE 12.4.

Relationship between irradiation dose and loss of active (filled squares) and passive (filled triangles) tension in rabbit skeletal muscle. Target analysis of these data revealed that the structure responsible for this loss was 3.2- to 3.4 -Md in size. Data are taken from ref. 43.

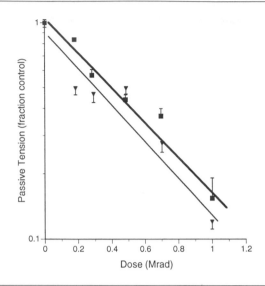

phide bonds) in a way that allowed the transfer of radiation energy between individual peptides (thus destroying the structure much more readily as a dimer than would be accomplished with isolated titin molecules).

Ultrastructural images revealed that myofibrillar alterations accompanied the cytoskeletal protein loss (Fig. 12.5). The classic signs of disruption—streaming of the Z-disk, loss of A-band register, and displacement of the A-band to extreme sides of the sarcomere—were observed in muscles subjected to irradiation. These micrographs are reminiscent of those obtained from muscle specimens subjected to intense eccentric exercise [27].

Taken together, the structural and mechanical data suggested a model in which the thick filaments are linked to the nearest Z-disks by elastic filaments made of titin (Fig. 12.6). Breakage of the elastic filaments by irradiation, for example, and possibly also by exercise, leads to thick filament misalignment on stretch or activation and a resulting loss in passive and active force generation capability.

Mechanical Properties of Titin. Quantification of the mechanical properties of the titin endosarcomeric cytoskeletal protein (and intermediate filament proteins) was reported by Wang and colleagues [112]. They mechanically

FIGURE 12.5.

Longitudinal electron micrograph of rabbit psoas muscle (a) at rest after irradiation and (b) 2 min after irradiation and activation. The loss of myofibrillar regularity, disruption of the Z-disk, and shifting of the A-bands after titin loss provide evidence for its role in stabilizing the contractile machinery of skeletal muscle. Reproduced from reference 44.

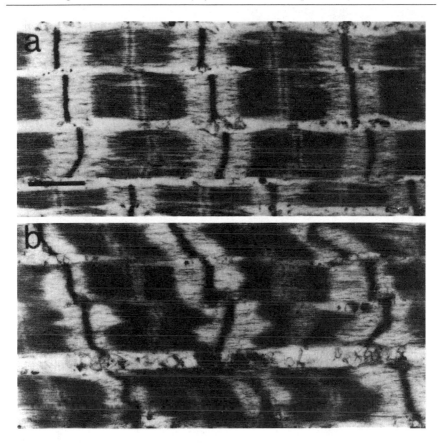

peeled back the surface membrane of a muscle fiber, leaving only the myofibrillar lattice intact. They then measured the relationship between sarcomere length and tension in the intact fiber, and they obtained a biphasic response in which the muscle was initially relatively compliant (at a sarcomere length designated SL_o), then stiffness increased until a yield point (at a sarcomere length designated SL_y) until, at very long lengths, it became much less stiff again (Fig. 12.7A). To determine the structural basis of this phenomenon, they labeled the titin molecule in various regions

FIGURE 12.6.

Schematic representation of the role of titin in maintaining positional stability of the thick filament. Titin provides a mechanical route of force transmission between the thick filament M-line and the adjacent Z-disk. Modified from ref. 26. Ninety percent of titin consists of 244 repeating copies of the FN3 and Ig domains. A special I-band region containing primarily the amino acids protein, glutamate, valine, and lysine (PEVK) appears to be the primary elastic region of the molecule. Drawn based on results in ref. 54.

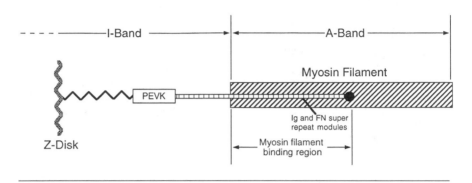

with two different monoclonal antibodies—one that labeled the portion of titin molecule located in the I-band and a second antibody that labeled titin in the A-band. By measuring the distance between either the A-band and M-line or I-band and Z-line, the authors measured the titin molecule strain in the A-band and I-band regions. They found that titin in the I-band region was strained to a much greater extent than titin in the A-band region (except at very long lengths). This suggested a mechanical model of titin as a two-part molecular spring with stiff A-band region in series with a more compliant I-band region. It was not clear whether the high stiffness in the A-band was a result of titin's intrinsic properties or whether it was a result of its association with the myosin filament. By selectively extracting thick filaments from the titin endosarcomeric lattice and again measuring titin strain in the region *that used to* contain the A-band, they found that the titin molecule had a relatively constant compliance along its entire 1μm-length, but that it was the *association* between titin and myosin that gave it the increased stiffness in the A-band (Fig. 12.7C). The explanation for the mechanical experiments that yielded a biphasic response was that, at very long lengths, a portion of the titin molecule "popped off" the thick filament. Furthermore, these authors extracted the complete myofibrillar apparatus, leaving only intermediate filament proteins (see below), and they demonstrated that intermediate filaments sustained significant loads only at very long sarcomere lengths (Fig. 12.7B). In the rabbit psoas muscle, these sarcomere lengths were 4.5 μm or greater, which is beyond actin-myosin filament overlap. Thus, it appears that, in normal rabbit psoas muscle, passive tension is sustained primarily by the titin molecule throughout the normal sarcomere length range but, at longer lengths, the titin molecule is further "recruited" by pulling off of the myosin filament. At extremely long lengths, the intermediate filament network may come into play as a structure that also sustains tension.

Cloning of the Titin Molecule. Fascinating insights into titin structure-function relationships were recently provided based on examination of the amino acid pattern predicted by the DNA sequence in the cloned titin molecule [54]. The primary structure was determined in the usual way—making complementary DNA (cDNA) copies of the messenger RNA encoding the synthesis of titin using reverse transcription. The cDNA was amplified, using the polymerase chain reaction (PCR), and was cloned for subsequent study. Because the titin molecule is so large, sequencing the entire molecule was accomplished by piecing together information from about 50 overlapping clones. The results were astounding! Titin, the largest protein known, is composed of a single chain of more than 27,000 amino acids with a molecular weight of about 3 million. This is at least 10 times the molecular weight of the average protein. Translation of a single titin molecule requires about 45 min, compared to 5 min for the average protein.

Titin Protein Motifs. Given titin's amino acid sequence, the various protein motifs within the molecule could be determined. Interestingly, about 90% of the titin protein consists of 244 repeating copies of the fibronectin type III (FN3) and immunoglobulin (Ig) domains (Fig. 12.6). This huge protein spans half of the sarcomere from the middle of the A-band (M-band) to the Z-band. Within this protein, several distinct zones were noticed. A super repeat pattern of Ig and FN3 motifs was repeated 11 times within the A-band region, which correlates exactly with the accessory proteins known to be arranged in 11 stripes across the myosin-containing A-band. In addition, a region within the I-band was defined containing primarily (70%) the amino acids proline (P), glutamate (E), valine (V), and lysine (K), which appeared to be the compliant region of the molecule and, thus, can be designated the PEVK region. To add further support to this idea, titins were compared between cardiac and skeletal muscle, and it was determined that PEVK region in cardiac muscle (which is known to be much stiffer than skeletal muscle) was only 163 amino acids long, whereas the PEVK region in the soleus muscle, which is about 10 times more compliant than that in cardiac muscle, was more than 2000 amino acids long. This finding may also provide a structural basis for the known difference in elasticity between different skeletal muscles. Whether all skeletal muscles are the same or whether systematic differences in passive elasticity between skeletal muscles can also be explained by differences in the PEVK region remains to be determined.

FIGURE 12.7.

Mechanical measurement of passive muscle fiber tension as a function of sarcomere length. (A) Passive tension, at an initial sarcomere length designated SL_o, is low but increases until the yield point at a sarcomere length designated SL_y. Squares, total passive tension; circles, passive tension of muscle, where all but intermediate filaments were extracted; triangles, passive tension of intact muscle with intermediate filament contribution subtracted. (B) Passive tension of only the intermediate filament lattice yields significant passive tension only at long sarcomere lengths. Ultrastructural analysis of titin

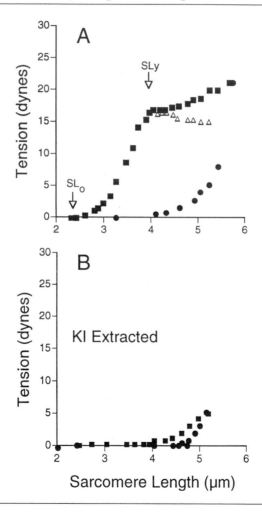

An alternative explanation of the biphasic mechanical response of titin to stretch was provided by Labeit and Kolmerer, based on this structural analysis [54]. They hypothesized that the initial, high-compliance portion of the stress-strain graph resulted from the unfolding of Ig domains in the *strain in the A-band and I-band regions suggests that it acts as a bimolecular spring. Throughout most of the normal sarcomere length range (lengths shorter than SL_y), titin strains primarily in the I-band region, whereas at long lengths, portions of the titin molecule are "recruited" off of the thick filament. (C) Proposed correlation of tension-segment strain curves to structural behavior, of the sarcomere matrix. Squares, passive tension of extracted muscle during loading; circles, passive tension of muscles during unloading. KI, potassium iodide. Data and schematic are taken from ref. 112.*

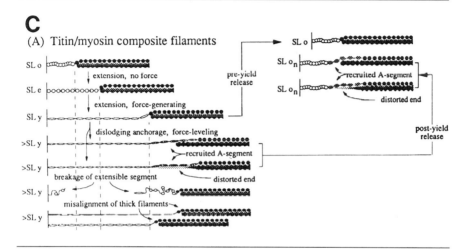

I-band, whereas the higher stiffness resulted from straining of the titin molecule itself. Distinguishing between this hypothesis and others requires further high-resolution molecular experimentation.

Determination of the structural origin of muscle passive tension and the factors that set resting sarcomere length is of great importance in modeling. Because muscle force is highly length dependent, relatively small sarcomere length changes can affect force generation significantly. Most current muscle models assume that muscle resting tension coincides with optimal sarcomere length and that this coincidence is the same for all muscles. Those with experience in contractile testing of muscle know that this is not the case. Some muscles are at optimal length with significant passive tension, whereas others are essentially slack while at optimal length. If differential titin isoform expression is responsible for setting muscle slack sarcomere length, it will be possible to generalize between muscles regarding this parameter after the various isoforms are known.

NEBULIN. *Molecular Ruler for Thin Filaments.* Electron microscopic studies of skeletal muscles across numerous species demonstrate that skeletal muscle thin filaments have a constant length. These filaments, containing actin, tropomyosin, and troponin, are longer than each of the individual molecules and thus require some type of polymerization and specific associations for assembly into the thin filaments observed by electron microscopy. Thus, it had been speculated that filament length regulation occurred with a template or ruler protein within the sarcomere. Nebulin, a family of giant endosarcomeric proteins with size variants from 600 to 900 kd, was proposed to serve as the thin filament length regulator [50, 53, 120].

Evidence that nebulin could regulate thin filament length came from immunoelectron microscopic studies showing that nebulin epitopes on the thin filament remained a fixed distance from the Z-line, regardless of stretch magnitude [50, 63, 78]. In addition, it was shown that a single nebulin molecule could span the entire length of the thin filament and, as the thin filament was extended, nebulin coextended by the same amount. Furthermore, separate studies performed by Kruger et al. and Labeit et al. have shown that nebulin isoform sizes are proportional to skeletal muscle thin filament length [50, 53]. This indirect evidence for nebulin as a thin filament length regulator is even more compelling in light of the observation that in some cardiac muscles in which thin filament lengths are not precisely regulated, nebulin is absent. Structurally, the data suggest that nebulin, tropomyosin, and troponin form a composite filament via lateral connections to actin and that nebulin aids in assembly and regulation of thin filament length.

Nebulin, as the name implies, has remained nebulous in terms of biophysical and biochemical characterization of the native protein. A region of the human nebulin transcript was cloned and sequenced, revealing an amino acid sequence containing highly conserved motifs of 35 residues repeating that approximately 200 times [53, 111]. Furthermore, a super-repeat motif of 245 residues exists that contains seven sets of the 35 residue modules [111]. Based on the super-repeat periodicity of the thin filament (38.5 nm, corresponding to one turn of the actin filament helix and composed of 7 actin monomers) that matches the nebulin repeat motif, it has been suggested that the repeating 35-residue motif is the basic structural unit of the nebulin-actin-binding domains [50, 53]. In addition, it appears that nebulin may interact with tropomyosin in the super-repeat region on actin [15, 111]. These molecular interactions between nebulin modules and actin subunits may facilitate nebulin's role as a thin filament regulator.

Functional Role of Nebulin. Currently, there is not general agreement on the role of nebulin during active muscle contraction. The observation that cloned nebulin fragments from the sarcomere thick and thin filament overlap region bind both to actin and mysoin led to the suggestion that nebulin may play a role in active muscle contraction. It has been proposed that nebulin may actually play a *regulatory* role in muscle contraction in a way that is similar yct distinct from that of tropomyosin and troponin. Root and Wang demonstrated that nebulin can regulate actin-myosin interaction via a calcium/calmodulin regulatory system in an in vitro motility assay [86]. These investigators studied actin-nebulin interactions by placing different regions of the nebulin molecule into an experimental chamber in which actin filaments were allowed to interact with myosin that was plated on coverslips. They found that the amino terminal region of nebulin (corresponding to the sarcomere overlap region) inhibited ATPase activity, preventing actin from being physically translated by myosin. However, the addition of calmodulin with calcium prevented this inhibition by reducing the binding affinity of nebulin fragments to actin and myosin. They thus hypothesized that nebulin prevents actomyosin interaction in resting muscles by controlling the position of the myosin head relative to actin but that this inhibition was removed upon activation by calcium and calmodulin. This type of study may provide a structural insight into the functional significance of actin-nebulin interactions on the thin filament of skeletal muscles.

The Extrasarcomeric Cytoskeleton

INTERMEDIATE FILAMENTS. As their name implies, intermediate filaments were first described based on their morphological appearance of intermediate size between actin microfilaments that are 6 nm in diameter and myosin filaments that are approximately 15 nm. The intermediate filaments (~10 nm in diameter) are abundant in, for example, smooth muscle. Thus, early studies attempting to show that the exosarcomeric lattice is composed of intermediate filaments would often make morphological comparisons between intermediate filaments isolated from gizzard smooth muscle and the filamentous system obtained from skeletal muscle (see Fig. 5B from ref. 113].

Early observation of muscle fiber ultrastructure suggested that adjacent myofibrils might have mechanical connections. One of the most compelling indirect arguments for this idea is that longitudinal electron micrographs of skeletal muscle usually demonstrate adjacent Z-bands and A-bands in nearly perfect register (Fig. 12.8). Because it is known that sarcomeres are arranged in series within the myofibril and that myofibrils are arranged in parallel, this aligned appearance suggests some type of connection between myofibrils. The exact location of the connection between adjacent myofibrils (e.g., Z-disk, M-band, etc.) was not implied by these observations.

Methods of Study. A difficulty in describing the muscle cytoskeleton in detail is the large number of proteins present, as well as the resolution of immunohistochemistry, even when the cytoskeleton is viewed using confocal microscopy. The typical study consists of measuring a particular antibody-staining pattern in muscle longitudinal sections and cross-sections and describing their codistribution with other proteins. In addition, in vitro binding assays are often used to determine which proteins are able to bind to each other (Table 12.2). Then, the structural information is integrated with

TABLE 12.2.
Binding between Major Proteins of Focal Adhesions Demonstrated in Vitro

Protein Studied	Proteins Found to Bind
Actin	α-Actinin, nebulin, vinculin, talin
Vinculin	Actin, talin, α-actinin, tensin, paxillin
α-Actinin	Actin, vinculin, extracellular matrix receptors
Talin	Vinculin, calpain, extracellular matrix receptors, actin
Dystrophin	Actin-, dystrophin-associated glycoproteins, syntrophins

binding information to produce a hypothetical arrangement of proteins (Fig. 12.9). For example, vinculin binds talin, α-actinin, and actin. Talin binds vinculin, as well as transmembrane integrins. Thus, with respect to these proteins, the modern models show talin and vinculin binding to one another, with vinculin binding to α-actinin and talin to the integrin (Fig. 12.9). Force would thus be transmitted from α-actinin in the Z-disk via the

FIGURE 12.8.
Longitudinal electron micrograph of a rabbit tibialis anterior skeletal muscle demonstrating regular array of A- and I-bands and adjacent Z-bands in nearly perfect register. This regularity between adjacent myofibrils indirectly suggests lateral connections between myofibrils.

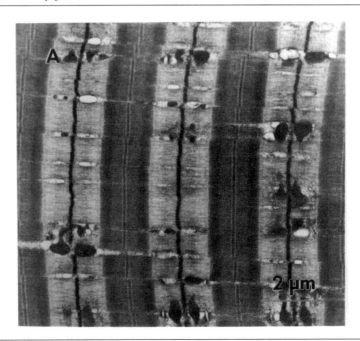

FIGURE 12.9.

Diagrammatic representation of the muscle fiber cytoskeletal lattice. Most of these relationships are hypothesized based on in vitro binding studies between proteins, deduced amino acid sequences from cDNA clones, and immunolabeling studies demonstrating colocalization. The variety of connections between structures provide a myriad of possible routes of force transmission from actomyosin interaction to the extracellular matrix.

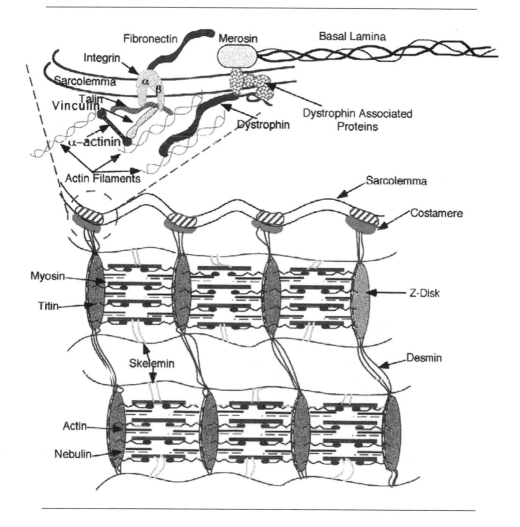

talin/vinculin complex to the integrin, which is directly connected to the endomysial collagen network. Of course, numerous studies are required to verify such a model.

Desmin Structure and Function. Desmin is the major component of the adult skeletal muscle intermediate filament system [55]. Traditional

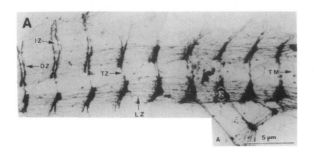

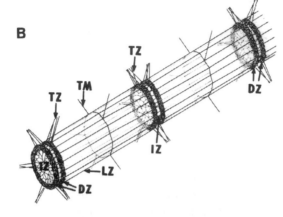

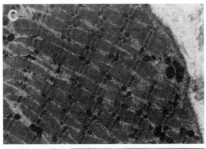

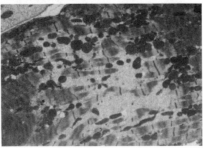

FIGURE 12.10.

(A) Electron micrograph of extracted intermediate filaments from rabbit skeletal muscle. Residue "clumped" on the filament network is an artifact of the extraction technique. Variability across the micrograph results from variable destruction of the intermediate filament lattice by the extracting solutions themselves. T_z, transverse filaments connecting Z-disk to Z-disk; TM, transverse filaments connecting M-line to M-line; LZ, longitudinal filaments connecting Z disk to Z-disk; IZ, internal filaments in the gaps of doublet Z-structures; DZ, doublet structure of highly disintegrated Z-structures. (B) Schematic diagram of muscle intermediate filament system. Reproduced from ref. 113. (C) Transmission electron micrograph of skeletal muscle from 10-wk-old desmin null mouse. Note lack of myofibrillar register and disorganized mitochondria. (Micrograph was provided courtesy of Dr. Yassemi Capetenaki, Department of Cell Biology, Baylor College of Medicine.

longitudinal electron micrographs are dominated by contractile filaments and fail to reveal major structures other than actin, myosin, and the Z-disk. Therefore, studies that have elucidated the nature of the muscular cytoskeleton require the use of extraction methods that selectively remove either the actin- or myosin-based filaments, or both. These extraction methods, involving the use of high ionic strength solutions (such as potassium iodide or other extraction solutions that are highly damaging to the tissue) also damage the intermediate filament system itself. Thus, many "residual filaments" that have been observed in previous ultrastructural studies have been interpreted as being damaged or fragmented contractile filaments. More recent studies, however, have demonstrated that this is, in fact, not the case. For example, Lazarides prepared sheets of Z-disk material from skeletal muscles and demonstrated selective peripheral localization of a protein linking adjacent Z-disks [55]. He named this protein desmin (Greek: desmos = "link") and hypothesized that the adjacent Z-disk connections provided mechanical stabilization to the muscle fiber itself. He also demonstrated the presence of α-actinin in the core region of the Z-disk, thus establishing the Z-disk to be composed of three major proteins: desmin, α-actinin, and actin. (Since that time, many more proteins have been localized to the Z-disk; see Table 12.1.) The three-dimensional nature of this intermediate filament system was further clarified in extraction studies performed by Wang and Ramirez-Mitchell, in which the intermediate filament lattice was shown to contain not only struts between adjacent Z-disks but also a Z-disk structure involving a doublet of rings of intermediate filaments (probably what was seen by Lazarides in his studies involving immunofluorescent detection of desmin), as well as longitudinal arrangements of intermediate filaments around the outside of the sarcomere [113]. These transverse and longitudinal filaments could serve to link adjacent myofibrils mechanically, as well as to provide mechanical continuity outside of the sarcomere along the myofibrillar length (Fig. 12.10A and B).

The significance of desmin in muscle development and subsequent function is suggested by the timing and influence of desmin expression during myogenesis. Early in myogenesis, the majority of cells that are destined to become myoblasts (presumptive myoblasts) contain vimentin without desmin. However, a small population of these cells becomes both vimentin- and desmin-positive, which represents the fact that these cells are now determined to be myoblasts [39, 48]. This desmin expression occurs before the expression of any contractile proteins. All postmitotic mononucleated myoblasts and multinucleated myotubes express both vimentin and desmin without exception. From this point on, cells may express desmin without myofibrillar proteins, but they never express myofibrillar proteins without desmin. At these later stages, desmin and vimentin intermediate filaments orient themselves to form bands that maintain the registry between I-Z-I bands of neighboring myofibrils. It is, therefore, believed in skeletal muscle that the desmin intermediate filament system is responsible for the precise registry of Z-bands between adjacent myofibrils and is a candidate for force transmission between these adjacent structures. The precise mechanics of such force transmission remains to be determined.

Desmin is a prototypical intermediate filament protein composed of a small head region (85 amino acids), an α-helical rod region (330 amino acids), and a tail region (45 amino acids). Interestingly, homology analysis of the desmin sequence reveals structural similarity with the myogenic regulatory factors, myoD, and myogenin [16, 20, 56]. These observations, along with the specific timing of desmin expression during myogenesis, raise questions regarding the role of desmin in muscle development. Is the role of desmin purely structural, organizing myofibrillar proteins, or might desmin be a causal factor in the myogenic program? To address this question, myoblasts were transiently transfected with a truncated desmin that was unable to polymerize into filaments [89]. This was a result of the lack of the desmin head region that is responsible for the polymerization and organization of desmin into filaments [14]. These authors found that, despite the lack of intact intermediate filaments, myoblasts fused and formed normal striated myofibrils and even began contracting spontaneously, which is normal for these cells. Another experiment addressed this question by creating a construct designed to express antisense desmin mRNA, thus interfering with filament formation by hybridizing with the desmin sense mRNA [56]. This experiment was performed in a stable cell line that not only failed to undergo differentiation, fusion, and myotube formation but even demonstrated inhibition of the myogenic regulators, myoD and myogenin. These data suggested that desmin was indeed necessary for normal myogenesis to take place. It is possible that the previous results, in which cells still developed somewhat normally, were obtained because the truncated desmin filaments were expressed in cells that had already differentiated [56, 89]. A similar result was obtained using a desmin null mutation within embryonic stem cell-derived embryoid bodies [114]. These authors also demonstrated lack of expression of myf5 and myosin heavy-chain.

The most recent and definitive experiments implemented the elegant experiment using transgenic animals completely lacking the desmin gene [57, 66]. Surprisingly, desmin null mice were viable and fertile, but the muscles of these mice showed numerous abnormalities reminiscent of diseased muscles, such as loss of myofibrillar regularity, abnormal placement of nuclei, and abnormal appearance of mitochondria (Fig. 12.10C). This study emphasizes the role that desmin must play in creating and/or maintaining the structural integrity of the myofibrillar lattice. In addition, even though desmin was absent throughout an animal's lifetime, myogenesis proceeded relatively normally. This may have been attributable to other proteins, such as vimentin, synemin, or even nestin substituting for desmin's normal function. Such a redundancy is relatively common in studies using knockout designs.

INTERMEDIATE FILAMENT-ASSOCIATED PROTEINS. Intermediate filament-associated proteins (IFAPs) bind to intermediate filaments and possess the ability to self-aggregate or coaggregate with other IFAPs. IFAPs are usually distributed throughout the cytoplasmic space during development but, as differentiation proceeds, they localize to specific structures within the cell. In differentiating skeletal muscle, three IFAPs, plectin, synemin, and paranemin, are distributed at the Z-disc periphery. All three proteins have been proposed to act as elements that cross-link intermediate filaments to the Z-disc [10, 83, 116]. Plectin has also been proposed as being involved in the anchoring of intermediate filaments to the sarcolemma [23]. However, these proposals are based on immunocytochemical localization studies and have not been supported by other, more direct, functional studies [22, 37, 83].

Plectin. Plectin, the most abundant and rather large IFAP, was recently cloned and sequenced by Wiche et al. [117], who showed it to be a 466-kd polypeptide chain with a structure similar to that of other intermediate filaments: a head domain, central α-helical-coiled rod domain and amino terminal tail domain. The rod domain consists of five subregions containing approximately 200 amino acids. Within this rod domain is a strong repeat of 10.4 residues that may be involved in self-association of plectin molecules. It has been suggested that the rod domain plays an important role in plectin-vimentin interactions at the level of the Z-disc and plectin-lamin B interactions at focal adhesion sites [23]. The globular carboxy terminal contains a strongly conserved repeat of about 335 residues based on 9 tandem repeats of a 19-residue motif, which is important in maintaining association between plectin and intermediate filaments [118]. By constructing rat cDNAs encoding truncated plectin mutants, the mutant proteins were distributed throughout the cell but failed to associate with intermediate filaments. A more complete understanding of the relationship between plectin structural domains and interaction with intermediate filaments will be important in understanding the role of plectin in muscle cell development and cell differentiation.

Synemin and Paranemin. Unlike plectin, the structure of synemin and paranemim remains unknown. Synemin (MW, 230 kd), first described by Lazarides and colleagues in chicken smooth muscle, and paranemin (MW, 280 kd) have been shown to colocalize with desmin and vimentin [10, 37]. This spatial colocalization between synemin/paranemin and desmin/vimentin occurs throughout the course of myogenesis and into the maturation phase of myotubes. It has been shown that during early muscle cell differentiation, desmin, vimentin, synemin, and paranemin are all expressed [83]. Like most intermediate filaments, synemin and paranemin is present early in myotube formation as wavy filaments in the cytoplasm, but as the myofiber matures they both migrate to the Z-disc periphery. At this stage synemin forms interlinked collars with desmin and vimentin in the Z-plane. However, as developing cells mature into adult muscle, paranemin is removed during the differentiation stage of both fast and slow muscle [83]. Recently, chicken synemin has been cloned and sequenced and revealed that the rod domain of synemin is most like that of intermediate filaments [5]. However, it is still unknown which structural features of the rod domain may aid in the interlinking of intermediate filaments. The role of paranemin, based on its absence in adult muscle, has been suggested as modulating the extent of intermediate filament cross-linking before skeletal muscle maturation [83]. It appears that paranemin may hinder maximal cross-linking of intermediate filaments during development until its loss in adult skeletal muscle.

Force Transmission via the Intermediate Filament Network. Given that muscle fibers contain an exosarcomeric mechanical linkage system, it is interesting to speculate about the path of force transmission that results from actomyosin interaction. When myosin interacts with actin, force is directly transmitted between molecules at their interface, and a tensile force is transmitted from the myosin filament via titin and actin to the Z-disk (Figs. 12.1A and 12.6). This force is transmitted longitudinally within the myofibril, between the sarcomere generating the force and its serial neighbor but also to adjacent parallel myofibrils, because adjacent Z-disks and M-lines are mechanically connected via the intermediate filament system. Thus, the force generated by a single sarcomere can easily be transmitted radially, as well as longitudinally (Fig. 12.1B).

Force Transmission after Muscle Injury. During muscle contraction, all sarcomeres in series within a fiber generate force at nearly the same time because of the longitudinal and radial arrangement of t-tubules and sarcoplasmic reticulum (for experiments demonstrating the time-course of activation, see ref. 34). A natural route of force transmission would be from one serial sarcomere to the next via activated contractile filaments. However, even in the case in which a serial sarcomere is inactive or damaged, longitudinal force might still be transmitted via the intermediate filament network, either longitudinally around the damaged sarcomere within the same myofibril or laterally to adjacent myofibrils. This arrangement provides a great deal of mechanical redundancy within the muscle cell and may be one reason why quantitative morphometric studies of muscle after injury have failed to produce a strong correlation between the area or volume fraction of injured tissue and loss in contractile performance [27, 59]. It can be seen by the argument presented above that a one-to-one correspondence between muscle function and muscle tissue injury does not necessarily exist.

Dynamic Nature of the Intermediate Filament Network. Muscle hypertrophy primarily occurs by the addition of new myofibrils within the fiber. This increase in number of myofibrils is the structural basis for the increased fiber diameter observed after muscle strengthening paradigms and is one reason that muscle fiber size is one of the most often-reported structural parameters in exercise studies. If myofibrils are interconnected as described above, how is a new myofibril inserted? The answer is not clear but must involve the remodeling of the intermediate filament network between adjacent myofibrils. In this regard, it is fascinating to note that there is a good deal of evidence for the dynamic nature of the intermediate filament network. For example, the nuclear intermediate filament meshwork is almost completely resorbed during each cell division cycle, permitting reorganization of the subcellar contents [33, 106]. Likewise we recently demonstrated in a rabbit muscle injury model that the intermediate filament protein desmin can be lost within 5 min of initiation of exercise [60]. We interpreted this finding to indicate, not so much direct structural damage to the myofibrillar lattice in response to high mechanical load; rather, we suggested that secondary proteolysis of the intermediate filaments occurred in preparation for muscle repair or remodeling. In this regard, it is fascinating that, based on the functional and structural similarities between extranuclear intermediate filaments and intranuclear lamins [65], it has been proposed that a major role of intermediate filaments is to regulate gene expression [99]. Similar remodeling was implied, based on measurement of actin and desmin content in fast rabbit muscle undergoing transformation to slow muscle as a result of chronic electrical stimulation. These authors demonstrated that the desmin:actin ratio increased significantly over the 3-wk stimulation period, as did the vimentin:actin ratio [2]. Because slow muscle fibers are known to have a greater volume fraction of Z-disk material [21], proteins associated with the Z-disk should increase in conjunction with the fiber type transformation. However, because the increased intermediate filament protein expression *preceded* the myosin heavy-chain isoform transformation, the possibility exists that the intermediate filament network represents the scaffold on which the newly formed sarcomeres will be assembled. Clearly, further studies are needed to determine the precise sequence of events, as well as the necessary and sufficient steps for such a process to occur.

FOCAL ADHESIONS. Having described the cytoskeletal protein arrangement within the myofibril (titin and nebulin) and those connections between myofibrils (intermediate filaments), we now focus on those connections between the intracellular proteins and the extracellular space. In other words, what is the path of force transmission from the outer boundary of the myofibrils to the extracellular matrix (Figs. 12.1C and D)? The discrete connections between the muscle fiber's inside and outside are made at specialized structures known as focal adhesions [46] and, in muscle in particular [73, 74], they have been termed "costameres" (Latin: costa = rib, mere = structure). The most significant point to be made with regard to these discrete structures is that force is transmitted from a muscle fiber to the extracellular space along the entire fiber length at the costameres, as well as at the muscle-tendon junction. It is an incorrect oversimplification to assume that muscle fibers generate force along their length and that force is transmitted only serially to the muscle-tendon junction.

Costamere Structure. The initial description of muscle focal adhesions was made using a monoclonal antibody to the protein vinculin. Vinculin had already been found in focal adhesions of smooth muscle [90] and fibroblasts [12] and was known to bind to numerous other proteins based on in vitro assays. Longitudinal micrographs of muscle cells revealed a punctate ap-

FIGURE 12.11

Longitudinal micrograph of avian skeletal muscle incubated with an antibody against vinculin. Note the discrete locations of vinculin along the fiber length. These types of micrographs provide evidence for the existence of "costameres" in skeletal muscle. (A) immohistochemical image with vinculin antibody; (B) phase micrograph showing position of vinculin relative to the Z-bands of the muscle fiber. Reproduced from ref. 74.

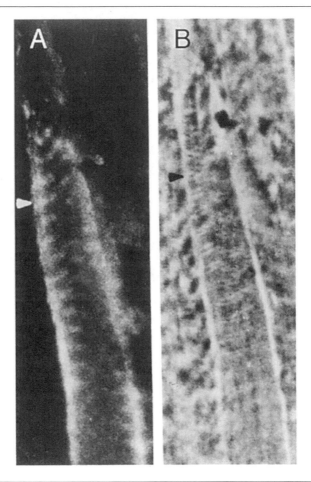

pearance of vinculin staining at a location just above the Z-band (Fig. 12.11). The periodicity of the vinculin pattern was shown, by comparison of phase contrast to immunohistochemical images, to remain in register with the Z-band, independent of sarcomere length. This provided indirect evidence of a connection between the Z-disk structure and the membrane surface. It would be simple if vinculin made the direct connection between myofibrils and transmembrane integrin receptors, but the actual situation is not nearly so simple. Currently, it is known that focal adhesions can be assembled from dozens of proteins, and certainly more will be discovered with time (Table 12.1).

Molecular Studies of Vinculin. Unfortunately, just because a protein *can* bind to another and because it *may be* colocalized with another, does not mean that the connections actually exist in vivo or demonstrate whether they are functionally important. To determine these latter conditions, more recent studies have implemented transgenic animals, in whom the effect of a particular protein is interrupted by forced expression of antisense mRNA that binds to the expressed RNA and prevents protein synthesis or by alteration of the gene expression pattern, using synthetic promoter systems or gene "knockouts." As an example of the type of information obtained from these studies, consider recent experiments with the vinculin protein. Decreased vinculin levels achieved using antisense vinculin mRNA caused mouse 3T3 fibroblasts to become more rounded with fewer focal adhesions and impaired cellular attachment [85]. This implicated vinculin in cell adhesion to the substrate. When cell proliferation was induced by serum, vinculin synthesis increased as one of the earliest responses [105], implicating vinculin in cell division and migration. These data point to a central role of vinculin in maintaining the integrity and function of focal adhesion sites. Future studies will be directed toward specific sites within the numerous molecules that interact at the focal adhesion sites. In this way, as has been accomplished for titin, regions of a molecule involved in structural integrity, binding, and regulation will be identified.

DYSTROPHIN AND THE DYSTROPHIN-ASSOCIATED PROTEINS. Dystrophin is lacking or abnormal in muscle from patients afflicted with muscular dystrophy [Table 12.3 and ref. 40]. Muscular dystrophy represents a family of approximately 10 disorders involving a primary myopathy. In other words, the problem with the muscle can be directly related to a problem within the muscle, as opposed to a problem with the peripheral or central nervous system. Symptoms of the disorder include false hypertrophy of the muscles (especially the calves), mental retardation, and quadriceps fermoris muscle atrophy. The disorder is X-linked and thus, primarily affects young males, with death usually occurring by age 14 secondary to respiratory muscle failure (in Duchenne muscular dystrophy (DMD)).

Dystrophin Structure. By creation of a fusion protein, it was determined that the protein product of the human DMD locus was missing during screening of a number of murine strains [41]. Then, a human cDNA clone representing a portion of the DMD transcript was isolated on the basis of its conserved sequence between mouse and human. This partial cDNA sequence was then used to isolate homologous cDNA sequences from mice and, ultimately, the entire 14-kB coding sequence of the human dytrophin gene was identified [49]. The dystrophin gene was shown

TABLE 12.3.
Involvement of Dystrophin-Associated Proteins in Muscle Disease

Clinical Diagnosis	Protein Deficiency
Congential muscular dystrophy (CMD)	Merosin deficiency
Severe child autosomal-recessive muscular dystrophy (SCARMD)	Dystrophin-associated glycoprotein deficiency
Duchenne muscular dystrophy (DMD)	Dystrophin deficiency
Becker muscular dystropy (BMD)	
Emery-Dreifuss muscular dystrophy (EDMD)	Emerin deficiency (gene product unknown)

to encode a 427-kd protein containing an actin-binding domain, a domain homologous to spectrin, and a cysteine-rich α-actinin binding domain (Fig 12.12). From the predicted amino acid sequence and homology with spectrin, it was hypothesized that this protein encoded a rod-shaped cytoskeletal protein [49]. The rod-shaped portion of the protein was highly homologous to spectrin and was thought to be localized in the subsarcolemal region [71], along with a complex of proteins known as the dystrophin-associated proteins (DAP (Fig. 12.13). It is interesting to note that many primary muscle diseases have now been traced to specific losses in one or more components of the DAP complex (Table 12.3) and points to the central role that many of these proteins must play in maintaining cell integrity and function [13].

Putative Functional Role of Dystrophin. Because dystrophic muscle demonstrates signs of degeneration and is more vulnerable to physical stress, dystrophin is believed to be important in maintaining muscle fiber integrity. However, the mechanism by which this is accomplished is not known.

FIGURE 12.12.
Schematic diagram of the dystrophin molecule (not to scale) based on analysis of the cDNA sequence. The four main domains of this molecule include an actin-binding domain (that connects dystrophin to the intracellular cytoskeletal lattice) and a spectrin-like domain (that presumably confers upon dystrophin its mechanical and structural properties), as well as a dystroglycan- and syntrophin-binding domain (that provides the interface to the extracellular matrix).

Amino Terminus   Carboxy Terminus

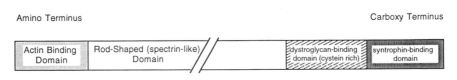

FIGURE 12.13.

Schematic representation of the dystrophin-associated glycoprotein complex. Many of these elements have numerical names based on their molecular mass, and their function is not yet clear. However, note that the four domains shown in Figure 12.12 are clearly represented. There is evidence that, within the cell, the dystrophin molecule exists as a dimer.

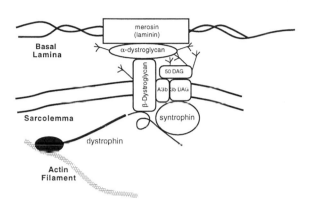

There is evidence that dystrophin may behave as a stabilizer of integral membrane ion channels or that it may stabilize folds in the membrane to prevent membrane disruption that could result from loading. Whatever the mechanism, it is clear that cells lacking the dystrophin gene product are more vulnerable to mechanical damage. This was demonstrated by Petrof et al., who stimulated muscle, using various paradigms, to determine whether the mechanical stress on the tissue was a greater determinant of damage, rather than the number of activations [77]. They speculated that mechanical stress would cause greater muscle damage to dystrophic tissue, compared to normal tissue, because the membranes would be less able to withstand the shear and tensile forces. This was, in fact, the case (Fig. 12.14). They further suggested that it was the stress on the tissue, rather than the number of contractions, that was the main factor causing damage. Petrof et al. suggested that the shear stress across the membranes was the main predictor of injury based on the observation that larger muscle fibers tended to be more easily damaged than smaller muscle fibers. Because the surface:volume ratio of a large muscle fiber is lower than a small muscle fiber, the authors suggested that the shear stress across the membrane produced by the myofibrils was causing the damage [77]. This was consistent with their observations comparing different sizes of muscle fibers contained in the extensor digitorum longus and diaphragm muscle fibers.

FIGURE 12.14.

Maximum tetanic tension generated by control diaphragm and dystrophic (mdx) diaphragm muscles after five maximal fused tetanic contractions (80 Hz for 700 ms), during which the muscle was lengthened at 0.5 L_o/s through a distance of 10% L_o over a 200-ms period. The larger force decline in the mdx muscle suggests that dystrophin played a structural role in maintaining muscle fiber integrity. This result was supported by other data presented in the original study. Data were taken from Table 2 of ref. 77.

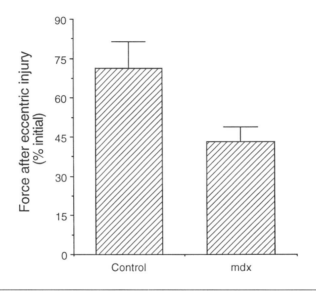

WHOLE MUSCLE FORCE GENERATION

Muscle Architecture Overview

Since the early anatomical studies of the 1600s, it has been known that muscle fiber arrangement varies widely between different skeletal muscles. Functional studies have since correlated the relationship between muscle force and excursion and the fiber arrangement within a muscle. To a first approximation, it has been demonstrated that a muscle's maximum tetanic tension is proportional to its physiological cross-sectional area (PCSA, see ref. 79) and a muscle's maximum shortening velocity is proportional to its muscle fiber length [9].

Physiological Cross-Sectional Area

Theoretically, PCSA is supposed to be proportional to the muscle's maximum tetanic tension. This value is almost never the cross-sectional area of the muscle measured in any of the traditional anatomical planes, as would be obtained using a noninvasive imaging method such as magnetic resonance imaging (MRI) or computerized tomography (CT) and, thus, PCSA must be determined indirectly. PCSA is supposed to represent the sum of the cross-sectional areas of all of the muscle fibers within the muscle and should, theoretically, be able to provide a check on whether our understanding of muscle fiber arrangement within a muscle is correct. When PCSA is directly proportional to maximum tetanic tension, it suggests that the individual muscle fibers are acting in parallel in a simple additive fashion. The value for PCSA in traditional muscle mechanical experiments is calculated using the following equation:

$$\text{PCSA (cm}^2) = \frac{\text{Muscle Mass (g)} \cdot \text{cosine } \theta}{\rho \text{ (g/cm}^3) \cdot \text{Fiber Length (cm)}}$$

where ρ represents muscle density (1.056 g/cm^3 for mammalian muscle) and θ represents surface pennation angle. This equation essentially represents muscle volume divided by fiber length. If the muscle were a cylinder, dividing volume by length would represent the cylinder cross-sectional area and should be a good estimate of force-generating potential. Because most muscles are spindle-shaped, the applicability of this equation is debatable. Thus, to compare predicted and measured maximum tetanic tensions, Edgerton and colleagues performed microdissection of individual guinea pig muscles after measuring maximum tetanic tension [79]. They found that PCSA and maximum tetanic tension were directly proportional (Fig. 12.15), with a proportionality constant of 22.5 N/cm^2. This was true for all muscles, except for the soleus, which contained a majority of slow fibers. The reason for this one exception has not been determined. These experimental results provide support for the mechanical model that muscles act as if the fibers were arranged in parallel. Whether muscle fibers are actually mechanically arranged in parallel or the experimental method is too gross to resolve the true interactions is not yet clear.

Architectural studies that report fiber length typically *measure* the length of a small bundle of fibers and equate it to fiber length. This is clearly an oversimplification that may not affect functional predictions made for the muscles but has significant implications in understanding the mechanics of force generation between muscle fibers contained in whole muscles and in understanding the distribution of muscle fibers within a motor unit.

Unfortunately, direct determination of muscle fiber length is technically difficult. In amphibian muscle, single fibers have been isolated and their contractile properties determined [19, 35, 47]. Even single mouse muscle fibers have been isolated [115]. Because the majority of the excellent mechanical studies were originally performed on amphibian muscles, this has led to the general idea that muscle fibers extend from one tendon plate to

FIGURE 12.15.

Comparison between measured maximum tetanic tension (P_o) and estimated P_o based on measurement of physiological cross-sectional area (PCSA) in guinea pig muscles. Note that PCSA and P_o are proportional for all muscles except the soleus, the one muscle with a preponderance of slow muscle fibers. MG-LG-PLT, medial and lateral heads of the gastrocnemius and plantaris; FHL, flexor hallucis longus; TA-TAA, tibialis anterior and tibialis anterior accessorius; TP, tibialis posterior, SOL, soleus; EDL, extensor digitorum longus. Data are taken from ref. 79.

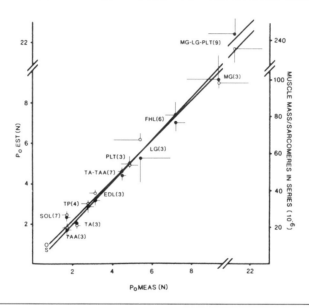

another. In several mammalian systems studied to date, this is clearly not the case (see below).

A second test of our understanding of muscle fiber arrangement within a whole muscle is based on the tenet that maximum muscle contraction velocity is proportional to muscle fiber length [29, 88, 91]. Unfortunately, although this is intuitively appealing, there is little experimental support for such an assertion. Gross mechanical and architectural studies comparing cat plantarflexors have supported this result in the case in which fiber lengths are very different between muscles [109, 110]. Also, measurement of cat semitendinosus muscle proximal and distal heads with separate and simultaneous stimulation provides approximate support for a proportionality between fiber length and maximum velocity [9]. However, it would be important to compare fiber length to maximum shortening velocity in a way analogous to the study of Powell et al. across a range of fiber lengths for

FIGURE 12.16.

Schematic diagram of muscle fiber arrangement in the cat sartorius muscle. Muscle fibers are arranged in series and probably are simultaneously activated to produce the functional equivalent of one long muscle fiber. These data are intriguing in light of the common notion that muscle fibers extend from one tendon plate to another and also require refined biomechanical models for adequate description. Drawn based on results in ref. 61.

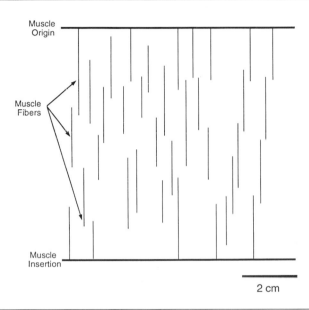

muscles with similar fiber type distributions [79]. As we will see in the next section, detailed measurements of single-muscle fiber lengths and orientation call into question such a simple view of muscle fiber arrangement.

Muscle Fiber Taper and Termination

Detailed measurement of muscle fiber lengths within intact whole muscles have revealed the seemingly paradoxical result that, in many muscles, fibers do not extend from one tendon plate to the other [61, 72]. The idea that series-fibered muscles exist (i.e., muscles contain fibers that are arranged end to end, in series within a fascicle) is not new, but the concept was revived with the report of Loeb et al. (Fig. 12.16), who documented this arrangement in the cat sartorius muscle [61]. They argued that the extreme length of the sartorius muscle (approximately 10 cm) necessitated such an arrangement because the conduction velocity along muscle fibers was not fast enough to activate the entire fiber simultaneously. Although the applicability of such

FIGURE 12.17.

Muscle fiber arrangement determined by glycogen depletion within seven different single motor units (MU) of the cat tibialis anterior muscle. Motor units 1–5 were physiologically typed as fast, and motor units 6 and 7 were physiologically typed as slow. The most proximal end of the muscle is defined as 0 mm, whereas the most distal portion of the muscle is denoted by the inverted "T" symbol. Fibers that taper at their end are shown as normal thin lines while fibers that end in blunted fashion are indicated by a right angle at the end of the line. Note that some muscle fibers actually begin and end with the muscle fascicle itself. Reproduced from ref. 72.

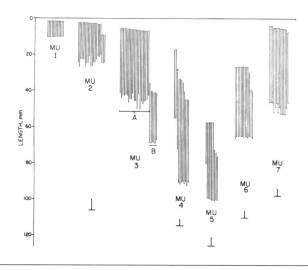

an argument is debatable, clearly a mechanical inefficiency would result if contracting sarcomeres were permitted to shorten rapidly against adjacent, compliant, inactivated sarcomeres. One can posit a rationale for such a series-fibered arrangement if the fibers so arranged are members of the same motor unit. In this way, multiple axons could innervate and simultaneously activate many fibers in series which would, in effect, behave as a single fiber. To test this idea, Edgerton and colleagues measured the length and distribution of muscle fibers within motor units, using the glycogen depletion method [72]. They demonstrated that not only did some of the fibers within a single unit *not* extend the entire fascicle length, but also many units had their origin or insertion completely in the center of the muscle belly (Fig. 12.17). This raises the general question as to how muscle fiber contractile force is transmitted to an external tendon, which may be quite a distance away from the fiber insertion site. In other words, the concept that all muscle fibers are arranged in bundles and transmit force along their length to the end regions, where they insert onto major tendon plates is no longer tenable (Fig. 12.1E). Despite the fact that muscle fiber insertion sites are highly specialized with respect to geometry and protein composition [97, 101, 102], the finding that many muscle fibers taper into almost a pointed end precludes force from being transmitted only at their tips, because the stress concentration at the small tapered fiber tip would be tremendous.

Lateral Force Transmission among Muscle Fibers

How else might muscle fibers transmit tension to the "outside world?" A creative experiment by Street showed that muscle force can be transmitted *laterally* between muscle fibers [92]. She dissected a single frog muscle fiber from one end of the muscle and left the surrounding fibers intact on the other end. While securing the bare end of the single muscle fiber and using a carefully placed electrode that activated only the single fiber, she measured the force generated by the single fiber (Fig. 12.18A). She then released the bare end of the single fiber and secured the remaining muscle fibers adjacent to the single fiber at the opposite end (Fig. 12.18B). It is important to note that now, the single fiber was totally free at the isolated end. Again, she activated the bare single fiber and measured an isometric force nearly equivalent to that measured when the bare end of the single fiber was secured! Note that this force was measured despite the fact that the bare single fiber was free to shorten. The interpretation of this experiment was that the physical interaction between adjacent fibers was sufficient so that the activated single fiber transmitted its force radially to adjacent fibers that were secured and that force was transmitted to the force-measuring end via these adjacent fibers. Either way, this experiment demonstrates the significant degree to which muscle fiber force can be transmitted outside of the fiber itself to neighboring muscle fibers. Note that this result was obtained in amphibian muscle, which has a relatively poorly developed endomysial connective tissue network. The situation for mammalian muscle would undoubtedly be more impressive where the endomysial connective tissue matrix is much more highly developed.

Based on our previous presentation of the specialized costameres that occur at regular intervals along the fiber's length, we suggest a model of force transmission in whole muscle, in which force is generated by the myofibrils and transmitted along and between myofibrils until it ultimately reaches the outside world by specialized adhesion receptors along the muscle length and at the fiber end (Fig. 12.1D and E). In this model, there is no problem with muscle fibers that taper or with fibers that terminate within the muscle itself, because force is transmitted all along the fiber length to the well-developed endomysial connective tissue matrix (Fig. 12.19) described by John Trotter [100, 103]. These striking pictures of the intramuscular connective tissue matrix are reminiscent of the well-defined endoneurial tubes that guide, nourish, and protect single axons. He also quantified the types of connections made by individual muscle fibers to the "outside world" and found that in no case did muscle fibers actually termi-

FIGURE 12.18.

Schematic arrangement of experimental measurements on frog muscle to determine magnitude of force transmitted laterally between fibers. Experimental condition is shown on left and tetanic tension resulting from single fiber stimulation shown at right. (A) Isolated fiber is secured at bare end and at end still containing surrounding fibers. (B) Isolated fiber secured only at end containing surrounding fibers. The surrounding fibers themselves are secured to the measuring device. Only the single fiber is activated in both cases, and isometric force generation is essentially identical. Based on the experiments of ref. 92.

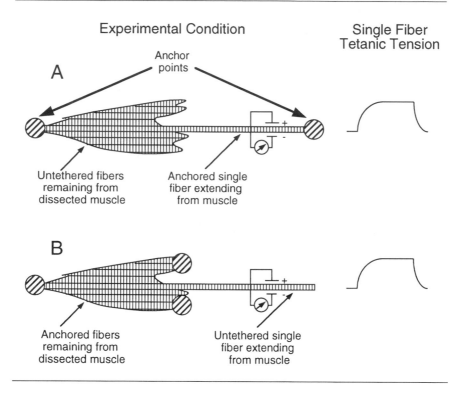

nate on one another (myomyous junction), even in the tapering regions of the fibers themselves. All connections observed were of the myotendinous type, even along the tapering region of the fiber.

It may be strategic to have a mechanically redundant muscle fiber force-generating system (i.e., one with numerous series and parallel connections) in the same way that is observed within the fiber in which mechanical redundancy is present so that sarcomeres can transmit force serially or radially. Lateral force transmission obviates the need for mechanical continuity along the fiber length for force generation to occur. Thus, if a fiber

FIGURE 12.19.

Endomysial connective tissue matrix image generated by scanning electron microscopy of a muscle whose fibers were removed by means of acid digestion. Micrograph courtesy of John Trotter, University of New Mexico, from ref. 103.

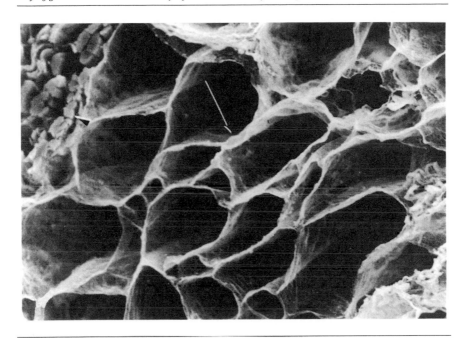

experiences focal injury, remaining fiber segments may still transmit tension to the outside world, effectively bypassing the injured region. Thus, force generation in muscle would result from a "volume" of myofibrils that generate and transmit force along multiple complex pathways and via a variety of filamentous systems. Future studies are required to define the pathway for force transmission within and between muscle fibers.

Physiological Significance of Varying Muscle Fiber Length

Several physiological and mechanical studies have been published that may represent manifestations of the significant variability in muscle fiber length that occurs within a muscle and even between motor units of different types within a muscle. For example, significant differences between fast and slow motor unit stiffness were reported for the cat peroneous tertius muscle [75]. Numerous other studies of motor units had been performed in which contractile properties were measured under isometric conditions [8, 11, 36]. It was previously shown that fast-contracting units (type FR and FF units) developed a higher tension and had lower endurance than slow units (type S

FIGURE 12.20.

Experimental measurement of motor unit stiffness obtained by applying a small (0.5-mm) stretch to the motor unit. (A) Comparison of stiffness of (left to right) passive muscle, 4 combined slow (S) units, and 1 fast-fatigable (FF) unit. Although FF unit force is higher, S unit stiffness is greater. (B) Comparison of stiffness of (left to right) passive muscle, 3 combined FR units, and 8 S units. Although fast-fatigue-resistant (FR) unit force is higher, S unit stiffness is greater by 46%. Reproduced from ref. 75.

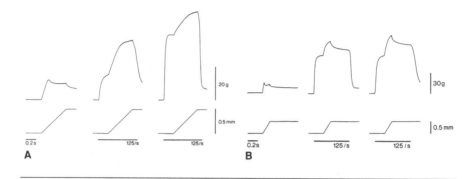

units) within the same muscles. However, Petit et al. applied small rapid stretches to the activated motor units and measured motor unit *stiffness* rather than isometric tension [75]. Stiffness was calculated as the change in force divided by the change in length (Fig. 12.20). They found that, while the fast units generated higher absolute isometric forces compared to slow units, the slow units had a stiffness that was over twice that of the faster units (Fig. 12.20). They subsequently demonstrated that the stiffness difference was indeed a result of cross-bridge properties by applying a second stretch to the stable population of cross-bridges formed after the stretch [76]. Alternatively, it is possible that the stiffness difference between units is a manifestation of shorter fibers within slow units that would appear to be stiffer because they undergo a greater strain for a given muscle deformation. In either case, the physiological effect of increased stiffness would be to provide increased stability against small positional perturbations. Huijing and Baan measured the length-tension properties of motor unit populations recruited at different thresholds [45]. They found that the width of the length-tension curves (which should be directly proportional to average fiber length) varied between low-threshold and high-threshold units, again suggesting that motor units of different types may be composed of muscle fibers of different lengths. (The possibility exists that this phenomenon was confounded by alterations in stimulation frequency that can occur with the type of activation method used.) We speculated that differential fiber length between fiber types could explain the selective damage to type fast glycolytic (FG) muscle fibers observed in the rabbit tibialis anterior after eccentric contractions based on a synthesis of the reports mentioned above [58]. In the rabbit tibialis anterior, differential FG fiber injury may have a simple geometrical explanation, namely, that FG fibers experience increased strain and injury because of their short fiber length. Clearly, sophisticated mechanical studies of motor units are required to unravel the answers to such questions. These types of provocative results warrant further study and present a considerable challenge to those who are currently generating biomechanical models of muscle. This is because whole muscles may have a level of organization that is much more complicated than that presented in classic anatomy and physiology texts. Although molecular studies of muscle are justifiably increasing in popularity, excellent physiological studies of whole muscles are needed to clarify many of the issues raised above.

SUMMARY

The actual path of force transmission in skeletal muscle from actomyosin interaction to tension at the tendinous insertion site is poorly understood. Within the muscle cell, endo- and exosarcomeric cytoskeletal proteins create series and parallel connections between contractile proteins resulting in a meshwork across which force can be transmitted in practically any direction with respect to the fiber axis. At the surface membrane, connections between the intermediate filament system, dystrophin, and specialized membrane complexes provide the route of force transmission to the extracellular matrix material. Finally, parallel and series connections between muscle fibers allow radial and longitudinal forces to converge on the connective tissue matrix. This complex pathway will certainly be the subject of future studies in muscle biology, biomechanics, and physiology.

ACKNOWLEDGMENTS

The UCSD Skeletal Muscle Physiology Laboratory was supported by the Department of Veterans Affairs Rehabilitation Research and Development Program, NIH Grant AR40050, Preferred Medical Products, and the Orthopaedic Research and Education Foundation. We thank Jim Tidball for helpful discussions. We also thank Drs. Robert Bloch, Maureen Price, Lars-Eric Thornell, and Kuan Wang for stimulating discussions and excellent presentations at the 1996 American College of Sports Medicine Meeting in Cincinnati, Ohio. We also thank Dr. Price and Dr. Roger Enoka for their helpful critique of this manuscript. Finally, we acknowledge Drs. Yassemi Capetenaki, Lars-Eric Thornell, and Denise Paulin for providing advance copies of their research manuscripts and Dr. Capetenaki for providing Figure 12.10C.

REFERENCES

1. Adams, M. E., M. H. Butler, T. M. Dwyer, M. F. Peters, A. A. Murnane, and S. C. Froehner. Two forms of mouse syntrophin, a 58kd dystrophin-associated protein, differ in primary structure and tissue distribution. *Neuron* 11:531–540, 1993.
2. Baldi, J. C., and P. J. Reiser. Intermediate filament proteins increase during chronic stimulation of skeletal muscle. *J. Muscle Res. Cell Motil.* 16:587–594, 1995.
3. Banus, M. G., and A. M. Zetlin. The relation of isometric tension to length in skeletal muscle. *J. Cell. Comp. Physiol.* 12:403–410, 1938.
4. Baron, M., M. Davison, P. Jones, and D. Critchley. The sequence of chick alpha-actinin reveals homologies to spectrin and calmodulin. *J. Biol. Chem.* 262:17623–17629, 1987.
5. Becker, B., R. M. Bellin, S. W. Sernett, T. W. Huiatt, and R. M. Robson. Synemin contains the rod domain of intermediate filaments. *Biochem. Biophys. Res. Commun.* 213:796–802, 1995.
6. Bennett, V. Ankyrins: Adaptors between diverse plasma membrane proteins and the cytoplasm. *J. Biol. Chem.* 267:8703–8706, 1992.
7. Blanchard, A., V. Ohanian, and D. Critcheley. The structure and function of alpha-actinin. *J. Muscle Res. Cell Motil.* 10:280–289, 1989.
8. Bodine, S. C., R. R. Roy, E. Eldred, and V. R. Edgerton. Maximal force as a function of anatomical features of motor units in the cat tibialis anterior. *J. Neurophysiol.* 6:1730–1745, 1987.
9. Bodine, S. C., R. R. Roy, D. A. Meadows, R. F. Zernicke, R. D. Sacks, M. Fournier, and V. R. Edgerton. Architectural, histochemical, and contractile characteristics of a unique biarticular muscle: the cat semitendinosus. *J. Neurophysiol.* 48:192–201, 1982.
10. Breckler, J., and E. Lazarides. Isolation of a new high molecular weight protein associated with desmin and vimentin filaments from avian embryonic skeletal muscle. *J. Cell Biol.* 92:795–806, 1982.
11. Burke, R. E., D. N. Levine, P. Tsairis, and F. E. Zajac. Physiological types and histochemical profiles in motor units of the cat gastrocnemius. *J. Physiol. (Lond.)* 234:723–748, 1973.
12. Burridge, K., and J. Feramisco. Microinjection and localization of a 130K protein in living fibroblasts: a relationship to actin and fibronectin. *Cell* 19:587–595, 1980.
13. Campbell, K. P. Three muscular dystrophies: loss of cytoskeletal-extracellular matrix linkage. *Cell* 80:675–679, 1995.
14. Cary, R. B., and M. W. Klymkowsky. Differential organization of desmin and vimentin in muscle is due to differences in their head domains. *J. Cell Biol.* 126:445–456, 1994.
15. Chen, M.-J. C., C.-L. Shih, and K. Wang. Nebulin as an actin zipper: a two-module nebulin fragment promotes actin nucleation and stabilizes actin filaments. *J. Biol. Chem.* 268:20327–20334, 1993.
16. Davis, R. L., H. Weintraub, and A. B. Lasser. Expression of a single transfected cDNA converts fibroblasts to myoblasts. *Cell* 51:987–1000, 1987.
17. Ebashi, S., A. Kodama, and F. Ebashi. Troponin. I. Preparation and physiological function. *J. Biochem.* 64:465–477, 1968.
18. Ebashi, S., K. Maruyama, and M. Endo. *Muscle Contraction: Its Regulatory Mechanisms.* New York: Springer-Verlag, 1980.
19. Edman, K. The relation between sarcomere length and active tension in isolated semitendinosus fibres of the frog. *J. Physiol. (Lond.)* 183:407–417, 1966.
20. Edmonson, D. G., and E. N. Olson. A gene with homology to the myc similarity region of myoD is expressed during myogenesis and is sufficient to activate the muscle differentiation program. *Genes Dev.* 3:628–640, 1989.
21. Eisenberg, B. R. Quantitative ultrastructure of mammalian skeletal muscle. L. D. Peachey, R. H. Adrian, and S. R. Geiger (eds.). *Skeletal Muscle.* Baltimore: American Physiological Society, 1983, pp. 73–112.
22. Foisner, R., F. E. Leichtfried, H. Herrmann, J. V. Small, G. Lawson, and G. Wiche. Cy-

toskeleton-associated plectin: in situ localization, in vitro reconstitution, and binding to immobilized intermediate filament proteins. *J. Cell Biol.* 106:723–733, 1988.

23. Fosiner, R., P. Traub, and G. Wiche. Protein kinase A and C-regulated interaction of plectin with lamin B and vimentin. *Proc. Natl. Acad. Sci. U. S. A.* 88:3812–3816, 1991.

24. Fowler, V. Identification and purification of a novel Mr 43,000 tropomyosin-binding protein from human erythrocyte membranes. *J. Biol. Chem.* 262:12792–12800, 1987.

25. Fowler, V. Tropomodulin: a cytoskeletal protein that binds to the end of erythrocyte tropomyosin and inhibits tropomyosin binding to actin. *J. Cell Biol.* 111:471–482, 1990.

26. Fridén, J., and R. L. Lieber. Structural and mechanical basis of exercise-induced muscle injury. *Med. Sci. Sports Exerc.* 24:521–530, 1992.

27. Fridén, J., M. Sjostrom, and B. Ekblom. A morphological study of delayed muscle soreness. *Experientia* 37:506–507, 1981.

28. Funatsu, T., and S. Ishiwata. Characterization of beta-actinin: a suppressor of the elongation at the pointed end of thin filaments in skeletal muscle. *J. Biochem.* 98:535–544, 1985.

29. Gans, C., and W. J. Bock. The functional significance of muscle architecture: a theoretical analysis. *Ergeb. Anat. Entwicklungsgesch. (Berl.)* 38:115–142, 1965.

30. Garfinkel, L. I., M. Periasamy, and B. Nadal-Ginard. Cloning and characterization of cDNA sequences corresponding to myosin light chains 1, 2, and 3, troponin-C, α-tropomyosin, and α-actin. *J. Biol. Chem.* 257:11078–11086, 1982.

31. Geiger, B. A 130K protein from chicken gizzard: its localization at the termini of microfilament bundles in cultured chicken cells. *Cell* 18:193–205, 1979.

32. Geiger, B., K. Tokuyasu, A. Dutton, and S. Singer. Vinculin, an intracellular protein localized at specialized sites where microfilament bundles terminate at cell membranes. *Proc. Natl. Acad. Sci. U. S. A.* 77:4127–4131, 1980.

33. Gerace, L., and G. Blobel. The nuclear envelope lamina is reversibly depolymerized during mitosis. *Cell* 19:277–287, 1980.

34. Gonzalez-Serratos, H. Inward spread of activation in vertebrate muscle fibers. *J. Physiol. (Lond.)* 212:777–799, 1971.

35. Gordon, A. M., A. F. Huxley, and F. J. Julian. The variation in isometric tension with sarcomere length in vertebrate muscle fibres. *J. Physiol. (Lond.)* 184:170–192, 1966.

36. Gordon, T., C. K. Thomas, R. B. Stein, and S. Erdebil. Comparison of physiological and histochemical properties of motor units after cross-reinnervation of antagonistic muscles in the cat hindlimb. *J. Neurophysiol.* 60:365–378, 1988.

37. Granger, B., and E. Lazarides. Synemin: a new high molecular weight protein associated with desmin and vimentin filaments in muscle. *Cell* 22:727–738, 1980.

38. Grove, B. K., V. Kurer, C. Lehner, T. C. Doetschman, J. C. Perriard, and H. M. Eppenberger. A new 185,000-dalton skeletal muscle protein detected by monoclonal antibodies. *J. Cell Biol.* 98:518–524, 1984.

39. Hill, C. S., S. Duran, Z. Lin, K. Weber, and H. Holtzer. Titin and myosin, but not desmin are linked during myofibrillogenesis in postmitotic mononucleated myoblasts. *J. Cell Biol.* 103:2185–2196, 1986.

40. Hoffman, E., and L. M. Kunkel. Dystrophin abnormalities in Duchenne/Becker muscular dystrophy. *Neuron* 2:1019–1029, 1989.

41. Hoffman, E. P., R. H. Brown, and L. M. Kunkel. Conservation of the Duchenne muscular dystrophy gene in mice and humans. *Science* 238:347–350, 1987.

42. Hofmann, P., M. Greaser, and M. Moss. C-protein limits shortening velocity of rabbit skeletal muscle fibers at low levels of calcium ion activation. *J. Physiol. (Lond.)* 439:701–715, 1991.

43. Horowits, R., E. S. Kempner, M. F. Bisher, and R. J. Podolsky. A physiological role for titin and nebulin in skeletal muscle. *Nature* 323:160–164, 1986.

44. Horowits, R., and R. J. Podolsky. The positional stability of thick filaments in activated skeletal muscle depends on sarcomere length: evidence for the role of titan filaments. *J. Cell Biol.* 105:2217–2223, 1987.

45. Huijing, P. A., and G. C. Baan. Stimulation level-dependent length-force and architectural characteristics of rat gastrocnemius muscle. *J. Electromyogr. Kinesiol.* 2:112–120, 1992.

46. Jockusch, B. M., P. Bubeck, K. Giehl, M. Kroemker, M. Rothkegel, M. Rüdiger, K. Schlüter, G. Stanke, and J. Winkler. The molecular architecture of focal adhesions. *Annu. Rev. Cell Dev. Biol.* 11:379–416, 1995.

47. Julian, F. J., and D. L. Morgan. The effect on tension of non-uniform distribution of length changes applied to frog muscle fibres. *J. Physiol. (Lond.)* 293:379–392, 1979.

48. Kaufman, S. J., and R. F. Foster. Replicating myoblasts express a muscle-specific phenotype. *Proc. Natl. Acad. Sci. U. S. A.* 85:9605–9610, 1988.

49. Koenig, M., A. P. Monaco, and L. M. Kunkel. The complete sequence of dystrophin predicts a rod-shaped cytoskeletal protein. *Cell* 53:219–228, 1988.

50. Kruger, M., J. Wright, and K. Wang. Nebulin as a thin length regulator of thin filaments of vertebrate skeletal muscles: correlation of thin filament length, nebulin size, and epitope profile. *J. Cell Biol.* 107:2199–2212, 1988.

51. Kuroda, M., and K. Maruyama. Gamma-actinin, a new regulatory protein from rabbit skeletal muscle. I. Purification and characterization. *J. Biochem.* 80:315–322, 1976.

52. Kuroda, M., T. Tanaka, and T. Masaki. Eu-actinin, a new structural protein of the Z-line of striated muscles. *J. Biochem.* 89:297–310, 1981.

53. Labeit, S., T. Gibson, A. Lakey, K. Leonard, M. Zeviani, P. Knight, J. Wardale, and J. Trinick. Evidence that nebulin is a protein-ruler in muscle thin filaments. *FEBS Lett.* 282:313–316, 1991.

54. Labeit, S., and B. Kolmerer. Titins: giant proteins in charge of muscle ultrastructure and elasticity. *Science* 270:293–296, 1995.

55. Lazarides, E. Intermediate filaments as mechanical integrators of cellular space. *Nature* 283:249–256, 1980.

56. Li, H., S. K. Choudhary, D. J. Milner, M. I. Munir, I. R. Kuisk, and Y. Capetanaki. Inhibition of desmin expression blocks myoblasts fusion and interferes with the myogenic regulators myoD and myogenin. *J. Cell Biol.* 124:827–841, 1994.

57. Li, Z., E. Colucci-Guyon, M. Picon-Raymond, M. Mericskay, S. Pourmin, D. Paulin, and C. Babinet. Cardiac lesions and skeletal myopathy in mice lacking desmin. *Dev. Biol.* 175:362–366, 1996.

58. Lieber, R. L., and J. Fridén. Selective damage of fast glycolytic muscle fibers with eccentric contraction of the rabbit tibialis anterior. *Acta Physiol. Scand.* 133:587–588, 1988.

59. Lieber, R. L., T. McKee-Woodburn, and J. Fridén. Muscle damage induced by eccentric contractions of 25% strain. *J. Appl. Physiol.* 70:2498–2507, 1991.

60. Lieber, R. L., L. E. Thornell, and J. Fridén. Muscle cytoskeletal disruption occurs within the first 15 minutes of cyclic eccentric contraction. *J. Appl. Physiol.* 80:278–284, 1996.

61. Loeb, G. E., C. A. Pratt, C. M. Chanaud, and F. J. R. Richmond. Distribution and innervation of short, interdigitated muscle fibers in parallel-fibered muscles of the cat hindlimb. *J. Morphol.* 191:1–15, 1987.

62. Magid, A., and D. J. Law. Myofibrils bear most of the resting tension in frog skeletal muscle. *Science* 230:1280–1282, 1985.

63. Maruyama, K., A. Matusno, H. Higuchi, S. Shimaoka, S. Kimura, and T. Shimuzu. Behavior of connectin (titin) and nebulin in skinned muscle fibres released after extreme stretch as revealed by immunoelectron microscopy. *J. Muscle Res. Cell Motil.* 10:350–359, 1989.

64. Masaki, T., and O. Takaiti. M-protein. *J. Biochem.* 75:367–380, 1974.

65. McKeon, F. D., M. W. Kirschner, and D. Caput. Homologies in both primary and secondary structure between nuclear envelope and intermediate filament proteins. *Nature* 319:463–468, 1986.

66. Milner, D. J., G. Weitzer, D. Tran, A. Bradley, and Y. Capetanaki. Disruption of muscle architecture and myocardial degeneration in mice lacking desmin. *J. Cell Biol.* 134:1255–1270, 1996.

67. Obinata, T., K. Maruyama, H. Sugita, K. Kohama, and S. Ebashi. Dynamic aspects of structural proteins in vertebrate skeletal muscle. *Muscle Nerve* 4:456–488, 1981.
68. Offer, G., C. Moos, and R. Starr. A new protein of the thick filaments of vertebrate skeletal myofibrils: extractions, purification and characterization. *J. Mol. Biol.* 74:653–676, 1973.
69. Ohashi, K., T. Mikawa, and K. Maruyama. Localization of Z-protein in isolated Z-disk sheets of chicken leg muscle. *J. Cell Biol.* 95:85–90, 1982.
70. Ohashi, K., M. Tsuneoka, and K. Maruyama. I-protein is localized at the junctional region of A-bands and I-bands of chicken fresh myofibrils. *J. Biochem.* 97:1323–1328, 1985.
71. Ohlendieck, K., J. M. Ervasti, J. B. Snook, and K. P. Campbell. Dystrophin-glycoprotein complex is highly enriched in isolated skeletal muscle sarcolemma. *J. Cell Biol.* 112:135–148, 1991.
72. Ounjian, M., R. R. Roy, E. Eldred, A. Garfinkel, J. R. Payne, A. Armstrong, A. W. Toga, and V. R. Edgerton. Physiological and developmental implications of motor unit anatomy. *J. Neurobiol.* 22:547–559, 1991.
73. Pardo, J. V., J. D. Siliciano, and S. W. Craig. Vinculin is a component of an extensive network of myofibril-sarcolemma attachment regions in cardiac muscle fibers. *J. Cell Biol.* 97:1081–1088, 1983.
74. Pardo, J. V., J. D. Siliciano, and S. W. Craig. A vinculin-containing cortical lattice in skeletal muscle: transverse lattice elements ("costameres") mark sites of attachment between myofibrils and sarcolemma. *Proc. Natl. Acad. Sci. U. S. A.* 80:1008–1012, 1983.
75. Petit, J., G. M. Filippi, C. Emonet-Dénand, C. C. Hunt, and Y. Laporte. Changes in muscle stiffness produced by motor units of different types in peroneus longus muscles of cat. *J. Neurophysiol.* 63:190–197, 1990.
76. Petit, J., G. M. Filippi, C. Gioux, C. C. Hunt, and Y. Laporte. Effects of tetanic contraction of motor units of similar type on the initial stiffness to ramp stretch of the cat peroneus longus muscle. *J. Neurophysiol.* 64:1724–1731, 1990.
77. Petrof, B. J., J. B. Shrager, H. H. Stedman, A. M. Kelly, and H. L. Sweeney. Dystrophin protects the sarcolemma from stresses developed during muscle contraction. *Proc. Natl. Acad. Sci. U. S. A.* 90:3710–3714, 1993.
78. Pierobon-Bormioli, S., R. Betto, and G. Salviati. The organization of titin (connectin) and nebulin in the sarcomeres: an immunocytolocalization study. *J. Muscle Res. Cell Motil.* 10:446–456, 1989.
79. Powell, P. L., R. R. Roy, P. Kanim, M. Bello, and V. R. Edgerton. Predictability of skeletal muscle tension from architectural determinations in guinea pig hindlimbs. *J. Appl. Physiol.* 57:1715–1721, 1984.
80. Price, M., and E. Lazarides. Expression of intermediate filament-associated proteins paranemin and synemin in chicken development. *J. Cell Biol.* 97:1860–1874, 1983.
81. Price, M. G. Skelemins: cytoskeletal proteins located at the periphery of M-discs in mammalian striated muscle. *J. Cell Biol.* 104.1325–1336, 1987.
82. Price, M. G., and R. H. Gomer. Skelemins, a cytoskeletal M-disc periphery protein, contains motifs of adhesion/recognition and intermediate filament proteins. *J. Biol. Chem.* 268:21800–21810, 1993.
83. Price, M. G., and E. Lazarides. Expression of intermediate filament-associated proteins paranemin and synemin in chicken development. *J. Cell Biol.* 97:1860–1874, 1983.
84. Ramsey, R. W., and S. F. Street. The isometric length-tension diagram of isolated skeletal muscle fibers of the frog. *J. Cell Comp. Physiol.* 15:11–34, 1940.
85. Rodriguez Fernandez, J. L., B. Geiger, D. Salomon, and A. Ben-Ze'ev. Suppression of vinculin expression by antisense transfection confers changes in cell morphology, motility and anchorage-dependent growth of 3T3 cells. *J. Cell Biol.* 122:1285–1294, 1993.
86. Root, D. D., and K. Wang. Calmodulin-sensitive interaction of human nebulin fragments with actin and myosin. *Biochemistry* 33:12581–12591, 1994.
87. Ruoslahti, E., and M. D. Pierschbacher. New perspectives in cell adhesion: RGD and integrins. *Science* 238:491–497, 1987.

88. Sacks, R. D., and R. R. Roy. Architecture of the hindlimb muscles of cats: functional significance. *J. Morphol.* 173:185–195, 1982.

89. Schultheiss, T., Z. Lin, H. Ishikawa, I. Zamir, C. J. Stoeckert, and H. Holtzer. Desmin/vimentin intermediate filaments are dispensable for many aspects of myogenesis. *J. Cell Biol.* 114:953–966, 1991.

90. Small, J. V. Geometry of actin-membrane attachments in the smooth muscle cell: the localisations of vinculin and alpha-actinin. *EMBO J.* 4:45–49, 1985.

91. Spector, S. A., P. F. Gardiner, R. F. Zernicke, R. R. Roy, and V. R. Edgerton. Muscle architecture and force-velocity characteristics of the cat soleus and medial gastrocnemius: Implications for motor control. *J. Neurophysiol.* 44:951–960, 1980.

92. Street, S. F. Lateral transmission of tension in frog myofibers: a myofibrillar network and transverse cytoskeletal connections are possible transmitters. *J. Cell Physiol.* 114:346–364, 1983.

93. Takahashi, K., F. Nakamura, A. Hattori, and M. Yamanoue. Paratropomyosin: a new myofibrillar protein that modifies the actin-myosin interaction in postrigor skeletal muscle. I. Preparation and characterization. *J. Biochem.* 97(4):1043–1051, 1985.

94. Thornell, L.-E., and M. G. Price. The cytoskeleton in muscle cells in relation to function. *Biochem. Soc. Trans.* 19:1116–1120, 1991.

95. Tidball, J., T. O'Halloran, and K. Burridge. Talin at myotendinous junctions. *J. Cell Biol.* 103:1465–1472, 1986.

96. Tidball, J. G. Myonexin: An 80-kDa glycoprotein that binds fibronectin and is located at embryonic myotendinous junctions. *Dev. Biol.* 142:103–114, 1990.

97. Tidball, J. G., and T. L. Daniel. Myotendinous junctions of tonic muscle cells: structure and loading. *Cell Tissue Res.* 245:315–322, 1986.

98. Tidball, J. G., G. Salem, and R. Zernicke. Site and mechanical conditions for failure of skeletal muscle in experimental strain injuries. *J. Appl. Physiol.* 74:1280–1286, 1993.

99. Traub, P., and R. L. Shoeman. Intermediate filament proteins: cytoskeletal elements with gene-regulatory function? *Int. Rev. Cytol.* 154:1–103, 1994.

100. Trotter, J. A. Interfiber tension transmission in series-fibered muscles of the cat hindlimb. *J. Morphol.* 206:351–361, 1990.

101. Trotter, J. A., K. Corbett, and B. P. Avner. Structure and function of the murine muscle-tendon junction. *Anat. Rec.* 201:293–302, 1981.

102. Trotter, J. A., S. Eberhard, and A. Samora. Structural connections of the muscle-tendon junction. *Cell Motil.* 3:431–438, 1983.

103. Trotter, J. A., and P. P. Purslow. Functional morphology of the endomysium in series fibered muscles. *J. Morphol.* 212:109–122, 1992.

104. Turner, C., J. Glenney, and K. Burridge Paxillin: a new vinculin-binding protein present in focal adhesions. *J. Cell Biol.* 111:1059–1068, 1990.

105. Ungar, F., B. Geiger, and A. Ben-Ze'ev. Cell contact- and shape-dependent regulation of vinculin synthesis in cultured fibroblasts. *Nature* 319:787–791, 1986.

106. Vikstrom, K. L., S.-S. Lim, R. D. Goldman, and C. G. Borisy. Steady state dynamics of intermediate filament networks. *J. Cell Biol.* 118:121–129, 1992.

107. Wallimann, T., T. Schlosser, and H. M. Eppenberger. Function of M-line-bound creatine kinase as intramyofibrillar ATP regenerator at the receiving end of phosphorylcreatine shuttle in muscle. *J. Biol. Chem.* 259:5238–5246, 1984.

108. Wallimann, T., D. C. Turner, and H. M. Eppenberger. Localization of creatine kinase isoenzymes in myofibrils. I. Chicken skeletal muscle. *J. Cell Biol.* 75:297–317, 1977.

109. Walmsley, B., J. A. Hodgson, and R. E. Burke. Forces produced by medial gastrocnemius and soleus muscles during locomotion in freely moving cats. *J. Neurophysiol.* 41:1203–1216, 1978.

110. Walmsley, B., and U. Proske. Comparison of stiffness of soleus and medial gastrocnemius muscles in cats. *J. Neurophysiol.* 46:250–259, 1981.

111. Wang, K., M. Knipfer, Q.-Q. Huang, A. van Heerden, L. Hsu, G. Gutierrez, Z.-L. Quian,

and H. Stedman. Human skeletal muscle nebulin sequence encodes a blueprint for thin filament architecture. *J. Biol. Chem.* 271:4304–4314, 1996.

112. Wang, K., R. McCarter, J. Wright, J. Beverly, and R. Ramirez-Mitchell. Viscoelasticity of the sarcomere matrix of skeletal muscles: The titin-myosin composite filament is a dual-stage molecular spring. *Biophys. J.* 64:1161–1177, 1993.

113. Wang, K., and R. Ramirez-Mitchell. A network of transverse and longitudinal intermediate filaments is associated with sarcomeres of adult vertebrate skeletal muscle. *J. Cell Biol.* 96:562–570, 1983.

114. Weitzer, G., D. J. Milner, J.-U Kim, A. Bradley, and Y. Capetenaki. Cytoskeletal control of myogenesis: a desmin null mutation blocks the myogenic pathway during embryonic stem cell differentiation. *Dev. Biol.* 172:422–439, 1995.

115. Westerblad, H., and D. G. Allen. The influence of intracellular pH on contraction, relaxation and $[Ca^{2+}]_i$ in intact single fibres from mouse muscle. *J. Physiol. (Lond.)* 466:611–628, 1993.

116. Wiche, G., and M. A. Baker. Cytoplasmic network arrays demonstrated by immunolocalization using antibodies to a high molecular weight protein present in cytoskeletal preparations from cultured cells. *Exp. Cell Res.* 138:15–29, 1982.

117. Wiche, G., B. Becker, K. Luber, G. Weitzer, M. J. Castanon, R. Hauptmann, C. Stratowa, and M. Stewart. Cloning and sequencing of rat plectin indicates a 466-kD polypeptide chain with a three-domain structure based on a central alpha-helical coiled coil. *J. Cell Biol.* 114:83–99, 1991.

118. Wiche, G., D. Gromov, A. Donovan, M. J. Castanon, and E. Fuchs. Expression of plectin mutant cDNA in cultured cells indicates a role of COOH-terminal domain intermediate filament association. *J. Cell Biol.* 121:607–619, 1993.

119. Wiche, G., R. Krepler, U. Artlieb, R. Pytela, and W. Aberer. Identification of plectin in different human cell types and immunolocalization at basal cell surface membranes. *Exp. Cell Res.* 155:43–49, 1984.

120. Wright, J., Q.-Q. Huang, and K. Wang. Nebulin is a full-length template of actin filaments in the skeletal muscle sarcomere: an immunoelectron microscopic study of it orientation and span with site-specific monoclonal antibodies. *J. Muscle Res. Cell Motil.* 14:476–483, 1993.

121. Yates, L. D., and M. L. Greaser. Quantitative determination of myosin and actin in rabbit skeletal muscle. *J. Mol. Biol.* 168:123–141, 1983.

13
Baroreflex Regulation of Blood Pressure during Dynamic Exercise

PETER B. RAVEN, Ph.D.
JEFFREY T. POTTS, Ph.D.
XIANGRONG SHI, Ph.D.

At the onset of dynamic exercise, arterial blood pressure (ABP) transiently decreases below preexercise pressures within the first 15–20 s and subsequently increases over the next 20–30 s of exercise to a level that exceeds resting blood pressure (Fig. 13.1). As exercise continues, mean arterial pressure increases linearly with increases in work rate, whereas systolic blood pressure increases markedly and diastolic blood pressure falls slightly (Fig. 13.2). The mechanisms that the human body uses to produce these characteristic changes in blood pressure have both intrigued and puzzled physiologists and exercise physiologists for over a century [21, 84]. Today, it is well accepted that there are two neural control mechanisms that are activated during exercise to mediate this characteristic response in ABP.

The first control mechanism is referred to as Central Command and involves descending neural signals from motor centers in the brain that recruit skeletal muscle to contract and, in a parallel fashion, activate brainstem centers that control autonomic neural outflow directed to the cardiovascular system. This mechanism is regarded as a feed-forward control system [39, 40, 56, 58, 76]. The second control mechanism originates from active skeletal muscle, in which metabolic and mechanical activation of receptors found in skeletal muscle elicit neural signals that are carried to cardiovascularly related sites in the brainstem by Groups III and IV muscle afferent fibers [19, 34, 43, 56, 58]. This mechanism is regarded as a feedback control mechanism. The efferent limb of this skeletal muscle reflex has also been shown to determine the degree of activation of the respiratory and cardiovascular systems [19, 41]. The cardiovascular response elicited by activation of skeletal muscle receptors has been referred to by McCloskey and Mitchell [34] as the "exercise pressor reflex." Another regulatory mechanism which involves sensing the level of ABP and central venous filling pressure by means of a group of mechanically sensitive receptors called arterial and cardiopulmonary baroreceptors, respectively [31, 33, 59], has only been accepted as playing a role in the control of ABP during exercise [45, 50, 51, 61,

FIGURE 13.1.

A schematic representation of the initial (0–30 s) hemodynamic responses during the onset of dynamic exercise. Note the initial (0 to 10 s) drop in MAP. Q_c, cardiac output; PRU, peripheral resistance units.

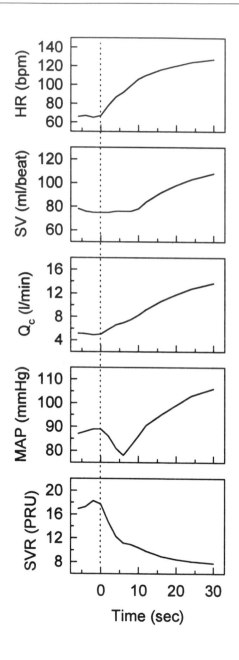

FIGURE 13.2.

A schematic representation of the overall hemodynamic responses to progressively increasing workload during dynamic exercise. HR and cardiac output (Q) increase linearly with increasing workload. SV reaches a plateau at approximately 40% of maximal oxygen uptake (VO₂) and SVR decreases with the progressively increasing workload. ABP is a resultant of the hemodynamic response, i.e., of the variables that result in the arterial pressure (pressure = resistance × flow). The systolic blood pressure (S) increases markedly and linearly with the increasing workload. Diastolic blood pressure (D) decreases slightly with increasing workload and, as a result, mean blood pressure (M) increases moderately with the increasing workload.

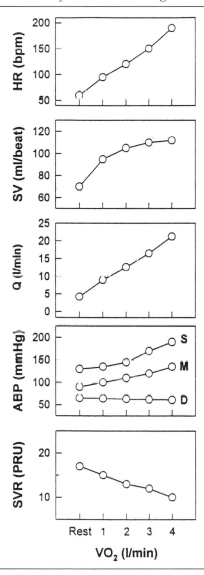

68]. At rest, these baroreceptor populations function as a classical negative feedback controller and are critical in the short-term, moment-to-moment regulation of ABP. Despite the intense investigation of baroreflex control of blood pressure over the past several decades [59], controversy rages on regarding the functional role of these baroreceptor populations during exercise. This debate has been fueled by the finding that after the onset of dynamic exercise, both heart rate (HR) and blood pressure increase in a somewhat parallel fashion. If the baroreflex system functions as a negative feedback control mechanism, then directionally analogous changes in HR and blood pressure should not occur, unless the baroreceptor reflex systems have been somehow altered or inhibited by the exercise.

The arterial blood pressure (ABP) is an outcome measure of three physiological variables, HR, stroke volume (SV), and total peripheral resistance (TPR), and their relationship is expressed as follows:

$$ABP = HR \times SV \times TPR \dots\dots\dots\dots\dots\dots\dots\dots\dots (I)$$

Arterial baroreflex function responds to changes in ABP by affecting the three physiological variables, HR, SV, and TPR. However, the resultant reflex changes have recently been shown to be greatly affected by the systemic arterial compliance [48]. Another set of baroreceptors, the cardiopulmonary baroreceptors, appears to have additional reflex control of TPR by primarily reflexly affecting limb vasculature, which in turn affects cardiac filling volumes [16]. In addition, cardiac filling appears to be directly responsive to arterial (carotid and aortic) baroreflex regulation of the venous capacitance [55, 69]. When humans are at rest, in either the supine or upright position, increases or decreases in mean ABP are sensed by the carotid and arotic baroreceptors and result in a reflex bradycardia and peripheral vasodilation and venodilation and a reflex tachycardia and peripheral vasoconstriction and venoconstriction, respectively [59]. The cardiopulmonary baroreceptors appear to be sensitive to changes in cardiac filling volume and reflexly cause peripheral vasodilation in the limbs during increases in central venous pressure (CVP, an indirect index of cardiac filling volume) and peripheral vasoconstriction in the limbs during decreases in CVP [33] (Fig. 13.3). The cardiopulmonary baroreceptor reflex (CPBR)-mediated responses have a selective range of response of approximately -4 mm Hg to $+2$ mm Hg that occurs without arterial baroreflex perturbation [67]. Despite the intense investigation of baroreflex control of blood pressure during rest, orthostasis and hypotension [59], which identify a reciprocal relationship between HR and vasomotor function with increases or decreases in mean arterial pressure (MAP), the absence of a reflex bradycardia and peripheral vasodilation in an exercise-induced increase in MAP and pulse pressure (Fig. 13.2) remains a

FIGURE 13.3.

These data identify the relationship between the changes in FVR that occur with decreases in CVP by 0 to − 20 torr LBNP and the increases in CVP induced by leg elevation (50 cm) plus LBPP (up to +20 torr). FVR, − 2.31 units/ mm Hg +44, R^2 = 0.96, N = 8. Modified from refs. 67 and 68.

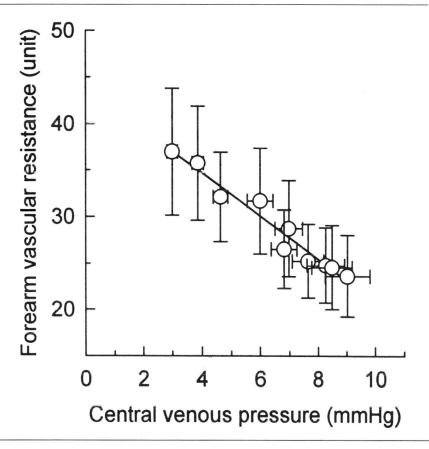

mystery that has intrigued many investigators over the years [2, 3, 5, 6, 8, 9, 11, 23, 25, 31, 38, 47, 54, 70, 72, 79, 80].

In this presentation we will summarize the information available to us concerning arterial and CPBR-mediated reflex regulation of ABP during dynamic exercise performed by humans. First, we will discuss the functional roles that the high-pressure carotid sinus and aortic baroreceptor reflexes play in the regulation of HR and arterial pressure during dynamic exercise. Secondly, we will discuss some of the findings from investigations that have examined the cardiovascular effects of selectively altering cardiopulmonary baroreceptors, with specific emphasis on regional changes in peripheral vascular resistance and efferent sympathetic nerve activity. Thirdly, we will attempt to summarize what is currently known of the functional interaction between the cardiopulmonary baroreflex and the carotid sinus baroreceptor reflex, both at rest and during dynamic exercise. Finally, we will conclude this presentation by discussing the potential interaction(s) that these three baroreceptor populations may have with "Central Command" and skeletal muscle reflexes. Where possible, we will integrate the data from animal models to provide a more in-depth and complete explanation of the neural mechanisms involved.

CAROTID BAROREFLEX

The carotid sinus baroreceptor reflex is a neural reflex arc consisting of unencapsulated free nerve-endings embedded in the walls of the internal carotid arteries at the carotid sinus bifurcation [59, 62]. These receptors are sensitive to mechanical deformation caused by changes in blood pressure in this region. When blood pressure increases, these receptors increase their firing rate and, in turn, alter the autonomic neural outflow to the heart and the peripheral circulation. These changes in sympathetic and parasympathetic efferent outflow will affect both the heart and the blood vessels in such a fashion as to return blood pressure to its original pressure. Thus, the carotid sinus baroreflex represents a rapidly responding mechanism that will always regulate blood pressure around some fixed value. This fixed value is the ABP (perfusion pressure), which is required to deliver oxygen and substrates to the major organ systems of the body (Fig. 13.4).

In 1957, Ernsting and Parry [12] developed a neck pressure/suction technique that, although cumbersome, allowed investigators to stimulate the carotid sinus baroreceptors selectively in humans while isolating the aortic and cardiopulmonary baroreceptors [23–28]. In 1966 Bevegard and Shephard [2] investigated the effects of neck suction during supine cycle ergometry. They reported a reflex decrease in HR and blood pressure that was similar during rest and exercise and concluded that the carotid baroreflex regulation of blood pressure was unaltered during exercise. Subsequently, throughout the 1970s several investigations using an infusion of the vasoactive drugs, phenylephrine and nitroprusside [3, 31, 47], as well as a more recent study using neck pressure and suction [70], evaluated the carotid and arterial (aortic and carotid) baroreceptor-mediated reflex control of HR by estimating changes in function from reflex changes in R-R interval. This approach of assessing baroreflex function consistently found that the sensitivity of the reflex to producing a change in HR was reduced during exercise. Unfortunately, these conclusions were biased by the nonlinear relation between HR and R-R interval [43, 68] in such a way that when baseline HR was elevated by exercise, the chronotropic changes to

FIGURE 13.4.

A schematic representation of the baroreflex function curve. A_1 is the difference between the response at threshold and the response at saturation, i.e., the responding range; A_2 is the coefficient of the slope of the function curve; A_3 is the point at which there is an equal depressor and pressor response to a given change in pressure, i.e., the centering point pressure; A_4 is the minimal response to the saturation pressure of the reflex, where no further response is elicited with a further increase in pressure. Thr. is the carotid sinus transmural pressure at the threshold of the reflex, and Sat. is the carotid sinus transmural pressure at the saturation of the reflex. The difference between Thr. and Sat. is the operating range of the reflex. The operating point of the reflex is the point at which the MAP is located on the reflex function curve.

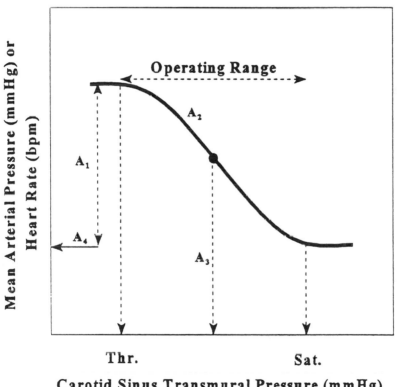

baroreflex activation were always less when these changes were expressed in R-R interval, compared to when they were expressed as a change in HR.

The concerns regarding these issues have been long-standing [43, 57] and have recently been readdressed by Potts et al. [49, 51] and Raven et al. [53]. In short, there are major methodological issues to be addressed when eval-

FIGURE 13.5.

A summary of the data from one subject from the experiments of Potts et al. [49, 51], demonstrating the reproducibility of the stimulus response to +40 torr NP and − 80 torr neck suction NS (left panel). On the right panel is the summary of the HR response data obtained from the same subject, using the [49, 51] protocol of Potts et al. of 5-s pulse at +40 and +20 torr NP and − 20, − 40, − 60, and − 80 torr NS within a discrete 10 s of breath hold at rest.

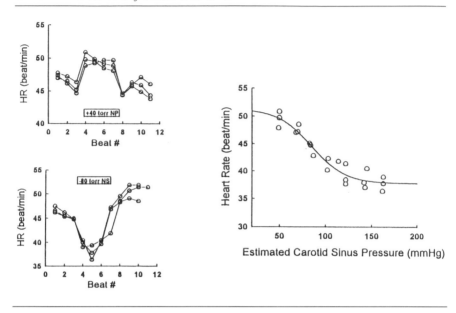

uating arterial baroreflex function during exercise, especially when one wishes to provide reproducible data from which he or she can describe a complete reflex function curve (Fig. 13.5). These issues include (a) sustained neck pressure or suction of greater than 5–10 s will compromise the selectivity of the carotid baroreflex response because the aortic baroreceptors will be activated and, subsequently, will counteract the reflex changes in ABP; (b) the use of vasoactive drugs (phenylephrine and nitroprusside) will activate both aortic and carotid baroreceptor regions, as well as prevent the evaluation of the vasomotor response of the reflex; (c) the use of changes in the R-R interval will bias the interpretation of the reflex response because of the nonlinear mathematical relationship between R-R interval and HR [43, 53, 57, 58]. (d) The effective neural response time of the carotid-cardiac baroreflex has been reported to remain unchanged during exercise, regardless of the baseline HR [49]. However, with increasing exercise intensity, HR increases (R-R interval decreases), and the interbeat interval begins to approach the neural latency of the baroreflex arc. As a result, the reflex chronotropic response to baroreflex activation is achieved over a larger number of heart beats during exercise, compared to those during rest. This effect of an elevation in baseline HR negates the use of pulse-synchronous changes in neck chamber pressure to evaluate carotid baroreflex function during exercise; (e) the increased sympathetic tone associated with exercise inhibits vagal neural transmissions that may modulate carotid cardiac reflex responses [83].

In order to account for these methodological concerns, Potts et al. [51] developed a 5-s period of neck pressure or suction (NP/NS) stimulus during a 10-s breath-hold period during rest and exercise over a range of NP/NS pressures from +40 to −80 torr. The advantages of such an approach include the following: (a) the breath hold removes the possibility of the reflex response being affected by respiration-related fluctuations in ABP, (b) the peak reflex response of HR and arterial pressure are unaffected by the baseline HR; (c) the brief period of stimulation obviated any counter response emanating from extracarotid (aortic and cardiopulmonary) baroreceptors; and importantly, (d) the reflex response is extremely reproducible, especially for HR, and enables the collection of data that fits the modeling procedures necessary to identify the established parameters of the reflex curve (Fig. 13.5) [20]. However, because the breath-hold maneuver cannot be sustained during heavy exercise without activating chemoreceptor and somatopressor reflexes, the workloads evaluated can only be light-to-moderate (25% $\dot{V}O_2$max and 50% $\dot{V}O_2$max). Another limitation is that the brief nature of the stimulus will result in an attenuation of the magnitude of the changes in arterial pressure (when used as an index of carotid vasomotor response), because a 20- to 40-s stimulus is required to establish the complete sympathetically mediated neural response [59]. Estimations of the carotid vasomotor reflex can be assessed from the mean blood pressure response to the NP/NS protocol, because the peak HR response occurs within the first 2 s and has returned to baseline levels at the time the peak blood pressure response occurs (Fig. 13.6). As the brief period of NP does not elicit significant changes in SV [??], the peak changes in blood pressure produced by this protocol are felt to be a function of changes in vasomotor tone and have been used successfully to model the carotid-vasomoter reflex [51].

Having accounted for most of the methodological problems described previously, Potts et al. [51] investigated the functional role of the carotid baroreflex at rest and during 25 and 50% $\dot{V}O_2$max. The investigators built the stimulus-response (S-R) function curves for the carotid baroreflex at rest and during exercise at mild and moderate work intensities. They found that the S-R function curves were systematically shifted to the higher levels of ABP associated with each exercise intensity. The data obtained clearly suggest that both the carotid-cardiac (HR) and the carotid-vasomotor (BP) reflex responses were reset to functionally operate at the prevailing pressure elicited by the exercise workload (Fig. 13.7). This is the first clear evi-

FIGURE 13.6.

The panels on the left and right illustrate the reflex HR (open circle) and blood pressure (closed circle) responses (represented as percent change from baseline) to 5 s of NP (+40 torr) and suction (− 80 torr), followed by 5 s of neck chamber pressure at 0 torr during a held expiration in a single subject at rest. There are three important points illustrated here: (a) During the first 5 s of NP/suction HR and blood pressure change (although apparently at different rates), the change in HR will alter cardiac output, which in turn can account for the change in blood pressure during this period, as SV remains constant [22]. (b) However, this does not explain the persistent change in blood pressure during the latter 5 s of the breath-hold period when HR has returned or is returning toward baseline. (c) The peak changes in HR occur consistently before the peak change in blood pressure (peak responses are indicated by the arrowheads). This phasic lag between the peak responses in HR and blood pressure indicates that changes in some variable other than cardiac output (i.e., PVR) must have occurred to produce the changes in blood pressure during the latter 5 s of this period. Also, although not illustrated here, these changes in blood pressure were not a function of the passive effects of the breath-hold maneuver.

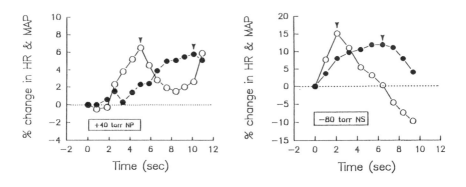

dence in humans that the carotid baroreflex was reset during dynamic exercise and that this reflex functioned to regulate HR and ABP with the same sensitivity as has been previously reported at rest. Subsequently, Papelier et al. [45] investigated greater exercise workloads and confirmed these initial findings.

The concept of the resetting of the baroreceptor at the onset of exercise has been tested earlier by DiCarlo and Bishop [8]. Intravenous infusion of nitroglycerin was used to attenuate the exercise-related increase in ABP while recording efferent renal sympathetic nerve activity (RSNA) in rabbits exercising on a treadmill. When the rabbits exercised during nitroglycerin infusion the level of RSNA evoked by exercise was increased. These data have been used as evidence that the arterial baroreceptor reflex was reset immediately on the start of exercise, which created a pressure error signal

FIGURE 13.7.

Parallel resetting. A schematic representation of the findings of Potts et al. [51] The significant increase in threshold and saturation pressures, with no change in the maximal gain of the reflex from rest to exercise, is evidence of resetting. This resetting occurred to the increased pressure of the exercise and upward to the greater response variable value induced by the exercise, and it is regarded as parallel resetting. The circle (●) represents the operating point of the reflex and the roman numerals (i, ii, iii) represent the progressive shift in operating point from rest to exercise.

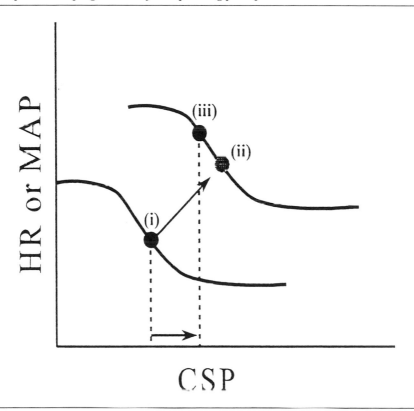

and resulted in the greater increase in RSNA. Furthermore, the short time-course of this effect suggests that resetting of the baroreflex may be mediated by a feed-forward mechanism, which does not require an error signal (i.e., "Central Command"). Clearly, the problem that remains is to delineate the mechanism(s) that is (are) responsible for the resetting of the arterial baroreflex at the onset of exercise.

Another finding arising from the modeling work of Potts et al. [51] is that the prestimulus steady state mean arterial blood pressure (the "operating" or "set" point pressure) is located very near the centering point of the baroreflex curve at rest; however, during exercise this point is reestablished above the centering point at a pressure near the threshold of the reflex curve (Fig. 13.7). It appears, therefore, that at rest the carotid baroreflex can alter the cardiac and vascular responses to both falls or rises in systemic pressure with an equal range of response, whereas during exercise the reflex will have a greater range of response when blood pressure rises. As the "exercise pressor reflex" has been demonstrated to produce a powerful hypertensive effect, the relocation of the operating pressure toward threshold provides an optimal position for buffering the hypertension produced by the "exercise pressor reflex" emanating from the working muscle. The ability of the arterial baroreflexes to buffer the "exercise pressor reflex" has been documented by Sheriff et al. [63]. If we hypothesize that increases in workload result in a shift in the operating point toward the threshold region of the reflex, then a point may be reached during exercise when the operating point actually falls below the threshold level of the baroreflex function curve. If this were to occur, then the baroreflex would be rendered inoperative to a hypotensive stimulus, and a much larger hypertensive stimulus would have to be delivered to the baroreflex in order to elicit a comparable reflex bradycardia or vasodilation. This may help to explain why Strange and coworkers [72] were able to report a significant augmentation of leg blood flow in response to -50 torr NS in humans cycling at 40% $\dot{V}O_2max$; yet, at the higher workload (88% $\dot{V}O^2max$), the -50 torr NS had no effect.

In contrast to the findings of Potts et al. [51] and Papelier et al. [45], Eiken and colleagues [11] have reported that the sensitivity of the carotid baroreflex was augmented during exercise. Furthermore, they found that the gain of the carotid baroreflex was also enhanced during exercise when lower body positive pressure (LBPP) was applied. The use of the LBPP was intended to restrict blood flow to the working muscle in order to activate the muscle chemoreflex. Unfortunately, these investigators used the 12-beat pulse-synchronous neck collar pressure procedure of Eckberg and Eckberg [10] which, although valid at rest, is inappropriate to use during exercise, because the interbeat interval begins to approach the latency of the baroreflex arc, as discussed previously. In addition, recent work by Williamson et al. [81] and Shi et al. [66] have demonstrated that application of LBPP to the lower extremity of resting humans may also activate mechanically sensitive muscle afferent fibers. These findings, in conjunction with the findings from McWilliam and colleagues [35–37], who reported that electrically induced muscle contractions that activated group III/IV muscle afferents inhibited carotid baroreflex-evoked bradycardia, suggest that application of LBPP in exercising humans would likely inhibit baroreflex function by activating both mechanically sensitive, as well as metabolically sensitive, skeletal muscle receptors [41].

Support for the findings in the exercising human of Potts et al. [51] and Papelier et al. [45] is present in the early findings of the elegant work of

Melcher and Donald [38] and Walgenbach and colleagues [79, 80]. In these studies, the investigators vascularly isolated the carotid sinus baroreceptors of the dog. They obtained the open-loop Stimulus-Response (S-R) relationship to stepwise increases of static pressure within the carotid sinuses and recorded the steady-state response of HR and blood pressure. This protocol was performed with the dog at rest, standing on the treadmill and at two levels of exercise (moderate and heavy). Although the approach of stimulating the carotid sinus was different between Potts et al. [51] and that of Donald and his colleagues [38, 79, 80], interpretations of the resultant data are similar. Melcher and Donald [38] found that the response curve relating HR and arterial pressure to changes in carotid sinus pressure (CSP) produced at rest and at two levels of exercise was functionally unchanged, i.e., maximal gain was unchanged. Furthermore, Raven et al. [53] recalculated the results of Melcher and Donald [38], using the logistic model of Kent et al. [20], and found that, regardless of the method of calculating gain, the transition from rest to moderate and heavy exercise was achieved without a change in the maximal gain of the carotid baroreflex. Consequently, we concluded as did Bevegard and Shephard [2] in 1966, that the carotid baroreflex is reset during the transition from rest to exercise to a new operating pressure without a change in the functional characteristics of the reflex and, therefore, is fully able to regulate blood pressure at the prevailing exercise blood pressure. The fundamental question remains as to what is (are) the mechanism(s) responsible for this resetting.

AORTIC BAROREFLEX

In general, the aortic baroreceptor-mediated changes in HR and blood pressure function in concert with the carotid baroreflexes. However, the operating range of aortic barorreceptor occurs over higher arterial pressures than those of the carotid baroreceptor [32, 59], and the aortic baroreceptor reflex accounts for two-thirds, whereas the CBR accounts for one-third of the complete arterial reflex response [13, 30, 32, 60].

In the investigation of Melcher and Donald [38], described previously, additional experiments were performed after acute bilateral vagotomy, which obviated the buffering effects of the aortic and cardiopulmonary baroreceptor-mediated reflexes. Even though the data confirmed that the functional ability of the carotid baroreflex was maintained during exercise, despite the absence of any vagal afferent input from the aortic and cardiopulmonary baroreceptors, the transition from rest to exercise resulted in an exercise blood pressure that was lower than the resting value. In addition, the carotid baroreflex operated at a lower arterial pressure range. Therefore, we suggest that both the aortic and the cardiopulmonary baroreceptors provide important afferent neural information that modulates carotid baroreflex function at rest and during exercise.

TABLE 13.1.
Cardiovascular Responses to Phenylephrine (PE) Infusion

	ΔHR (beats/min)	ΔMAP (mm Hg)	ΔCVP (mm Hg)	$\Delta HR \Delta MAP$ (beats/min/mm Hg)
PE				
Resting	-12.7 ± 1.9	11.8 ± 0.4	3.6 ± 0.4	-1.10 ± 0.19
Exercise	-12.9 ± 1.9	11.3 ± 0.8	2.8 ± 0.4	-1.15 ± 0.15
P	NS	NS	NS	NS
PE + LBNP + NP				
Resting	-10.2 ± 1.8	14.0 ± 0.6	0.2 ± 0.3	-0.74 ± 0.13
Exercise	-10.5 ± 1.6	12.4 ± 0.9	0.9 ± 0.2	-0.86 ± 0.12
P	NS	NS	NS	NS

From ref. 68. Values are means $\pm$ SE. ΔHR, change in HR; ΔMAP, change in MAP; ΔCVP, change in CVP; LBNP = lower body negative pressure, NP is neck pressure

A number of technical and human subject concerns make it very difficult to isolate the aortic baroreceptor reflex in humans. Mancia et al. [30] provided an experimental approach which, by selectively and nonselectively stimulating the carotid baroreceptors, could be used to calculate the individual contributions of the carotid and extracarotid baroreceptors to the control of HR at rest. Ferguson et al. [13] and Sanders et al. [60] developed a sophisticated modification of the protocol and were able to provide evidence indicating a greater relative contribution of the aortic baroreceptor reflex in the regulation of HR and sympathetic nerve activity at rest. Subsequently, Shi et al. [64, 65] used a further modification of this protocol to investigate the relative contribution of the aortic and carotid baroreflex control of HR in endurance-trained and untrained subjects at rest. They found that the sensitivity of the aortic baroreflex control of HR was reduced in endurance-trained subjects, compared to age-matched sedentary controls. Further, they found that the reduction in aortic baroreflex sensitivity could completely account for the well-reported attenuation in overall arterial baroreflex function found in highly trained endurance athletes [52, 71]. And recently, Shi et al. [68] has provided similar information on the role of the aortic baroreflex control of HR during exercise (Table 13.1). Baroreflex gain was estimated from (a) the ratio of the change in HR to the change in MAP (ΔHR/ΔMAP) during phenylephrine (PE) infusion and (b) aortic-HR function during PE plus lower-body negative pressure (LBNP) and NP during rest and 25% $\dot{V}O_2$max supine bicycle exercise. LBNP and NP were used to counteract the PE-induced increase in CVP and carotid sinus pressure (CSP), respectively.

It was concluded that the gain of the isolated aortic-HR reflex was the same during exercise as it was during rest. Unfortunately, because of the use of vasoactive drugs no information about the aortic-vasomotor reflex was obtained. Furthermore, they were unable to establish the operating range of the reflex and, hence, it was unclear whether classical resetting of the aortic baroflex had occurred during the transition from rest to exercise.

CARDIOPULMONARY BARORECEPTOR REFLEX

In a series of elegant studies Johnson et al. [16] used LBNP to decrease central blood volume and cardiac filling volume progressively, thereby selectively unloading the cardiopulmonary baroreceptors, and they defined a range of LBNP from 0 to −20 torr, which selectively stimulated the cardiopulmonary baroreflex. This has been confirmed in a number of subsequent investigations in which LBNP between 0 to −20 torr only elicited increases in FVR without changes in HR [33, 46, 66, 67]. Recently, the selective unloading of the cardiopulmonary baroreceptors by low levels (0 to −20 torr) of LBNP has been challenged by Taylor et al. [73]. In these experiments, magnetic resonance imaging (MRI) of the ascending and descending aortic was used to describe a change in the two-dimensional image area of the aortic arch during −5, −10, −15, and −20 torr LBNP. Although changes in image area were not significant at −5 and −10 torr and were only significantly different at −15 torr and −20 torr, the investigators concluded that because a significant relationship existed between the decrease in image area and the amount of LBNP between 0 and −20 torr that the aortic baroreceptors were involved in the FVR to the LBNP. These findings challenge the use of LBNP between 0 and −20 torr to unload the cardiopulmonary baroreceptor selectively. This conclusion is in contrast to the direct aortic arch catheterization investigations of Johnson et al. [16] and, more recently, those of Jacobsen et al. [15], who found no change in MAP and pulse pressures or in aortic dp/dt during 0 to −20 torr LBNP while right atrial pressure decreased and forearm vascular resistance [15, 16] and muscle sympathetic nerve activity increased [15]. It is possible that two-dimensional area images are altered by LBNP because of the footward forces pulling the heart downward within the thoracic cavity, thereby changing the three-dimensional configuration of the heart and great vessels without altering mechanical wall stress. Indeed, the lack of change in calculated aortic arch transmural pressures estimated from the data of the Johnson et al. [16] and Jacobsen et al. [15] with the lack of a significant tachycardiac response found by all three investigations [15, 16, 73] during LBNP levels of 0 to −20 would suggest that the high pressure baroreceptor reflexes are not involved in the increased FVR.

More recently, Shi et al. [67], using both leg elevation plus LBPP and LBNP to increase (+2 mm Hg) and decrease (−4 mm Hg) total venous pressure, respectively, have described an operating range and response range of reflex changes in FVR, (ΔFVR) by the cardiopulmonary baroreceptors. By adding in additional data points from a previous investigation that

FIGURE 13.8.

A model of the FVR and the CVP relationship during LBNP (up to − 20 torr) and passive leg elevation of 50 cm and leg elevation plus LBPP of +20 torr in a group of eight exercise-trained individuals. The solid line indicates the S-R relationship derived from logistic modeling [20]. The dashed line denotes the first-order differential or gain of the S-R curve. Baseline CVP was 6.9 mm Hg (i.e., operational point), a gain of − 2.08 unit/mm Hg. The operating range, i.e., the CVP difference between threshold (+1.14 mm Hg) and saturation (+10.1 mm Hg) pressure was 9.27 mm Hg. The response range, i.e., the difference between maximal and minimal forearm vascular resistance responses was 18.8 peripheral resistance units. The central point was 5.8 mm Hg and corresponded to the maximal gain of − 2.54 unit/mm Hg.

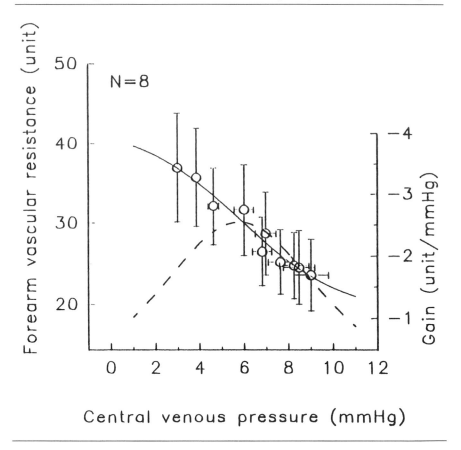

Central venous pressure (mmHg)

loaded the cardiopulmonary baroreceptors, using leg elevation plus LBPP to raise CVP [67], we modeled the resultant data according to the mathematical growth curve model of Kent et al. [20] (Fig. 13.8).

Although the concept that the CBR has the classic properties of a baroreflex and that its function is to regulate cardiac filling pressures appears to be important at rest, it also would be important to define the reflex function in investigations of its role during dynamic exercise.

In the early work using the exercising dog model, in which the carotid sinuses were vascularly isolated and the vagi were sectioned [38], it was evident that the neural afferent information obtained from the cardiopulmonary baroreceptor was important in establishing the operating range of the carotid baroreceptor. Indeed, one could suggest that in the absence of information about cardiac filling pressures, the arterial baroreceptor reflex regulates arterial pressure at a lower systemic pressure during exercise. Furthermore, the tonic activity from the cardiopulmonary reflex may play a greater role in circulatory regulation after endurance training. DiCarlo and Bishop [7] used intrapericardial injections of procaine to anesthetize vagal afferent nerve traffic emanating from the heart wall of a rabbit and found significant increases in resting blood pressure and RSNA in endurance-trained but not sedentary rabbits. These results suggest that the attenuation in arterial baroreflex function, which accompanies endurance exercise training [52], may result from an enhanced inhibitory influence of cardiac afferents.

Mack et al. [29] used LBNP of −10 and −20 torr to unload the cardiopulmonary baroreceptors selectively while human subjects were bicycling at an average workload of 77 watts. They found that MAP and HR were unchanged when −10 torr LBNP was applied during exercise while cardiac output (Q_c) and SV decreased and FVR increased in proportion to the amount of LBNP. It was concluded that the elevated MAP was regulated and was not the consequence of differential changes in Q_c or FVR. In addition, the authors further concluded that during exercise the cardiopulmonary baroreflex was actively involved in regulating the cardiac filling pressure during exercise, as has been established at rest [46]. An additional interpretation of the data of Mack et al. [29] is to suggest that if the cardiopulmonary baroreflex is operating to regulate cardiac filling pressure, then it must have been reset to the higher cardiac filling pressures of exercise to regulate the increased cardiac filling volumes produced by exercise.

INTERACTION BETWEEN THE ARTERIAL AND CARDIOPULMONARY BARORECEPTORS

At rest Pawelczyk and Raven [46] demonstrated a significant augmentation of the carotid baroreflex gain when cardiopulmonary baroreceptors were selectively unloaded by 0 to −20 torr LBNP. More recently Shi et al. [66] has demonstrated a significant attenuation of the carotid baroreflex gain by selectively increasing CVP (+4 mm Hg) using venous infusions of Dextran in resting humans. In addition, Shi et al. [66] confirmed the inhibitory nature of somatic afferents on carotid baroreflex function reported by McWilliam

FIGURE 13.9.
(Upper panel) A summary of the HR responses to the 5 s NP/NS protocol of Potts et al. [50] of one individual during 25% V̇O$_2$ peak cycling exercise. LBNP reduced CVP, −1.8 mm Hg (——) and −4.0 mm Hg (----). (Lower panel.) Represents the increase in gain of the carotid-cardiac reflex during exercise: control (solid line); low level LBNP decreased CVP −1.8 mm Hg (dashed line), and high level LBNP decreased CVP −4.0 mm Hg (dotted line).

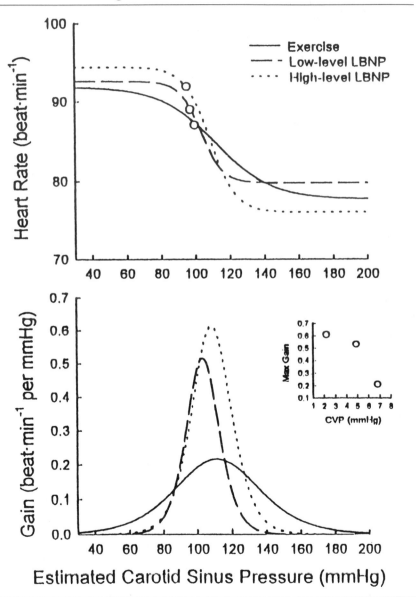

et al. [35–37] in unanesthetized decerebrate cats. In these investigations, Shi et al. [66] used +30 torr LBPP on resting human subjects and found a decreased maximal gain of the carotid baroreflex even though the increase in central venous pressure (CVP) was only +2 mmHg, an increase in CVP at which no effect on CBR function was observed [66]. These findings suggest that LBPP +30 torr had activated intramuscular pressure-sensitive receptor and via the III/IV [36, 37] neural afferents emanating from the skeletal muscle inhibited, via integration within the central nervous system, the CBR function. Williamson et al. [81] in humans and others using animals [17, 18, 44] have demonstrated that by increasing pressure in the legs a pressure sensitive pressor reflex from the skeletal muscle is activated.

Subsequently, Potts et al. [50] tested the hypothesis that the interaction that has been reported between the carotid baroreflex and the cardiopulmonary baroreceptor at rest [46] may also be present during exercise. This investigation used LBNP between 0 and −35 torr to unload the cardiopulmonary baroreceptors and produce equivalent changes in CVP during both rest and semirecumbent bicycle exercise of 25% of $\dot{V}O_2$max. The carotid-cardiac baroreflex function curve was obtained during each level of CVP at rest and exercise, and the maximal gain of the reflex was calculated. The data indicated that when the cardiopulmonary baroreceptors were unloaded at rest, the carotid-cardiac baroreflex gain was augmented (Fig. 13.9). Importantly, it was also found that low-levels of LBNP (−18 torr) during exercise significantly increased carotid-cardiac baroreflex gain without affecting the level of HR or ABP. This indicates that this enhancement of baroreflex gain during exercise was mediated by deactivating cardiopulmonary baroreceptors selectively. This finding demonstrates that cardiopulmonary baroreceptors continue to exert a tonic inhibition of carotid baroreflex sensitivity during exercise, as has been previously reported at rest. Therefore, it would appear from these investigations that the carotid baroreflex regulation of HR is facilitated during exercise when cardiac filling pressures are reduced. This type of facilitatory interaction between carotid and cardiopulmonary baroreceptors can enhance the regulation of ABP during conditions that produce central hypovolemia, such as exercise of prolonged duration or exercise performed in hyperthermic environments. Both of these conditions result in a reduction and a redistribution of the stressed blood volume of the circulation produced by an increase in thermoregulatory demands.

INTERACTION OF CENTRAL COMMAND AND SKELETAL MUSCLE REFLEXES ON ARTERIAL BAROREFLEX FUNCTION DURING EXERCISE

The precise mechanism(s) mediating the changes in baroflex function, as previously outlined during exercise, remain unknown; however, there are several potential candidates. Two attractive possibilities are the descending cortical influences of Central Command [42, 76, 77] and peripheral muscle input carried by Group III/IV afferent fibers [19, 41]. Both of these neural pathways are activated during volitional exercise and may act at the level of the brainstem to modulate baroreflex function during exercise.

Although an exact location for Central Command has not yet been identified, Waldrop and Porter [77] have suggested that the hypothalamic locomotor region (HLR) may be the putative site for Central Command. Furthermore, Waldrop and Stremel [78] have performed single-unit extracellular recording from neurons in the HLR and have found that these neurons respond directly to electrically induced muscle contraction. In addition, direct electrical stimulation of the posterior hypothalamus by Coote et al. [4], as well as microinjections of gammo-aminobutyric acid (GABA) antagonists into the posterior hypothalamus by Bauer et al. [1], have been shown to blunt baroreflex function in anesthetized cats. Together, these data suggest that this region of the brain may serve as an integrative area for cardiovascular control during exercise.

A series of studies by McWilliam and colleagues have examined the specific role of group III/IV muscle afferent on carotid baroreflex control of HR in unanesthetized decerebrate cats [35–37]. They isolated the carotid sinus regions so that they could rapidly change carotid sinus pressure (CSP) and thereby compared the reflex bradycardia to an increase in CSP with the bradycardia produced by the same level of baroreflex activation, accompanied by somatic afferent activity produced by electrical stimulation of L7–S1 ventral roots. They found that when somatic afferents were activated the reflex bradycardia to the same increase in CSP was attenuated. This finding suggested that the sensitivity of the carotid baroreflex was reduced by somatic afferent activation. Although the mechanism mediating this effect was not discussed by these investigators, Toney and Mifflin [74, 75] have recently conducted two studies that suggest that convergence of carotid baroreceptor and somatic afferent projections at the level of the Nucleus Tractus Solitarius (NTS) produces a time-dependent inhibition of barosensitive NTS neuronal discharge. This finding may provide insight into the mechanism by which somatic afferents alter baroreflex function. Although these studies have indicated a specific region in the brainstem where these two reflex pathways may interact, there are clearly a number of other potential brainstem sites where somatic and baroreceptor afferent projects may converge and interact. Clearly, further research is required in this area before we completely understand the mechanisms involved in the central integration of these two reflex pathways.

Since Central Command and somatic and baroreceptor afferents are all activated during exercise, a central neural site(s) must exist to integrate these neural inputs in order to generate the appropriate cardiovascular response. The ventrolateral medulla (VLM) has been identified as a potential integrating site. Nolan et al. [42] recorded from neurons in the VLM, which altered their discharge properties to induce muscle contraction electrically and stimulated Central Command (caudal hypothalamic stimulation). As the cells were also found to have a basal cardiovascular rhythm of baroreflex origin [76] it is likely that integration of Central Command, peripheral feedback from skeletal muscle, and arterial baroreceptors occurs in the VLM.

SUMMARY

From the work of Potts et al. [49, 51] Papelier et al. [45] and Shi et al. [68] it is readily apparent that the arterial (aortic and carotid) baroreflexes are reset to function at the prevailing ABP of exercise. The blood pressure of exercise is the result of the hemodynamic (cardiac output and TPR) responses, which appear to be regulated by two redundant neural control systems, "Central Command" and the "exercise pressor reflex" [58]. Central Command is a feed-forward neural control system that operates in parallel with the neural regulation of the locomotor system [39, 40, 58] and appears to establish the hemodynamic response to exercise [56]. Within the central nervous system it appears that the HLR may be the operational site for Central Command [78]. Specific neural sites within the HLR have been demonstrated in animals to be active during exercise [78]. With the advent of positron emission tomography (PET) and single-photon emission computed tomography (SPECT), the anatomical areas of the human brain related to Central Command are being mapped [14, 82]. It also appears that the Nucleus Tractus Solitarius and the ventrolateral medulla may serve as an integrating site as they receive neural information from the working muscles via the group III/IV muscle afferents as well as from higher brain centers [42, 76]. This anatomical site within the CNS is now the focus of many investigations in which arterial baroreflex function, Central Command and the "exercise pressor reflex" appear to demonstrate inhibitory or facilitatory interaction [76].

The concept of whether Central Command is the prime mover in the resetting of the arterial baroreceptors to function at the exercising ABP or whether the resetting is an integration of the "exercise pressor reflex" information with that of Central Command is now under intense investigation. However, it would be justified to conclude, from the data of Bevegard and Shepherd [2], Dicarlo and Bishop [8], Potts et al. [49, 51], and Papelier et al. [45] that the act of exercise results in the resetting of the arterial baroreflex. In addition, if, as we have proposed, the cardiopulmonary baroreceptors primarily monitors and reflexly regulates cardiac filling volume, it would seem from the data of Mack et al. [29] and Potts et al. [50] that the cardiopulmonary baroreceptor is also reset at the beginning of exercise. Therefore, investigations of the neural mechanisms of regulation involving Central Command and cardiopulmonary afferents, similar to those being undertaken for the arterial baroreflex, need to be established.

ACKNOWLEDGMENTS

The production of this review chapter was supported in part by funds from the National Institutes of Health—National Heart Lung Blood Institute, Grant #HL 45547 and the Life Sciences Division of the National Aeronautics and Space Administration of the United States of America under the NSCORT-NAGW #3853.

REFERENCES

1. Bauer, R. M., M. B. Vela, T. Simon, and T. G. Waldrop. A GABAEergic mechanism in the posterior hypothalamus modulates baroreflex bradycardia. *Brain Res. Bull.* 20:633–641, 1988.
2. Bevegard, B. S., and J. T. Shepherd. Circulatory effects of stimulating the carotid arterial stretch receptors in man at rest and during exercise. *J. Clin. Invest.* 45:132–142, 1966.
3. Bristow, J. D., E. B. Brown, Jr., D. J. C. Cunningham, et al. Effect of bicycling on the baroreflex regulation of pulse interval. *Circ. Res.* 28:582–592, 1971.
4. Coote, J. H., M. Hilton, and J. F. Perez-Gonzalez. Inhibition of the baroreceptor reflex on stimulation in the brainstem defense center. *J. Physiol. (Lond.)* 288:549–560, 1979.
5. Cunningham, D. J. C., E. Strange-Petersen, T. G. Pickering, and P. Sleight. Effect of hypoxia, hypercapnia and asphyxia on the baroreceptor cardiac reflex at rest and during exercise in man. *Acta Physiol. Scand.* 86:456–465, 1972.
6. Daskalopoulos, D. A., J. T. Shepherd, and S. C. Walgenbach. Cardipulmonary reflexes and blood pressure in exercising sino-aortic denervated dogs. *J. Appl. Physiol.* 57(5):1417–1421, 1984.
7. DiCarlo, S. E., and V. S. Bishop. Exercise training enhances cardiac afferent inhibition of baroreflex function. *Am. J. Physiol.* 258:H212–H220, 1990.
8. DiCarlo, S. E., and V. S. Bishop. Onset of exercise shifts operating point of arterial baroreflex to higher pressures. *Am. J. Physiol.* 262:H303–H307, 1992.
9. Ebert, T. J. Carotid baroreceptor reflex regulation of forearm vascular resistance. *J. Physiol.* 337:655–664, 1983.
10. Eckberg, D. L., and M. J. Eckberg. Human sinus node responses to repetitive, ramped carotid baroreceptor stimuli. *Am. J. Physiol.* 242:H638–H644, 1982.
11. Eiken, O., V. A. Convertino, D. F. Doerr, et al. Characteristics of the carotid baroreflex in man during normal and flow-restricted exercise. *Acta Physiol. Scand.* 144:325–331, 1992.
12. Ernsting J., and D. J. Parry. Some observations of the effects of stimulating the stretch receptors in the carotid artery in man. *J. Physiol. (Lond.)* 137:454P–456P, 1957.
13. Ferguson, D. W., F. M. Abboud, and A. L. Mark. Relative contribution of aortic and carotid baroreflexes to heart rate control in man during steady-state dynamic increases in arterial pressure. *J. Clin. Invest.* 76:2265–2274, 1985.
14. Fink, G. R., L. Adams, J. D. G. Watson, et al. Hypernea during and immediately after exercise in man: evidence of motor control involvement. *J. Physiol. (Lond.)* 489:663–675, 1995.
15. Jacobsen, T. N., B. J. Morgan, U. Schjerrer, et al. Relative contributions of cardiopulmonary and sino-aortic baroreflexes in causing sympathetic activation in the human skeletal muscle circulation during orthostatic stress. *Cir. Res.* 73:367–378, 1993.
16. Johnson, J. M., L. B. Rowell, M. Niederberger, and M. M. Eisman. Human splanchnic and forearm vasoconstrictor responses to reductions in right atrial and aortic pressure. *Circ. Res.* 34:515–524, 1974.
17. Julius, S. The blood pressure seeking properties of the central nervous system. *J. Hypertens.* 6:177–185, 1988.
18. Julius, S., R. Sanchez, S. Malayan, et al. Sustained blood pressure elevation to lower body compression in pigs and dogs. *Hypertension* 4:782–788, 1982.
19. Kaufman, M. P., and H. V. Forster. Reflexes controlling circulatory, ventilatory and airway

responses to exercise. *Handbook of Physiology, Sect 12: Exercise: Regulation and Integration of Multiple Systems.* Bethesda, MD: American Physiological Society. 1996, pp. 381–447.

20. Kent, B. B., J. W. Drane, B. Blumenstein, and J. W. Manning. A mathematical model to assess changes in the baroreceptor reflex. *Cardiology* 57:295–310, 1973.

21. Krogh, A., and J. Lindhard. A comparison between voluntary and electrically induced muscular work in man. *J. Physiol. (Lond.)* 51:182–201, 1917.

22. Levine, B. D., J. A. Pawelczyk, J. C. Buckey, et al. The effect of carotid baroreceptor stimulation on stroke volume. *Clin. Res.* 38:333A, 1990.

23. Ludbrook, J. Reflex control of blood pressure during exercise. *Ann. Rev. Physiol.* 45: 155–168, 1983.

24. Ludbrook, J., I. B. Faris, J. Iannos, and G. G. Jamieson. Sine-wave evocation of the carotid baroreceptor reflex in conscious rabbits. P. Sleight (ed.) *Proceedings of the Oxford Baroreceptor Workshop.* Oxford, England: Oxford University Press, 1980.

25. Ludbrook, J., I. B. Faris, J. Iannos, G. G. Jamieson, and W. J. Russell. Lack of effect of isometric handgrip exercise on response of the carotid sinus baroreceptor reflex in man. *Clin. Sci. Mol. Med.* 55:189–194, 1978.

26. Ludbrook, J., G. Mancia, and A. Zanchetti. Does the baroreceptor-heart rate reflex indicate the capacity of the arterial baroreceptors to control blood pressure? *Clin. Exp. Pharmacol. Physiol.* 7:499–503, 1980.

27. Ludbrook, J., G. Mancia, A. Ferrari, and A. Zanchetti. Factors influencing the carotid baroreceptor response to pressure changes in a neck chamber. *Clin. Sci. Mol. Med.* 51:347S–349S, 1977.

28. Ludbrook, J., G. Mancia, A. Ferrari, and A. Zanchetti. The variable-pressure neck-chamber method for studying the carotid baroreflex in man. *Clin. Sci. Mol. Med.* 53:165–171, 1977.

29. Mack, G. W., H. Nose, and E. R. Nadel. Role of cardiopulmonary baroflexes during dynamic exercise. *J. Appl. Physiol.* 65:1827–1832, 1988.

30. Mancia, G., A. Ferrari, L. Gregorini, et al. Circulatory reflexes from carotid and extra carotid baroreceptor areas in man. *Circ. Res.* 41(3):309–315, 1977.

31. Mancia, G., G. Grassu, G. Bertinieri, A. Ferrari, and A. Zanchetti. Arterial baroreceptor control of blood pressure in man. *J. Auton. Nerv. Syst.* 11:115–124, 1984.

32. Mancia, G., and A. L. Mark. Arterial baroreflexes in humans. *Handbook of Physiology, Sect 2: The Cardiovascular System.* Bethesda, MD: American Physiological Society, 1983, pt. 2, vol. 3, pp. 755–793.

33. Mark, A. L., and G. Mancia. Cardipulmonary baroreflexes in humans. *Handbook of Physiology, Sect 2: The Cardiovascular System.* Bethesda, MD: American Physiological Society, 1983, pt. 2, vol. 3, pp. 795–813.

34. McCloskey, D. I., and J. H. Mitchell. Reflex cardiovascular and respiratory responses originating from exercising muscle. *J. Physiol. (Lond.)* 224:173–186, 1972.

35. McMahon, S. E., and P. N. McWilliam. Changes in R-R interval at the start of muscle contraction in the decerebrate cat. *J. Physiol. (Lond.)* 447:549–562, 1992.

36. McWilliam, P. N., and T. Yang. Inhibition of cardiac vagal component of baroreflex by group III and IV afferents. *Am. J. Physiol.* 260:H730–H734, 1991.

37. McWilliam, P. N., T. Yang, and L. X. Chen. Changes in the baroreceptor reflex at the start of muscle contraction in the decerebrate cat. *J. Physiol. (Lond.)* 436:549–558, 1991.

38. Melcher, A., and D. E. Donald. Maintained ability of carotid sinus baroreflex to regulate arterial pressure during exercise. *Am. J. Physiol.* 241:H838–H849, 1981.

39. Mitchell, J. H. Cardiovascular control during exercise: central and reflex neural mechanisms. *Am. J. Cardiol.* 55:33D–41D, 1985.

40. Mitchell, J. H. Neural control of the circulation during exercise. *Med. Sci. Sports Exerc.* 22:141–154, 1990.

41. Mitchell, J. H., and R. F. Schmidt. Cardiovascular reflex control by afferent fibers from skeletal muscle receptors. *Handbook of Physiology, Sect 2: The Cardiovascular System.* Bethesda, MD: American Physiological Society, pt. 2, vol. 3, 1983, pp. 623–658.

42. Nolan, P. C., J. A. Pawelczyk, and T. G. Waldrop. Neurons in the ventrolateral medulla receive input from descending "central command" and feedback from contracting muscles. *Physiologist* 35:240, 1992.

43. O'Leary, D. S. Heart rate control during exercise by baroreceptors and skeletal muscle afferents. *Med. Sci. Sports Exerc.* 28(2):210–217, 1996.

44. Osterziel, K. J., S. Julius, and D. O. Brant. Blood pressure elevation during hindquarter compression in dogs is neurogenic. *J. Hypertens.* 2:411–417, 1984.

45. Papelier, Y., P. Escourrou, J. P. Gauthier, and L. B. Rowell. Carotid baroreflex control of blood pressure and heart rate in man during dynamic exercise. *J. Appl. Physiol.* 77:502–507, 1994.

46. Pawelczyk, J. A., and P. B. Raven. Reductions in central venous pressure improve carotid baroreflex responses in humans. *Am. J. Physiol.* 257:H1389–H1395, 1989.

47. Pickering, T. G., B. Gribbin, E. S. Peterson, et al. Effects of autonomic blockade on the baroreflex in man at rest and during exercise. *Circ. Res.* 30:177–185, 1972.

48. Potts, J. T., T. Hatanaka, and A. A. Shoukas. Effect of arterial compliance on carotid sinus baroreceptor reflex control of the circulation. *Am. J. Physiol.* 270:H988–H1000, 1996.

49. Potts, J. T., and P. B. Raven. Effect of dynamic exercise on human carotid-cardiac baroreflex latency. *Am. J. Physiol.* 268:H1208–H1214, 1995.

50. Potts, J. T., X. Shi, and P. B. Raven. Cardiopulmonary baroreceptors modulate carotid baroreflex control of heart rate during dynamic exercise in humans. *Am. J. Physiol.* 268: H1567–H1576, 1995.

51. Potts, J. T., X. R. Shi, and P. B. Raven. Carotid baroreflex responsiveness during dynamic exercise in humans. *Am. J. Physiol.* 265:H1928–H1938, 1993.

52. Raven, P. B., and J. A. Pawelczyk. Chronic endurance exercise training: a condition of inadequate blood pressure regulation and reduced tolerance to LBNP. *Med. Sci. Sports Exerc.* 25:713–721, 1993.

53. Raven, P. B., J. T. Potts, X. Shi, and J. A. Pawelczyk. Baroreceptor mediated reflex regulation of blood pressure during exercise. B. Saltin and N. Secher (eds.). *Exercise and the Circulation in Health and Disease.* Champaign, IL: Human Kinetics Publishers, 1997.

54. Robinson, B. F., S. E. Epstein, G. D. Beiser, and E. Braunwald. Control of heart rate by autonomic nervous system: studies in man on the interaction between baroreceptor mechanisms and exercise. *Circ. Res.* 19:400–410, 1996.

55. Rothe, C. F. Venous system: physiology of the capacitance vessels. *Handbook of Physiology, Sect. 2: The Cardiovascular System.* Bethesda, MD: American Physiological Society, 1983, pt. 2, pp. 397–452.

56. Rowell, L. B. What signals govern the cardiovascular response to exercise? *Med. Sci. Sports Exerc.* 12:307–315, 1980.

57. Rowell, L. B. Circulatory adjustments to dynamic exercise. L. B. Rowell (ed.). *Human Circulation: Regulation during Physical Stress.* New York: Oxford University Press, 1986, pp. 213–256.

58. Rowell, L. B., D. S. O'Leary, and D. L. Kellogg, Jr. Integration of cardiovascular control systems in dynamic exercise. L. B. Rowell and J. T. Shepherd (eds.). *Handbook of Physiology, Sect 12: Exercise: Regulation and Integration of Multiple Systems.* New York: Oxford University Press, 1996, chap. 17, II, pp. 770–840.

59. Sagawa, K. Baroreflex control of systemic arterial pressure and vascular bed. *Handbook of Physiology, Sect. 2: The Cardiovascular System.* Bethesda, MD: American Physiological Society, pt. 2, vol. 3, pp. 453–496.

60. Sanders, J. S., D. W. Ferguson, and A. L. Mark. Arterial baroreflex control of sympathetic nerve activity during elevation of blood pressure in normal man: dominance of aortic baroreflexes. *Circulation* 77(2):279–288, 1988.

61. Scherrer, U., S. L. Pryor, L. A. Bertocci, and R. G. Victor. Arterial baroreflex buffering of sympathetic activation during exercise-induced elevations in arterial pressure. *J. Clin. Invest.* 86:1855–1861, 1990.

62. Sheehan, D., J. H. Mulholland, and B. Safiroff. Surgical anatomy of the carotid sinus nerve. *Anat. Rec.* 80:431–442, 1941.

63. Sheriff, D. D., D. S. O'Leary, A. M. Scher, and L. B. Rowell. Baroreflex attenuates pressor response to graded muscle ischemia in exercising dogs. *Am. J. Physiol.* 258:H305–H310, 1990.

64. Shi, X., J. M. Andersen, J. T. Potts, B. H. Foresman, S. A. Stern, and P. B. Raven. Aortic baroreflex control of heart rate during hypertensive stimuli: effect of fitness. *J. Appl. Physiol.* 74:1555–1562, 1993.

65. Shi, X., C. G. Crandall, J. T. Potts, J. W. Williamson, B. H. Foresman, and P. B. Raven. A diminished aortic cardiac reflex during hypotension in aerobically fit young men. *Med. Sci. Sports Exerc.* 25:1024–1030, 1993.

66. Shi, X., B. H. Foresman, and P. B. Raven. Interaction of central venous pressure, intramuscular pressure and carotid baroreflex function. *Am. J. Physiol. (Heart. Circ. Physiol.)* 272, 1997.

67. Shi, X., K. M. Gallagher, S. A. Smith, K. H. Bryant, and P. B. Raven. Diminished forearm vasomotor response to central hypervolemic loading in aerobically fit individuals. *Med. Sci. Sports Exerc.* 28(12)1388–1395, 1996.

68. Shi, X., J. T. Potts, P. B. Raven, and B. H. Foresman. Aortic cardiac reflex during dynamic exercise. *J. Appl. Physiol.* 78(4):1569–1574, 1995.

69. Shoukas, A. A., and K. Sagawa. Control of total systemic vascular capacity by the carotid sinus baroreceptor reflex. *Circ. Res.* 33:22–33, 1973.

70. Staessen, J., R. Fiocchi, R. Fagard, et al. Progressive attenuation of the carotid baroreflex control of blood pressure and heart rate during exercise. *Am. Heart J.* 114.765–772, 1987.

71. Stegemann, J., A. Busert, and D. Brock. Influence of fitness on the blood pressure control system in man. *Aerosp. Med.* 45:45–48, 1974.

72. Strange, S., L. B. Rowell, N. J. Christensen, B. Saltin. Cardiovascular responses to carotid sinus baroreceptor stimulation during moderate to severe exercise in man. *Acta Physiol. Scand.* 138:145–153, 1990.

73. Taylor, J. A., J. R. Halliwill, T. E. Brown, et al. Non-hypotensive hypovolemia reduces ascending aortic dimensions in humans. *J. Physiol. (Lond.):* 483:289–298, 1995.

74. Toney, G. M., and S. W. Mifflin. Time-dependent inhibition of hindlimb somatic afferent inputs to nucleus tractus solitarius. *J. Neurophysiol.* 72(1):63–71, 1994.

75. Toney, G. M., and S. W. Mifflin. Time dependent inhibition of hindlimb somatic afferent transmission within nucleus tractus solitarius: an in vivo intracellular recording study. *Neuroscience* 68(2):445–453, 1995.

76. Waldrop, T. G., F. L. Eldridge, G. A. Iwamoto, and J. H. Mitchell. Central neural control of respiration and circulation during exercise. *Handbook of Physiology, Sect 12: Exercise: Regulation and Integration of Multiple Systems.* Bethesda, MD: American Physiological Society, 1996, pp. 333–380.

77. Waldrop, T. G., and J. P. Porter. Hypothalamic involvement in respiratory and cardiovascular regulation. J. A. Dempsey and A. I. Pack (eds). *Regulation of Breathing.* New York: Marcel Dekker, 1995, pp. 315–394.

78. Waldrop, T. G., and R. W. Stremel. Muscular contraction stimulates posterior hypothalamic neurons. *Am. J. Physiol.* 256:R348–R356, 1989.

79. Walgenbach-Telford, S. Arterial baroreflex and cardiopulmonary mechanoreflex function during exercise. I. H. Zucker and J. P. Gilmore, (eds.). *Reflex Control of the Circulation.* 1991, pp. 765–793.

80. Walgenbach, S. C., and D. E. Donald. Inhibition by carotid baroreflex of exercise-induced increases in arterial pressure. *Clin. Res.* 52:253–262, 1983.

81. Williamson, J. W., J. H. Mitchell, H. L. Olesen, et al. Reflex increase in blood pressure induced by leg compressions. *J. Physiol. (Lond.)* 475:351–357, 1994.

82. Williamson, J. W., A. C. L. Nobrega, R. McCall, et al. Activation of the insular cortex during dynamic exercise in humans. *J. Physiol. (Lond.)* 1997.

83. Yang, T., J. B. Senturia, and M. N. Levy. Antecedent sympathetic stimulation alters time course of chronotropic response to vagal stimulation in dogs. *Am. J. Physiol.* 266:H1339–H1347, 1994.

84. Zuntz, N., and J. Geppert. Uber die Natur der normalen Atemreize und den Ort ihrer Wirkung. *Arch. Ges. Physiol.* 38:337–338, 1886.

14
Physical Activity, Adolescence, and Health: An Epidemiological Perspective

DEBORAH J. AARON, Ph.D.
RONALD E. LAPORTE, Ph.D.

During the past few years three has been much discussion in the lay press and among health promoters concerning the declining activity and fitness levels of our youth, especially teenagers. The expressed view has been that we have become a nation of "couch potatoes" in which our youth spend considerably more time playing video games, surfing the Internet, and watching television than exercising. Furthermore, many have the opinion that this level of "inactivity" has produced, and will continue to produce, a nation of overweight teenagers, whose future is bleak because of their risk for obesity and, subsequently, chronic disease, such as noninsulin-dependent diabetes mellitus and coronary heart disease (CHD).

There are several perceptions that have contributed to this view of inactivity in our youth and the impending epidemic of noncommunicable disease as they age. We would like to ask the reader to agree or disagree with each of these beliefs and then tally the number of statements with which you agree:

Agree	Disagree		
_____	_____	1.	Teenagers are inactive.
		2.	Active teenagers have a better CHD risk profile than inactive teenagers.
_____	_____	3.	It is important to be active during adolescence to reduce the risk of subsequent CHD and other chronic diseases in adulthood.
_____	_____	4.	Active teenagers will become active adults.
_____	_____	5.	The active teenager is the most physically fit teenager.
_____	_____	6.	Teenagers who participate in athletics will develop a healthy life-style in which they are less likely to drink alcohol, smoke, or use drugs.
_____	_____	7.	The major health problems of youth are smoking, AIDS, alcohol consumption, illicit drug use, violence, and teenage pregnancy.
_____	_____	8.	There are few risks associated with activity in youth.

_____ _____ 9. Greater physical activity (PA) levels and fitness will protect against injuries.

_____ _____ 10. The optimal way to reduce injury risk in youth is to improve presport screening and provide better training and equipment.

In the current report, we will address each of these perceptions. We contend that these are health myths, as the above statements are unproven or false. Before beginning to address each of these perceptions, it is important to provide some background information. The direct links between exercise and disease are generally made with epidemiological investigations assessing PA and its relationship to various health conditions. Surprisingly, though, few epidemiological studies in children have actually evaluated the relationship of PA to health, despite the widespread belief in the importance of PA to the health of children.

In this chapter we will review what is known about the benefits and risks of PA to the health of children and, in particular, to that of adolescents. The literature is reviewed and data are presented from our Adolescent Injury Control Study (AICS) to address the issues related to the benefits and risks of PA. The AICS was a 4-yr prospective study of the incidence and determinants of physician-treated injuries in a population-based cohort of 1245 adolescents. It was initiated in August 1989 in a metropolitan school district near Pittsburgh, Pa. The objectives of the study were to (a) determine the incidence of adolescent injury and (b) to determine the injury risks associated with exposure to increasing amounts and increasing intensity of PA, independent of potential confounders. The study group consisted of students 12–16 yr of age and was comprised of similar numbers of males ($n = 641$) and females ($n = 604$). The racial composition of the study was Caucasian (73%), African-American (24%), and Hispanic or Asian (3%). Extensive PA data was collected during the 4 yr of the study, using a questionnaire that has been shown to be reproducible and valid in this population [3]. AICS provided a unique opportunity to study the epidemiology of PA in adolescents and to examine its relation to health benefits and injury risk.

We have recently argued that review papers can "increase" their shelf life if the review tables are put onto the Internet and updated regularly [16]. Tables that summarize the literature reviewed in his manuscript can be found on the World Wide Web (http://www.pitt.edu/~debaaron/PA/review.html).

TEENAGERS ARE INACTIVE

Given the emphasis placed on increasing the PA level of adolescents, there are no population-based data to indicate that activity levels have decreased from those of 10 or 20 yr ago. In addition, there are relatively few data on the current activity level of adolescents.

The primary source for adolescent PA data in the United States is the Youth Risk Behavior Survey (YRBS), conducted periodically by the Centers for Disease Control and Prevention. The YRBS [35] is a national survey of high school students in Grades 9–12 and was designed to measure the prevalence of health risk behaviors in this age group. Included in the YRBS are a number of questions to assess participation in vigorous activity, light-to-moderate activity, physical education class, and competitive sports. The overall results of the 1995 YRBS survey [60] indicated that 10.4% of adolescents are inactive, 63.7% participate in vigorous activity at least 3 times/week, and 50.3% participate in school-sponsored competitive athletics. When compared to the Healthy People 2000 Goals [59] for activity levels in adolescents, these data indicate that U.S. adolescents meet the goal for inactivity and are very close to meeting the goal for participation in vigorous activity. In addition, there has been no significant change in the participation in vigorous activity from 1991 to 1995, although the number of students participating in school-sponsored competitive sports has significantly increased from 1991 to 1995. There are several subgroups of adolescents who are far from reaching the 2000 Goals, specifically, African-American females and older females. It is interesting to note that the increased participation in competitive sports was most evident among these subgroups.

Two other studies provide additional information, because they report quantitative data on the PA of adolescents. Past-year activity was assessed by questionnaire, and the frequency and duration of participation were quantified. The National Children and Youth Fitness Study (NCYFS) assessed past-year activity in a national sample of 6478 students in the 7th through 12th grades [49]. The AICS assessed past-year activity in a population-based cohort of 1245 students in the 7th through 9th grades [4]. Although conducted a number of years apart, these two studies report surprisingly similar results. The median time spent in leisure time PA during the past year was 12–13 hr/wk in the NCYFS sample and 12.6 hr/wk in the AICS population.

The results from the YRBS, NCYFS, and AICS indicate that, consistently, the PA levels of adolescents are quite high. It is important to note that adolescent PA levels are considerably greater than those seen in adults, in whom the health benefits of PA have been documented. Thus, there are no strong data to indicate that teenagers are inactive or are becoming inactive.

ACTIVE TEENAGERS HAVE A BETTER CHD RISK FACTOR PROFILE THAN INACTIVE TEENAGERS

The association of PA to cardiovascular risk factors is equivocal in adolescents [44]. In general, no significant differences in blood lipid and blood pressures levels are found between active and inactive adolescents [6, 8, 32, 40, 41, 43, 51, 56, 58]. However, interpreting the results of these studies is difficult, because different measures of PA were used, and many studies suffer from small, nonrandom samples. In addition, selection bias may have occurred in some studies that compared athletes to sedentary children, in that those with a high-risk profile, e.g., obesity, smoking, or high blood pressure, may be unwilling or unable to be physically active. Another difficulty in trying to examine the PA-CHD risk factor relationship among adolescents is that pubertal changes have a profound impact on most of the CHD risk factors and may override any PA-risk factor relationship.

One would think that of all the associations, the PA-obesity relationship would be high. However, even here, the association is not strong. Although some cross-sectional studies have found an inverse relationship between PA and body mass index (BMI) or skinfold measurements [32, 40, 58], others have found no associations [6, 43, 51]. However, even if a relationship was found it is not possible to determine the direction of the relationship. Does low PA lead to increased body fatness, or does obesity lead to decreased PA? This question can only be answered by a longitudinal study. Two recent longitudinal studies in young children have reported a significant inverse association between PA and indices of body fatness [34, 46]. We have prospectively examined the relationship of PA to weight gain as part of AICS [2]. After controlling for age, race, and change in height, no association was found between PA and weight gain during adolescence, as the 2-yr weight gain was similar between activity groups.

A different approach to address the association of PA to risk factors is to investigate the effect of increasing PA (training studies) on the risk factors. Training studies in healthy adolescents generally show no effect of increasing PA on lipid levels or blood pressure [14, 28, 39, 47]. In contrast, initiating an exercise program has been shown to decrease blood pressure in hypertensive adolescents [27], decrease of body fat in obese adolescents [13, 52], and improve lipid profiles in high-risk adolescents [19, 52].

We thus conclude that there is very little evidence to suggest that adolescents who are physically active have a better CHD risk factor profile than their less active counterparts.

IT IS IMPORTANT TO BE ACTIVE DURING ADOLESCENCE TO REDUCE THE RISK OF SUBSEQUENT CHD AND OTHER CHRONIC DISEASES IN ADULTHOOD

There is currently no evidence that physical activity levels in adolescence have any association with adult chronic disease. Several studies have attempted to relate historical participation in competitive athletics during college to current disease status. In a study of male former college athletes, postcollege habitual PA and not competitive athletics in college predicted a low risk for CHD [48]. In contrast, participation in college athletics was found to decrease the risk of breast and reproductive cancers in women [22]. However, college age individuals, especially intercollegiate athletes, are not representative of the general population of adolescents. Clearly, these studies provide no direct evidence that high levels of PA during the adolescent years will decrease the risk of adult chronic disease.

ACTIVE TEENAGERS WILL BECOME ACTIVE ADULTS

One widely held perception is that active children become active adults. Therefore, some individuals involved in health promotion believe that interventions to change the PA patterns of adolescents will have long-term benefits. Yet, it is difficult to find data to support the contention that adult PA patterns are established during youth. The evidence to date has come primarily from retrospective studies [15, 17, 50] or studies that began tracking PA in college students, when patterns may be established [45, 48].

Prospective studies of the relationship between adolescent and adult PA are sparse and limited by small sample sizes or the assessment of PA. Glenmark et al. [26] assessed PA in a small sample of adolescents (age 16 yr) and then again in adulthood (age 27 yr). The results indicated that adolescent PA was a significant predictor of PA in adult women but not in men. In a large study of 3297 subjects [37], PA was assessed in subjects when they were 13 yr olds and again when they were 36 yr old. Above-average ability at games and a high energy level at age 13 were found to be predictive of PA level at age 36. However, the two measures of adolescent PA reflected a categorical rating by teachers during school hours. It is questionable as to whether this is an unbiased or representative assessment of PA.

Thus, there is very little support for the belief that physically active adolescents will be active adults.

THE ACTIVE TEENAGER IS THE MOST PHYSICALLY FIT TEENAGER

Overall, the association between PA and aerobic fitness is not strong. Studies generally report low correlations between habitual PA and aerobic fitness ($r = 0.01$–0.30) in adolescents [6, 7, 20, 23, 51, 57, 58] or no significant difference in VO_2max between active and inactive adolescents [33, 62]. The lack of association between PA and aerobic fitness is consistent with results seen in adults [38]. It is likely that factors such as genetics [11] and normal growth and maturation [31] are much more strongly related to fitness than PA levels in adolescence.

TEENAGERS WHO PARTICIPATE IN ATHLETICS WILL DEVELOP A HEALTHY LIFE-STYLE IN WHICH THEY ARE LESS LIKELY TO DRINK, SMOKE, OR USE DRUGS

A report from the President's Council on Physical Fitness and Sports states that by participating in athletics, youngsters are less likely to get involved with drugs and alcohol [61]. However, there are limited data to support this statement. The few studies that have examined this statement have been cross-sectional in nature, and the results are inconsistent. In AICS, we had the opportunity to follow 437 individuals who were "clean" in the first year of the study (no reported alcohol, cigarette, or drug use) for a period of 3-yr [1]. After 3 yr of follow-up, the cumulative incidence of the initiation of adverse health behaviors were: cigarette smoking, 15%; alcohol use, 27%; and marijuana use, 6%. There was little evidence that PA levels or participation in competitive athletics reduced the likelihood of engaging in these behaviors. There are some evidence in females that activity reduced the risk of smoking. The cumulative proportion of female students initiating cigarette use was 10, 23, and 22% for the high-, moderate-, and low-activity groups, respectively. However, there was also evidence that more active boys were more likely to drink than those who were not active. Males who participated in competitive athletics were significantly more likely than nonathletes to initiate alcohol use (44 vs 17%, $P < 0.01$). We thus see little evidence that PA and competitive athletics are related to high-risk behaviors in a manner consistent with health promotion.

THE MAJOR HEALTH PROBLEMS OF YOUTH ARE SMOKING, AIDS, ALCOHOL CONSUMPTION, ILLICIT DRUG USE, VIOLENCE, SUICIDE, AND TEENAGE PREGNANCY

Indeed, these are major health problems. However, another major health problem among the youth of America are injuries. Injuries rank as No. 1 of the 10 leading causes of death among teenagers. Morbidity data follow the same pattern, and more than one-half of all nonfatal injuries are related to sports and recreation. Why do we not pay more attention to sports and recreation injuries?

One possibility is that sports and recreation injuries are viewed as acceptable forms of ill health, whereas alcohol poisoning, drug overdose, and suicide are viewed as unacceptable. Most people would freely answer questions regarding injuries from sports. However, few are likely to answer honestly to questions about drug overdoses or suicide attempts, as those actions are socially unacceptable. Sports injuries are in many ways a "red badge of courage"! There needs to be the recognition that all forms of morbidity are "unacceptable," even injuries from sports. Clearly, adolescent sports injuries are very serious and costly but are neglected and apparently acceptable.

THERE ARE FEW RISKS ASSOCIATED WITH PA IN YOUTH

Regular participation in sports and recreation has been recommended as a primary health goal of our nation for adolescents [59]. It is, however, important to view this health goal cautiously, because sports and recreation may be a primary source of morbidity and mortality for this age group. Data from Gallagher et al. [24] demonstrate the magnitude of sports-related injury in adolescents. In the age group from 13–19 yr, 1 male in 8 and 1 female in 11 will have a sports-related injury each year that is of sufficient severity so as to be seen at an emergency room or require hospitalization. Any factor that produces a 15% hospital rate per year should be seriously examined.

There has been limited epidemiological research directly relating PA and injury. The population research evaluating sports and recreational injury has been primarily descriptive in nature [5, 9, 10, 12, 18, 21, 25, 29, 30, 36, 42, 53–55]. Much of the research has been sport-specific, e.g., the incidence of injuries in runners [10] or football players [5]. As Kraus and Conroy [36] and Blair et al. [10] have pointed out, there are major limiting factors to the previous research. One problem is that researchers often report injuries exclusively among runners or football players. The difficulty with this approach is that it does not take into account the injury risk among the non-participants. Therefore, we know little concerning the relative risk of sports participation. The second problem is that most of the research has not quantified the "exposure" or the "dose" of activity. We know little concerning the injury risk per "activity hours," nor do we know much about the relationship between intensity of sports and recreation and subsequent risk of injury during adolescence.

Despite the paucity of research, it is clear that the incidence of sports and recreation injuries is extremely high. The range of incidence for injuries requiring some form of hospital attention are from 3/100 to 20/100 per yr. A teenager has an incidence of injury that is annually measured in double-digit percentages, in contrast to most other end points, at which incidence is measured in rates per 10,000 or per 100,000. Because sports injuries are often thought of as being benign, both parent and child accept the risk for injury as an unavoidable part of sports participation. Thus, it is somewhat surprising that sports-related injuries in adolescents have not been investigated using classic epidemiological techniques to evaluate incidence and to determine the role of PA upon injury risk. Injuries are actually much easier to evaluate than other chronic conditions. The quantification and classification of injuries, especially relatively serious injuries, are well-defined. The onset of serious injury is typically abrupt, and the circumstances surrounding the onset are easily defined. Injuries occur in sufficient numbers for researchers to use a prospective study design.

Because of the paucity of information about the relationship of PA to adolescent injuries, the AICS was initiated. AICS was a population-based prospective study of adolescent injuries designed to (a) determine the incidence of adolescent injury and (b) determine the injury risks associated with exposure to increasing amounts and increasing intensity of PA, independent of potential confounders.

The 3-yr of injury surveillance yielded a total of 1076 injuries for an annualized rate of 34/100/yr. Forty-six percent of the cohort experienced at least one physician-treated injury during the 3 yr of surveillance, and 8% of the students suffered three or more injuries. Thirteen percent of the cases involved reinjuring a previous injury. The emergency department was the most frequent site of medical care, accounting for 56% of all cases, followed by the offices of primary care physicians (24%) and specialists (18%), as well as hospitalization settings (2%). There was one injury-related fatality during the study.

All medically treated injuries were classified as being sports or nonsports related. Sports and recreation were the primary causes of adolescent injury throughout each of the 3 yr and accounted for 55% of all the injuries. Clearly, sports and recreation are a primary contributor to physician visits and hospitalization in adolescents. Male sports injuries occurred most frequently in an unsupervised environment (55%), but female sports injuries were most common in the supervised environment of interscholastic athletics (48%). Twenty-six percent of male sports injuries occurred in interscholastic sports. Physical education class, which is mandatory in Pennsylvania schools, accounted for a significantly greater number of female sports injuries (16%) than male sports injuries (7%).

GREATER PA AND FITNESS LEVELS WILL PROTECT AGAINST INJURIES

If one went to a physician with a healthy child and the physician said "I would like to prescribe a drug that we think will be beneficial to your child. However, the drug has no proven health benefits, and there is a 15% chance that taking the drug will result in the child having to see a physician again because of a detrimental effect." Would we permit our children to take this drug? With the promotion of increased activity, especially vigorous activity, we readily allow our children to take the "exercise prescription." We do so primary because of our poor understanding of both the risks and benefits of activity among children.

In AICS we found a dose-response relationship between PA levels and injury risk. In both males and females, there was an increased risk of injury with increased PA (Fig. 14.1). This relationship was even stronger when we examined the injury risk of participating in competitive sports (Fig. 14.2). This makes perfect sense when viewed from the Haddon perspective of injury and energy transfer. Activity involving an increase in exposure to en-

FIGURE 14.1.

Relationship of habitual leisure time PA to sports injury risk in adolescents.

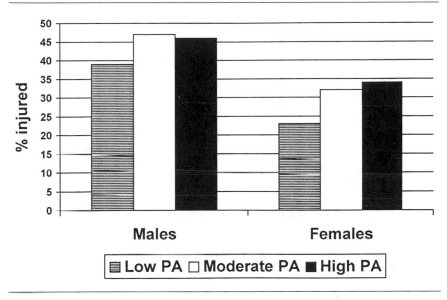

ergy transfer has an increased risk of injury. The magnitude of this effect is large. We have estimated that males have a 4-fold greater risk of injury when they are engaged in competitive athletics compared to other time periods, i.e., when they are not participating in competitive athletics. For females, there is a 5.5-fold increased risk. This must be put into the context of risk factors for disease. The individual risk factors for CHD, smoking, hypertension and hyperlipidemia, each increase risk by a factor of 3–5. There are major efforts to reduce exposure to these CHD risk factors. Competitive athletics are related to injury in a magnitude as great, if not greater, yet few people talk about reducing exposure to activity in order to reduce injury risk. Engaging in competitive sports thus appears to be a potent risk factor for adolescent injury.

THE OPTIMAL WAY TO REDUCE INJURY RISK IN YOUTH IS TO IMPROVE PRESPORT SCREENING AND PROVIDE BETTER TRAINING AND EQUIPMENT

There is little evidence that any of the above-mentioned events is the best means to reduce the risk of injury in adolescents. There have been very few randomized clinical trials of sports injury prevention, yet they would be easy to conduct. There is no concrete information about whether these costly interventions have any effect.

FIGURE 14.2.

Relationship of participation in competitive athletics to sports injury risk in adolescents.

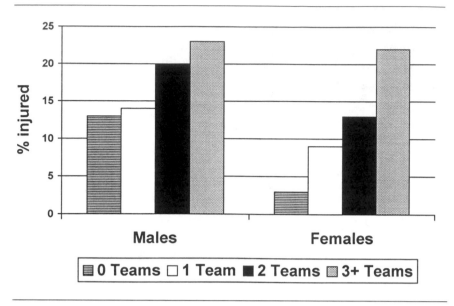

The easiest method to reduce sports injury is to reduce exposure to sport. At first approximation, this may not seem very palatable, as most believe that being active in youth is beneficial to health. Perhaps we should, however, examine the reduction of exposure as a means of reducing sports injuries.

Based on our data from AICS, if there were 1000 male children participating in competitive athletics, training for about 13 wk, for 13.5 hr/wk (a total of 175,500 hr in athletics), we would predict 40 injuries would occur. During a similar period of 175,500 hr not engaged in competitive athletics, we would expect 7 injuries to occur.

Obviously, the "banning" of competitive athletics to reduce injuries in sport is an absurd idea. Youth engage in sport in part to have "fun" and sports are a widely accepted part of growing up. In addition, there are benefits of sport participation (e.g., companionship and socialization) that are unrelated to health or fitness. These benefits are difficult to measure and, possibly, could be equal to the cost saved from reducing exposure to sport. However, we should begin to take more seriously the risk-benefit ratio of sport and its relation to other activities of health promotion. Reducing the exposure by 20% would be an enormous savings for the morbidity of children, as well as financial saving of health care dollars. A 20% reduction in time spent in com-

TABLE 14.1.

Approaches to Reduce Exposure to Competitive PA by 20%, Resulting in a Decreased Number of Sports-Related Injuries in Adolescents

No. of Participants	Length of Season (wk)	hr/ wk	Total Exposure (hr/season)	Expected Injuries	Approaches to ↓ No. of Sports-Related Injuries
1000	13	13.5	175,500	40	
800	13	13.5	140,400	32	Reduce participants
1000	11	13.5	148,500	33	Reduce length of season
1000	13	11.0	143,000	33	Reduce practice/game time

petitive sports would reduce the number of injuries from 40 to 32–33, preventing approximately 18% of the injuries in males. This could be accomplished in three ways; reducing the number of participants, reducing the length of the season, or reducing the practice/game time (Table 14.1). A reduction in exposure would not have to be applied to all sports. The most dangerous sports (based on the relative risk of injury) could be targeted. Reduction of exposure is a major approach for injury control, as it has been proven to be effective in many other forms of injury control.

CONCLUSIONS

Many of our beliefs about exercise and health in children are myths., There are no conclusive data indicating that an "active child is a healthy child" or that an "active child will be an active and healthy adult." However, many of us have participated in sports as our children do and have enjoyed it and have been willing to "pay the price" in terms of injury risk. With the global rise in medical care costs, however, can we continue to pay the price, particularly when the health benefits are unproved? We think not.

Of the adolescents from age 12–16 from our AICS cohort, 1 in every 11 was seen in an emergency room or hospital annually for a sports-related injury. Our incidence rates are consistent with other reports on sports-related morbidity in adolescents. Based on our prospective data, we estimate that there will be 6 hospitalizations, 187 emergency room visits, and 136 physician visits per 1000 adolescents from ages 12–18 in Western Pennsylvania annually. A conservative estimate of the direct costs of injuries to this school district can be calculated by applying an estimated cost of $200 per injury to the observed annual rate of 350 injuries/yr. This projects to an annual cost to this school district of approximately $70,000, with no consideration for rehabilitation costs or follow-up physician visits. Clearly, adolescent injuries are an enormous burden of morbidity, mortality, and cost on our society today, and most of these injuries can likely be prevented.

There are several things that need to be considered. The first is true knowledge of the risks involved. A parent and child should be required to sign an informed consent before the child participates in as in-depth a manner as those participating in medical research studies. School districts and local areas should appraise their policies about physical activity in adolescence based on science. There need to be considerably more epidemiological studies, case-control, prospective, and clinical trials to assess the risk:benefit ratio of exercise in children. It is likely that the general message that our teenagers are inactive and all should exercise a lot more is wrong.

There are other reasons for promoting activity that should be considered and balanced with health. For example, participation in athletics is thought to improve socialization. Physical activity and exercise in youth is natural; however, it is not very safe. We need to establish approaches toward safety and identify for whom PAs can have health benefits that outweigh the risk of injury as well as what type of activity we are discussing. There is a need for more epidemiological studies to describe the epidemiology of and determine the risk factors for sports injuries in adolescents. Finally, controlled clinical trials of sports injury prevention should be undertaken, based on the results of these epidemiological studies.

REFERENCES

1. Aaron, D. J., S. R. Dearwater, R. Anderson, T. Olsen, A. M. Kriska, and R. E. LaPorte. Physical activity and the initiation of high-risk health behaviors in adolescents. *Med. Sci. Sports Exerc.* 27:1639–1645, 1995.
2. Aaron, D. J., S. R. Dearwater, A. M. Kriska, et al. Are activity and/or fitness related to weight gain in adolescents? Data from the AIC Study. *Med. Sci. Sports Exerc.* 24:S124, 1992.
3. Aaron, D. J., A. M. Kriska, S. R. Dearwater, J. A. Cauley, K. F. Metz, and R. E. LaPorte. Reproducibility and validity of an epidemiologic questionnaire to assess past year physical activity in adolescents. *Am. J. Epidemiol* 142:191–201, 1995.
4. Aaron, D. J., A. M. Kriska, S. R. Dearwater, et al. The epidemiology of leisure physical activity in an adolescent population. *Med. Sci. Sports Exerc.* 25:847–853, 1993.
5. Alley, R. H. Head and neck injuries in high school football. *J. Am. Med. Assoc.* 188:418–422, 1964.
6. Anderson, L. B., P. Henckel, and B. Saltin. Risk factors for cardiovascular disease in 16–19-year-old teenagers. *J. Intern. Med.* 225:157–163, 1989.
7. Armstrong, N., J. Balding, P. Gentle, et al. Peak oxygen uptake and physical activity in 11- to 16-year olds. *Pediatr. Exerc. Sci.* 2:349–358, 1990.
8. Armstrong, N., J. Williams, J. Balding, P. Gentle, and B. Kirby. Cardiopulmonary fitness, physical activity patterns, and selected coronary risk factor variables in 11- to 16-year olds. *Pediatr. Exerc. Sci.* 3:219–228, 1991.
9. Beartrais, A. L., D. M. Fergusson, and F. T. Shannon. Childhood accidents in New Zealand birth cohort. *Aust. Paediatr.* 18:238–242, 1981.
10. Blair, S. N., H. W. Kohl, and N. N. Goodyear. Rates and risks for running and exercise injuries: studies in three populations. *Res. Q. Exerc. Sport* 58:1–8, 1987.
11. Bouchard, C., R. Lesage, G. Lortis, et al. Aerobic performance in brothers, dizygotic and monozygotic twins. *Med. Sci. Sports Exerc.* 18:639–646, 1986.
12. Boyce, W. T., L. W. Springer, S. Sobolewski, et al. Epidemiology of injuries in a large, urban school district. *Pediatrics* 74:342–349, 1984.

13. Brownell, K. D., and F. S. Kaye. A school-based behavior modification, nutrition education, and physical activity program for obese children. *Am. J. Clin. Nutr.* 35:277–283, 1982.

14. Bryant, J. G., H. L. Garrett, and M. S. Dean. The effects of an exercise programme on selected risk factors to coronary heart disease in children. *Soc. Sci. Med.* 19:765–766, 1984.

15. Bucher, C. A. National adult fitness survey: some implications. *J. Health Phys. Educ. Rec.* 45:25–28, 1974.

16. Chang, Y.-F., E. Portuese, and R. E. LaPorte. Increasing the shelf-life of review papers (letter). *Br. Med. J.* 312:513, 1996.

17. Dishman, R. K. Supervised and free-living physical activity: no differences in former athletes and nonathletes. *Am. J. Prev. Med.* 4:153–160, 1988.

18. Feldman, K. W., C. A. Woodward, K. C. Hodgson, et al. Prospective study of school injuries: incidence, types, related factors, and initial management. *Can. Med. Assoc. J.* 129:1279–1283, 1983.

19. Fisher, A. G., and M. Brown. The effects of diet and exercise on selected coronary risk factors in children. *Med. Sci. Sports Exerc.* 14:171, 1982.

20. Forth, C. D., and A. W. Salmoni. Relationships among self-reported physical activity, aerobic fitness and reaction time. *Can. J. Sport Sci.* 17:88–90, 1988.

21. Freide, A. M., C. V. Azzana, S. S. Gallagher, et al. The epidemiology of injuries to bicycle riders. *Pediatr. Clin. North Am.* 32:141–152, 1985.

22. Frisch, R. E., G. Wyshad, N. L. Albright, et al. Lower prevalence of breast cancer and cancers of the reproductive system among former college athletes compared to non-athletes. *Br. J. Cancer* 52:885–891, 1985.

23. Fuchs, R., K. E. Powell, N. K. Semmer, et al. Patterns of physical activity among German adolescents: the Berlin-Bremen Study. *Prev. Med.* 17:746–763, 1988.

24. Gallagher, S. S., K. Finison, B. Guyer, and S. Goodenough. The incidence of injuries among 87,000 Massachusetts children and adolescents: results of the 1980–91 statewide childhood injury prevention program surveillance system. *Am. J. Public Health* 74:1340–1346, 1984.

25. Garrick, J. G., and R. K. Requa. Injuries in high school sports. *Pediatrics* 61:465–469, 1978.

26. Glenmark, B., G. Hedberg, and E. Jansson. Prediction of physical activity level in adulthood by physical characteristics, physical performance and physical activity in adolescence. an 11-year follow-up study. *Eur. J. Appl. Physiol.* 69:530–538, 1994.

27. Hagberg, J. M., D. Goldring, A. A. Ehsani, et al. Effect of exercise training on the blood pressure and hemodynamic features of hypertensive adolescents. *Am. J. Cardiol.* 52:763–768, 1983.

28. Hunt, H. F., and J. R. White. Effects of ten weeks of vigorous daily exercise on serum lipids and lipoproteins in teenage males. *Med. Sci. Sports Exerc.* 12:93, 1980.

29. Jaketa, S. Student accidents in Hawaii's public schools. *J. Sch. Health* 54:208–209, 1984.

30. Johnson, C. J., A. P. Canter, V. K. Harlein, et al. Injuries resulting in fractures in Seattle public schools during the year 1969–70. *J. Sch. Health* 42:454–457, 1972.

31. Kemper, H. C. G. Sources of variation in longitudinal assessment of maximal aerobic power in teenage boys and girls: The Amsterdam Growth and Health Study. *Hum. Biol.* 63:533–547, 1991.

32. Kemper, H. C. G., J. Snell, R. Verschuur, et al. Tracking of health and risk indicators of cardiovascular disease from teenager to adult: Amsterdam Growth and Health Study. *Prev. Med.* 19:642–655, 1990.

33. Kemper, H. C. G., and R. Verschuur. Longitudinal study of coronary risk factors during adolescence and young adulthood: the Amsterdam Growth and Health Study. *Pediatr. Exerc. Sci.* 2:359–371, 1990.

34. Klesges, R. C., L. M. Klesges, L. H. Eck, and M. L. Shelton. A longitudinal analysis of accelerated weight gain in preschool children. *Pediatrics* 95:126–130, 1995.

35. Kolbe, L. J. An epidemiological surveillance system to monitor the prevalence of youth behaviors that most affect health. *Health Educ.* 9:44–48, 1990.

36. Kraus, J. K., and C. Conroy. Mortality and morbidity from injuries in sports and recreation. *Annu. Rev. Public Health* 5:163–192, 1984.

37. Kuh, D. J. L., and C. Cooper. Physical activity at 36 years: patterns and childhood predictors in a longitudinal study. *J. Epidemiol. Community Health* 46:114–119, 1992.

38. Lamb, K. L. and D. A. Brodie. Leisure-time physical activity as an estimate of physical fitness: a validation study. *J. Clin. Epidemiol.* 44:41–52, 1991.

39. Linder, C. W., R. H. DuRant, and O. M. Mahoney. The effect of physical conditioning on serum lipids and lipoproteins in white male adolescents. *Med. Sci. Sports Exerc.* 15:232–236, 1983.

40. Macek, M., D. Bell, J. Rutenfranz, et al. A comparison of coronary risk factors in groups of trained and untrained adolescents. *Eur. J. Appl. Physiol.* 58:577–582, 1989.

41. Macek, M., J. Rutenfranz, K. Lange Andersen, et al. Favorable levels of cardiovascular health and risk indicators during childhood and adolescence. *Eur. J. Pediatr.* 144:360–367, 1985.

42. Manheimer, D. I., J. Dewey, G. D. Mellinger, and L. Covoa. 50,000 child-years of accidental injuries. *Public Health Rep.* 81:519–533, 1966.

43. Marti, B., and E. Vartiainen. Relationship between leisure time exercise and cardiovascular risk factors among 15-year-olds in eastern Finland. *J. Epidemiol. Community Health* 43:228–233, 1989.

44. Montoye, H. J. Physical activity, physical fitness, and heart disease risk factors in children. *The Academy Papers: Effects of Physical Activity on Children*. Champaign, IL: Human Kinetics, 1986, pp. 127–152.

45. Montoye, H. J., W. D. VanHuss, H. W. Olson, et al. The longevity and morbidity of college athletes. Phi Epsilon Kappa Fraternity, 1957.

46. Moore, L. L., U. S. Nguyen, K. J. Rothman, L. A. Cupples, and R. C. Ellison. Preschool physical activity level and change in body fatness in young children: the Framingham Children's Study. *Am. J. Epidemiol.* 142:982–988, 1995.

47. Nizankowska-Blaz, T., and T. Abramowicz. Effects of intensive physical training on serum lipids and lipoprotein. *Acta Paediatr. Scand.* 72:357–359, 1983.

48. Paffenbarger, R. S., R. T. Hyde, A. L. Wing, and C. H. Steinmetz. A natural history of athleticism and cardiovascular health. *J. Am. Med. Assoc.* 252:491–495, 1984.

49. Ross, J. G., C. O. Dotson, G. G. Gilbert, et al. After physical education: physical activity outside of school physical education programs. *J. Phys. Educ. Rec. Dance* 56:77–81, 1985.

50. Sallis, J. F., M. E. Hovell, C. R. Hofstetter, et al. A multivariant study of determinants of vigorous exercise in a community sample. *Prev. Med.* 18:20–34, 1989.

51. Sallis, J. F., T. L. Patterson, M. J. Buono, et al. Relation of cardiovascular fitness and physical activity to cardiovascular disease risk factors in children and adults. *Am. J. Epidemiol.* 127:933–941, 1988.

52. Sasaki, J., M. Shindo, H. Tanaka, M. Ando, and K. Arakawa. A long-term aerobic exercise program decreases the obesity index and increases the high density lipoprotein cholesterol concentration in obese children. *Int. J. Obes.* 11:339–345, 1987.

53. Sheps, S. B., and G. D. Evans. Epidemiology of school injuries: a two year experience in municipal health department. *Pediatrics* 79:69–75, 1987.

54. Shively, R. A., W. A. Grana, and D. Ellis. High school sports injuries. *Physician Sports Med.* 9:46–50, 1981.

55. Sibert, J. R., G. B. Maddocks, and B. M. Brown. Childhood accidents: an epidemic of epidemic proportions. *Arch. Dis. Child.* 56:225–235, 1981.

56. Suter, E. and M. R. Hawes. Relationship of physical activity, body fat, diet, and blood lipid profiles in youths 10–15 yr. *Med. Sci. Sports Exerc.* 25:748–754, 1993.

57. Taylor, W., and T. Baranowski. Physical activity and cardiovascular fitness, and adiposity in children. *Res. Q. Exerc. Sport* 62:157–163, 1991.

58. Tell, G. T., and O. D. Vellar. Physical fitness, physical activity, and cardiovascular disease risk factors in adolescents: the Oslo Youth Study. *Prev. Med.* 17:12–24, 1988.

59. U.S. Department of Health and Human Services. *Healthy People 2000: National Health Promotion and Disease Prevention Objectives*. Washington, DC: GPO. 1991.

60. U.S. Department of Health and Human Services. *Physical Activity and Health: A Report of the Surgeon General*. Atlanta: US Department of Health and Human Services, Centers for Disease Control and Prevention, National Center for Chronic Disease Prevention and Health Promotion, 1996, pp. 186–200.

61. Vidmar, P. The role of the federal government in promoting health through the schools: report from the President's Council on Physical Fitness and Sports. *J. Sch. Health* 62:129–130, 1992.

62. Weymans, M., and T. Reybrouch. Habitual level of physical activity and cardiorespiratory endurance capacity in children. *Eur. J. Appl. Physiol.* 58:803–807, 1989.

15
Perception of Physical Exertion: Methods, Mediators, and Applications

ROBERT J. ROBERTSON, Ph.D.
BRUCE J. NOBLE, Ph.D.

The perception of exertion is defined as the subjective intensity of *effort, strain, discomfort,* and/or *fatigue* that is experienced during physical exercise. Scientific and clinical inquiry regarding the perceptual milieu associated with physical exertion was first undertaken in the 1960s by Gunnar A. V. Borg, a Swedish psychologist. Borg studied perceptions experienced during exercise using an adaptation of Stevens' law that states that human sensation grows as a power function of a physical stimulus [71]. An outgrowth of Borg's early work was the development and validation of a series of psychophysical category scales to quantify exertional perceptions associated with a wide range of physical activities. A distinguishing feature of these category scales is that they are easily administered and interpreted, facilitating interindividual comparisons of sensory processing during exercise. Versions of Borg's scales have been adapted for use in clinical and research settings throughout many parts of the world.

Since Borg's pioneering work, the discipline of *perceived exertion* has focused on three primary areas: (a) development and validation of perceptual scaling methodology; (b) laboratory experiments to identify physiological and psychological mediators of the effort sense; and (c) clinical, sports, and pedagogical applications. Research in these three areas has proceeded more or less in concert, undertaken by physiologists, psychologists, clinicians, and physical educators. This chapter presents a synthesis of both experimental and clinical research in the areas of perceived exertion methods, mediators, and applications.

GLOBAL MODEL

At the outset, an examination of the many factors that influence the perceived intensity of exertion during dynamic exercise may help to place the field of study in a global perspective. The global explanatory model, presented in Figure 15.1, describes a variety of physiological, psychological, and performance factors that shape the perception of physical exertion [171]. The model expresses exertional perception as a "gestalt-like" response that incorporates information from both internal and external en-

407

FIGURE 15.1.
Global explanatory model of perceived exertion. Reproduced from ref. 171.

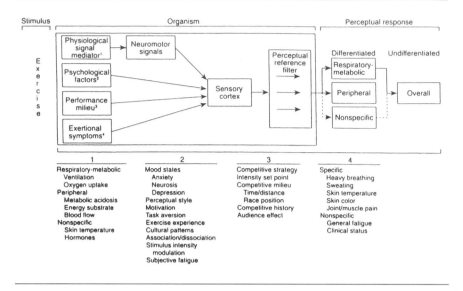

vironments. To appreciate the gestalt properties of the exertional milieu, it is necessary to distinguish between perception and sensation. Sensation involves direct stimulation of a sensory end organ. Perception, on the other hand, involves both pure sensation and a complex of internal and external stimuli for which there may be no direct link with sensory end organs. The global model uses perception, as opposed to sensation, as its organizing conceptual framework in explaining the exertional milieu associated with physical exercise. The model is a fourth-generation conceptualization that has been derived from previous explanatory models developed by Noble et al. [167] and Robertson [201]. Perceptual responsiveness is explained sequentially by interpreting the model from left to right. Physiological responses to an exercise stimulus serve as the initial mediators that shape the intensity of the perceptual signal. The effect of these signal mediators is to alter tension-producing properties of skeletal muscle. An increase in peripheral and/or respiratory muscle tension during exercise is brought about by a greater discharge of central feedforward commands arising from the motor cortex. Corollary pathways carrying a copy of these central commands terminate in the sensory cortex. These corollary discharges are subsequently interpreted as perceptual signals of exertion. The final mediating step in the exertional process occurs when the signal arising from the sensory cortex is matched with the contents of the perceptual cognitive reference filter. As the signal passes through the reference filter it is fine tuned, its intensity modulated according to a matrix of past and present events that reflect the individuals psychological characteristics and perceptual style. The resulting perceptual response can be differentiated to the active limbs and respiratory system, or it can appear as an undifferentiated rating for the overall body.

SCALING METHODOLOGY

The validity of clinical, sports, and pedagogical applications of exertional perceptions is directly dependent on the use of appropriate scaling methodology. The next two sections briefly describe category and ratio scaling methods and examine the importance of Borg's range model in the assessment and interpretation of perceived exertion responses during dynamic exercise. For a detailed discussion of the psychophysical concepts underlying the validation of perceived exertion rating scales and specific guidelines for the development of scaling instructions and perceptual anchoring procedures, the reader is referred to chapter 3 in Noble and Robertson's text on perceived exertion [171].

Category Scales

The assessment of exertional perceptions in either clinical or experimental settings is most frequently undertaken using category scaling procedures [171]. From a psychophysical standpoint, a category scale requires that the sensory response continuum be partitioned into equal intervals. Scale categories are labeled with a finite set of numbers. Two or more of the numerical categories are directly linked to adjectives called verbal descriptors. The distance between each category is presumed to correspond to equal sensory response intervals.

The category rating scales that are most commonly used to assess exertional perceptions in experimental, clinical, and/or occupational settings are listed below in chronological order of development: (a) Borg's 21 partition scale—1962; (b) Borg's 15-partition scale (i.e., the RPE scale)—1962; (c) the University of Pittsburgh 9-partition scale—1969; (d) Borg's 10-partition Category-Ratio (CR-10) scale—1980; and (e) Fleishman's 7-partition scale (Occupational Effort Index)—1979. Of these, the RPE scale, the Pittsburgh scale, and the CR-10 scale are most frequently cited in the perceived-exertion literature [171]. The numerical format and associated verbal descriptors for these three scales are presented in Figure 15.2. Fleishman's Occupational Effort Index is considered later in Ergonomic Applications of Perceived Exertion.

Each of the three scales presented in Figure 15.2 has been validated by correlating RPE with heart rate (HR) and/or VO_2 responses during cycle and treadmill tests or during water immersion arm/leg ergometry. In these validation experiments, exercise intensity was either progressively incre-

FIGURE 15.2.

Perceived exertion category scales: (a) fifteen-category Borg scale to rate perceptions of exertion (RPE); (b) category-ratio scale of perceived exertion; (c) nine-category Pittsburgh scale of perceived exertion.

(a)	Fifteen category scale to rate perceptions of exertion (RPE)	(b)	Category-ratio scale of perceived exertion (CR-10)	
6	No exertion at all	0	Nothing at all	
7	Extremely light	0.5	Very, very weak	(just noticeable)
8		1	Very weak	
9	Very light	2	Weak	(light)
10		3	Moderate	
11	Light	4	Somewhat strong	
12		5	Strong	(heavy)
13	Somewhat hard	6		
14		7	Very strong	
15	Hard (heavy)	8		
16		9		
17	Very hard	10	Very, very strong	(almost max)
18		●	Maximal	
19	Extremely hard			
20	Maximal exertion	(c)	Pittsburgh perceived exertion scale	
		1		
		2	Not at all stressful	
		3		
		4		
		5		
		6		
		7		
		8	Very, very stressful	
		9		

mented or presented in random order. Test-retest scale reliability has been determined for short, long, and intermittent exercise protocols using correlational analysis. The validity correlations for the three RPE category scales in Figure 15.2 were statistically significant, ranging from $r = 0.56–0.94$. Test-retest reliability coefficients ranged from $r = 0.78–0.91$. As such, the 15-category Borg RPE scale, the 9-category Pittsburgh scale, and the C-R 10 scale are valid and reliable psychophysical instruments to measure exertional perceptions during dynamic exercise [12, 15, 16, 19, 171, 200, 204, 218, 223].

Ratio Scales

Ratio scaling procedures that have been used in perceived-exertion experiments are termed magnitude estimation and magnitude production [171]. In open-magnitude scaling, the rater estimates how many times greater the exertion is perceived to be, as compared to the amount of exertion associated with a standard exercise intensity. The perceptual response is taken as any number expressed as a multiple of the numeric standard. Magnitude production scaling procedures require the rater to adjust exercise intensity to produce a predetermined level of perceived exertion. The perceptual response is expressed in measurement units that describe mode-specific exercise intensity, i.e., power output, muscular force, oxygen uptake. In general, ratio scaling validation experiments indicate that the perception of muscular effort during short, long, and intermittent exercise bouts grows as a positively accelerating function of cycle ergometer power output with an average psychophysical exponent of 1.6 [22].

Based on these initial findings, as well as those on a number of follow-up investigations, both magnitude estimation and magnitude production are valid ratio scaling procedures to assess exertional perception in experimental settings involving static and dynamic muscular contractions [176].

Scale Section

Selection of the appropriate type of scale to measure exertional perceptions is primarily dependent on a priori decisions about psychophysical comparisons and interpretations of test responses. Numerically formatted category scales (i.e., Borg 15- and Pittsburgh 9-partition scales) are recommended for use during graded-cycle and treadmill tests in which: (a) exercise intensity is progressively incremented; (b) psychological responses that are of experimental importance distribute as a linear function of exercise intensity; and (c) clinical, physiological, and perceptual responses are to be used conjunctively to assess exercise tolerance and prescribe exercise intensity [171]. It is recommended that the CR-10 scale and magnitude estimation-production procedures be used when it is of interest to: (a) compare perceptual responses between various experimental pertubations in which the physiological reference for comparison falls on an exponential curve and (b) determine how perception of exertion grows as a function of physiological responses that change exponentially with increasing exercise intensity.

BORG'S PSYCHOPHYSICAL RANGE MODEL: CORNERSTONE OF CATEGORY SCALING

The validity of category rating scales to assess interindividual differences in perceived exertion is based on the assumptions presented in Borg's range model of human sensory responses to external physical stimuli (Fig. 15.3) [137]. The range model describes the conceptual framework necessary to establish stimulus-response congruence throughout the entire relative metabolic range during dynamic exercise. The principal assumptions that comprise this conceptual framework are as follows. (a) For any given stimulus range (i.e., rest-to-peak exercise intensity), there exists a corresponding and equal perceived-exertion range. (b) For all clinically normal individuals, both the perceptual range and the intensity of the perceptual signals at the low and high ends of the stimulus range are equal.

FIGURE 15.3.

Borg's psychophysical range model, depicting the equality between exercise stimulus and perceptual response continua.

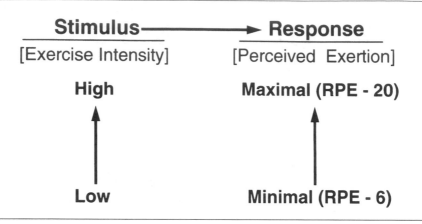

The scaling rationale inherent in the above assumptions holds that as exercise intensity increases from very low to maximal levels, there is a *corresponding* and *equal* increase in perceptual intensity from "no exertion" to "maximal exertion." In this case, any two clinically normal individuals can respond with a perceptual rating that falls at 50% of their perceptual response range, even though the absolute power output (i.e., exercise stimulus) associated with that perceptual rating is higher for the individual with the comparatively higher maximal aerobic power. Comparison of perceived-exertion responses between individuals differing in level of maximal aerobic power is, therefore, possible.

The importance of the range model in assessing RPE using category scaling methodology was first described by Borg in 1962 [13]. Borg's pioneering development of the range model provided the theoretical underpinnings upon which his original 21- and 15-partition category scales were validated. All subsequent perceived exertion category scales have been developed, validated, and implemented according to the basic tenants of the range model. In this regard, the range model specifies the content of the instructions to the rater concerning use of a category scale to transpose feelings of exertion into numerical ratings. The range model also defines procedures to establish the low and high perceptual scale anchors. It is during these anchoring procedures that the subjective correspondence between stimulus (i.e., exercise intensity) and response (i.e., perceived exertion) ranges is cognitively established. The individuals perceptual range is then the same width as the stimulus range, and the intensity of exertional perceptions at the low and high end of the response continuum corresponds directly with exercise intensities that are extremely low and extremely high.

In summary, when clear and unequivocal scaling instructions and anchoring procedures are used, the range model subjectively equates minimal and maximal perceptual intensities between individuals who otherwise may vary in physiological, psychological, and physical activity attributes. The intensity of a perceptual signal at any point in the exercise stimulus range is then determined by its relative position within the response range, as defined by the minimal and maximal rating scaling categories [137].

EFFORT CONTINUA

Perceptual responses during exercise are influenced by an array of exertional symptoms, i.e., strain, fatigue, discomfort, pain, etc. Systematic quantification of these exertional symptoms increases the clinical sensitivity of perceptually based exercise testing and exercise prescription [16]. Such clinical applications are based on the assumption that perceived-exertion responses during dynamic exercise have corollary physiological mediators. The functional interdependence of perceptual and physiological responses during dynamic exercise provides an empirical rationale for the clinical application of subjective estimates of physical exertion. This rationale is an outgrowth of Borg's original thesis that the subjective response to an exercise stimulus involves three main effort continua that can be characterized as: *physiological, perceptual,* and *performance* [14]. The effort continua depict the relation between physiological demands of exercise performance and the perception of exertion associated with that performance. The functional link between the three effort continua indicates that perceptual responses provide much of the same information about exercise performance as do selected physiological responses. Decisions concerning the intensity and duration of exercise performance can then be based on the functional interaction between the perceptual and physiological continua [107, 240]. Each of the effort continua are influenced by such factors as psychological mood states, clinical status, and exercise mode [15].

EXERTIONAL SYMPTOMS AND PHYSIOLOGICAL SUBSTRATA

The effort sense is a complex psychophysical process that integrates a large number of exertional symptoms, each of which is presumed to be linked to an underlying physiological mediator [124]. The linguistic expression of these exertional symptoms forms a "perceptual reality," allowing for a more global measurement of the physiological and psychological factors that are rate-limiting during dynamic exercise [26].

One of the most pronounced symptoms of exertional intolerance is the sensation of fatigue [239]. Weiser et al. [239], using key cluster analysis, identified three subsets of fatigue during cycle ergometer exercise, i.e., leg fatigue, general fatigue, and cardiopulmonary fatigue. These three fatigue subclusters evidenced a modest but significant interrelation, i.e., $r = 0.26$–0.82. Horstman et al. [107] independently validated Weiser's exertional symptom classification, demonstrating that during submaximal (80% VO_2peak) cycle ergometry, fatigue in the legs (i.e., aches, cramps, muscular and articular pain, and heaviness) and the cardiorespiratory system (i.e., dyspnea) were strong predictors of submaximal endurance exercise.

Weiser and Stamper [240] developed a psychophysical model that describes the sensory link between subjective symptoms and physiological mediators during dynamic exercise. This model uses a pyramidal format to categorize sensory events that extend from specific physiological substrata to a global report of exertional perceptions for the overall body. The model positions exertional symptom clusters within a vertical sensory pathway. The base of the pyramid contains the underlying *physiological substrata*. These physiological processes mediate the intensity of subjective symptoms of fatigue and exertional intolerance during cycle exercise. The next level in ascending order contains *discrete symptoms* (i.e., shortness of breath, muscle aches, and weariness) that have their origins in the underlying physiological substrata. These discrete symptoms are grouped into fatigue subclusters, i.e., cardiopulmonary, leg, and general fatigue. The subclusters combine at the *ordinate* level of sensory processing to form a primary symptom cluster labeled bicycling fatigue. The *superordinate* level is positioned at the peak of the pyramid. Here, the primary symptom clusters are integrated into a global report of fatigue for the overall body.

Perceptual signals that are differentiated according to their specific physiological mediators provide a more precise measure of the physiological and/or pathological processes that shape the "exertional context" during exercise [179, 204, 205, 208]. Pandolf et al. [175, 179] modified Weiser's theoretical model (i.e, see paragraph above) to include the concept of differentiated exertional signals. This modification redefines the subordinate level of sensory processing by adding two differentiated clusters, i.e., local muscular exertion and cardiopulmonary exertion. These clusters are directly related to the physical exertion cluster at the ordinate level. Exertional symptoms can then be differentiated according to physiological mediators that are specific to either the active muscles and joints or the cardiopulmonary and aerobic metabolic systems.

A number of nonspecific symptom clusters (i.e., task aversion and motivation) that are described in Weiser's model directly reflect psychological traits. Nonspecific psychological symptom clusters are located at the ordinate level of sensory processing. These symptom clusters interact to form a "perceptual style," which systematically influences exertional perceptions at all levels of subjective reporting. As such, the symptom clusters labeled task aversion and motivation in Weiser's original model can be combined into a single conceptual classification, termed the "perceptual-cognitive reference filter." This filter contains a catalogue of "sensory context" reflecting a broad range of psychological and cognitive processes. Although these psychological constructs are not necessarily related to underlying physiological substrata, they nevertheless systematically account for individual differences in perceived exertion during physical exercise. From an operational standpoint, the perceptual-cognitive reference filter is positioned at the subordinate level of sensory processing. The filter modulates the intensity of sensory signals as they travel from their physiological/neuromotor origins to conscious expression of both differentiated and undifferentiated exertional perceptions. A more detailed description of the situational and dispositional psychological components that comprise the perceptual-cognitive reference filter are presented later in this chapter.

PERCEPTUAL SIGNAL INTEGRATION AND DOMINANCE

During dynamic exercise, RPE can be anatomically regionalized to the active limbs and shoulders, as well as to the chest, yielding differentiated sensory signals [175, 178, 204]. Two methodological questions are frequently asked with respect to differentiated perceptual ratings: (a) What is the mode of *integration* of the differentiated signals as their separate sensory intensities converge to form the undifferentiated report of exertion for the overall body? (b) Which differentiated perceptual signal is the most intense for a given exercise task and/or performance setting, hence, *dominating* the integration process?

Exertional responsiveness during dynamic exercise appears at both the ordinate and superordinate level of perceptual processing [171]. The responses at the ordinate level are anatomically differentiated and, hence, are closely linked to underlying physiological substrata. The undifferentiated perceptual response for the overall body appears at the superordinate level and is the net integration of the various differentiated signals. The flow of the perceptual signal as it courses from underlying physiological substrata to conscious expression at both the ordinate and superordinate levels of reporting was described in a first-generation model developed by Kinsman and Weiser [125] and, later, in second- and third-generation models presented by Pandolf et al. [179] and Noble and Robertson [171], respectively. Each differentiated rating of perceived exertion is assumed to carry a specific intensity weighting. Those differentiated perceptual signals arising from the body regions predominantly involved in the exercise or occupational task have the highest intensity weighting [174, 204, 240], i.e., they dominate the sensory integration process. Normally, signal integration and sensory dominance are examined as interrelated neurological events, wherein both processes are of primary importance in the functional expression of the undifferentiated perceptual response for the overall body.

The mode of integration of differentiated perceptual signals appears to depend on: (a) the exercise type; (b) the anatomical origin of the differentiated signals, i.e., arms, legs, shoulders, and chest; and (c) the performance/environmental medium, i.e., air or water. The functional link between signal integration and sensory dominance is most clearly demonstrated during cycle ergometer exercise, in which muscle mass per unit of external work is standardized. During cycle ergometry, the differentiated signal from the legs is typically more intense (i.e., dominant) than that from either the chest or the overall signal [41, 71, 89, 179, 204]. As an example, Robertson et al. [204] used a cycle ergometer paradigm wherein power output was held constant (840 kg/min) while pedal rate varied (40, 60, and 80 rev/min). At each pedal rate, the legs rating was more intense than the arms rating. The undifferentiated rating for the overall body was a weighted average of the differentiated legs and chest ratings. These data indicate that during cycling, peripheral signals from involved limbs dominate the perceptual integration process.

When pronounced perceptual signals arise from two discrete sources, such as occurs during wheelbarrow pushing, the intensity of the undifferentiated rating is higher than that of either of the differentiated ratings [89]. During maximal treadmill running, the intensity of the undifferentiated rating is equal to or greater than the dominant differentiated rating, irrespective of the number of regional signals involved [89, 107].

A number of experiments have examined the mode of signal integration and sensory dominance during prolonged (60–180 min) submaximal cycle ergometer [116], arm ergometer [210], and arm-plus-leg ergometer [178] exercise undertaken at 60–70% VO_2peak. In addition, Noble et al. [167] and Ueda et al. [232] determined the mode of perceptual signal integration during swimming, using multiple regression techniques. In the paradigms involving cycle-only exercise, the legs rating was always more intense than the chest rating, thereby dominating the perceptual-integration process. For those paradigms using arm ergometry or combined arm and leg ergometry, the perceptual signal from the arms was always dominant. In each of these submaximal exercise paradigms, the undifferentiated rating of perceived exertion for the overall body appeared as a weighted average of the anatomically differentiated ratings.

Differentiated perceptual responsiveness has also been assessed during intermittent exercise, water immersion ergometry, and hand-weighted bench stepping [206], yielding reasonably similar results between investigations. Swank and Robertson demonstrated that during high-intensity (90% VO_2peak), intermittent cycle ergometer exercise, the leg perceptual rating was more intense than the chest rating [228]. The chest and overall body ratings were similar for each intermittent exercise bout. Robertson et al. examined differentiated perceptual responsiveness during combined arm and leg water immersion ergometry [199]. The perceptual rating for the arms was consistently more intense (i.e., dominant) than the legs rating over a wide range of power outputs and pedal-crank rates. The undifferentiated rating for the overall body appeared as a weighted average of the differentiated arms and legs signals. A similar mode of signal integration and dominance was observed during hand-weighted bench stepping undertaken at 70% of mode specific VO_2peak [206].

Two investigations have assessed differentiated ratings of perceived exertion during treadmill walking while the subject is manually transporting external payloads [4, 202]. The payloads were carried by a waist belt, head pack, frontal yolk and transverse yoke. For all load carriage modes, the perceptual rating for the legs dominated the integration process. When the payload was transported by waist belt, the undifferentiated rating for the overall body was a weighted average of the differentiated legs and chest ratings.

Dominance of anatomically differentiated sensory signals also persists during the abatement of exertional responsiveness after maximal treadmill exercise [209]. Robertson et al. reported that the rating of perceived exertion for the legs was more intense than the rating for the chest when determined over a 12-min supine postexercise period [209]. The undifferentiated rating for the overall body approximated a weighted average of the differentiated regional ratings during the recovery period.

Pandolf et al. [179] and Pimental and Pandolf [186] found that when light external loads were carried at slow and moderate walking speeds, the intensities of the local (i.e., legs) and central (i.e., chest) differentiated signals did not differ from those of the undifferentiated rating for the overall body. When heavier external loads were transported, the central ratings were more intense than the local ratings. These responses suggest the presence of a differentiation threshold (DT) for ratings of perceived exertion during manual load transport. The DT marked the walking speed at which the intensities of the peripheral and respiratory-metabolic perceptual signals were first reported to be different from the overall signal of exertion. At speeds faster than the DT, the chest signal was the dominant factor in mediating the overall perception of exertion during manual load transport.

Robertson et al. arrived at a different conclusion regarding the presence of a DT for perceived exertion ratings during manual load transport [209]. At walking speeds of less than 6.44 km/hr while the subject is transporting a payload equivalent to 7.5% of body weight and at walking speeds less than 4.83 km/min while transporting a payload equivalent to 15% of body weight, ratings of perceived exertion were the same for the legs, chest, and overall body. These speeds marked the DT for the two different payload conditions. At speeds faster than the DT, exertion was perceived to be more intense in the legs than in the overall body and less intense in the chest than in the overall body. Once the DT is reached or exceeded, the mode of perceptual integration and emergence of the dominant signal appear to be an interactive function of the weight of the payload and the locomotor speed.

Experimental findings suggest that the mode of perceptual integration and the dominant sensory signal should be identified separately for physical activities that vary in type, metabolic intensity, and number of involved anatomical regions.

PHYSIOLOGICAL MEDIATORS OF EXERTIONAL PERCEPTIONS

Physiological responses to an exercise stimulus mediate the intensity of exertional perceptions by acting either individually or collectively to alter tension producing properties of peripheral and respiratory skeletal muscle. The underlying physiological events that mediate perceptual signals of exertion are classified as *respiratory-metabolic, peripheral* and *nonspecific* [171]. It should be noted that the terms peripheral and respiratory-metabolic, respectively, are used to replace the previously used terms local and central when one is classifying physiological mediators of the effort sense. This contemporary nomenclature is consistent with the recommendations advanced by Noble and Robertson in their text on perceived exertion [171].

Respiratory-Metabolic Perceptual Signals

Respiratory-metabolic signals of perceived exertion include ventilatory (V_E) drive, oxygen consumption (VO_2), carbon dioxide production, HR, and blood pressure [112, 153, 176, 178, 204].

VENTILATORY DRIVE. The sensory link between V_E and respiratory effort has been established by both simple and multiple regression analyses. Correlation coefficients ranging from $r = 0.61$–0.94 have been reported between RPE and both V_E and respiratory rate (RR) [17, 69, 115, 170, 180, 212, 213, 217, 221, 230]. Breathlessness was found to be a strong independent predictor of RPE in young women with mild asthma [244]. Pulmonary ventilation and RR consistently accounted for the greatest amount of variance in a stepwise multiple-regression model to predict RPE during treadmill and cycle ergometer exercise in neutral and hot environments [170, 212].

The strongest evidence in support of ventilatory drive as a physiological mediator of respiratory-metabolic exertional signals has been found when V_E was experimentally manipulated to determine whether RPE demonstrated a corresponding change. When V_E drive was experimentally perturbed by hypnosis [159], induced erythrocythemia [208], hypoxia [144, 201], hyperoxia [182], and variations in cycle pedaling frequency [205] and testing mode [86], RPE exhibited corresponding changes. That is, RPE either increased or decreased in conjunction with experimentally induced increases or decreases in V_E drive.

As an example, Robertson et al. [203] used $NaHCO_3^-$ ingestion to attenuate ventilatory buffering of metabolic acidosis during combined arm and leg exercise. It was expected that the perceptual signal arising from the chest would also be attenuated after an alkalotic shift in blood pH. At a power output equivalent to 80%, VO_2peak, V_E, and RPE-chest were lower ($P < 0.01$) under alkalosis, as compared to under a placebo condition (Fig. 15.4). Because metabolic acidosis is limited at lower exercise intensities,

FIGURE 15.4.

*Effect of induced alkalosis on ratings of perceived exertion in the chest (RPE-CHEST)
and for the overall body (RPE-OVERALL) during arm and leg exercise. At a given
%VO₂max, means that are connected by an * are significantly (P < 0.01) different.
Reproduced from ref. 208.*

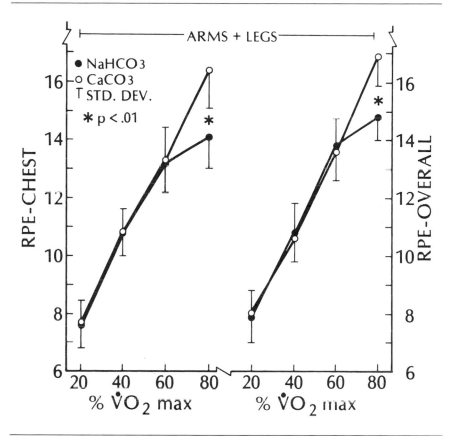

neither V_E nor RPE-chest differed between acid-base condition at power
outputs ranging from 20 to 60% VO₂peak.

The role of RR and tidal volume (TV) in mediating the intensity of perceptual signals of exertion has been examined using experimental perturbations involving variations in cycle ergometer pedaling frequency and
blood pH. Under these experimental conditions, RPE changed in direct
correspondence with increases or decreases in RR, whereas TV was unaffected by the perturbations [204, 205]. Adjustments in RR during dynamic
exercise appear to be one of the primary physiological mediators of respiratory-metabolic signals of perceived exertion [201].

RESPIRATORY GASES. The demand for breathing is regulated, in a large part, by the metabolic requirements for tissue oxidation (VO_2) and carbon dioxide excretion (VCO_2). These two determinants of pulmonary gas exchange serve as physiological mediators for the respiratory-metabolic signal of exertion.

Correlation coefficients for the relation between VO_2 and RPE range from $r = 0.76$ to $r = 0.97$ for both intermittent and continuous arm and leg exercise [69, 93, 212, 213, 221, 230]. The role of aerobic metabolism in mediating respiratory-metabolic perceptions of exertion is more clearly defined by the relative (i.e., $\%VO_2max$) than the absolute VO_2 [11, 178, 208, 212]. As an example, Robertson et al. found that, at a constant submaximal VO_2, RPE was lower when a subject breathing normoxic, as compared to hypoxic, gas mixtures [208]. On initial inspection, VO_2 and RPE appeared to be independent responses. However, VO_2max is attenuated during acute hypoxia exposure. Therefore, the absolute VO_2 that serves as a reference point represents a lower relative aerobic metabolic rate under normoxic than simulated altitude conditions. The perceptual responses were apparently mediated by the relative level of VO_2. Confirmation of this assumption occurred when RPE was expressed as a function of $\%VO_2max$. Using a constant $\%VO_2max$ as a reference, RPE was the same between normoxic and hypoxic conditions.

Several investigations have not found a functional interdependence between RPE and $\%VO_2max$, rejecting the relative metabolic rate as a perceptual signal mediator. Notable among these investigations are those that examined perceptual responses under selected conditions of heat and cold stress [189, 230]. Possibly, the relation between RPE and $\%VO_2max$ is distorted when heat flux is altered by changes in environmental temperature.

Investigations by Cafarelli and Noble [43] and Robertson et al. [203] have established a functional link between *carbon dioxide excretion* VCO_2 and perceptual signals of exertion during dynamic exercise. These investigations concluded that at relatively high exercise intensities, a greater ventilatory drive secondary to the increased demand for CO_2 excretion intensifies respiratory-metabolic signals of perceived exertion.

CARDIOVASCULAR RESPONSES. The findings of investigations that examined the role of HR in mediating the respiratory-metabolic signal of exertion are inconsistent. Evidence suggesting that HR mediates the intensity of perceptual signals of exertion has primarily been derived from correlational data. Initial experiments to validate the Borg scale yielded a correlation of $r = 0.85$ between HR and RPE responses to progressively incremented cycle ergometer power outputs. Correlation coefficients ranging from $r = 0.42–0.94$ have been found between HR and RPE for a wide range of exercise modalities [16, 69, 77, 89, 93, 140, 212, 218, 230]. However, it is recognized that correlational data do not infer causality. A considerable amount of experimental evidence demonstrates a lack of correspondence between HR and RPE when one or the other variable has been experimentally manipulated during dynamic exercise. The literature reviews of Robertson [208] and Pandolf [176] provide a more detailed description of these experimental findings. When experimental evidence is examined collectively, it can be concluded that HR does not appear to function as an important physiological mediator for respiratory-metabolic signals of exertion.

Central nervous system regulation of vascular smooth muscle may mediate respiratory-metabolic perceptions of exertion through as yet undefined neurophysiological pathways [176]. In this regard, a relation between scaled perceptual responses and systemic blood pressure has been found by some investigators [114, 177] and not by others [184, 222].

Peripheral Perceptual Signals

Peripheral physiological mediators influence the intensity of perceptual signals arising from exercising muscles in the limbs, trunk, and upper torso.

BLOOD PH. During high-intensity dynamic exercise, acidotic shifts in blood pH are thought to mediate peripheral perceptions of exertion in active limbs [130, 203]. Robertson et al. [203] manipulated blood pH via oral administration of either $NaHCO_3$ or $CaCO_3$ (i.e., a placebo) during separate arm and leg exercise trials (Fig. 15.5). During arm exercise at 80% VO_2peak, RPE-arms was lower under the alkalotic than under the comparatively more acidotic placebo condition. RPE-arms was not affected by blood acid-base shifts during leg exercise. RPE-legs was lower under alkalosis during leg exercise but did not differ from the placebo condition during arm exercise. Shifts in blood pH during high-intensity exercise (i.e., 80% VO_2peak) would appear to mediate peripheral exertional perceptions arising from active muscle. A casual link between the intensity of exertional perceptions and blood pH shifts has also been demonstrated during recovery from maximal treadmill exercise [209].

BLOOD LACTIC ACID. Experimental investigations that manipulated blood lactic acid concentration [HLa] to determine whether corresponding changes occurred in perceived exertion provide both refuting and supporting evidence for a peripheral mediating effect of metabolic acidosis. A substantial number of psychophysiological experiments have demonstrated that perturbation of blood [HLa] does not yield corresponding changes in the intensity of scaled exertional perceptions [1, 2, 10, 74, 77, 139, 156, 182, 209, 212, 220, 224, 245]. In contrast, several lines of experimental evidence support blood [HLa] as a physiological mediator for ratings of perceived exertion [24, 28, 58, 69, 70, 89, 108, 166]. Noble et al. [166] found that blood [HLa] and RPE-legs increased as a positively accelerating function of power output during progressive cycle ergometer exercise. The exponents of the functions for blood [HLa] (2.2) and RPE-legs (1.65) were reasonably similar, suggesting a psychophysiological link between these variables. Similar power functions for the relation between blood [HLa] and RPE have been reported by Borg et al. [28]. Additionally, for a given blood [HLa], RPE did

FIGURE 15.5.

*Effect of induced alkalosis on ratings of perceived exertion for the arms (RPE-A) and legs (RPE-L) during separate arm and leg exercise. At a given %VO₂max, means that are connected by an * are significantly (P < 0.01) different. Reproduced from ref. 203.*

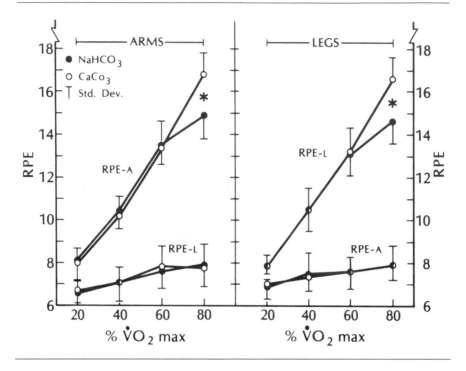

not differ between arm and leg exercise, between cycle and treadmill exercise, between pre- and posttraining and between incremental and constant treadmill exercise [70, 227].

It appears that blood [HLa] is linked to the intensity of peripheral exertional perceptions through its collateral relation with exercise intensity during progressively incremented test protocols. That is, both RPE and blood [HLa] serve as specific cases of a more generalized psychophysiological response that reflects the relative intensity of exercise [24, 28, 166].

MUSCLE LACTIC ACID. Evidence linking muscle lactic acid and the intensity of peripheral exertional perceptions is limited and inconsistent. Lollgen et al. [139] found muscle lactate to be independent of pedal frequency when cycle ergometer power output was held constant. In contrast, RPE distributed as a parabolic function of pedal frequency, being lowest at 60 and 80 rev/min. Noble et al. [166] reported that RPE-legs and muscle [HLa] increased as positively accelerating functions of power output during progressive cycle exercise. Owing to the extremely limited availability of experimental evidence, the role of muscle lactate in mediating the intensity of exertional perceptions must be interpreted cautiously.

SELECTED PERIPHERAL MEDIATORS. A number of selected physiological processes are also thought to mediate the intensity of peripheral exertional perceptions. A greater percentage of fast-, rather than slow-twitch, fibers in limb muscle has been associated with higher RPE during cycle ergometry in some [136, 166] but not other investigations [139]. Disruption of nutritive blood flow to exercising limbs, as occurs during high-intensity isometric and isotonic muscular contractions, increases the magnitude of perceived exertion [44, 226]. The decline of blood-borne glucose pools during the mid- to later stages of endurance exercise has been shown to initiate fatigue and, in turn, intensify perceptions of exertion arising from involved limb muscles [33, 51, 55, 155, 164, 210]. In contrast, a number of investigations have found that the intensity of peripheral exertional perceptions during prolonged exercise is independent of alterations in blood glucose concentration [80, 84, 110, 173]. Finally, results of laboratory experiments are neither consistent nor strongly supportive of plasma fatty acids and glycerol as mediators of exertional perception during long-term exercise [47, 54, 110, 231].

Nonspecific Mediators

The class of mediators termed nonspecific consists of physiological processes involved in hormonal regulation, temperature regulation, and pain reactivity.

CATECHOLAMINES AND β-ENDORPHINS. Evidence supporting blood catecholamine (CAT) level as a hormonal mediator of exertional perceptions is suggestive but not totally consistent. During multistage treadmill exercise, RPE correlated positively with both norepinephrine ($r = 0.63$) and epinephrine ($r = 0.54$) [220]. In addition, both RPE and vanillylmandelic acid (urinary index of CAT secretion) were attenuated at a given submaximal power output after a 5-wk exercise training program [63]. These findings suggest that CAT secretion may mediate the intensity of perceived exertion, especially at exercise intensities that exceed the lactate inflection point, i.e., 50–70% VO$_2$max [45, 85]. In contrast, several investigations have shown that the intensity of exertional perceptions was independent of CAT levels when hormonal response to exercise was manipulated by carbohydrate supplementation [80] and by alterations in exercise mode [50, 107].

The morphine-like action of β-endorphins is thought to exert an analgesic effect during high-intensity exercise, consequently mediating the intensity of exertional perceptions associated with localized muscular pain and discomfort. Farrell et al. [79] observed that RPE was lowest under exercise conditions in which plasma β-endorphins were highest, suggesting a link between these variables. In contrast, Droste et al. [64] and Kraemer et al. [131] reported that RPE did not correlate with exercise-induced increases in β-endorphins that were sampled from systemic circulation.

BODY CORE (T_c) AND SKIN TEMPERATURE (T_s). T_c and ratings of perceived exertion increase as metabolic heat production increases during dynamic muscle contractions. However, experimental evidence does not support a causal relation between physiological factors that regulate T_c and the intensity of exertional perceptions. Correlations between T_c and RPE are consistently low ($r = 0.14$–0.20) and not statistically significant [115, 230]. A correspondence was not noted between T_c and RPE during exercise involving hot [127, 189], neutral [56], and cold [230] environments; arm and leg ergometry [188, 230]; eccentric muscle training [127]; thermal acclimation [189]; and varying stages of the menstrual cycle [225].

Correlational evidence that links T_s with RPE during exposure to hot and cold environments is both limited and inconsistent. Noble et al. [170], using stepwise multiple-regression models, reported that T_s accounted for significant variance in RPE under hot environmental conditions. By contrast, Toner et al. [230] did not find a significant correlation between T_s and RPE during arm and leg exercise in cold water. In general, evidence derived from investigations during which environmental temperature was experimentally manipulated supports T_s as a mediator of exertional perceptions under both hot and cold conditions [10, 127, 147, 170, 187, 189].

Thermal sensation and thermal comfort are related to a number of physiological indices of thermal strain. Therefore, both of these thermal measures may also influence exertional perceptions during exercise under hot and cold ambient conditions.

Thermal sensation is related to skin ($r = 0.73$) and ambient ($r = 0.72$) temperature but is independent of metabolic rate, muscle temperature, and rectal temperature [88, 115, 180, 230]. It is possible that thermal sensation is a catalyst for the mediating effect of T_s on perceived exertion during exercise in hot environments. In contrast, Toner et al. [230] did not find a correlation between thermal sensation and RPE during cold-water immersion. Thermal comfort is related to skin sweat ($r = 0.66$) and to conductance (i.e., blood flow; $r = 0.56$) but is independent of metabolic rate and of muscle, T_s, T_c, and ambient temperature [88, 115, 143]. The perceptual mediating effect of the thermal comfort-discomfort continuum may mirror the extent to which the onset of sweat production and cutaneous vasodilation (i.e., skin redness) are an uncomfortable index of heat stress.

PAIN RESPONSIVENESS. Borg et al. (28) reported that RPE and ratings of pain intensity in the legs were strongly correlated ($r = 0.91$). The physiological basis of pain sensation during exercise appears to involve localized muscular ischemia [52]. Local muscle soreness also appears to mediate the intensity of differentiated exertional perceptions during swimming [172].

An increase in blood lactate concentration as a precursor of exercise-induced pain has been proposed by Borg et al. [28] but was rejected by Ljunggren et al. [136].

Neurophysiological Pathways for Exertional Perceptions

PERIPHERAL SIGNALS. The final common pathway for peripheral and, quite possibly, nonspecific signals of perceived exertion involves both a central feedforward and a combined feedforward-feedback neurophysiological mechanism [38]. In a feedforward mechanism, a copy of efferent commands from the central motor cortex is simultaneously transmitted via corollary pathways to the sensory cortex for interpretation and conscious expression as exertional perception [36, 37, 40, 113, 138]. A feedback mechanism transmits signals from peripheral receptors in muscle, joints, tendons, and skin to the sensory cortex. A functional interaction is proposed between the feedforward and feedback loops. Such an interactive mechanism provides for a precise adjustment of the sensory response according to the level of force production in contracting muscle [37, 42, 91, 113, 149, 150]. The reader is referred to Cafarelli's comprehensive research review for a more detailed explanation of the final common neurophysiological pathway for peripheral exertional sensations [39].

RESPIRATORY-METABOLIC SIGNALS. During exercise, ventilatory drive and alveolar ventilation increase in order to meet tissue oxidative requirements and to buffer metabolic acidosis. Static and dynamic inspiratory muscle tension must increase to produce a greater pulmonary ventilation [119]. As inspiratory muscle tension increases, so does the magnitude of respiratory effort sensation. The intensity of respiratory effort is related to those factors that directly influence inspiratory muscle contractile properties: (a) pattern of tension development, (b) functional weakening of the inspiratory muscle; and (c) inspiratory muscle fatigue [3, 73, 87, 112, 118, 119, 120–122].

Experimental evidence supports a link between sensory signals of respiratory exertion and the magnitude of centrally generated motor efferent commands. A greater number of motor commands must be discharged centrally when inspiratory muscle tension is increased to meet an increased ventilatory drive or to compensate for intercostal muscular weakening and fatigue. The neurophysiological signal for respiratory effort is transmitted to the sensory cortex by corollary discharges that diverge from these descending motor commands [90, 123, 149]. Peripheral afferent feedback from muscle spindle primaries, stretch receptors (lungs) and joint receptors (chest wall) may help to scale and calibrate central motor outflow commands [21, 90, 119, 122, 150]. The afferent signals are integrated centrally with information derived from efferent motor commands [121, 150]. In this manner, the respiratory-metabolic and peripheral exertional signals share a final common neurophysiological pathway [171].

PSYCHOLOGICAL MEDIATORS OF EXERTIONAL PERCEPTIONS

A broad range of situational and dispositional psychological factors systematically influences the intensity of exertional perceptions in both clinical and sports settings [158, 171].

Situational Factors

Situational factors that systematically influence the intensity of exertional perceptions are specific to a given time, physical activity setting, or exercise mode. They are most closely aligned with "state" personality characteristics, as defined according to traditional psychological disciplines. Situationally specific factors during dynamic exercise include hypnosis, expected duration of exercise, anticipated performance outcome, self-presentation, and attentional focus.

Morgan [157] was among the earliest investigators to examine the potentiating influence of psychological factors in explaining individual differences in perceived exertion. In these early studies, hypnotic perturbation was used to determine the importance of psychological inputs to the effort sense. At a constant-cycle ergometer power output, subjects increased their RPE when hypnotic suggestion indicated that they were pedaling up a steep hill, suggesting a situationally specific effect on perceptual responsiveness [157, 159]. However, a more recent experiment by Kraemer et al. [132] failed to confirm this finding.

A number of performance-related psychological factors appear to systematically influence the perceptual response during dynamic exercise. In general, when it anticipated that exercise duration is to be extended beyond original expectations or that less-than-positive performance outcomes are possible, perceptual signals of exertion intensify [195, 246].

The desire to present oneself to the audience in a socially acceptable manner interacts with the perceptual experience during a competitive exercise performance [100, 196]. Individuals designated as high self-constructors have a desire to impress others and, as such, rate exertional perceptions lower than those of low self-constructors [30]. In addition, the gender of the experimenter may influence RPE responses. Boutcher et al. [30] reported that males rated their exertional perceptions comparatively higher in the presence of a female experimenter during heavy exercise. It is of note that these psychosocial influences appear to be most salient at low- and moderate-exercise intensities. At high intensities, when physiological mediators are very potent, psychosocial influence is dampened.

Certain individuals routinely focus their attention on external cues (i.e., settings and events) when formulating a sensory response, ultimately attenuating exertional perceptions [183]. A similar response has been reported by Fillingim and Fine [81], in which exercise-related symptoms were lower when attention was focused on external environmental cues rather than on internal cardiorespiratory cues. Investigations by Johnson and Siegel [111] and Boutcher and Trenske [32] also support the hypothesis that an external attentional focus reduces internal symptomatology, attenuating exertional signals during dynamic exercise.

A number of investigations do not support situational factors as perceptual mediators. Exertional perceptions (RPE) were not altered when highly trained subjects exercised in the presence of a coactor [229], when untrained subjects exercised at high intensity in the presence of a coactor [100], and when photo slides were used to distract attentional focus [82]. In addition, music either did not alter RPE [53, 111] or lowered RPE at peak exercise intensities. It was suggested that music affects exertional perceptions owing to its emotional impact, rather than acting as a distracter from internal sensation [32].

Dispositional Factors

Dispositional factors that influence perceptual signals of exertion are enduring psychological traits that predictably shape an individual's behavioral response over a wide range of psychosocial and environmental settings. In traditional psychology, these enduring factors are termed trait characteristics. Dispositional traits that are thought to systematically influence the perceived intensity of exertional strain during dynamic exercise are sensory augmentation-reduction, locus of control, sex role typology, cognitive style, self-efficacy, and Type A personality [171].

Robertson et al. [198] observed that individuals classified as sensory augmenters according to a kinesthetic figural aftereffect test rated perceived exertion to be higher than those classified as sensory reducers during cycle ergometer exercise. Although experimental validation is as yet equivocal, it is thought that individuals with an external locus of control rate their perception of exertion higher than those exhibiting internal control [129]. Feminine-typed women and feminine-typed men rate perceptions of physical exertion higher than those typed as masculine or androgynous for their respective genders [105, 171]. Finally, the higher an individual's self-efficacy, the lower appears to be the RPE during short-term cycle ergometer exercise [148].

Morgan [157] found RPE to be positively correlated with extroverted personality characteristics in university students. It was proposed that extroverts suppress somatic pain and discomfort, i.e., the higher the extroversion, the lower the RPE. However, Williams and Eston [241] could not confirm this finding.

Morgan and Pollock [160] identified two divergent cognitive strategies that differentiated elite marathoners from recreational long-distance runners. Marathoners were found to use an association strategy whereby attention was given to internal sensory cues during training and/or competition. Recreational runners used a dissociation strategy in which internal bodily signals were dampened, using distractive thinking. Extending, this conceptualization, Schomer [214] compared exertional perceptions that were determined during a training session between highly experienced marathoners and minimally experienced marathoners. A strong positive relation was found between associative cognitive strategies and the intensity of exertional perceptions while training.

Individuals with the Type A behavior pattern are often time conscious, hard driving, and under certain circumstances outwardly hostile [171]. Carver et al. [46] demonstrated that fatigue ratings during exercise were lower in Type A than in Type B subjects. Three other investigations have examined the relation between Type A personality and the intensity of exertional perceptions [57, 62, 194]. *The findings of these investigations do not support a Type A-RPE relation, possibly owing to variations in the exercise protocols used and in procedures to measure both Type A behavior and perceived exertion. This conclusion notwithstanding, the link between the Type A behavior pattern and the intensity of exertional perceptions remains an attractive hypothesis, meriting continued investigation.*

PERCEPTUALLY BASED GRADED EXERCISE TESTING

Ratings of perceived exertion are frequently used as an *adjunct* to standard physiological and clinical responses during a graded exercise test (GXT). Measurement of perceived exertion during exercise testing is an easily applied procedure, requiring no bioelectrical instrumentation or extensive scaling expertise on the part of the subject, patient, athlete, and/or physical education student [171].

Test Termination Criteria

One of the most common and perhaps earliest application of RPE in a clinical setting involves the use of perceptual responses to guide the progression of a GXT and to signal the impending point of test termination. In this context RPE serves two very important methodological functions. First, when the terminal RPE (i.e., the highest scale category) is reported, it provides subjective confirmation that clinical and/or physiological end points of the GXT have been achieved. Second, the intensity of perceived exertion at a given time during testing indicates the point within the functional metabolic range to which the evaluation has progressed. When RPE reaches 15–17 on the Borg scale, preliminary procedures to safely terminate the test should be initiated [171].

Aerobic and Anaerobic Tests

The perceptually based Sjostrand physical work capacity (PWC) test systematically increases power output until a predetermined submaximal end point is attained. RPE is measured at the end of each 3-min stage [15, 18]. The power output (PO) at a criterion RPE of 15 (PO_{R15} on the Borg scale is determined. Upon completion of an aerobic training program, the same test protocol is again used to determine the PO_{R15}.) A pretraining to posttraining increase in PO at a criterion RPE of 15 indicates an improvement in cardiorespiratory fitness [18]. The physiological rationale underlying the perceptually based Sjostrand protocol holds that as functional aerobic power increases, a higher-power output can be performed at a given criterion RPE.

The perceptually based Sjostrand protocol has been validated by correlating PO derived for a criterion RPE with PO derived for a criterion HR. The validity coefficients ranged from $r = 0.60$ to $r = 0.75$ [13, 29]. In addition, PO at an RPE of 17 (PO_{R17}) correlated reasonably well ($r = 0.50$) with performance on such field criteria as running, skiing, lumber work, and military activities [13].

An alternative perceptually based submaximal cycle ergometer protocol uses a constant-power output, performed for a 6 to 8 min period. RPE is determined during the last minute of exercise. The rationale underlying this test protocol is that, at a fixed power output, the dependent measure (i.e., RPE) will be comparatively lower after a training program, indicating an improvement in aerobic fitness.

The perceptually based run test reverses the system of classifying independent and dependent variables that is customarily used in treadmill testing [14, 207]. Running speed is self-selected according to perceptual preference, thereby becoming a dependent variable [14, 207]. Total time to perform three separate test distance (600–1200 m) at a self-selected pace is recorded and converted to running speed [29, 68]. RPEs from the three test trials are then plotted as a function of their respective running speeds. The running speed that is equivalent to a criterion RPE (i.e., V_{R15}) is then identified. The faster the V_{R15}, the higher the individual's level of aerobic fitness is. An increase in V_R after completion of an aerobic training program indicates that functional aerobic power has improved [171].

The run test has been validated for distances between 600 and 1200 m using runners, general sports participants, and nonexercisers. Correlations between V_R and cycle ergometer physical work capacity and between 1500 m run and predicted VO_2max ranged from $r = 0.57$–0.74, indicating acceptable test validity [21, 29]. The test-retest reliability coefficient was $r = 0.93$.

A more detailed description of perceptually based exercise tests, including those that assess anaerobic power [20] and those that use a flexible feedback protocol [23] can be found in Noble and Robertson's text on perceived exertion [171].

Training Adaptations

RPE determined during a GXT can be used to monitor training outcomes. This is accomplished by measuring RPE at a fixed metabolic (i.e., VO_2) reference point during testing. As functional aerobic power increases over the course of training, the reference submaximal VO_2 represents a progressively lower relative metabolic rate. Because the intensity of the perceptual signal is linked to the relative metabolic rate (i.e., $\%VO_2max$), RPE is also lower at the fixed reference point. A number of investigations have reported such an attenuation of exertional perceptions after therapeutic and competitive aerobic training regimes when comparisons were made at a fixed metabolic rate [70, 72, 96, 128, 134, 179].

Perceptual Preference

Consideration of perceptual preference when selecting a GXT protocol helps to eliminate the influence of patient motivation on end point criteria. Perceptual preference is expressed as the exercise conditions that are associated with the lowest RPE. Moffatt and Stamford [156] noted that both men and women preferred a cycle ergometer protocol that incremented pedal rate, as opposed to brake resistance. Under test conditions in which cycle ergometer brake resistance is progressively incremented, it is often practical to select a pedal rate that is metabolically optimal and perceptually preferable. For most individuals, pedal rates that fall within a range of 60–80 rev/min have the highest metabolic efficiency, whereas rates approximating 40 and 120 rpm have the lowest efficiency [50]. In general, RPE is lowest at the midrange pedal rates and highest at the extremes of the range [181, 204, 224]. Pedal rates ranging from 60 to 80 rpm are, therefore, both perceptually preferable and metabolically optimal for most individuals. In addition, self-selected test protocols have been shown to be physiologically valid for treadmill evaluation [151].

An important consideration when incorporating a self-selected training pace into an exercise prescription is to ensure that the perceptually preferred intensity elicits a physiological response that falls within the stimulus zone to improve cardiorespiratory fitness [61]. Investigations by Farrell et al. [79] and Dishman et al. [61], involving a self-selected training pace, suggest that this is a reasonable expectation. In both investigations the self-selected exercise intensities ($65–75\% VO_2peak$) fell within the cardiorespiratory training zone. A common finding was that the RPE corresponding to the preferred training intensities ranged from 9 to 14 on the Borg scale. These numerical categories were generally associated with the verbal scale descriptors "very light" to "somewhat hard" and seemed compatible with the notion of a preferred exercise intensity that is subjectively tolerable over prolonged training periods.

Perceived exertion responses at preferred exercise intensities seem largely independent of aerobic fitness level. Dishman et al. [61] instructed a group of physically active and a group of physically inactive young men to select a cycle ergometer intensity that was subjectively preferable during a 20-min training bout. RPE was similar between groups despite a 25- to 50-watts greater absolute power output in the trained than in the untrained subjects. It is of note that exertional symptoms (i.e., task aversion, general fatigue, local fatigue) did not differ between groups, suggesting a contributory role of these subjective responses in the selection of preferred training intensities for prolonged, steady-state exercise.

Clinical Assessment

Tests of functional aerobic power are routinely administered to patients who are taking cardioactive medications. The pharmacological action of these medications can alter hemodynamic responses to GXTs. On the other hand, RPE is largely independent of cardioactive medications, making it ideal to monitor test progression [56, 70, 190, 222, 235].

An objective of diagnostic exercise testing is to *discriminate* between normal and pathological responses during a physical challenge. Diagnostic discriminate function analysis uses normal perceptual responses to an exercise test as a clinical reference. Perceptual responsiveness during a GXT has proven to be a useful diagnostic criterion for discriminate function analysis of coronary artery disease [27, 96, 117, 161, 190], chronic obstructive pulmonary disease [49, 135, 141, 215], psychiatric disorders [27], neuromuscular dysfunction [8, 211], and selected atherogenic risk factors [109]. The underlying assumption is that when there is either a clinical or physiological discrimination between pathological and normal responses to a GXT, there is a corresponding perceptual discrimination.

Methodological Considerations

A number of methodological factors pertaining to test administration and/or interpretation can influence perceptual responses during an exercise evaluation. These are:

1. The volume of muscle mass activated by a specific test mode [212, 213, 219].
2. Individual differences as a function of gender [27, 102, 168], chronological age [5], menstruation [225], and pregnancy [188]
3. Test conditions such as sleep deprivation [78, 146] and environmental temperature [191].
4. Interaction between protocol and exercise mode [69, 95].

When the above factors are not controlled, both intra- and interindividual comparisons of test responses may be difficult. A detailed explanation of the systematic effect of these testing methods on perceptual responses and suggested approaches to control their confounding influence are described by Noble and Robertson [171].

PERCEPTUALLY BASED EXERCISE PRESCRIPTION

Determination of exercise training intensity for clinical and competitive purposes can be based on both physiological and perceptual (i.e., RPE) responses to a GXT. Because these test responses are functionally related, RPE is used for both the *prescription* and the *regulation* of exercise intensity [165]. A perceptually regulated exercise prescription assumes that a predetermined aerobic metabolic rate can be attained and maintained by using a target RPE in a manner analogous to that for a target HR [60, 206]. In this prescriptive procedure, both RPE and VO_2 (or metabolic equivalents (METS)) are determined at the end of each stage of a GXT, as well as at the point of maximal exertion, i.e., denoting functional aerobic power. The prescribed percentage (i.e., 50–85%) of VO_2max that is to be achieved during a given training or therapeutic session is then calculated, using these test responses. The target training range is determined by plotting the RPE responses obtained during the GXT as a function of corresponding VO_2 responses. The target RPE range that is equivalent to the prescribed $\%VO_2$ max is then identified from this plot. During a given training session, exercise intensity is titrated until the target RPEs that have been estimated during the GXT are subjectively produced to achieve the requisite physiological overload stimulus. Using this procedure, perceptual regulation of exercise intensity ensures that the prescribed relative metabolic rate (i.e., $\%VO_2$max or $\%$METSmax) falls within the stimulus zone to improve cardiorespiratory fitness [171].

Perceptual Estimation-Production Paradigm

A perceptually based exercise prescription assumes a target RPE that has been *estimated* during a GXT can be used to regulate exercise intensity by *producing* a similar level of exertion during training or rehabilitative therapy. Perceptual regulation of exercise intensity is considered physiologically and clinically valid when HR, VO_2 rate-pressure-product, or ECG criteria do not differ when comparisons are made at similar levels of exertion between a GXT (i.e., estimation trial) and an individual training session (i. e., production trial). A number of laboratory and field-based experiments have examined the physiological and clinical validity of the perceptual estimation-production paradigm in prescribing and regulating exercise intensity [9, 35, 48, 65, 66, 75, 92, 162, 163, 221, 234]. Self-regulation of exercise intensity using RPE was physiologically valid when production trials were administered in random order and when perceptual scaling instructions were periodically reinforced by a special feedback procedure. Although some inconsistencies exist, these experiments generally agree that a target RPE estimated during a GXT can be produced during a training session in order to regulate exercise intensity.

RPE at Lactate and Ventilatory Inflection Points

The lactate and ventilatory inflection points serve as physiological markers upon which a perceptually regulated exercise prescription can be developed [101, 103]. RPE at the lactate and ventilatory inflection points ranges from 12 to 14 on the Borg scale for arm, leg and combined arm, and leg exercise [58, 192, 193]. The comparative stability of RPE at the lactate and ventilatory inflection points holds for men and women of varying age and training experience and also persists from one training session to the next [31, 34, 58, 95, 104, 193]. The relative metabolic rates (i.e., 50–80% VO_2max) that typically define the lactate and ventilatory inflection points fall within the training zone for cardiorespiratory conditioning. Therefore, the regulation of exercise intensity by producing an RPE that corresponds to these points provides an appropriate overload stimulus to improve functional aerobic power and can be considered a physiologically valid prescriptive procedure. Specific procedures to use the lactate and ventilatory inflection points as prescriptive anchors are described by Noble and Robertson [171].

Cross-Modal Prescription Using RPE

Exercise conditioning programs in both clinical and competitive settings often use a circuit training format, wherein a different activity is undertaken at each exercise station. The regulation of exercise intensity during circuit training necessitates a cross-modal prescriptive procedure [171]. Robertson et al. [206] examined the validity of a perceptually based cross-modal exercise prescription using treadmill, stationary cycle, and hand-weighted bench-stepping exercise. When compared at 70% of mode-specific VO_2peak, RPE for the overall body was the same between a treadmill reference test and both the cycling and hand-weighted bench-stepping tests. Therefore, a perceptually based cross-modal exercise prescription is physiologically valid when exercise intensity is set equal to the relative VO_2. A target RPE-O that is equivalent to the prescribed %VO_2peak can be derived during graded treadmill exercise and generalized to a variety of modes ranging from leg-only exercise (e.g., cycling) to combined arm and leg exercise (e.g., hand-weighted bench stepping).

A perceptually regulated exercise prescription assumes that generalizing a target RPE from a GXT to a constant-intensity submaximal training bout is physiologically valid procedure. Central to this prescription procedure is the expectation that a target RPE estimated during a load- or grade-incremented test protocol transfers in a numerically invariant form to prolonged steady-state exercise. In general, the assumption of invariant transfer properties of target training RPEs appears valid. As an example, Dishman [60] used HR response as a physiological criterion to validate a field-based walk-jog training program that was regulated by target RPEs. When the target RPE was produced during training, the actual attained HR was within +3 beats/min of the expected value. In contrast, when exercise intensity was regulated by a target HR, the actual training response was 18–23 beats/min greater than the prescribed value, an error margin that is unacceptable in the presence of certain clinical conditions.

Special Prescription Issues

A number of special issues should be considered in the development and implementation of a perceptually regulated exercise prescription. Among these are: (a) walk-run trading functions [169, 171], (b) anginal pain/discomfort [25, 26], (c) cardioactive medications [56, 70, 94, 216, 222, 235], (d) preferred training intensity [50, 59, 152], and (e) intermittent vs. concentric muscle contraction [102].

In addition, RPE can be used independently or in conjunction with HR responses to indicate (a) when it is necessary to adjust the intensity of a training stimulus [191] and (b) the magnitude of physiological adaptation to an aerobic training program involving cardiac and hypertensive patients, as well as clinically normal participants [72, 96, 104, 134]. Both RPE and HR at a given training intensity will decrease as functional aerobic power increases, reflecting a positive training adaptation.

PEDIATRIC APPLICATIONS OF PERCEIVED EXERTION

A growing number of clinical investigations have examined the perception of physical exertion in children and adolescents ranging in age from 4 to 16 yr. The Borg RPE scale presented in its original adult format and the developmentally indexed Children's Effort Rating Table (CERT, ref. 243) have been partially validated for use with normal and clinically involved males and females in this age range. In general, the 15-category Borg RPE scale has been the primary instrument of choice in these initial investigations, with an almost exclusive emphasis on the undifferentiated perceptual response for the overall body. These initial investigations have focused on (a) physiological validity of RPE responses, using HR and/or PO as criterion measures, (b) the critical age threshold below which a perceived exertion rating scale cannot be effectively applied to pediatric population subsets, and (c) scale format, i.e., numerical categories and verbal descriptors.

Validity and Reliability of the RPE Scale for Use with Children

The Borg RPE scale has been validated for pediatric population subsets by correlating perceptual responses with measures of HR and PO during dynamic exercise. These perceptual validation studies indicated that the relation between RPE (15-category Borg scale) and HR obtained for a series of sequentially ordered POs ranged from $r = 0.55-0.94$ for healthy male and female subjects (7–9 yr old) [5, 6, 133, 155]. Validity coefficients for RPE expressed as a function of HR during combined arm and leg (68–92% VO_2peak) exercise ranged from $r = 0.58-0.82$ for selected subsets of pediatric patients, i.e., obese, muscular dystrophy/atrophy, spina bifida, cerebral palsy. A summary of validation experiments involving children and adolescents, in which RPE (Borg scale) was determined for progressively incremented exercise intensities has been compiled by Bar-Or [6].

Validation of the Borg scale for use with pediatric subjects has also been undertaken by correlating RPE with PO during both leg and arm plus leg ergometer protocols. Correlation coefficients ranged from $r = 0.74$–0.93 for healthy male and female children and adolescents, ages 9–15 yr old [133, 237].

Although somewhat limited, data generally indicate that the Borg RPE scale is valid for use with both normal and clinically involved male and female pediatric subjects. Scale validity was usually higher for normal, as compared to clinically involved, children and adolescents.

Test-retest reliability of the Borg scale, when applied to clinically normal as well as obese children and adolescents undergoing cycle ergometer exercise, is quite high and consistent with response reproducibility in adults. Reliability coefficients for RPE determined during both progressive incremental test protocols ranged from $r = 0.86$–0.92 for males and females, ages 9–15 yr old [6, 133, 237]. It is of note that test-retest reliability of the Borg scale, when used with obese and normal weight pediatric subjects (9–15 yr old), improves as the relative exercise intensity increases. Bar-Or [6], using an incremental cycle protocol, found that the test-retest reliability coefficient for RPE (Borg scale) was $r = 0.59$ when exercise intensity was 20% VO_2peak. However, at 80% VO_2peak, the reliability coefficient increased to $r = 0.89$. This discrepancy may reflect a comparative insensitivity of the Borg scale to assess exertional perceptions in pediatric subjects at lower exercise intensities and/or inadequate perceptual anchoring procedures for the lowest scale category.

Validity of the RPE scale for use with pediatric subjects may vary depending on whether the physiological criteria (i.e., VO_2 and/or PO) are expressed in absolute or relative units. Bar-Or observed that RPE (Borg scale) determined for selected subsets of pediatric subjects was related to the absolute but not the relative VO_2 or PO [6, 67]. In addition, when comparisons were made at an absolute PO, obese boys and girls responded with a higher RPE than nonobese subjects. When comparisons were made at a given reference %VO_2peak, no between-group differences were observed. These responses likely reflected the higher maximal aerobic power in the nonobese than obese subjects. That is, the reference VO_2 and/or PO represented a comparatively higher relative metabolic stress for obese subjects [6]. Few investigations have compared RPE responses between pediatric and adult subjects using absolute and/or relative exercise intensity as a reference point [238]. Bar-Or observed that when such comparisons are made, children assign a lower RPE at a given absolute or relative exercise intensity than adults. [5].

When examined collectively, both the correlational and interprotocol investigations summarized above strongly suggest that the Borg RPE scale is a valid psychophysical instrument to assess perceptions of exertion in normal and clinically involved pediatric population subsets.

Development and Validation of the CERT

A number of pediatric exercise specialists have noted that the standard Borg scale format has a number of methodological and cognitive limitations when applied to children and adolescents. Williams et al. [243] observed that pediatric subjects—particularly those younger than 11 yr old—cannot cognitively assign numbers to words or phrases that describe exercise-related feelings. Many younger children also have difficulty interpreting certain verbal scale descriptors that are semantically more advanced than their present level of reading comprehension. The verbal descriptors that comprise the standard Borg scale format may exacerbate this problem of reading comprehensive when they are used to assess exertional perceptions in children.

In response to the foregoing methodological and cognitive limitations, a developmentally indexed scale to assess exertional perceptions has been developed. This scale is called the CERT. The CERT is presented as a partition scale having numerical categories ranging from 1 to 10, with verbal descriptors assigned to each category. The objective in developing this scale was to incorporate a comparatively narrow range of numerical partitions and corresponding verbal descriptors into a developmentally indexed category rating scale appropriate for use with normal and clinically involved pediatric population subsets. It was also expected that the CERT responses would evidence a more consistent relation with submaximal exercise HR than is typically the case when the standard Borg scale format is used with pediatric subjects. CERT responses were expected to approximate a linear relation with HR responses within the range of 100–200 beats/min during dynamic exercise.

Experimental validation of the CERT used a psychophysiological estimation/production paradigm. Male and female children (8–11 yr) initially underwent a progressively incremented Sjostrand cycle ergometer protocol wherein they estimated their exertional perceptions at the end of each successive exercise stage, using the CERT. In a subsequent cycle ergometer test, PO was self-selected to produce exertional perceptions equivalent to CERT categories 5, 7, and 9. Scale validation criteria were HR and PO responses during the production trial [75]. During the cycle production trial, the PO equivalent to CERT values of 5, 7, and 9 correlated significantly with the PO determined at the same CERT categories during the estimation trial, i.e., $r = 0.84$, 0.87, and 0.91, respectively [76]. HR correlations between the estimation and production trials yielded validity coefficients of $r = 0.65$, 0.78, and 0.79 ($P < 0.01$) for CERT categories 5, 7, and 9, respectively. Although an explanation is not readily available, both PO and HR at CERT categories 5, 7, and 9 were 13–18% ($P < 0.01$) lower in the production than in the estimation trials. As a follow-up experiment, Lamb [133] validated the CERT for use with healthy 5th grade boys and girls (mean age, 9.6 yr). In this validation experiment, CERT category responses during a progressive cycle ergometer protocol correlated strongly with both HR ($r = 0.96$) and PO ($r = 0.98$) for the mixed gender sample.

Critical Age Threshold

The chronological age below which children have difficulty comprehending and applying category scaling methodology to estimate their perception of exertion has not been clearly defined. A number of investigations have described this "critical age" threshold in somewhat general terms. Ward et al. [238] and Williams et al. [243] reported that children from 8 to 14 yr old were capable of using the Borg RPE scale to produce predetermined (i.e., target) exercise intensities. In contrast, Bar-Or [5] maintained that children younger than 16 yr of age were less competent in using the Borg RPE scale than individuals who were more than 18 yr of age. In a comparatively limited sample of Japanese children, the critical age threshold appeared to be 9 yr. Japanese children younger than 9 yr were unable to use the RPE scale effectively [155]. Lamb [133] found that 5th grade male and female students (mean age, 9.6 yr) understood and were able to apply the CERT while perceptually regulating exercise intensity.

Children of kindergarten age have a tendency to use only certain scale categories while avoiding others. Williams et al. [242] reported that kindergarten students consistently reported CERT categories 3 (easy), 7 (hard), and 8 (very hard) during a step test while carrying supplemental weights, even though the payload was systematically varied. It would appear that very young children are unable to match the full perceptual response range with a corresponding exercise stimulus range during dynamic activities.

Special Considerations

Certain perceived responses during dynamic exercise that are reasonably consistent in normal and clinically involved adult population subsets are not always reproducible in children and adolescents. Most notably, these inconsistencies involve (a) the sensitivity of RPE as a marker of training adaptations, (b) the RPE:HR ratio, and (c) the reproducibility of RPE at the ventilatory and/or lactate threshold.

Bar-Or and Inbar [7] demonstrated that RPE at a given submaximal HR declined after 8 wk of aerobic training or heat acclimatization in children 8–10 yr old. The magnitude of this posttreatment decrease in RPE at a fixed physiological reference was greater in children than in adults exposed to a comparable training and environmental intervention [7].

In selected groups of clinically normal adults, RPE (Borg scale) can be multiplied by a factor of 10 to approximate the submaximal HR during steady-state cycle ergometer exercise [171]. This RPE:HR ratio normally holds for protocols involving young, healthy male subjects exercising under thermoneutral environmental conditions. However, the RPE × 10 calculation does not approximate exercise HR in either normal weight or obese children during dynamic exercise [5].

A substantial number of investigations have shown that RPE at the ventilatory (VT) or lactate threshold (LT) is reasonably constant (i.e., 12–14 on the Borg scale) for male and female adults varying in aerobic fitness and competitive training experience [31, 58, 227]. In contrast, consistency in perceptual responsiveness at the VT does not appear to hold for children. Mahon and Marsh [142] determined the VT during two separate testing sessions, using a mixed-gender sample (mean age, 10.4 yr). The VO_2 at the VT did not differ between tests. However, RPE was lower ($P < 0.05$) during the second, as compared to the first, test (i.e., 11.4 vs. 12.4 on the Borg scale). Large interindividual variability in RPE at the VT (i.e., 6–19) was noted despite between-test consistency in the physiological marker (VO_2) of the VT. The difference in RPE between the two separately determined VTs was in part attributed to a greater comfort and familiarity with the perceptual scaling procedures and testing protocol during the second evaluation session.

ERGONOMIC APPLICATIONS OF PERCEIVED EXERTION

Ergonomic application of exertional perceptions has focused on: (a) development and validation of rating scales that are unique to occupational settings; (b) intra- and interindividual perceptual responsiveness during various industrial, military, and household activities; and (c) perceptual and metabolic congruence during selected work and exercise tasks undertaken in air and water environmental mediums.

Scale Development and Validation

The majority of investigations involving ergonomic assessment of exertional perceptions have used either the Borg 15-category RPE scale or the Borg CR-10 scale. In addition, three category scales have been specifically developed and validated for use in occupational and/or household settings. A common characteristic of these uniquely formatted ergonomic scales is that they have comparatively few numerical categories, facilitating their use in both simple and complex motor tasks that involve different anatomical regions and varying levels of muscle mass activation.

The most widely used of the ergonomic perceptual scales is the Occupational Effort Index developed by Hogan and Fleishman [83]. The Occupational Effort Index assesses perceptual strain associated with a wide range of job tasks and also predicts the metabolic cost of performing these tasks. Response validity of the Occupational Effort Index was established by determining scale sensitivity to individual differences in muscular strength, aerobic fitness, gender, and exercise training responses.

The Occupational Effort Index has a seven category numerical format. These seven numerical categories each have corresponding verbal descriptors that are the same as those that appear in the original 15-category Borg scale. In this configuration, the 6–20 numerical categories of the Borg scale are reduced by approximately one-half, producing a scale with partitions ranging from 1 to 7. The Occupational Effort Index has been validated against energy cost measurements derived for 24 different manual materials handling tasks. When averaged over all tasks, the validity correlation between effort rating and energy cost was $r = 0.88$. The interclass correlation to determine rater agreement was $r = 0.83$ [106].

Two other perceived exertion category scales have been specifically developed for ergonomic applications. In the first of these, Varghese et al. modified the Borg CR-10 scale, producing a category format having numerical partitions from 1 to 5 and corresponding verbal descriptors ranging from "very light" to "very heavy" [236]. This scale is primarily intended to assess exertional perceptions associated with household activities such as cleaning and storing water. In the second of these scales, Marley et al. used a unique adaptation of the Borg 15-category RPE format to study the perceived effort of drilling task [145]. In this adaptation, a silhouette of a human figure is displayed in tandem with the standard 15-category format. The silhouette directs the raters attention to specific anatomical sites from which perceptual signals of exertion are expected to arise and their respective intensities subsequently rated.

The three specially devised ergonomic scales of perceived exertion described above have a common objective in measuring the effort of occupational and/or household tasks and, in turn, grouping these tasks according to their shared perceptual and physiological strain.

Ergonomic Applications

Ergonomic application of exertional perceptions has been undertaken in occupational, military, and home settings. The majority of these ergonomic investigations examined perceptual responses for the overall body during manual work tasks [99, 197, 233, 236]. In addition, a number of experiments also scaled perceptual signals of exertion that were specifically differentiated to those anatomical sites (i.e., arms, hands, legs, shoulders, chest) involved in task execution [97, 98, 126, 145, 154, 185]. The use of such differentiated exertional ratings increases measurement sensitivity when determining the intensity of perceptual strain that is specific to the body region involved in the work task.

One of the earliest laboratory assessments of perceived exertion during simulated manual occupational tasks was undertaken by Gamberale et al. [89]. In this investigation, differentiated RPE for the limbs was compared between trials involving a standard cycle ergometer protocol, wheelbarrow pushing, and manual load lifting. Subsequent application of ratings of perceived exertion in occupational settings was quantified the perceptual strain associated with such work tasks as asbestos removal, lumber work, manual materials handling, driving screws, and cardiopulmonary resuscitation [97–99, 145, 154, 185, 197, 233]. The objective of these investigations was to use perceptual and metabolic criteria to identify ergonomically appropriate (a) anatomical work positions, (b) protective work clothing, (c) manual lifting techniques, and (d) work rates for a specified time period. Those work conditions having the least intense perceptions of exertion was considered subjectively optimal for performance of a given occupational task. Such perceptually based studies provided ergonomic data on which manual occupational tasks could be modified in order to better match worker's attributes (i.e., perceptual and physiological) with both the psychological and physical demands of the task.

Military applications of exertional perceptions have focused on manual load carriage systems for use in field conditions [4, 179, 186, 207]. In these investigations, payloads were transported by pack frame, frontal and transverse yokes, and utility belts. The experimental objective was to identify peak payloads that could be manually transported during thermally stressful military operations using perceptually optimal and metabolically efficient load carriage systems.

Many tasks undertaken in the home setting on a daily basis evoke low-to-moderate levels of perceptual and physiological strain. Ergonomic investigations have examined the exertional perceptions associated with such household tasks as cleaning, cooking, storing foodstuffs, and transporting materials [4, 236]. The perceptual and metabolic data derived from these investigations provide information with which household appliances, fixtures, and structures can be designed according to ergonomic and human factors criteria.

Perceptual-Metabolic Congruence

Establishing perceptual and metabolic congruence is of ergonomic interest when identifying optimal performance intensities (i.e., locomotor speed, pedal, and/or crank rate) for exercise tasks undertaken in air and water environmental mediums [4, 98, 154, 186, 199, 202]. Two recent investigations by Robertson et al. help to explain perceptual-metabolic congruence in an ergonomic context [199, 202]. In the first of these, differentiated RPE and VO_2 responses were determined in young women during treadmill walking while they were transporting payloads equivalent to 0, 7.5, and 15% of total body weight [202]. The intensity of the legs and chest RPE did not differ at comparatively slow walking speeds. At higher speeds, RPE-legs was more intense than RPE-chest, denoting a differentiation threshold. Of note was that for each payload condition, the differentiation threshold occurred at the same level of metabolically efficiency, i.e., $VO_2 = 10.5$ ml/m. The second of these investigations examined the link between perceptual preference (i.e., lowest RPE) and gross metabolic efficiency during combined arm and leg water immersion ergometry [199]. In general, ratings of perceived exertion were lowest and metabolic efficiency highest for a pedal crank rate of 40 rev/min at power outputs of 50, 100, and 150 watts. The findings of these ergonomic investigations support perceptual and metabolic congruence during selected exercise tasks undertaken in both air and thermoneutral water.

CONCLUSIONS

This chapter presents a critical review of experimental and clinical research in the area of perceived exertion. Specific consideration is given to: (a) category and ratio scaling methodology, (b) physiological and psychological perceptual mediators, and (c) clinical, pediatric, and ergonomic applications of perceived exertion. It is suggested that future experimental and clinical investigations in the discipline of perceived exertion focus on (a) development and validation of population-specific category and ratio scales, (b) identification of physiological, neuromuscular, and psychological perceptual mediators, (c) development and validation of perceptually based exercise testing and exercise prescription techniques, and (d) quantification of individual differences in perceived exertion responsiveness with respect to clinical status, ethnic/cultural origin, and developmental age.

REFERENCES

1. Allen, P. D., and K. B. Pandolf. Perceived exertion associated with breathing hyperoxic mixtures during submaximal work. *Med. Sci. Sports* 9:122–27, 1977.
2. Allen, W. K., D. R. Seals, B. F. Hurley, A. A. Ehsani, and J. M. Hagberg. Lactate threshold and distance-running performance in young and older endurance athletes. *J. Appl. Physiol.* 58:1281–1284, 1985.
3. Bakers, J. H., and S. M. Tenney. The perceptions of some sensations associated with breathing. *Respir. Physiol.* 10:85–92, 1970.
4. Balogun, J. A., R. J. Robertson, F. L. Goss, M. A. Edwards, R. C. Cox, and K. F. Metz. Metabolic and perceptual responses while carrying external loads on the head and by yoke. *Ergonomics* 29:1623–1635, 1986.
5. Bar-Or, O. Age related changes in exercise prescription. G. Borg (ed). *Physical Work and Effort.* New York: Pergamon Press, 1977, pp. 255–266.
6. Bar-Or, O. Rating of perceived exertion in children and adolescents: clinical aspects. G. Ljunggren and S. Dornic (eds.). *Psychophysics in Action.* Berlin: Springer-Verlag, 1989. pp. 105–113.
7. Bar-Or, O., and O. Inbar. Relationship between perceptual and physiological changes during heat acclimitization in 8–10 year old boys. H. Lavalee and R. Shepard (eds.). *Frontiers of Activity and Child Health.* Quebec: Pelicon, 1977, pp. 205–214.
8. Bar-Or, O., and S. L. Reed. Ratings of perceived exertion in adolescents with neuromuscular disease. G. Borg and D. Ottoson (eds.). *The Perception of Exertion in Physical Work.* London: Macmillan, 1986, pp. 137–48.

9. Bayles, C. M., K. F. Metz, R. J. Robertson, F. L. Goss, J. Cosgrove, and D. McBurney. Perceptual regulation of prescribed exercise. *J. Cardiopulmon. Rehab.* 10:25–31, 1990.

10. Bergh, U., U. Danielsson, L. Wennberg, and B. Sjodin. Blood lactate and perceived exertion during heat stress. *Acta Physiol. Scand.* 126:617–618, 1986.

11. Berry, M. J., A. Weyrich, R. Robergs, and K. Krause. Ratings of perceived exertion in individuals with varying fitness levels during walking or running. *Eur. J. Appl. Occup. Physiol.* 58(5):494–499, 1989.

12. Borg, G. Interindividual scaling and perception of muscular force. *Kung. Fysiogaf. Sallskap. Lund Forhandling* 31:117–25, 1961.

13. Borg, G. Physical performance and perceived exertion. *Studia Psychogia et Paedagogica,* Lund, Sweden: Geerup, 1962, vol. 11, pp. 1–35.

14. Borg, G. Perceived exertion as an indicator of somatic stress. *Scand. J. Rehabil. Med.* 2:92–98, 1970.

15. Borg, G. The perception of physical performance. R. J. Shepard (ed.). *Frontiers of Fitness.* Springfield, IL: Charles C Thomas, 1971, pp. 280–294.

16. Borg, G. Perceived exertion: a note on "history" and methods. *Med. Sci. Sports* 5:90–93, 1973.

17. Borg, G. *Perception of Panting during Ergometer Work.* Reports from the Institute of Applied Psychology, No. 73. Stockholm: University of Stockholm, 1976.

18. Borg, G. Subjective effort in relation to physical performance and working capacity. H. L. Pick (ed). *Psychology: From Research to Practice.* New York: Plenum Press, 1978, pp. 333–361.

19. Borg, G. Psychophysical bases of perceived exertion. *Med. Sci. Sports Exerc.* 14:377–381, 1982.

20. Borg, G. Ratings of perceived exertion and heart rates during short-term cycle exercise and their use in a cycling strength test. *Int. J. Sports Med.* 3:153–158, 1982.

21. Borg, G. Some Characteristics of a Simple Run Test and Its Correlation with a Bicycle Ergometer Test of Physical Work Capacity. Reports from the Institute of Applied Psychology, No. 625. Stockholm: Univ. of Stockholm, 1984.

22. Borg, G., and H. Dahlstrom. Psykofysisk undersokning avarbete pacykelergometer. *Nord. Med.* 62:1383, 1959.

23. Borg, G., B. Edgren, and G. Marklund. A Flexible Work Test with a Feedback System Guiding the Test Course. Reports from the Institute of Applied Psychology, No. 8. Stockholm, Univ. of Stockholm, 1970.

24. Borg, G., P. Hassmen, and M. Lagerstrom. Perceived exertion related to heart rate and blood lactate during arm and leg exercise. *Eur. J. Appl. Physiol.* 56:679–85, 1987.

25. Borg, G., A. Holmgren, and I. Lindblad. Perception of Chest Pain during Physical Work in a group of patients with angina pectoris. Reports from the Institute of Applied Psychology, No. 81, Stockholm: Univ. of Stockholm, 1980.

26. Borg, G., A., and I. Lindblad. The Determination of Subjective Intensities in Verbal Descriptions of Symptoms. Reports from the Institute of Applied Psychology, No. 75. Stockholm: Univ. of Stockholm, 1976.

27. Borg, G., and H. Linderholm. Exercise performance and perceived exertion in patients with coronary insufficiency, arterial hypertension and vasoregulatory asthenia. *Acta Med. Scand.* 644 (Suppl.) 187:17–26, 1970.

28. Borg, G., G. Ljunggren, and R. Ceci. The increase of perceived exertion, aches and pains in the legs, heart rate and blood lactate during exercise on a bicycle ergometer. *Eur. J. Appl. Physiol. Occup. Physiol.* 54:343–49, 1985.

29. Borg, G., and M. Ohlsson. A Study of Two Variants of a Simple Run-Test for Determining Physical Work Capacity. Reports from the Institute of Applied Psychology, No. 61. Stockholm: Univ. of Stockholm, 1975.

30. Boutcher, S. H., L. A. Fleischer-Curtian, and S. D. Gines. The effects of self-presentation on perceived exertion. *J. Sports Exerc. Psychol.* 10:27–80, 1988.

31. Boutcher, S. H., R. L. Seip, R. K. Hetzler, E. F. Pierce, D. Snead, and A. Weltman. The ef-

fects of specificity of training on rating of perceived exertion at the lactate threshold. *Eur. J. Appl. Physiol.* 59:365–369, 1989.

32. Boutcher, S. H., and M. Trenske. The effects of sensory deprivation and music on perceived exertion and affect during exercise. *J. Sport Exerc. Psychol.* 12:167–76, 1990.

33. Burgess, M. L., R. J. Robertson, J. M. Davis, and J. M. Norris. RPE, blood glucose and carbohydrate oxidation during exercise: effects of glucose feedings. *Med. Sci. Sports Exerc.* 23:353–359, 1991.

34. Burke, E. J. Perceived exertion: Subjectivity and objectivity in work assessment. G. Borg and D. Ottoson (eds). *The Perception of Exertion in Physical Work.* London: Macmillan, 1986, pp. 149–159.

35. Burke, E. J., and M. L. Collins. Using perceived exertion for the prescription of exercise in healthy adults. R. C. Cantu (ed.). *Clinical Sports Medicine.* Toronto: Collamore Press, D. C. Health, 1983, pp. 93–105.

36. Cafarelli, E. Peripheral and central inputs to the effort sense during cycling exercise. *Eur. J. Appl. Physiol.* 37:181–189, 1977.

37. Cafarelli, E. Effect of contraction frequency on effort sensations during cycling at a constant resistance. *Med. Sci. Sports* 10:270–275, 1978.

38. Cafarelli, E. Peripheral contributions to the perception of effort. *Med. Sci. Sports Exerc.* 14:382–389, 1982.

39. Cafarelli, E. Force sensation in fresh and fatigued human skeletal muscle. (ed.) *Exerc Sport Sci. Rev.* 16:139–168, 1988.

40. Cafarelli, E, and B. Bigland Ritchie. Sensation of static force in muscles of different length. *Exp. Neurol.* 65:511–525, 1979.

41. Cafarelli, E., W. S. Cain, and J. C. Stevens. Effort of dynamic exercise: Influence of load, duration and task. *Ergonomics* 20:147–158, 1977.

42. Cafarelli, E., J. Liebesman, and J. Kroon. Effect of endurance training on muscle activation and force sensations. *Can. J. Physiol. Pharmacol.* 73:1765–1772, 1995.

43. Cafarelli, E., and B. J. Noble. The effect of inspired carbon dioxide on subjective estimates of exertion during exercise. *Ergonomics* 19:581–589, 1976.

44. Cain, W. S., and J. C. Stevens. Constant effort contractions related to the electromyogram. *Med. Sci. Sports* 5:121–127, 1973.

45. Carton, R. L., and E. C. Rhodes. A critical review of the literature on rating scales for perceived exertion. *Sports Med.* 2:1298–1222, 1985.

46. Carver, C. S., A. E. Copleman, and D. C. Glass. The coronary-prone behavior pattern and the suppression of fatigue on a treadmill test. *J. Personality Soc. Psychol.* 33:460–466, 1976.

47. Casal, D., and A. Leon. Failure of caffeine to affect substrate utilization during prolonged running. *Med. Sci. Sports Exerc.* 17:174–179, 1985.

48. Ceci, R., and R. Hassmen. Self-monitored exercise at three different RPE intensities in treadmill vs. field running. *Med. Sci. Sports Exerc.* 29.732–738, 1991.

49. Chida, M., M. Inase, M. Ichioka, I. Miyazato, and F. Marumo. Ratings of perceived exertion in chronic obstructive pulmonary disease—a possible indicator for exercise training in patients with this disease. *Eur. J. Appl. Physiol.* 62:390–393, 1991.

50. Coast, J. R., R. H. Cox, and H. G. Welch. Optimal pedalling rate in prolonged bouts of cycle ergometry. *Med. Sci. Sports Exerc.* 18:225–230, 1986.

51. Coggan, A. R., and E. F. Coyle. Reversal of fatigue during prolonged exercise by carbohydrate infusion or ingestion. *J. Appl. Physiol.* 63:1–8, 1987.

52. Coldwell, L. S., and R. P. Smith. Pain and endurance of isometric muscle contractions. *J. Engineer. Psychol.* 5:25–32, 1966.

53. Copeland, B. L., and B. D. Franks. Effects of types and intensities of background music on treadmill endurance. *J. Sports Med. Phys. Fitness* 31:100–103, 1991.

54. Costill, D., G. Dalsky, and W. Fink. Effects of caffeine ingestion on metabolism and exercise performance. *Med. Sci. Sports* 10:155–158, 1978.

55. Coyle, E. F., A. R. Coggan, M. K. Hemmert, and J. L. Ivy. Muscle glycogen utilization dur-

ing prolonged strenuous exercise when fed carbohydrate. *J. Appl. Physiol.* 61:165–172, 1986.

56. Davies, C. T., and A. J. Sargeant. The effects of atropine and practolol on the perception of exertion during treadmill exercise. *Ergnomics* 22:1141–1146, 1979.

57. DeMeersman, R. E. Personality, effort perception and cardiovascular reactivity. *Neuropsychobiology* 19:192–194, 1988.

58. DeMello, J. J., K. J. Cureton, R. E. Boineau, and M. M. Singh. Ratings of perceived exertion at the lactate threshold in trained and untrained men and women. *Med. Sci. Sports Exerc.* 19:354–362, 1987.

59. Dishman, R. K. Contemporary sport psychology. *Exer. Sport Sci. Rev.* 10:120–159, 1982.

60. Dishman, R. K. Prescribing exercise intensity for healthy adults using perceived exertion. *Med. Sci. Sports Exerc.* 26(9):1087–1094, 1994.

61. Dishman, R. K., R. P. Farquhar, and K. J. Cureton. Responses to preferred intensities of exertion in men differing in activity levels. *Med. Sci. Sports Exerc.* 26:783–790, 1994.

62. Dishman, R. K., R. E. Graham, R. G. Holly, and J. G. Tieman. Estimates of type A behavior do not predict perceived exertion during graded exercise. *Med. Sci. Sports Exerc.* 23:1276–1282, 1991.

63. Docktor, R., and B. Sharkey. Note on some physiological and subjective reactions to exercise and training. *Percept. Mot. Skills* 32:233–234, 1971.

64. Droste, C., M. Greenlee, M. Schreck, and H. Roskamm. Experimental pain thresholds and plasma beta-endorphin levels during exercise. *Med. Sci. Sports Exerc.* 23:334–341, 1991.

65. Dunbar, C. C., and C. Goris, D. W. Michielle, and M. I. Kalinski. Accuracy and reproducibility of an exercise prescription based on ratings of perceived exertion for treadmill and cycle ergometer exercise. *Percept. Mot. Skills* 78:1335–1344, 1994.

66. Dunbar, C. C., R. J. Robertson, R. Baun, M. F. Blandin, K. Metz, R. Burdett, and F. L. Goss. The validity of regulating exercise intensity by ratings of perceived exertion. *Med. Sci. Sports Exerc.* 24:94–99, 1992.

67. Eakin, B. L., K. M. Finta, G. A. Serwer, and R. H. Beekman. Perceived exertion and exercise intensity in children with or without structural heart defects. *J. Pediatr.* 120:90–93, 1992.

68. Edgren, B., and G. Borg. The Reliability and Stability of the Indicators in a Simple Run Test. Reports from the Institute of Applied Psychology, No. 57, Stockholm: Univ. of Stockholm, 1975.

69. Edwards, R. H. T., A. Melcher, C. M. Hesser, O. Wigebtz, and L. G. Ekelund. Physiological correlates of perceived exertion in continuous and intermittent exercise with the same average power output. *Eur. J. Clin. Invest.* 2:108–114, 1972.

70. Ekblom, B., and A. N. Goldbarg. The influence of physical training and other factors on the subjective rating of perceived exertion. *Acta Physiol. Scand.* 83:399–406, 1971.

71. Ekblom, B., Lovgren, O, Alderin, M., Fridstrom, M., and Satterstrom, G. Effect of short-term physical training on patients with rheumatoid arthritis: I. *Scand. J. Rheumatol.* 4:80–86, 1975.

72. Ekelund, L. G., J. A. Blumenthal, M. C. Morey, and C. C. Ekelund. The effect of nonselective and selective betablockade on perceived exertion during treadmill exercise in mild hypertensive type A and B males and the interaction with aerobic training. G. Borg and D. Ottoson (eds.) *The Perception of Exertion in Physical Work.* London: Macmillan 1986, pp. 191–198.

73. El-Manshawi, A., K. J. Killian, E. Summers, and N. L. Jones. Breathlessness during exercise with and without resistive loading. *J. Appl. Physiol.* 61:896–905, 1986.

74. Essig, D., D. L. Costill, and P. J. Van Handel. Effects of caffeine ingestion on utilization of muscle glycogen and lipid during leg ergometer cycling. *Int. J. Sports Med.* 1:86–90, 1980.

75. Eston, R. G., B. L. Davies, and J. G. Williams. Use of perceived effort ratings to control exercise intensity in young healthy adults. *Eur. J. Appl. Physiol.* 56:222–224, 1987.

76. Eston, R. G., K. L. Lamb, A. Bain, A. M. Williams, and J. G. Williams. Validity of a perceived exertion scale for children: a pilot study. *Percept. Mot. Skills,* 78:691–697, 1994.

77. Eston, R. G., and J. G. Williams. Exercise intensity and perceived exertion in adolescent boys. *Br. J. Sports Med.* 20:27–30, 1986.

78. Faria, I. E., and B. J. Drummond. Circadian changes in resting heart rate and body temperature, maximal oxygen consumption and perceived exertion. *Ergonomics* 25:381–386, 1982.

79. Farrell, P. A., W. K. Gates, M. G. Maksud, and W. P. Morgan. Increases in plasma B-endorphin/B-lipotropin immunoreactivity after treadmill running in humans. *J. Appl. Physiol. Respir. Environ. Exerc. Physiol.* 52:1245–1249, 1982.

80. Felig, P., A. Cherif, A. Minagawa, and J. Wahren. Hypoglycemia during prolonged exercise in normal men. *N. Engl. J. Med.* 306:895–900, 1982.

81. Fillingim, R. B., and M. A. Fine. The effects of internal versus external information processing on symptom perception in an exercise setting. *Health Psychol.* 5:115–123, 1986.

82. Fillingim, R. B., D. L. Roth, and W. E. Haley. The effects of distraction on the perception of exercise-induced symptoms. *J. Psychosom. Res.* 33:241–248, 1989.

83. Fleishman, E., D. Gebhardt, and J. Hogan. The perception of physical effort in job tasks. D. Ottoson (ed.). *The Perception of Exertion in Physical Work.* London: Macmillan Press, 1986, pp. 225–242.

84. Foster, C., D. L. Costill, and W. J. Fink. Effects of pre-exercise feedings on endurance performance. *Med. Sci. Sports* 11:1–5, 1979.

85. Frankenhaeuser, M., B. Post, B. Nordheden, and H. Sjoeberg. Physiological and subjective reactions to different physical work loads. *Percept. Mot. Skills* 28:343–349, 1969.

86. Franklin, B. A., L. Vander, D. Wrisley, and M. Rubenfire. Aerobic requirements of arm ergometry: implications for exercise testing and training. *Phys. Sports Med.* 11:81–90, 1983.

87. Fuller, D., J. Sullivan, and R. Fregosi. Expiratory muscle endurance performance after exhaustive submaximal exercise. *J. Appl. Physiol.* 80(5):1495–1502, 1996.

88. Gagge, A. P., A. J. Stolwijk, and B. Saltin. Comfort and thermal sensations and associated physiological responses during exercise at various ambient temperatures. *Environ. Res.* 2:209–229, 1969.

89. Gamberale, F. Perception of exertion, heart rate, oxygen uptake and blood lactate in different work operations. *Ergonomics* 15:545–554, 1972.

90. Gandevia, S. C., K. J. Killian, and E. J. Campbell. The effect of respiratory muscle fatigue on respiratory sensations. *Clin. Sci.* 60:463–466, 1981.

91. Gandevia, S. C., and D. I. McCloskey. Sensations of heaviness. *Brain* 100:345–354, 1977.

92. Glass, S. C., R. G. Knowlton, and M. D. Becque. Accuracy of RPE from graded exercise to established exercise training intensity. *Med. Sci. Sports Exerc.* 24:1303–1307, 1992.

93. Goslin, B. R., and S. C. Rorke. The perception of exertion during load carriage. *Ergonomics* 29:077–686, 1986.

94. Grimby, G., and U. Smith. Beta-blockade and muscle function. *Lancet* 2(8103):1318–1319, 1978.

95. Gutin, B., K. F. Ang., and K. Torrey. Cardiorespiratory and subjective responses to incremental and constant load ergometry with arms and legs. *Arch. Phys. Med. Rehabil.* 69:510–513, 1988.

96. Gutmann, M. C., R. W. Squires, M. L. Pollock, C. Foster, and J. Anholm. Perceived exertion-heart rate relationship during exercise testing and training in cardiac patients. *J. Cardiac Rehabil.* 1:52–59, 1981.

97. Hagen, K. B., and K. Harms-Ringdahl. Ratings of perceived thigh and back exertion in forest workers during repetitive lifting using squat and stoop techniques. *Spine* 19(22):2511–2517, 1994.

98. Hagen, K. B., K. Harms-Ringdahl, and J. Hallen. Influence of lifting technique on perceptual and cardiovascular responses to submaximal repetitive lifting. *Eur. J. Appl. Physiol.* 68:477–482, 1994.

99. Hagen, K. B., T. Vik, N. E. Myhr, P. A. Opsahl, and K. Harms-Ringdahl. Physical workload, perceived exertion, and output of cut wood as related to age in motor-manual cutting. *Ergonomics* 36(5):479–488, 1993.

100. Hardy, C. J., E. G. Hall, and P. H. Prestholdt. The mediational role of social influence in the perception of exertion. *J. Sport Exerc. Psychol.* 8:88–104, 1986.

101. Haskvitz, E. M., R. L. Seip, J. Y. Weltman, A. D. Rogol, and A. Weltman. The effect of training intensity on ratings of perceived exertion. *Int. J. Sports Med* 13:377–383, 1992.

102. Henriksson, J., H. G. Knuttgen, and F. Bonde-Peterson. Perceived exertion during exercise with concentric and eccentric muscle contractions. *Ergonomics* 15:537–544, 1972.

103. Hetzler, R. K., R. L. Seip, S. H. Boutcher, E. Pierce, D. Snead, and A. Weltman. Effect of exercise modality on ratings of perceived exertion at various lactate concentrations. *Med. Sci. Sports Exerc.* 23:88–92, 1991.

104. Hill, D. W., K. J. Cureton, S. C. Grisham, and M. A. Collins. Effect of training on the rating of perceived exertion at the ventilatory threshold. *Eur. J. Appl. Physiol.* 56:206–211, 1987.

105. Hochstetler, S. A., W. J. Rejeski, and D. L. Best. The influence of sex-role orientation on ratings of perceived exertion. *Sex Roles* 12:825–835, 1985.

106. Hogan, J. C., and E. A. Fleishman. An index of the physical effort required in human task performance. *J. Appl. Psychol.* 64:197–204, 1979.

107. Horstman, D., Morgan, W., Cymerman, A., and Stokes, J. Perception of effort during constant work to self-imposed maximum. *Percept. Mot. Skills* 48:1111–1126, 1979.

108. Horstman, D. H., R. Weiskopf, and S. Robinson. The nature of the perception of effort at sea level and high altitude. *Med. Sci. Sports* 11:150–154, 1979.

109. Hughes, J. R., R. S. Crow, D. R. Jacobs, Jr., M. B. Mittelmark, and A. S. Leon. Physical activity, smoking and exercise-induced fatigue. *J. Behav. Med.* 7:217–230, 1984.

110. Ivy, J. L., D. L. Costill, W. J. Fink, and R. W. Lower. Influence of caffeine and carbohydrate feedings on endurance performance. *Med. Sci. Sports* 11.1:6–11, 1979.

111. Johnson, J., and D. Siegel. Active vs. passive attentional manipulation and multidimensional perceptions of exercise intensity. *Can. J. Sports Sci.* 12:41–45, 1987.

112. Jones, N. L. Dyspnea in exercise. *Med. Sci. Sports Exerc.* 16:14–19, 1984.

113. Jones, L. A., and I. W. Hunter. Force and EMG correlates of constant effort contractions. *Eur. J. Appl. Physiol. Occup. Physiol.* 51:75–83, 1983.

114. Juhani, I., S. Pekka, and A. Timo. Strain while skiing and hauling a sledge or carrying a backpack. *Eur. J. Appl. Physiol.* 55:597–603, 1986.

115. Kamon, E., K. Pandolf, and E. Cafarelli. The relationship between perceptual information and physiological responses to exercise in the heat. *J. Hum. Ergol. Tokyo* 3:45–54, 1974.

116. Kang, J., R. J. Robertson, F. L. Goss, S. G. DaSilva, P. Visich, R. R. Suminski, A. C. Utter, and B. G. Denys. Effect of carbohydrate substrate availability on ratings of perceived exertion during prolonged exercise of moderate intensity. *Percept. Mot. Skills* 82:495–506, 1996.

117. Karlsson, J., H. Astrom, A. Holmgren, C. Kaijser, and E. Orinius. Angina pectoris and blood lactate concentration during graded exercise. *Int. J. Sports Med.* 5(6):348–351, 1984.

118. Killian, K. J. The objective measurement of breathlessness. *Chest* 88(suppl):84S–90S, 1985

119. Killian, K. J. Breathlessness—the sense of respiratory muscle effort. G. Borg and D. Ottoson (eds.). *Perception of Exertion in Physical Work.* London: Macmillan, 1986, pp. 71, vol. 46, 82.

120. Killian, K. J., D. Bucens, and E. Campbell. Effect of breathing patterns on the perceived magnitude of added loads to breathing. *J. Appl. Physiol.* 52:578–584, 1982.

121. Killian, K. J., and E. J. Campbell. Dyspnea and exercise. *Annu. Rev. Physiol.* 45:465–479, 1983.

122. Killian, K. J., S. C. Gandevia, E. Summers, and E. J. M. Campbell. Effect of increased lung volume on perception of breathlessness, effort and tension. *J. Appl. Physiol. Respir. Environ. Exerc. Physiol.* 57:686–691, 1984.

123. Killian, K. J., and N. L. Jones. The use of exercise testing and other methods in the investigation of dyspnea. *Clin. Chest Med.* 5:99–108, 1984.

124. Kinsman, R., P. Weiser, and D. Stamper. Multidimensional analysis of subjective symptomatology during prolonged strenuous exercise. *Ergonomics* 16:211–226, 1973.

125. Kinsman, R. A., and P. C. Weiser. Subjective symptomatology during work and fatigue. E. Simonson and P. L. Weises (eds.). *Psychological Aspects of Fatigue.* Springfield, IL: Charles C Thomas, 1976, pp. 336–405.

126. Kirk, J., and D. A. Schneider. Physiological and perceptual responses to load-carrying in female subjects using internal and external frame backpacks. *Ergonomics* 35(4):445–455, 1992.

127. Knuttgen, H. G., E. R. Nadel, K. B. Pandolf, and J. F. Patton. Effects of training with eccentric muscle contractions on exercise performance, energy expenditure and body temperature. *Int. J. Sports Med.* 3:13–17, 1982.

128. Knuttgen, H. G., L. D. Nordesjo, B. Ollander, and B. Saltin. Physical conditioning through interval training with young male adults. *Med. Sci. Sports* 5:220–226, 1973.

129. Kohl, R. M., and C. H. Shea. Perceived exertion: influences of locus of control and expected work intensity and duration. *J. Hum. Mov. Studies* 15:225–272, 1988.

130. Kostka, C. E., and E. Cafarelli. Effect of pH on sensation and vastus lateralis electromyogram during cycling exercises. *J. Appl. Physiol.* 52:1181–1185, 1982.

131. Kraemer, W. J., J. E. Dziados, L. J. Marchitelli, S. E. Gordon, E. A. Harman, R. Mello, S. J. Fleck, P. N. Frykman, and N. T. Triplett. Effects of different heavy-resistance exercise protocols on plasma B-endorphin concentrations. *J. Appl. Physiol.* 74(1):450–459, 1993.

132. Kraemer, W. J., R. V. Lewis, N. T. Triplett, L. P. Koziris, S. Heyman, and B. J. Noble. Effects of hypnosis on plasma proenkephalin peptide F and perceptual and cardiovascular responses during submaximal exercise. *Eur. J. Appl. Physiol. Occup. Physiol.* 65(6):573–578, 1992.

133. Lamb, K. L. Children's rating of effort during cycle ergometry: an examination of the validity of two effort rating scales. *Pediatr. Exerc. Sci.* 7:407–421, 1995.

134. Lewis, S., P. Thompson, N. H. Areskog, P. Vodak, M. Marconyak, R. DeBusk, S. Mellen, and W. Haskell. Transfer effects of endurance training to exercise with untrained limbs. *Eur. J. Appl. Physiol.* 44:25–34, 1980.

135. Linderholm, H. Perceived exertion during exercise in the discrimination between circulatory and pulmonary disorders. G. Borg and D. Ottoson (eds.). *Perception of Exertion in Physical Work.* London: Macmillan, 1986, 199–206.

136. Ljunggren, G., R. Ceci, and J. Karlsson. Prolonged exercise at a constant load on a bicycle ergometer: ratings of perceived exertion and leg aches and pain as well as measurements of blood lactate accumulation and heart rate. *Int. J. Sports Med.* 8:109–116, 1987.

137. Ljunggren, G., and S. Dornic. *Psychophysics in Action.* Berlin: Springer-Verlag, 1989, pp. 8–9.

138. Lloyd, A. R., S. C. Gandevia, and J. P. Hales. Muscle performance, voluntary activation, twitch properties and perceived effort in normal subjects and patients with the chronic fatigue syndrome. *Brain* 114:85–98,1991.

139. Lollgen, H., T. Graham, and G. Sjogaard. Muscle metabolites, force and perceived exertion bicycling at varying pedal rates. *Med. Sci. Sports Exerc.* 12:345–351, 1980.

140. Lollgen, H., H. V. Ulmer, and G. von Nieding. Heart rate and perceptual responses to exercise with different pedalling speed in normal subjects and patients. *Eur. J. Appl. Physiol.* 37:297–304, 1977.

141. Mahler, D. A., and M. B. Horowitz. Perception of breathlessness during exercise in patients with respiratory disease. *Med. Sci. Sports Exerc.* 26(9):1078–1081, 1994.

142. Mahon, A. D., and M. L. Marsh. Reliability of the rating of perceived exertion at ventilatory threshold in children. *Int. J. Sport Med.* 13(8):567–571, 1992.

143. Marcus, P., and P. Redman. Effect of exercise on thermal comfort during hypothermia. *Physiol. Behav.* 22:831–835, 1979.

144. Maresh, C. M., M. R. Deschenes, R. L. Seip, L. E. Armstrong, K. L. Robertson, and B. J. Noble. Perceived exertion during hypobaric hypoxia in low- and moderate-altitude natives. *Med. Sci. Sports Exerc.* 25:945–951, 1993.

145. Marley, R. J., and J. E. Fernandez. Psychophysical frequency and sustained exertion at varying wrist postures for a drilling task. *Ergonomics* 38(2):303–325, 1995.

146. Martin, B. J., and G. M. Gaddis. Exercise after sleep deprivation. *Med. Sci. Sports Exerc.* 13:220–223, 1981.

147. Maw, G. J., S. H. Boutcher, N. A. S. Taylor. Ratings of perceived exertion and affect in hot and cool environments. *Eur. J. Appl. Physiol.* 67:174–179, 1993.

148. McCauley, E., and K. S. Courneya. Self-efficacy relationships with affective and exertion responses to exercise. *J. Appl. Soc. Psychol.* 22:312–326, 1992.

149. McCloskey, D. I. Kinesthetic sensibility. *Physiol. Rev.* 58:763–820, 1978.

150. McCloskey, D. I., S. Gandevia, E. K. Porter, and J. G. Colebatch. Muscle sense and effort: motor commands and judgements about muscular contractions. *Adv. Neurol.* 39:151–167, 1983.

151. McConnell, T. R., and B. A. Clark. Treadmill protocols for determination of maximum oxygen uptake in runners. *Br. J. Sports Med.* 22:3–5, 1988.

152. Michael, E. D., and L. Eckard. The selection of hard work by trained and non-trained subjects. *Med. Sci. Sports* 4:107–110, 1972.

153. Mihevic, P. M., J. A. Gliner, and S. M. Horvath. Perception of effort and respiratory sensitivity during exposure to ozone. *Ergonomics* 24:365–374, 1981.

154. Mital, A., Foononi-Fard, and M. L. Brown. Physical fatigue in high and very high frequency manual materials handling: perceived exertion and physiological indicators. *Hum. Factors* 36(2):219–231, 1994.

155. Miyashita, M., K. Onodera, and I. Tabata. How Borg's RPE-scale has been applied to Japanese. G. Borg and D. Ottoson (eds.) *Perceptual Exertion in Physical Work.* London: Macmillan, 1986, pp. 27–34.

156. Moffatt. R. J., and B. A. Stamford. Effects of pedalling rate changes on maximal oxygen uptake and perceived effort during bicycle ergometer work. *Med. Sci. Sports* 10:27–31, 1978.

157. Morgan, W. P. Psychological factors influencing perceived exertion. *Med. Sci. Sports* 5:97–103, 1973.

158. Morgan, W. P. Psychological components of effort sense. *Med. Sci. Sports Exerc.*, 26(9): 1071–1077, 1994.

159. Morgan, W. P., K. Hirta, G. A. Weitz, and B. Balke. Hypnotic perturbation of perceived exertion: ventilatory consequences. *Am. J. Clin. Hypn.* 18:182–90, 1976.

160. Morgan, W. P., and M. L. Pollock. Psychological characterization of the elite distance runner. *Ann. N. Y. Acad. Sci.* 301:382–403, 1977.

161. Myers, J. N. Perception of chest pain during exercise testing in patients with coronary artery disease. *Med. Sci. Sports Exerc.* 26(9):1082–1086, 1994.

162. Myles, W. S. Sleep deprivation, physical fatigue, and the perception of exercise intensity. *Med. Sci. Sports Exerc.* 17:580–584, 1985.

163. Myles, W. S., and D. Maclean. A comparison of response and production protocols for assessing perceived exertion. *Eur. J. Appl. Physiol.* 55:585–587, 1986.

164. Nieman, D. C., K. A. Carlson, M. E. Brandstater, R. T. Naegele, and J. W. Blankenship. Running endurance in 27-h-fasted humans. *J. Appl. Physiol.* 63:2502–2509, 1987.

165. Noble, B. Clinical applications of perceived exertion. *Med. Sci. Sports Exerc.* 14:406–411, 1982.

166. Noble, B. J., G. Borg, I. Jacobs, R. Ceci, and P. Kaiser. A category-ratio perceived exertion scale: relationship to blood and muscle lactates and heart rate. *Med. Sci. Sports Exerc.* 15:523–529, 1983.

167. Noble, B. J., W. J. Kraemer, J. G. Allen, J. S. Plank, and L. A. Woodard. The integration of physiological cues in effort perception: Stimulus strength vs. relative contribution. G. Borg and D. Ottoson (eds.). *The Perception of Exertion in Physical Work.* London: Macmillan, 1986, pp. 83–96.

168. Noble, B. J., and C. M. Maresh, and M. Ritchey. Comparison of exercise sensations be-

tween males and females. J. Borms, M. Hebbelnick, and A. Venerando (eds.). *Women and Sport.* Basel: S. Karzer, 1981, pp. 175–179.

169. Noble, B. J., K. F. Metz, K. B. Pandolf, C. W. Bell, E. Cafarelli, and W. E. Sime. Perceived exertion during walking and running: II. *Med. Sci. Sports* 5:116–120, 1973.

170. Noble, B. J., K. F. Metz, K. B. Pandolf, and E. Cafarelli. Perceptual responses to exercise: A multiple regression study. *Med. Sci. Sports* 5:104–109, 1973.

172. O'Connor, P. J., W. P. Morgan, and J. S. Raglin. Psychobiologic effects of 3 d of increased training in female and male swimmers. *Med. Sci. Sports Exerc.* 23(9):1055–1061, 1991.

173. Okano, G., H. Takeda, I. Morita, M. Katoh, Z. Mu, and S. Miyake. Effect of pre-exercise fructose ingestion on endurance performance in fed men. *Med. Sci. Sports. Exerc.* 20:105–109, 1988.

174. Pandolf, K. B. Influence of local and central factors in dominating rated perceived exertion during physical work. *Percept. Mot. Skills* 46:683–698, 1978.

175. Pandolf, K. B. Differentiated ratings of perceived exertion during physical exercise. *Med. Sci. Sports Exerc.* 14:397–405, 1982.

176. Pandolf, K. B. Advances in the study and application of perceived exertion. *Exerc. Sport Sci. Rev.* 11:118–158, 1983.

177. Pandolf, K. B. Local and central factor contributions in the perception of effort during physical exercise. G. Borg and D. Ottoson (eds.). *The Perception of Exertion in Physical Work.* London: Macmillan, 1986, pp. 97–110.

178. Pandolf, K. B., D. S. Billings, L. L. Drolet, N. A. Pimental, and M. N. Sawka. Differentiated ratings of perceived exertion and various physiological responses during prolonged upper and lower body exercise. *Eur. J. Appl. Physiol.* 53:5–11, 1984.

179. Pandolf, K. B., R. L. Burse, and R. F. Goldman. Differentiated ratings of perceived exertion during physical conditioning of older individuals using leg-weight loading. *Percept. Mot. Skills* 40:563–574, 1975.

180. Pandolf, K. B., E. Cafarelli, B. J. Noble, and K. F. Metz. Perceptual responses during prolonged work. *Percept. Mot. Skills* 35:975–985, 1972.

181. Pandolf, K. B., and B. J. Noble. The effect of pedaling speed and resistance changes on perceived exertion for equivalent power outputs on the bicycle ergometer. *Med. Sci. Sports* 5:132–136, 1973.

182. Pederson, P. K., and H. G. Welch. Oxygen breathing, selected physiological variables and perception of effort during submaximal exercise. G. Borg (ed.). *Physical Work and Effort.* New York: Pergamon Press, 1977, pp. 385–400.

183. Pennebaker, J. W., and J. M. Lightner. Competition of internal and external information in an exercise setting. *J. Pers. Soc. Psychol.* 39:165–174, 1980.

184. Perkins, R. K., J. E. Sexton, R. D. Solberg-Kassel, and L. H. Epstein. Estimates of Type A behavior do not predict perceived exertion during graded exercise. *Med. Sci. Sports Exerc.* 23(11):1283–1288, 1991.

185. Pierce, E. F., N. W. Eastman, R. W. McGowan, and M. L. Legnola. Metabolic demands and perceived exertion during cardiopulmonary resuscitation. *Percept. Mot. Skills* 74:323–328, 1992.

186. Pimental, N., and Pandolf, K. Energy expenditure while standing or walking slowly uphill or downhill with loads. *Ergonomics* 222:963–973, 1979.

187. Pivarnik, J. M., T. R. Grafner, and E. S. Elkins. Metabolic, thermoregulatory, and psychophysiological responses during arm and leg exercise. *Med. Sci. Sports Exerc.* 20:1–5, 1988.

188. Pivarnik, J. M., W. Lee, and J. Miller. Physiological and perceptual responses to cycle and treadmill exercise during pregnancy. *Med. Sci. Sports Exerc.* 23(4):470–475, 1990.

189. Pivarnik, J. M., and L. C. Senay. Effect of endurance training and heat acclimation on perceived exertion during exercise. *J. Cardiopulm. Rehabil.* 6:499–504, 1986.

190. Pollock, M. L., A. S. Jackson, and C. Foster. The use of the perception scale for exercise prescription. G. Borg and D. Ottoson (eds.). In *The Perception of Exertion in Physical Work.* London: MacMillan, 1986, pp. 161–178.

191. Pollock, M. L., J. H. Wilmore, and S. M. Fox. *Exercise in Health and Disease: Evaluation and Prescription for Prevention and Rehabilitation.* Philadelphia: W. B. Saunders, 1984.
192. Prusaczyk, W. K., K. J. Cureton, R. E. Graham, and C. A. Ray. Differential effects of dietary carbohydrate on RPE at the lactate and ventilatory thresholds. *Med. Sci. Sports Exerc.* 24(5):568–575, 1992.
193. Purvis, J. W., and K. J. Cureton. Ratings of perceived exertion at the anaerobic threshold. *Ergonomics* 24:295–300, 1981.
194. Rejeski, W. D., D. Morley, and H. Miller. Cardiac rehabilitation: coronary-prone behavior as a moderatory of graded exercise. *J. Card. Rehabil.* 3:339–346, 1983.
195. Rejeski, W. J., and P. M. Ribisl. Expected task duration and perceived effort: an attributional analysis. *J. Sport Psychol.* 2:227–36, 1980.
196. Rejeski, W. J., and B. Sanford. Feminine-type females: The role of affective schema in the perception of exercise intensity. *J. Sport Psychol.* 6:197–207, 1984.
197. Rissanen, S., J. Smolander, and V. Louhevaara. Work load and physiological responses during asbestos removal with protective clothing. *Int. Arch. Occup. Environ. Health* 63:241–246, 1991.
198. Robertson, R., R. Gillespie, E. Hiatt, and K. Rose. Perceived exertion and stimulus intensity modulation. *Percept. Mot. Skills* 45:211–218, 1977.
199. Robertson, R., F. Goss, T. Michael, N. Moyna, P. Gordon, P. Visich, J. Kang, T. Angelopoulos, S. DaSilva, and K. Metz. Metabolic and perceptual responses during arm and leg ergometry in water and air. *Med. Sci. Sports Exerc.* 27(5):760–764, 1995.
200. Robertson, R., F. Goss, T. Michael, N. Moyna, P. Gordon, P. Visich, J. Kang, T. Angelopoulos, S. DaSilva, and K. Metz. Validity of the Borg Perceived Exertion Scale for use in semirecumbent ergometry during immersion in water. *Percept. Mot. Skills* 83:3–13, 1996.
201. Robertson, R. J. Central signals of perceived exertion during dynamic exercise. *Med. Sci. Sports Exerc.* 14:390–396, 1982.
202. Robertson, R. J., C. J. Caspersen, T. G. Allison, G. S. Skrinar, R. A. Abbott, and K. F. Metz. Differentiated perceptions of exertion and energy cost of young women while carrying loads. *Eur. J. Appl. Physiol.* 49:69–78, 1982.
203. Robertson, R. J., J. E. Falkel, A. L. Drash, A. M. Swank, K. F. Metz, S. A. Spungen, and J. R. LeBoeuf. Effect of blood pH on peripheral and central signals of perceived exertion. *Med. Sci. Sports Exerc.* 18:114–122, 1986.
204. Robertson, R. J., R. L. Gillespie, J. McCarthy, and K. D. Rose. Differentiated perceptions of exertion: Part 1. Mode of integration of regional signals. *Percept. Mot. Skills* 49:683–689, 1979.
205. Robertson, R. J., R. L. Gillespie, J. McCarthy, and K. D. Rose. Differentiated perceptions of exertion: Part II. Relationship to local and central physiological responses. *Percept. Mot. Skills* 49:691–697, 1979.
206. Robertson, R. J., F. L. Goss, T. E. Auble, R. Spina, D. Cassinelli, E. Glickman, R. Galbreath and K. Metz. Cross-modal exercise prescription at absolute and relative oxygen uptake using perceived exertion. *Med. Sci. Sports Exerc.* 22:653–659, 1990.
207. Robertson, R. J., F. L. Goss, and K. F. Metz. Ratings of perceived exertion (RPE) in cardiac rehabilitation: application and validation. J. P. Broustet (ed.). *Proceedings of the Vth World Congress on Cardiac Rehabilitation.* Andover, Hampshire, England: Intercept Limited, 1993, pp. 151–159.
208. Robertson, R. J., and K. F. Metz. Ventilatory precursors for central signals of perceived exertion. G. Borg and D. Ottoson (eds). *The Perception of Exertion in Physical Work.* London: Macmillan, 1986, pp. 111–121.
209. Robertson, R. J., P. A. Nixon, C. J. Casperson, K. F. Metz, R. A. Abbott, and F.L. Goss. Abatement of exertional perceptions following high intensity exercise: physiological mediators. *Med. Sci. Sports Exerc.* 24:346–353, 1992.
210. Robertson, R. J., R. T. Stanko, F. L. Goss, R. J. Spina, J. J. Reilly, and K. D. Greenawalt. Blood glucose extraction as a mediator of perceived exertion during prolonged exercise. *Eur. J. Appl. Physiol.* 61:100–105, 1990.

211. Rodriquez, A. A., and J. C. Agre. Physiologic parameters and perceived exertion with local muscle fatigue in postpolio subjects. *Arch. Phys. Med. Rehabil.* 72:305–308, 1991.
212. Sargeant, A. J., and C. T. Davies. Perceived exertion during rhythmic exercise involving different muscle masses. *J. Hum. Ergol. (Tokyo)* 2:3–11, 1973.
213. Sargeant, A. J., and C. T. Davies. Perceived exertion of dynamic exercise in normal subjects and patients following leg injury. G. Borg (ed.). *Physical Work and Effort.* New York: Pergamon Press, 1977, pp 345–356.
214. Schomer, H. Mental strategies and the perception of effort of marathon runners. *Int. J. Sport Psychol.* 17:41–59, 1986.
215. Silverman, M., J. Barry, H. Hellerstein, J. Janos, and S. Kelson. Variability of the perceived sense of effort in breathing during exercise in patients with chronic obstructive pulmonary disease. *Am. Rev. Respir. Dis.* 137:206–209, 1988.
216. Sjoberg, H., M. Frankenhaeuser, and H. Bjurstedt. Interactions between heart rate, psychomotor performance and perceived effort during physical work as influenced by beta-adrenergic blockade. *Biol. Psychol.* 8:31–43, 1979.
217. Skinner, J. S., G. Borg, and E. R. Buskirk. Physiological and perceptual reactions to exertion of young men differing in activity and body size. B. D. Franks (ed.). *Exercise and Fitness.* Chicago: Athletic Institute, 1969, pp. 53–66.
218. Skinner, J. S., R. Hustler, V. Bersteinova, and E. R. Buskirk. The validity and reliability of a rating scale of perceived exertion. *Med. Sci. Sports* 5:97–103, 1973.
219. Skinner, J. S., R. Hustler, V. Bersteinova, and E. R. Buskirk. Perception of effort during different types of exercise and under different environmental conditions. *Med. Sci. Sports* 5:110–155, 1973.
220. Skrinar, G. S., S. P. Ingram, and K. B. Pandolf. Effect of endurance training on perceived exertion and stress hormones in women. *Percept. Mot. Skills* 57:1239–1250, 1983.
221. Smutok, M. A., G. S. Skrinar, and K. B. Pandolf. Exercise intensity: Subjective regulation by perceived exertion. *Arch. Phys. Med. Rehabil.* 61:569–574, 1980.
222. Squires, R. W., J. L. Rod, M. L. Pollock, and C. Foster. Effects of propranolol on perceived exertion after myocardial revascularization surgery. *Med. Sci. Sports Exerc.* 14:276–280, 1982.
223. Stamford, B. A. Validity and reliability of subjective ratings of perceived exertion during work. *Ergonomics* 19:53–60, 1976.
224. Stamford, B. A., and B. J. Noble. Metabolic cost and perception of effort during bicycle ergometer work performance. *Med. Sci. Sports* 6:226–231, 1974.
225. Stephenson, L. A., M. A. Kolka, and J. E. Wilderson. Perceived exertion and anaerobic threshold during the menstrual cycle. *Med. Sci. Sports Exerc.* 14:218–222, 1982.
226. Stevens, J. C., and A. Krimsley, Build-up of fatigue in static work: role of blood flow. G. Borg (ed.). *Physical Work and Effort.* New York: Pergamon Press, 1977, pp. 145–156.
227. Stoudemire, N., L. Wideman, K. Pass, C. McGinnes, G. Gaesser, and A. Weltman. The validity of regulating blood lactate concentration during running by ratings of perceived exertion. *Med. Sci. Sports Exerc.* 28:490–495, 1996.
228. Swank, A., and R. Robertson. Effect of induced alkalosis on perception of exertion during intermittent exercise. *J. Appl. Physiol.* 67(5):1862–1867, 1989.
229. Sylva, M., R. Boyd, and M. Mangum. Effects of social influence and sex on rating of perceived exertion in exercising elite athletes. *Percept. Mot. Skills* 70:591–594, 1990.
230. Toner, M. M., L. L. Drolet, and K. B. Pandolf. Perceptual and physiological responses during exercise in cool and cold water. *Percept. Mot. Skills* 62:211–220, 1986.
231. Trice, I., and E. M. Haymes. Effects of caffeine ingestion on exercise-induced changes during high-intensity, intermittent exercise. *Int. J. Sport Nutr.* 5:37–44, 1995.
232. Ueda, T., T. Kurokawa, K. Kikkawa, and T. Choi. Contribution of differentiated ratings of perceived exertion to overall exertion in women while swimming. *Eur. J. Appl. Physiol.* 66:196–201, 1993.
233. Ulin, S. S., T. J. Armstrong, S. H. Snook, and W. M. Keyserling. Perceived exertion and

discomfort associated with driving screws at various work locations and at different work frequencies. *Ergonomics* 36(7):833–846, 1993.

234. Van Den Burg, M., and R. Ceci. A comparison of a psychophysical estimation and a production method in a laboratory and a field condition. G. Borg and D. Ottoson (eds.). *Perception of Exertion in Physical Work.* London: Macmillan, 1986, pp. 35–46.

235. Van Herwaarden, C. L., R. A. Binkhorst, J. F. Fennis, and A. Van 'T Laar. Effects of propranolol and metroprolol on haemodynamic and respiratory indices and on perceived exertion during exercise in hypertensive patients. *Br. Heart J.* 41:99–105, 1979.

236. Varghese, M. A., P. N. Saha, and N. Atreya. A rapid appraisal of occupational workload from a modified scale of perceived exertion. *Ergonomics* 37(3):485–491, 1994.

237. Ward, D. and O. Bar-Or. Usefulness of RPE scale for exercise prescription with obese youth. *Med. Sci. Sports Exerc. (suppl)* 19:15, 1987.

238. Ward, D., J. Jackman, and F. Galiano. Exercise intensity reproduction: children versus adults. *Pediatr. Exerc. Sci.* 3:209–218, 1991.

239. Weiser, P. C., R. A. Kinsman, and D. A. Stamper. Task specific symptomatology changes resulting from prolonged submaximal bicycle riding. *Med. Sci. Sports* 5:79–85, 1973.

240. Weiser, P. C., and D. A. Stamper. Psychophysiological interactions leading to increased effort, leg fatigue, and respiratory distress during prolonged, strenuous bicycle riding. G. Borg (ed.). *Physical Work and Effort.* New York: Pergamon Press, 1977, pp. 401–416.

241. Williams, J. G., and R. G. Eston. Does personality influence the perception of effort? The results from a study of secondary schoolboys. *Phys. Educ. Rev.* 9:94–99, 1986.

242. Williams, J. G., R. Eston, and B. Furlong. CERT: a perceived exertion scale for young children. *Percept. Mot. Skills* 79:1451–1458, 1994.

243. Williams, J. G., R. G. Eston, and C. Stretch. Use of rating of perceived exertion to control exercise intensity in children. *Pediatr Exerc. Sci.* 3:21–27, 1991.

244. Yorio, J. M., R. K. Dishman, W. R. Forbus, K. J. Cureton, and R. E. Graham. Breathlessness predicts perceived exertion in young women with mild asthma. *Med. Sci. Sports Exerc.* 24:860–867, 1992.

245. Young, A. J., A. Cymerman, and K. B. Pandolf. Differentiated ratings of perceived exertion are influenced by high altitude exposures. *Med. Sci. Sports Exerc.* 14:223–228, 1982.

246. Zohar, D., and G. Spitz. Expected performance and perceived exertion in a prolonged physical task. *Percept. Mot. Skills* 52:975–984, 1981.

Index

Page references followed by *t* or *f* indicate tables or figures, respectively.